汉英双解实用中医词汇

CHINESE-ENGLISH BILINGUAL GLOSSARY OF TRADITIONAL CHINESE MEDICINE

王宝祥　董雪梅　主编

科 学 出 版 社

1993

(京) 新登字 092 号

内容简介

本书汇集中医词目约 4000 条,概括了中医基础理论及临床各科的内容,基本符合医疗和教学的要求。同时,本书还收编了常用中草药约 300 余种,药物名称均以汉、英、拉丁文三种形式给出。书中还附有标准中医门诊病案、住院病案书写格式,病案书写格式均以汉英两种文字排出。

该书将中医词目,常用中草药,病案书写集于一书,内容丰富,使用方便。本书是以汉英两种形式编写,所以对开展高层次中医药国际交流与合作具有较强的实用性。

汉英双解实用中医词汇

王宝祥　董雪梅　主编

责任编辑　徐津津

科学出版社出版

北京东黄城根北街 16 号
邮政编码:100717
化学工业出版社印刷厂印刷
新华书店北京发行所发行　各地新华书店经销

*

1993 年 10 月第 一 版　　开本:850×1168　1/32
1993 年 10 月第一次印刷　　印张:25
印数:1—4 000　　　　　　字数:800 000
ISBN 7-03-003528-3/R・181
定价:21.80

顾　问	林子强	欧阳基		
主　编	王宝祥	董雪梅		
英文主译	董雪梅			
中文副主编	于维萍	母建华	薛一涛	
英文副主编	左连君	张培华		
编　委	于维萍	王宝祥	尹洪安	左连君
	母建华	吕润凯	李文基	林子强
	张　宏	张培华	董雪梅	董雪萍
	蔡　蔚	蔡剑前	薛一涛	
主　审	王永安	吕同杰	李玉林	余昌正
	周次清	蔡剑前	J·布莱克	

（均以姓氏笔划为序）

Advisors　LinTzichiang，J. P.
　　　　　OuYangji
Editor—in—Chief　Wang Bao xiang
　　　　　　　　　Dong Xue mei
English Editor—in—Chief　Dong Xue mei
Associate Editors—in—Chief of TCM
Yu Weiping　Mu Jianhua　Xue Yitao
Associate Editors—in—Chief of English
　Zuo Lianjun　Zhang Peihua
Editors　YuWeiping　WangBaoxiang　Yin Hong an
　　　　Zuo Lianjun　MuJianhua　Lu Run kai
　　　　Li Wenji　Lin Tzi chiang　Zhang Hong　Zhang Peihua
　　　　Dong Xue mei　Dong Xue ping　Cai Wei
　　　　Cai Jian qian　Xue Yi tao
Chief Revisors
　　　　Wang Yong an　LuTongjie　Li Yu lin
　　　　Yu Chang zheng　Zhou Ci qing　J・Black
　　　　Cai Jian qian

目 录

前言

序

用法说明

词汇正文 ……………………………………………………（ 1 ）

附录1　中医病案书写格式 ……………………………………（691）

附录2　常用中草药名称 ………………………………………（710）

附录3　药用衡量折算表 ………………………………………（726）

附录4　天干地支 ………………………………………………（727）

附录5　二十四节气 ……………………………………………（728）

条目汉语拼音音节索引 …………………………………………（729）

前　言

　　1991年10月，北京金秋时节，世界卫生组织与中华人民共和国国家中医药管理局共同举办了世人瞩目的国际传统医药大会。来自42个国家和地区的政府官员与传统医药界专家、同仁共商发展大计，提出"人类健康需要传统医学"的口号，发表了《北京宣言》，并将每年的10月18日定为世界传统医药日。

　　作为与会者置身于这一令人激动、振奋的情景之中，共同的事业增进了不同肤色，不同语言，不同信仰的同仁、朋友之间的友谊与了解，也更加坚定了我们编写本词汇的信心。

　　任何事物都有一个逐渐发展的过程，水平有一个逐渐提高的过程。探讨中医英译是手段，目的是将中医药介绍给各国学者，使之了解发源于中国古代哲学思想的中医理论体系。随着高科技发展，借助现代化方法、手段对中医药进行微观研究，揭示事物本质，并已获得大量科研数据；治疗研究采用了西医病名，诊断，疗效标准与西医统一；中医论文在国际专业会议上交流，在西医杂志上发表，并得到西医理解。展望医学发展的未来，中医药学得到世界的瞩目，且不可忽视对中医哲理的领悟。

　　本书集中医基础理论、临床各科词目、国家中医药管理局医政司颁发的《中医内外妇儿科病证诊断疗效标准》中八十一个病证及其辨证分类、中医病案书写格式于一书，这将有助于中国与各国中医药学者从事高层次的学术交流。中医英译形式力求保持中医药学的特色与内涵，并使用世界卫生组织发布的标准中医名词英译，使中医英译逐步实现规范化、标准化。

　　本书承蒙世界卫生组织传统医学顾问、中国科学院学部委员、中国中医研究院教授陈可冀先生亲自作序。承蒙澳洲中医药针灸联合会会长林子强教授，山东大学美国现代文学研究所教授、美国印第安那大学终身教授欧阳基先生，山东中医学院教授、美国康乃尔大学客座教授、主诊王永安先生，著名中医教授、学者吕同杰先生、周次清先生、蔡剑前女士、余昌正先生、李玉林先生，英语专家J·布莱克先生审阅，并提出许多宝贵意见，在此一并表示衷心感谢！

　　本书可作为海内外各国中医院校师生从事教学、医疗、科研的工具书，可作为各国对中医药感兴趣的人们的参考书。

　　中医药学源远流长，部分专业术语英译难度较大，敬希海内外广大读者对本词汇欠妥之处予以指正。

　　愿中国传统医药学为全人类的健康长寿作出贡献！

编　者
于山东济南
1992. 8.

Introduction

In October, 1991, the golden season of autumn in Beijing, an international conference on traditional medicine, which focussed the world attention, Was jointly held by WHO and the State Administration of Traditional Chinese Medicine of P. R. China with government officials, specialists and colleagues in the field of traditional medicine from 42 countries and regions taking part to discuss the future development of the traditional medicine. The conference put forward the slogan "Mankind needs traditional medicine to maintain health", adopted a "Beijing Declaration", and agreed to make every October 18 "The Day of Traditional medicine".

As participants of the conference, we were merged in the inspiring and exciting atmosphere. The common cause promoted friendship and understanding among friends and colleagues of different races with different beliefs. This further strengthens our confidence in writing this book.

Things develop gradually and usually become improved step by step. The approach to translate TCM theories to English is the medium of introducing them to foreign scholars, thus, enabling them to understand the TCM theoretical system formed on the basis of the ancient chinese philosophy. Along with the high—science and tech development, large amount of data has been gained by microcosmic Study of TCM to reveal its nature by using modern methods. The names of disease diagnostic and therapeatic criteria that coincide with those of western medicine have been adopted in the therapeutic study. TCM theses are exchanged at international conferences, published in the western medicine journals and have gained understanding of western doctors. Looking into the future of medical development, TCM is eyed on all over the world, hence, the importance of understanding its philosophic theory can not be neglected.

This book collects entries, including basic theories and clinical subject, the diagnostic criteria and types of differentiation of 81 kinds of diseases as well as the standard forms of medical record—writing in traditional Chinese medicine issued by the State Administration of Traditional Chinese Medicine of P. R. China. This will aid in academic exchange in higher level among the scholars from China and different countries.

Striving to maintain the characteristics and original intention of traditional Chinese medicine in English translation, using the standard English translation on the words of TCM issued by WHO, so as to make English translation on TCM standard ization and criterions.

We are deeply indebted to Mr. Chen keji, consultant on traditional medicine to WHO, academic member of the Chinese Academy of Science, professor of Chinese Academy of TCM, for his foreword.

We express special appreciation to Mr. Lin Tzichiang, national president of Federation of Chinese Medicine and Acupuncture Societies, Australia, to Mr. Ou yongji, professor of Institute for studies in Modern American Literature of Shandong University, professor of Indiana University, U.S.A, to Mr. Wang Yongan, professor of Shandong College of TCM, visiting professor of Kernel University, U.S.A, to famous professors of TCM: Lu Tongjie, Zhou Ciqing, Caijiangqian, Yu Changzheng, Li Yulin, to Mr. J. Black, English teacher, for their valuable, instructive suggestions.

This book will be a book in TCM teaching, clinical management and scientific research for teachers and students of TCM colleges of the world, of also meet the needs for those who are interested in TCM.

TCM, Which dates back to ancient time, has an unique and profound theoretical system. Certain parts of its terminology have particular denotations, so is difficult to translate. Inaccuracies in the book, therefore, are unavoidable, we sincerely hope that our friends in TCM circle and all the readers will oblige us with timely corrections.

May traditional Chinese medicine make agreat contribution to mankind to maintain health and enjoy a long happy life.

The Editors

Jinan, Shandong Province

August, 1992

序

  我国是伟大的文明古国,有光彩夺目的中华民族文化,中医药学也是其中的组成部分;作为炎黄子孙,我们以有这样宝贵的、优秀的文化而骄傲。

  任何科学,都应是国际性的,医学科学也不例外;民族性也很重要,但是与国际性相对而言的。我国今天正处在历史发展的伟大时代,我们这一代人负有继往开来的重任。我们不仅要面向全中国,让中医药学继续为全国人民健康贡献力量,同时,还应当面向全世界,让中医药学走向世界,为全世界人民的健康服务。

  中医药学有自己独特的理论和经验,在不少医药学理论、概念,以及学术用语的语义特征上,有自己的特色,常常与现代医学有明显的差异或不同;例如中医学中的"肝藏",和现代医学的"liver"概念有明显不同;中医学中"痰"和现代医学中的"sputum"也不同;中医学中的"手三阴"的"手",并非"hand"所能概括,还包括"arm"在内;所以,要将中医药学介绍给全世界,中医药学名词术语的英汉语对译,是一项十分艰巨而繁重的任务,有待规范化或标准化。

  我很高兴看到《汉英双解实用中医词汇》的编纂,本书就中医基础、临床各科、针灸、气功、中药名词,以及由国家中医药管理局公布的《中医病案书写规范》,都作了汉英对排对译,很是实用。有些词语的英译与国内一些学者的译法不完全一致,但却有益于今后的进一步交流、统一和提高。我认为本书对中医药学教学、科研、医疗方面都是很好的参考用书,对主编及主译者的毅力表示赞赏。是为序。

陈可冀

一九九二年六月

于北京西苑

Foreword

Our country, one of the great ancient civilized countries in the world, has its dazzlingly brilliant Chinese culture, of which traditional Chinese medicine (TCM) is a component part (Being Descendant of the Chinese nation). We take pride for having such a valuable and splendid culture.

Any branches of sciences should be of the international, so is medical science. Although national character is also of importance, yet it is only comparative to the international. Our country is now in the great era of historical development; the generation of us takes on the heavy responsibilities of carrying forward the cause and forging ahead into the future. It is not only for us to face the whole China and continue to make TCM serve the Chinese people's health, but to face the whole world and make use of it to serve the health of the people world over.

TCM has its own distinctive thoeries and experience. In many of the thoeries, conceptions as well as the meanings of its terms, it has its own peculiarity, and is often obviously different from those of modern medicine. e. g. the conception of "liver" in TCM is quite different from that in modern medicine, and so is "sputum". The word "hand" in "three yin of the hand" means more than its usual meaning, which also includes the "arm" etc. Therefore, it is arduous and strenuous for us to translate TCM terms from Chinese into Englsh while tryiny to introduce it to the whole world. And such a work needs to be normalized and standardized.

I'm pleased to see the compilation and publication of this Chinese — English Bilingual Glossary of Traditional Chinese Medicine. It compiles with English translation all the basic TCM thoeries, clinical terms of each department, acupuncture and moxibustion, qigong, and traditional pharmacy as well as "the standard forms of medical record—writing in traditional Chinese medicine" issued by the State Administration of TCM. Hence it is very practical in use. Though it is not identical in English translation for other scholars at home, yet it is valuable for furthering the exchanges, standardization and improvement in this field. I think it would be a good reference book in TCM teaching, scientific research as well as clinical management, and I appreciate the willpower of the chief editors and translators to accomplish this book. For all this I write this foreword.

Chen Keji

Xi yuan, Beijing

June, 1992

用 法 说 明

一、本词典收入中医基础、临床各科、针灸及气功等词条约4000条。以汉语拼音字母顺序排列，同音异调的汉字按声调顺序排列；多字词条按第一个汉字的汉语拼音字母音调排列；第一个汉字的音调相同者，按第二个汉字的汉语拼音字母顺序和音调排列，依次类推。

二、每一词条的主要部分是本词与释义，均作中、英文双重解释。

三、每一词条的编排次序是汉语词条本词及汉语拼音，汉语的释义；然后是英文词条本词（大写体，排黑体字母）及其英文释义。一义多词者，均收入同一义词条中，在汉语拼音后，将同义词条收入括号内。

四、汉语拼音均注调号，采用标准中国普通话发音及音调。

五、一项词条含有多条不同的释义时，各条释义分别列出，前面标以1、2、等数码，并分别作中、英文双重解释。

六、英语释义的文字，如已含有词条本词内容，则不另行释义。

七、对少数中医专业词条及文字的特定含义，使用目前国内外已约定成俗的音译，以保持其中医特色。如将"气"译为qi；将"阴、阳"分别译为yin, yang；将"气分、血分"分别译为qifen, xuefen；将"痹"译为bi；将"阳明"译为yangming；将"营卫"译为yingwei，等等。本书采用了世界卫生组织针灸穴名标准化英语译名及其缩写。如将肺经译为 Lung Meridian；三焦经译为 Triple Energizer Meridian；督脉译为 Governor Vessel，缩写为 GV，等等。

八、本词典附录一，收编了国家中医药管理局医政司（1991.5）颁发的中医病案书写格式，均以汉文、英文对排形式，以便查阅、使用。

九、本词典附录二，收入三百味常用中草药，以其作用功效为排列顺序。每一味中草药药名均用汉字、汉语拼音、拉丁文（大写体）及英文（斜体）四种形式。

Guide to the Use of This Book

1. This book has collected about 3800 entries of basic theory, various clinical branches of TCM, acupuncture and moxibustion as well as Qigong. The Chinese headwords are arranged in alphabetic order of the Chinese phonetic symbols; headwords with the same pronuciation but different tones are arranged in the order of the four tones while those with two Chinese characters or more arranged according to alphabetical of the Chinese phonetic symbols of the first Chinese character; when the tones of the first Chinese character are the same, then see the alphabetic order and tones of the second Chinese character and so on and so forth.

2. The major parts of each entry consists of headword and its explanation, both in Chinese and English.

3. Arrangement of the entries: The first item is the headword in Chinese, attached with Chinese phonetics, then the Chinese explanation. The corresponding terms in English are printed in capital letters, followed by English explanation. Terms with the same meaning are collected in brackets under the same entry following the Chinese phonetics of the headword.

4. All the Chinese characters are marked with tones according to the pronunciation and intonation of the standard Chinese Putonghua.

5. The various meanings of a Chinese headword are marked off by Arabic numerals (1. 2. 3. etc.) with English corresponding terms and explanations.

6. If the English corresponding term is just the same with its explanation, then the Chinese explanation is not again translated into English.

7. A small number of headwords or words which have their specific meaning in TCM are translated in a way which is established by usage both at home and abroad, ie, "qi","yin,yang", "qifen, xuefen", "bi", "yangming", "yingwei" etc. The standard acupuncture nomenclature issued by Regional WorKing Group on the standardization of Acupuncture Nomenclature, WHO Regional Office for the Western Pacific, are also used, ie, "Lung Meridian"; "Triple Energizer Meridian"; "Governor Vessel, GV", etc.

8. In appendix I, the standard forms of medical record-writing in TCM issued by the Department of Medical Affairs of State Administration of TCM(May, 1991).

9. Appendix II, 300 Kinds of common Chinese materia Medica which are arranged in the order of their effect, each of which is written first in Chinese, followed by Chinese phonetics, then in Latin (printed in capital letter), and in English (prihted in Italic type).

阿是穴 【ā shì xué】(不定穴)即无具体名称,也无固定位置,而是以压痛点或其它反应点做为腧穴的穴位。

Ah Shih Point, Pressure Pain Point, Adventitious Point a point without fixed title and location, but selected by eliciting pressed pain and other response at the tender site, which is a category of acupuncture points.

癌 【ái】(恶性肿瘤)肿块凹凸不平,边缘不齐,坚硬不移,形如岩石,溃后血水淋漓,臭秽难闻,不易收敛。

Cancer a malignant tumour featuring uneven surface, indistinct margin, stony hard and immovable, which when rupture occurs, would discharge smelly bloody fluid. It is a very stubborn disease.

艾灸补泻 【ài jiǔ bǔ xiè】(火补火泻)火力由小到大,渐渐深入,待火自然燃尽,灼伤皮肉者为补法,具温阳补虚之功效,如用口吹其火,使其速燃,使受术者觉烫,不待烧及皮肉即移去艾炷者为泻法,具祛寒散结之功效。

Reinforcing or Reducing by Cone Moxibustion two different treatments, reinforcing treatment requests the burning of the cone from weak to strong gradually and applies heat to points or certain locations of the human body until a local scar is formed, it reinforces yang qi and prevents collapse while the reducing one requests a quick and strong burning of the cone by poffing air on it, making the patient feel fairly hot and removing the cone before a scar is formed, it relieves the stagnation of qi and blood by expelling pathogenic coldness.

艾绒 【ài róng】将干燥艾叶磨碎制成的粗药末,是灸治所用的主要材料。

Moxa Wool chief material for moxibustion, made of dry moxa leaves ground into wool.

艾条(卷) 【ài tiáo (juǎn)】用艾绒卷成的圆柱形长条,根据有无药物含

Moxa Stick a cylinder made of dry moxa; it is classified into two types:

量，分清艾条与药艾条两种。一般长二十厘米，直径一点五厘米，可燃烧一小时左右，多用于悬灸。

one is pure moxa stick and the other is medicinal moxa stick in which other herbal medicine is mixed; about 20 cm in length and 1.5 cm in diameter, enough to burn for about one hour, generaly used in hanging moxibustion.

艾炷 【ài zhù】艾绒制成的圆锥形艾团，用拇指、食指、中指捏成三种大小不同的艾炷，最小的艾炷形如麦粒；中等艾炷如半个枣核；大艾炷形如拇指上端，直接灸使用两种小艾炷；间接灸使用大艾炷。

Moxa Cones cones of dry moxa wool. Place a small amount of moxa wool on a board, knead and shape it into a cone usually with the thumb, index and middle fingers in three sizes. The smallest is as big as a grain, the medium size is about half a date stone, and the largest is the size of the upper part of the thumb. The two smaller cones are suitable for direct moxibustion, while the largest for indirect moxibustion.

艾炷灸 【ài zhù jiǔ】将艾炷置于穴位点燃的一种灸法，有直接灸与间接直接灸两种方法。

Moxa Cone Moxibustion a method of moxibustion with a moxa cone burning on the selected point directly or indirectly.

嗳腐 【ài fǔ】嗳气而气味酸腐而臭，多因脾胃虚弱，饮食不节，食物不化，停滞肠胃所致。

Eructation with Foul Odour a symptom caused by the asthenia of the spleen and the stomach or immoderate diet leading to the accumulation of indigested food in the stomach and intestines.

嗳气 【ài qì】（嗌气）指气从胃中上逆有声，其声沉长的症状，多因脾胃虚弱或胃有痰、火、食滞，使胃失和降所致，也有因肝气上逆而嗳气者。

Eructation the noisy belching of gas from the stomach through the mouth, due to asthenia of the spleen and stomach, or failure of descending of stomach-qi resulting from the accumulation of phlegm, fire and indigested food in the stomach. It could

溢奶 【ài nǎi】因小儿吮乳汁过多，胸膈不快，胃满而溢出。

安神 【ān shén】治疗神志不安，心悸失眠的方法，通常分为重镇安神和养心安神两种。

安中 【ān zhōng】中指中气，即脾胃之气，用药物来调整安定脾胃之气的方法，即称为安中，一般指"和胃"和"调和肝胃"等法。

按摩 【àn mó】1.又称推拿，在人体一定部位上，运用各种按摩手法和进行特定的肢体活动来防治疾病的方法。2.正骨八法之一，包括按法和摩法，用以舒筋散瘀和消肿。

暗产 【àn chǎn】指受孕一月之内而流产者，多因肝郁，恼怒或房事不节所致。

熬 【áo】将药物加入适量的水或辅料，用小火慢慢煎煮，或浓缩成膏状物。

also be caused by failure of descending of liver-qi.

Milk Vomiting　　a disorder seen in the case of overfeeding in infants.

Tranquilization　　a treatment for restlessness, palpitation and insomnia; either by the application of smoothing medicine (minerals) or reinforcing the mental system.

Regulation of the Middle-Energizer　　a treatment for the disorder of middle-energizer (qi of the spleen and stomach), generally referring to the regulation of stomach-qi, or the regulation of interaction between the liver and stomach.

Massage　　1. also called Chinese tuina, a method of prevention and treatment of diseases by applying various massage manipulation, or by passive movements of the body. 2. One of the eight manipulations of bonesetting, used for relaxing the muscles, dissipating blood stasis, and promoting subsidence of swelling.

Abortion within the First Month of Pregnancy　　early miscarriage due to stagnation of liver-qi, anger, or frequent sexual intercourses.

Stewing　　a method of processing medicinal herbs by boiling with proper amount of water or other liquid adjuvants by low fire to concentrate it as an extract.

八法 【bā fǎ】八种治疗方法，即汗、吐、下、和、温、清、消、补。

Eight Medical Treatments generally referring to the eight comprehensive principles of Chinese traditional therapy, including diaphoresis, inducing emesis, purgation, reconciliation (regulating the functions of the internal organs), warming, Purifying resolution and invigoration.

八纲 【bā gāng】八种辨证纲领，即阴、阳、表、里、寒、热、虚、实。

Eight Principal Syndromes the eight aspects for different diagnosis, including yin and yang, superficies and interior, cold and heat, asthnia and sthenia.

八纲辨证 【bā gāng biàn zhèng】辨证的基本方法之一，把疾病复杂的临床表现用阴、阳、表、里、寒、热、虚、实八个纲领进行分析归纳，以说明病变的部位、性质以及正邪盛衰等情况，对疾病作出诊断。

Diagnosis in accordance with Eight Principal Syndromes one of the basic methods of differential diagnosis, based on the analysis and comprehension of the complicated clinical manifestations through the Eight Principal Syndromes—— yin and yang, superficies and interior, cold and heat, asthenia and sthenia, to determine the nature and site of pathological changes and the conflict between the body resistance and the pathogenic factors.

八会 【bā huì】指脏、腑、筋、髓、血、骨、脉、气等的精气会聚的地方。

Eight Convergent Points the points where the essential substances of the zang, fu, tendons, marrow, blood, bones, vessels and qi gather.

八廓 【bā kuò】将外眼分为八个部

Eight Walls the eight parts divid-

位,因它有如城廓护土之意,故为八廓。

八谿 【bā xī】 即肘关节、腕关节、膝关节、踝关节左右侧共八处。

拔火罐 【bá huǒ guàn】 一种治疗的方法,用竹筒、陶瓷或玻璃制成的小罐或宽口瓶作为火罐,拨罐时,先将点燃的酒精棉球在火罐内燃片刻,然后迅速将火罐倒扣在一定的体表部位上,使火罐借助冷却后火罐的空气减少所产生的负压,使火罐紧吸在皮肤表面上,引起局部充血,留罐时间每次约十分钟左右,适用于治疗疼痛、痹证,消化系统疾病及某些呼吸系统疾病。

白 【bái】 五色之一,即白色,它与五行中的金,五脏中的肺以及与虚证、寒证有密切关系。

白崩 【bái bēng】 阴道突然流出大量白色稀薄液体的一种病证。可因忧思过度,劳伤心脾或虚冷劳极伤于胞脉所致。

白带 【bái dài】 阴道分泌的白色粘液,正常情况下,白带量少色淡,无

ed into the external eyeball, which was served as a wall to protect eyes.

Eight Crevices the joints referring to the elbows, wrists, knees and ankles.

Cupping a therapy in which the operator clamps a cotton ball soaked with 95% alcohol with the forceps or nippers, ignites it and put it into the cup, and immediately take it out and place the cup on the selected region, the air inside the cup has become lesser dense than outside, and the skin becomes congested with violet-coloured blood stasis formation, usually the cup is sucked in place for 10 minutes. It is suitable for the treatment of pains, bi-syndromes and the diseases of the digestive and respiratory system.

White a colour which is matched with metal (in the Five Elements) and lung (in the Five Zang-organs), and is closely related to the asthenia syndrome and cold syndrome.

Leukorrhagia with whitish discharge profuse discharge of whitish and thin fluid from the vagina, probably resulting from great sorrow, impairment of the heart and spleen by overstrain, or impairment of bao vessel by asthenic cold and overstrain.

Leukorrhea a whitish viscid discharge from the vagina. It is consid-

臭;如白带增多,颜色和臭味改变,多属病态。

ered as normal when discharge is scanty, colourless and odourless, and as pathological when it becomes profuse with alterations in colour and odour.

白癜风 【bái diàn fēng】(白驳风)因风邪袭表,气血失和,血不荣肤所致,以局部皮肤色素脱色而呈白色为特征的一种皮肤病。白斑边缘清楚,其中的毛发也变白,表面光滑,不痛不痒。

Vitiligo a skin disease characterized by circumscribed areas of depigmentation of the skin, due to the attack of pathogenic wind to the superficies and incoordination between qi and blood leading to the lack of nourishment of the skin. The patches have a hyperpmented border, with discoloured hair and smooth surface but without pain or itching.

白喉 【bái hóu】因感受时行疫毒所致的一种急性传染病,表现为咽部疼痛,扁桃体出现白点,逐渐形成边界清楚的灰白色假膜,并迅速向周围漫延,不易剥脱,如强行剥脱则易出血,若延至喉部,则引起呼吸道阻塞的症状。

Diphtheria an acute infectious disease caused by an epidemic and virulent factor; marked by sorethroat, with spots appearing over the tonsile with gradual formation of grapy-white pseudo membrane which is clearly outlined, spread rapidly, bleeds easily when it is forcibly removed. Obstruction of the respiratory tract may occur when the larynx is involved.

白厚滑苔 【bái hòu huá tāi】舌苔白厚而光滑。常是寒湿之邪侵袭机体的表现,表证见此舌苔,多是风寒兼湿的表现;里证见此舌苔,则是脾胃寒湿的表现。

Whitish, Thick and Smooth Tongue Fur a sign usually signifying the attack of pathogenic cold-damp factors to the body. It occurring in superficie-syndrome suggests the involvement of superficies by wind-cold and damp factors, while that occurring in interior-syndrome suggests the presence of the pathogenic

白睛 【bái jīng】（白眼）包括球结膜与巩膜，属肺，谓气轮。

白痢 【bái lì】粪便以白色粘液或脓液为主的痢疾，多因湿热病邪滞于气分所致。

白漏 【bái lòu】阴道流出白色稀薄液体，淋漓不断的病证，多因脾肺气虚所致。

白霉苔 【bái méi tài】舌苔白而有糜点如饭粒，常见胃中热极，津液腐化所致。

白膜侵睛 【bái mó qīn jīng】因肝肺热盛或阴虚火旺所致的角膜病变，表现为黑、白交界处出现灰白色小滤泡，患眼刺痛羞明流泪。

白内障 【bái nèi zhàng】（圆翳内障）因肝肾不足或肝经风热上攻而成，症见瞳内有圆形白色翳障，而瞳神外观无异常。

cold-damp factors in the spleen and stomach.

Bulbar Conjunctiva and Sclera both of them belong to the lung and named as qi-wheel.

Dysentery with whitish stool dysentery characterized by the discharge of mucous and purulent stool, which is caused by the stagnation of pathogenic damp-heat factors in qifen.

Leukorrhagia a condition with continuous discharge of whitish, thin fluid from the vagina, usually due to deficiency of the spleen-qi and lung-qi.

Whitish and Mould-Like Tongue Fur a sign caused by the excessive accumulation of heat in the stomach and the putrefaction of body fluid.

Phlyctenular Keratitis a corneal disease due to hyperactivity of the liver-heat and the lung-heat of yin deficiency and excessive pathogenic fire; manifested as the formation of a small, gray, circumscribed lesion at the corneal limbus, accompanied with pain, photophobia and lacrimation.

Cataract a condition caused by asthenia of the liver and kidney, or the attack of pathogenic wind-heat in the liver meridian upward to eyes; manifested as opacity of the crystalline lens of eyes but with normal appearance of the pupil.

白粘腻苔 【bái nián nì tāi】舌苔表面复盖着层厚浊粘液,常是体内有痰湿之邪的反映,多属寒证。

Whitish-Greasy Tongue Fur a sign usually signifying the accumulation of the pathogenic phlegm-damp inside the body and attributive to cold-syndrome.

白㾦 【bái pēi】(白疹,晶瘖) 一种细小的白色小泡状皮疹,常分布于颈、项、胸腹等处,多见于湿温病,是湿热之邪郁阻气分的反映。

Sudamina Crystallina whitish vesicles distributed over the skin of the neck, chest and abdomen, mostly seen in damp-warm disease when the pathogenic damp-heat factors are stagnated in qifen.

白刃疔 【bái rèn dīng】鼻孔内生小白泡,顶硬根突,堵塞鼻孔,多由肺经火毒凝聚所致。

White Boil white boil which is developing in the nasal cavity and obstructing the nostril, caused by accumulation of the pathogenic fire factor in the lung meridian.

白苔 【bái tāi】舌苔色白,其厚薄及湿润度的变化反映不同的病变,苔白而薄是正常舌苔,苔白而干者,多因津液不足引起。

Whitish Tongue Fur a sign which suggests different pathological changes according to the thinkness and moisture of the fur. A thin whitish fur is normal, while a thin whitish and dry fur suggests insufficiency of body fluid.

白秃疮 【bái tū chuāng】因接触传染所致的头部霉菌性皮肤病,初起时头皮上呈散在性白色屑斑,逐渐漫延成片,瘙痒,久则发枯脱落,形成秃斑。

Tinea Capitis fungal infection of the scalp, marked by scattered, whitish desquamation on the scalp with itching and gradual formation of irregular patches of baldness.

白屑风 【bái xiè fēng】因风邪侵入毛孔,郁久血燥,肌肤失养所引起的一种皮肤病,多见于青年人,好发于头皮,呈弥漫而均匀的糠秕干燥白屑,痒甚,搔痒时白屑脱落,毛发易脱,相当于脂溢性皮炎。

Seborrheic Dermatitis a skin disease due to invasion of pathogenic wind factor through the hair follicles and stagnation of it leading to blood-dryness and lack of nourishment of the skin; mostly seen in the young, occurring on the scalp with exfoliation of dry and whitish scale-

白浊 【bái zhuó】小便白色而混浊的一种病证,多因湿热下注膀胱所致。

Whitish and Turbid Urine a condition due to the attack of pathogenic damp-heat factors to the urinary bladder.

百合病 【bǎi hé bìng】古病名,因情志抑郁或大病之后,心肺阴虚而内热所致的病证。

"Bulbus Lilii" Syndrome referring to the depressive state of psychosis, due to pathogenic heat factor retained in the interior caused by the deficency of the heart-yin and lung-yin after emotional depression or serious illness.

百日咳 【bǎi rì ké】(奶嗽、时行顿咳)一种流行于冬春季节的传染病,以五岁以下婴儿多见,临床以阵发性、痉挛性咳嗽和痉咳后伴有特殊的吸气性回声为特征。

Whooping Cough infectious disease occurring frequently in winter andspring, mostly seen in children under five year of ages; characterizedby paroxysmal spasmodic cough with an inspiratory wheezing sound.

百晬嗽 【bǎi zuì sòu】(胎嗽,百晬咳)指新生儿出生百日之内,患咳嗽、气急、痰涎壅盛等症,包括一般感冒和新生儿肺炎等疾病。

Neonatal Cough a disease occurring in infants under the age of hundred days, manifested as productive cough and shortness of breath; seen in common cold, neonatal pneumonia, etc.

斑 【bān】指发于皮肤表面的片状块,多因热病,热郁阳明,迫及营血,外发于肌表所致。

Macule a discolored patch on skin that is not elevated above the surface, due to retention of the pathogenic heat factor in yangming involving yingfen and xuefeng and dispersing to the superficies.

斑痧 【bān shā】身发紫斑,头晕眼花,恶心呕吐为主症的一种病证,常因痧毒入于腠理,留滞血分,内攻脏腑所致。

Eruptive Sha-syndrome a disease characterized by purplish rashes over the body, dizziness, nausea and vomiting; due to retention of pathogenic sha factor in xuefen in-

斑秃 【bān tū】（油风）指在短期内发生头发成片脱落，皮肤光泽或伴有搔痒的一种疾病，多由血虚生风，风盛火燥，发失濡养所致。

斑疹 【bān zhěn】指热病过程中发于肌肤表面的片点状的斑块或疹子，成片状，抚之不碍手者称为斑；形如粟米，高于皮肤之上，抚之碍手者称为疹。

半表半里证 【bàn biǎo bàn lǐ zhèng】外邪侵犯半表半里引起的证候，常表现为寒热往来、胸胁胀满、心烦喜呕、不思饮食、口苦咽干、眼花、脉弦等。

半刺 【bàn cì】古代针刺手法之一，其特点为浅刺出针快，常用于治疗感冒发热、咳嗽痰多、气喘等疾病。

半身不遂 【bàn shēn bù suí】一侧肢体瘫痪的病状，多见于中风后遗症。

volving the viscera.

Alopecia Areata patchy loss of hair on the scalp occurring in a short time associated with itching; caused by deficiency of blood with production of pathogenic wind factor and fire-dryness factor leading to poor nourishment of the hair.

Eruption visible efflorescent spot or patch on the skin occurring in febrile disease. That not elevated above the surface is macule, while the elevated above the surface is papule.

Half-Superficies and Half-Interior a syndrome due to attack of the exogenous factors to the part between the superficies and the interior of the body, manifested as alternating episodes of chills and fever, oppressed feeling over the chest and hypochondrium, restlessness, nausea and vomiting, loss of appetite, dry throat, bitter taste in the mouth, wiry pulse, etc.

Half-Puncture one of the ancient acupuncture manipulations, with its characteristics of shallowly puncturing, and quickly withdrawing is usually applied for the treatment of common cold with fever, cough with excessive phlegm, asthma, etc.

Hemiplegia paralysis of one side of the body, commonly seen in the sequelae of apoplexy.

半身汗出 【bàn shēn hàn chū】只有一侧躯干和肢体出汗而另侧无汗的病状,多因气血失调,痰湿阻滞经络所致。

Hemihidrosis a morbid state of sweating only from one side of the body and limbs, caused by the disorder of qi and blood, and the retention of pathogenic damp-phlegm in the meridians and collaterals.

半身麻木 【bàn shēn má mù】身体半边或上下半身麻木的症状。

Hemianesthesia numbness or loss of sensation of one side, or the upper or lower part of the body.

半肢风 【bàn zhī fēng】以偏瘫或截瘫为主症的疾病。

Half-part of the Body Involved due to Apoplexy a morbid condition marked by hemiplegia or paraplegia as the major symptom.

包煎 【bāo jiān】某些粉末状、粘性较强及有绒毛的药物,煎药时宜用纱布包好入煎,以防止落液混浊,糊锅或刺激咽喉,如旋复花、车前子、灶心土等。

Medicine Decocted with Wrappings some powder-like, sticky and villous drugs should be wrapped in a piece of gauze for decoction so that the decoction will not be turbid, irritating to the throat, or burnt at the bottom of the pot; e. g. British inula flower, Asiatic plantain seed and burnt clay-lining of kitchen range.

胞 【bāo】1. 子宫。2. 胎盘的简称。3. 膀胱。4. 眼睑。

Bao 1. uterus 2. placenta 3. urinary bladder 4. eyelid.

胞痹 【bāo bì】(膀胱痹)因风寒湿邪久客膀胱,膀胱气化失常所致的病证,症见小腹胀满、疼痛拒按、小便艰涩不利。

Bladder-Bi a condition due to hypofunction of the bladder caused by the prolonged stay of pathogenic wind-cold-damp factors, manifested as distention, pain and tenderness over the lower abdomen, and dysuria.

胞寒不孕 【bāo hán bù yùn】因肾阳不足;或风寒客于胞中,以致胞宫寒冷,难以摄精受孕的病症。

Sterility due to Retention of Cold Factor in the Uterus a condition caused by the insufficiency of kidney-yang or the attack of pathogenic

胞系了戾 【bāo xì liǎo lì】指膀胱排尿障碍，表现为下腹隐隐胀疼，想小便而不能畅通排出，多因膀胱由热邪所迫所致。

胞衣不下 【bāo yī bù xià】（胎衣不下）指胎儿娩出后，胎盘超出半小时以上未能排出，多因分娩后出血大虚，无力继续排出所致。

胞肿 【bāo zhǒng】俗称眼皮肿，指胞睑肿胀，除由眼睑疾患引起外，还可发生于多种眼病及全身疾病。

胞阻 【bāo zǔ】指妊娠期间发生小腹部疼痛或阴道流血的症候，多因胞脉气血运行失畅，或血虚胞脉失养所致。

薄皮疮 【báo pí chuāng】因风热壅滞肌肤所致。体表生疮，溃流脓血后，脓腔呈空壳状，仅留一层薄皮。

豹文刺 【bào wén cì】古代针刺手法之一，在患处前后，左右刺中血脉，放出瘀血，用以治疗经络瘀阻等病。

wind-cold factors to the uterus resulting in coldness of the uterus with failure to recept the sperm.

Dysfunction of Bladder　a morbid state usually due to the pathogenic heat factor attacking the bladder, manifested as distending pain over the lower abdomen and dysuria.

Retention of Placenta　failure to expel the placenta more than half an hour after childbirth, due to over consumption of qi and blood during labour.

Edema of Eyelids　a morbid condition caused by eyelid disorder and various eye disorders or somatic diseases.

Embarrassment of the Fetus　abdominal pain or vaginal bleeding during pregnancy caused by the impediment of qi and blood flow in the bao meridian, or deficiency of blood with failure to nourish the bao meridian.

Thing-Covering Boil　due to stagnation of wind-heat in the skin and muscle, marked by the formation of a small cavity covered with a layer of thin skin after the drainagae of pus.

Bao Wen Puncture　one of the ancient acupuncture manipulations, by puncturing the points around the affected part and letting the blood stasis out, applied for the treatment of the obstruction of meridians.

暴崩 【bào bēng】指妇女由于暴怒伤肝；或跌扑闪挫，伤及冲任，迫血妄行，症见非经期而突然经血暴下如注。

暴聋 【bào lóng】指突然发生的耳聋。

暴厥 【bào jué】指突然昏厥。

暴盲 【bào máng】平日素无他疾，突然目盲不见物，眼眶和瞳神外观正常，多因肝气上逆，气滞血瘀；或元气大虚所致，多见于急性视神经炎、视网膜中央动脉栓塞、眼底出血、视网膜脱离等。

暴痫 【bào xián】指骤然发作的痫证。

暴瘖 【bào yīn】即突然失音，常见于声带急性炎症、水肿等。

暴注 【bào zhù】指突然发生的剧烈的泄泻。

悲则气消 【bēi zé qì xiāo】指悲伤过度，使肺气运行不畅，肺气消耗的病症。

背痛 【bèi tòng】症见背部板滞，疼痛，牵连肩项，兼有恶寒等，因风寒侵袭足太阳经，经脉涩滞所致的证

Sudden Onset of Metrorrhagia profuse uterine bleeding occurring at irregular intervals, due to impairment of the liver by a rage, or damage of the thoroughfare or conception maridians with impediment of the blood circulation by trauma.

Sudden Deafness deafness onsets suddenly.

Sudden Syncopy syncope occurs suddenly.

Sudden Onset of Blindness a condition of sudden loss of vision with normal appearance of eyes, due to adverse rising of liver-qi, stagnation of qi and blood, or exhaustion of primordial qi; usually seen in cases of acute optic neuritis, embolism of retinal central artery, retinal bleeding, retinal detachment, etc.

Sudden Epilepsy epilepsy with sudden onset.

Sudden Onset of Aphonia a sudden loss of voice, seen in the acute inflammation and edema of the vocal cord.

Sudden Diarrhea severe diarrhea with sudden onset.

Sorrow may Lead to the Consumption of Qi a morbid condition due to oversadness, in which the circulation of lung-qi is impeded and the consumption of lung-qi ensues.

Backache a condition caused by the blockage of the foot-taiyang meridian after involved by

背恶寒 【bèi wù hán】指背部自觉寒冷感,多见于外感证初期,症兼发热头痛、脉浮;亦见于阳气不足,阴寒里盛,症兼肢冷、脉沉细等。

Chilly Sensation of the Back a symptom mostly seen in the early stage of superficies syndome resulting from exogenous pathogenic factors, usually accompanied with fever, headache and floating pulse; also seen in the insufficiency of yang qi and sthenia of yin cold in the interior, usually accompanied with cold limbs, sunken and small pulse, etc.

焙 【bèi】把药物放在净瓦片上或锅上,用微火加热焙干,但不使药物烧焦。

Heating in Soft Fire a method of processing medicinal herb by baking thd drug in a pan or clean tile in a soft fire to make it dry but not charred.

奔豚 【bēn tún】古病名,多因肾脏阴寒之气上逆或肝经气火冲逆所致,症见气从小腹上冲胸咽或伴有腹痛,往来寒热等。

Ben-Tun Syndrome the ancient name for a disease due to adverse rising of yin-cold qi from the kidney or of the pathogenic fire factor of liver meridian; manifested as the subjective feeling of an air flow rushing upward from the lower abdomen to the throax and throat, accompanied with abdominal pain or alternating episodes of chills and fever.

贲门 【bēn mén】七冲之一,即胃的上口,连结胃与食管。

Chardia one of the seven important openings, the upper opening of the stomach, connecting with esophagus.

本草 【běn cǎo】我国历代记载药物

Medicinal Works the ancient

的著作，著名的如李时珍所编《本草纲目》。

works on materia medica, such as the wellknown "Compendium of Materia Medica" written by Li Shizhen.

崩漏 【bēng lòu】(崩中漏下) 经血非时而下，或量多如注，或量少而淋漓不净，或崩与漏交替出现，辨证分类 1. 血热证。2. 脾虚证。3. 肾虚证 (肾阴虚，肾阳虚)。4. 血瘀证。

Metrorrhagia uterine bleeding occurring at completely irregular intervals, marked by profuse bleeding or prolonged, scanty flow, or marked by both above. Types of differentiation 1. syndorme of blood-heat 2. syndrome of the spleen deficiency 3. syndrome of the kidney deficiency 4. syndrome of blood stasis.

鼻 【bí】五官之一，是嗅觉器官，被认为是肺的门户，和脾、胆等脏腑也有密切的关系。

Nose one of the five sense organs, serving as the organ of the sense of smell. It is considered as the orifice to the lung and is related to the functions of the spleen and gallbladder.

鼻疮 【bí chuāng】鼻上生疮，状如粟粒，甚则鼻外色红发肿，痛如火灸，多因肺经热毒上炎而成。

Rhinal Furuncle pyogenic infection of the nose, marked by miliary induration, erythema, swelling and burning pain; usually due to flaming up of pathogenic heat factor of the lung meridian.

鼻疔 【bí dīng】疔生于鼻孔内，红肿胀痛；或生小白泡，堵塞鼻窍，多因肺经火毒凝聚而成。

Boil in Nasal Cavity circumscribed inflammation of the mucous membrane lining the nasal cavity, marked by redness, swelling, pain, or by small white blisters blocking the nasal aperture; usually caused by the accumulation of pathogenic fire factor in the lung meridian.

鼻风 【bí fēng】指新生儿因鼻塞不能吃奶，多因感受风寒所致。

Nasal Wind a disorder hindering milk sucking in newborn caused by the attack of the pathogenic wind-

鼻干燥 【bí gān zào】鼻干无涕,多因肺燥、肺虚、阴血不足等所致

鼻疳 【bí gān】因乳食不调,上焦积热,壅滞肺中所致。症见鼻中赤痒、连唇生疮、肌肤枯瘦、手足潮热,或鼻下两旁微烂、脓汁浸淫。

鼻疽 【bí jū】疽生于鼻柱上,多因肺火薰蒸,热毒凝聚而成,初起坚硬色紫,局部发热跳痛,逐渐酿脓。

鼻孔 【bí kǒng】七窍之一,指鼻下部的两个孔道。

鼻衄 【bí nù】(鼻衄血)指鼻中出血,多因肺热上壅,迫血妄行;或胃热薰蒸;或肝火偏旺;或肺肾阴虚;或头风,伤酒所致。

鼻塞 【bí sāi】(鼻窍不利、鼻窒)鼻塞不通,多因风寒或风热引起肺气不宣所致。常伴有其他表证。

cold.

Dryness of Nasal Cavity   a condition resulting from the lung dryness and deficiency of yin-blood leading to the lung-asthenia.

Infantile Malnutrition Involving the Nose   a type of infantile malnutrition due to improper feeding and accumulation of pathogenic heat in the upper energizer and the lung, manifested as redness and itching of the nose, boils over the lips, emaciation, feverish sensation of the feet and hands, or paranasal lesions with purulent discharge.

Pusture on Nose Bridge   a condition caused by the hyperactivity of lung-fire leading to local accumulation of pathogenic heat factor; manifested as indurated, purplish nodule on the nose bridge, local heat, bursting pain and pustulation.

Nares   one of the seven orifices, the external orifices of the nose

Epistaxis   bleeding from the nose, due to abnormal rushing up of the lung-heat forcing the blood out of the vessels, or attack of stomach-heat, or hyperactivity of liver-fire, or deficiency of lung-yin and kidney-yin, or attack of pathogenic wind factor to the head, or overdrinking.

Stuffy Nose   a condition caused by inhibition of lung-qi resulting from the attack of pathogenic wind-cold

鼻痔 【bí zhì】(鼻瘜肉) 鼻内生长瘜肉，因风寒袭肺，津液壅塞所致，症见鼻塞，嗅觉减退。

鼻渊 【bí yuān】因风寒和风热或胆移热于脑，或兼气虚所致的病证，症见鼻塞、不闻香臭、涕色黄臭、头晕、头痛、健忘等，相当于鼻窦炎。

鼻针疗法 【bí zhēn liáo fǎ】针刺方法之一，对毫针斜刺外鼻部周围的穴位，主要用于治疗关节炎、神经痛及咳喘病等。

鼻肿 【bí zhǒng】鼻忽然肿胀，疼痛异常，多因肺经火毒凝聚而成。

闭 【bì】 1. 见"闭证"。2. 指大便或小便不通。

闭经 【bì jīng】(经闭) 指女子年逾十八周岁，月经未至者，为原发性闭经；或正常月经周期建立后，又停经三个月以上者，为继发性闭经。辨证

or wind-heat factors, usually accompained with other manifestations of superficies-syndrome.

Nasal Polyp　　a protruding growth from the mucosa of the nose, which is caused by the attack of pathogenic wind-cold factors to the lung leading to the accumulation of fluid in the nose, accompanied with stuffy nose and anosmia.

Sinusitis　　a condition due to attack of pathogenic wind-cold or wind-heat factors and gallbladder heat to the brain, or associated with deficiency of qi; manifested as stuffness of the nose, anosmia, yellowish and foul nasal discharge, accompanied with dizziness, headache, amnesia.

Nose Acupuncture　　a type of acupuncture treatment by puncturing the points around the nose with filiform needles, usually applied for the treatment of arthritis, neuralgia, asthmatic cough, ect.

Swelling of Nose　　a morbid condition of sudden appearance of a swollen nose, accompanied with intense pain caused by the attack of pathogenic fire from the lung meridian to the nose.

Blockage　　1. Sthenia-type Coma 2. Retention of Feces or Urine.

Amenorrhea　　a disorder referring to the woman of eighteen year-old has no menstruation, considering primary amenorrhea; or stopping

分类 1. 肾阴虚证 2. 气血虚弱证 3. 痰湿阻滞证 4. 阴虚内热证 5. 寒凝证 6. 气滞血瘀证。

menstruation for three months after the regular circle, considering secondary amenorrhea. Types of differentiation 1. syndrome of deficiency of the kidney-yin 2. syndrome of insufficiency of both qi and blood 3. syndrome of obstruction of phlegm-dampness 4. syndrome of internal heat caused by deficiency of yin 5. syndrome of cold stagnation 6. syndrome of qi stagnation leading to blood stasis.

闭证 【bì zhèng】由于邪气内陷，闭阻心窍所致，以神昏为主症，伴有牙关紧闭、两手握拳、痰涎壅盛、脉弦滑或洪数为主要临床表现的证候。

Blockage sthenia-type coma, a syndrome with coma as the major symptom, due to mental disorder resulting from the retention of the pathogenic factors, accompanied with lockjaw, clenching of fists, salivation and profuse expectoration, wiry and smooth pulse or bounding and fast pulse, etc.

闭气 【bì qì】（闭息）指吸气后停闭呼吸，为延长吸气之意。

Closing Qi also called closing breathing, referring to stopping breathing for a moment, so as to make inhaling long and deep.

痹 【bì】1. 泛指邪气闭阻肢体、经络、脏腑所引起的多种疾病。2. 指风寒湿邪侵袭肢体经络而导致肢节疼痛、麻木、屈伸不利的证候。3. 闭阻不通的病理。

Bi 1. referring to the diseases due to blocking of extremities, meridians and viscera by pathogenic factors. 2. a syndrome marked by arthralgia, numbness and dyskinesia of the limbs; due to attack of the meridians of the limbs by pathogenic wind, cold and damp factors. 3. an obstructive disorder.

痹气 【bì qì】由于阳虚、寒盛,使营卫失调、血行不畅,致气血闭阻不通的病理。主要见于痛证。

痹证 【bì zhèng】指风寒湿邪侵袭肢体经络而导致肢节疼痛、麻木、屈伸不利的证候。

髀 【bì】1. 指股部的代称。2. 指股部的上半部分。

髀枢 【bì shū】指骨关节。

砭石 【biān shí】我国石器时代产生和使用的,最古的医疗工具之一,专用于刺割患部。以治疗各种疼痛,刺破皮下小血管放血或切开脓包等。

便秘 【biàn bì】指大便干燥秘结,排出困难;或排便次数少,二、三天以上不大便。多因气虚推动无力,或阴虚血少,大肠燥结,或胃中实热,气滞不行所致。

便脓血 【biàn nóng xuè】指大便带脓血,是痢疾的常见症状。

便溏 【biàn táng】指大便稀薄不成形,常伴有食欲不佳、疲乏、腹隐痛、脉濡弱等,多因脾虚不能运化水谷精微

Impediment of Qi   a morbid state usually seen in painful conditions, which is due to the deficiency of yang and domination of cold factor leading to the imbalance of ying-wei qi, and obstruction of qi and blood circulation.

Bi-syndrome   a syndrome marked by arthralgia, numbness and dyskinesia of the limbs; due to attack of the meridians of the limbs by pathogenic wind, cold and damp factors.

1. The Thigh 2. The Upper of The Thgh

Hip Joint.

Stone Needle   a medical instrument used in the Stone of China for relieving pain, letting out blood and perforating an abscess by local cutting with it.

Constipation   a condition of infrequency or difficulty in defecation with discharge of dry and impacted feces due to inhability of promoting peristalsis resulting from the deficiency of qi, or dryness of the large intestine resulting from the deficiency of yin and blood, or stagnation of qi resulting from the retention excessive heat in the stomach.

Purulent and Bloody Stool   a sign commonly seen in dysentery.

Loose Stool   a disorder accompanied with poor appetite, fatigue, dull abdominal pain, and floating, slow and

和水湿所致。

便血 【biàn xuè】指排出血便的病证，因火邪热毒迫血妄行；或湿毒蕴结大肠；或脾胃阳虚；或风邪结于阴分所致。

变证 【biàn zhèng】疾病由简单变复杂，从轻证变重证的证候变化。

辨斑疹 【biàn bān zhěn】通过观察斑疹出现的部位、分布情况、颜色及伴随症状来判断病情的一种方法。

辨疮疡 【biàn chuāng yáng】通过观察疮疡红肿情况、皮肤颜色、肿块硬度、疼痛及感觉情况、脓液的清稀、发病的缓急、病程的长短来辨别疮疡的属性。

辨络脉 【biàn luò mài】望诊内容之一，通过观察浅表的小血管的色泽和充盈度，结合皮肤的冷暖，帮助了解脏腑气血病变。

weak pulse which is usually due to disorder of transportation of food and water resulting from the hypofunction of the spleen.

Hematochezia the discharge of bloody stool, due to extravasation of blood caused by the attack of pathogenic fire and virulent heat factors, accumulation of virulent damp in the large intestine, deficiency of spleen-yang and stomach-yang, or accumulation of pathogenic wind factor in yinfen.

Deteriorated Case the condition of patient which is changing from simple to complex and from mild to severe during the course of a disease.

Differentiation of Macules a differentiating method of a disease through the observation of the location, distribution and colour of the macules and the associated symptoms.

Differentiation of Sore a method of differentiating the nature of a sore according to redness and swelling of the lesion, the colour of the skin, the consistency of the mass, the local feeling and pain, the thickness of the pus, and the onset and duration of the disease.

Inspection of Luo-Vessel a method of physical examination by observing the colour and capacity of the superficial small vessels and by feeling the temperature of skin, so as to understand the disorders of qi, blood and

辨证 【biàn zhèng】将四诊所搜集的临床资料,运用脏腑、经络、病因等基础理论,加以分析归纳而作出诊断。

辨证论治 【biàn zhèng lùn zhì】将四诊所搜集的临床资料,运用脏腑、经络、病因等基础理论,加以分析,归纳,从而作出诊断和定出治疗措施。

辨证求因 【biàn zhèng piú yīn】通过分析疾病的症状和体征,从而找出它的病因和病机的一种方法。

标本 【biāo běn】标本是个相对概念,临床上应用标本关系,辨别病证的主次、本末、轻重、缓急、以确定治疗原则。

标本同治 【biāo běn tóng zhì】当疾病发展到标证与本证均对病人有危害时,则应采取标本兼顾的治法。

zang, fu organs.

Differential Diagnosis clinical observation for making a diagnosis based on the analysis and comprehension of the clinical data collected by the four methods of examination with the basic theories of zang, fu, meridians and pathogeny.

Treatment Based on the Differential Diagnosis making a diagnosis and selecting the treatment based on the analysis and comprehension of the clinical data collected by the four methods of examination with the basic theories of zang-fu, meridians and pathogeny.

Differential Diagnosis Aiming at the Etiology a diagnostic method or the determination of etiology and pathogenesis of a disease through the analysis of symptoms and signs.

Primary and Secondry Symptoms andsigns two conceptions existing with opposite relation, such as major and minor, primary and secondary, mild and severe, insidious and acute; the differentiation between them would be helpful to determine the therapeutical principle in clinical practice.

Treatment of the Primary and Secondary Symptoms simultaneously a principle of treatment should be applied when the primary aspects and the secondary ones are equally harmful to the patient.

瘭疽 【biāo jū】(燎疽)(1) 指疽发于手指端或足趾端者。(2) 泛指发生于体表的疽由外伤感染,毒入肌肤、筋脉所致;或由脏腑火毒凝结而成。

Felon (1) a purulent infection or abscess involving the pulp of the distal phalanx of the finger or toe. (2) broadly, the suppurative lesions on the body surface caused by injury, complicated by infection or accumulation of virulent fire factor in the viscera.

表寒 【biǎo hán】感受风寒之邪所致的一种证候,症见恶寒发热、无汗、身体疼痛、舌苔薄白而润、脉浮紧等。

Cold-Syndrome of Superficies a type of syndrome caused by the attack of pathogenic wind-cold factors, characterized by chillness, fever, anhidrosis, general aching, thin and whitish, moist fur on the tongue, floating and tense pulse, etc.

表寒里热 【biǎo hán lǐ rè】(外寒内热)表寒证与里热证并见,多因患者素有里热,复外感风寒;或在表的风寒未解。入里化热所致。临床上既见表寒的证候又并见里热的证候。

Cold in the Superficies and Heat in the Interior a morbid condition resulting from the exposure to pathogenic wind-cold factor in a person with pre-existing pathogenic heat in the interior, or from the pathogenic wind-cold factor in the exterior which invades the interior and transforms into heat factor; manifested clinically as both exterier cold and internal heat-symptoms and signs.

表解里未和 【biǎo jiě lǐ wèi hé】在表的病变已消失,在里的病变尚存在。多因里有痰饮、食滞、瘀血或伤阴等所致。

Superficies Subsided while Interior Unrelieved a morbid condition mostly caused by retention of phlegm, accumulation of indigested food and blood stasis in the body or damage of yin.

表里 【biǎo lǐ】是八纲辨证辨别疾病的部位和病势深浅的两个纲领。一般以病变在皮毛、经络属表,病较轻浅;病变在脏腑属里,病较深重。

Superficies and Interior two principal aspects for estimating the site and severity of a disease. In general, a disease involving the skin, hair and

表里传 【biǎo lǐ chuán】即疾病在互为表里的两经相传。如太阳与少阴、阳明与太阴、少阳与厥阴都是互为表里，若疾病由太阳传入少阴，即为表里传。

表里俱寒 【biǎo lǐ jù hán】表寒证与里寒证并见。因外感风寒，内为生冷寒滞所伤；或平时已有脾肾阳虚，复感受风寒之邪所致。

表里俱热 【biǎo lǐ jù rè】即表里同见热性的证候，多因外邪化热充斥表里，或内原有积热又感温邪所致。

表里俱实 【biǎo lǐ jù shí】肌表和脏腑均表现为邪气盛的病证，临床上既可见表实的证候又并见里实的证候。

表里俱虚 【biǎo lǐ jù xū】既有卫外的

meridians is considered as a mild form impairing the superficies, while that involving the viscera as a more serious form impairing the interior.

Transmission from Superficies to Interior　the progress of a disease which involves the superficial meridian first and then the corresponding interior meridian, e. g., from taiyang to shaoyin, from yang ming to taiyin, from shaoyang to jueyin.

Cold both in Superficies and Interior　simultaneous occurrence of superficial and internal cold-syndrome resulting from the exposure to pathogenic cold factor and damage by indigested food or drugs of cold nature, or from the exposure to wind-cold factors in a person whose spleen-yang and kidney-yang are deficient.

Heat both in Superficies and Interior　a morbid condition caused by the exogenous pathogenic factors transforming to heat which accumulates in both the superficies and the interior, or the attack of pathogenic warm factor to the body with retention of heat.

Excess both in Superficies and Interior　a morbid state with hyperactivity of pathogenic factors in both zang-fu organs and the superficies; manifested clinically as the symptoms of excess syndrome both in the superficies and interior.

Deficiency both in Superficies and Inte-

阳气不足，又有脏腑气血虚衰的证候。

表里双解【biǎo lǐ shuāng jiě】表里同病时，既治表证又治里证的一种治法。

表里同病【biǎo lǐ tóng bìng】1. 指既有恶寒发热、头痛等表证，又有胸满、腹痛、腹泻等里证。2. 指表里出现同一类性质的病。

表热【biǎo rè】感受风热阳邪而出现的一种证候。

表热里寒【biǎo rè lǐ hán】《外热内寒》表热证与里寒证并见。多因素有脏腑虚寒，复兼外感风热；或外邪未解而过服寒凉，使脾胃阳气不足所致。

表实【biǎo shí】表证一种，多因外邪侵入后，正邪相争于肌表，腠理密闭所表现出的证候。除有表证的症状外，常以恶寒、无汗、头痛、身痛、脉

rior   a morbid condition with deficiency of the protective yang-qi and also of qi, blood and zang-fu organs.

Expelling Pathogenic Factors both in the Superficies and Interior   a treatment for the case with both superficies-syndrome and interior-syndrome.

Syndromes Appearing both in Superficies and Interior.   1. a condition in which the superficies-syndrome (chillness, fever, headache, etc.) and the interiors-syndrome (chest fullness, abdominal pain, diarrhea, etc.) appear at the same time. 2. a condition in which the same nature of disorder appears in both the superficies and the interior.

Heat-Syndrome of Superficies   a type of superficies-syndrome caused by the attack of pathogenic wind-heat, and yang factors.

Heat in Superficies and Cold in Interior   a morbid condition resulting from the exposure to pathogenic wind-heat in person whose viscera are in an asthenia-cold state, or from the insufficiency of yang-qi of the spleen and stomach due to excessive intake of food or drugs of cold nature when the exogenous factor is not eliminated.

Sthenia-Syndrome of Superficies   a type of superficies-syndrome caused by the conflict between the healthy qi and the pathogenic factors in the su-

浮有力为特点。

表邪 【biǎo xié】在表的病邪，多指六淫邪气在表，常见发热、恶风寒，或鼻塞咳嗽等症。

表邪内陷 【biǎo xié nèi xiàn】由于正气不足，邪气亢盛，致在表的病邪陷入于里的病证。症见不恶寒、高热神昏、谵妄等。多属病情恶化的一种表现。

表虚 【biǎo xū】表证的一种，是正邪相争于肌表而卫外的阳气不足，腠理不密而出现的一种证候。除有表证的症状外，以自汗或汗出恶风、脉浮缓无力等为特征。

表证 【biǎo zhèng】病邪在浅表的证候，多见于外感病的初期。症见恶寒发热、头痛、鼻塞咳嗽、舌苔薄白、脉浮等。

perficies when the superficies is strong; characterized by chillness, anhidrosis, headache, general aching and floating-vigorous pulse.

Pathogenic Factors Involving the Superficies referring to the six exogenous pathogenic factors attacking the superficies, leading to symptoms as fever, chilliness, stuffy nose, cough, etc.

Superficial Pathogenic Factors Invading the Interior a morbid condition indicative of the deterioration of disease, caused by insufficiency of healthy-qi and hyperactivity of the pathogenic factors invading the interior from the superficies; marked by high fever not accompanied with chilliness, loss of consciousness, delirium, etc; It is the characteristics of worse condition.

Asthenia-Syndrome of Superficies a type of superficies-syndrome caused by the conflication between the healthy-qi and the pathogenic factors in the superficies when the protective yang-qi is debilitated and the superficies is weakened; characterized by spontaneous perspiration, aversion to wind while sweating and floating, slow and weak pulse.

Superficies-Syndrome a syndrome caused by the attack of pthogenic factors to the superficies, seen in the early stage of diseases due to exogenous pathogenic factors; manifested as

表证入里 【biǎo zhèng rù lǐ】表证化热，病势向里发展，症见不恶寒反恶热、心烦口渴、小便黄赤、舌苔黄燥。

冰瑕翳 【bīng xiá yì】翳生于风轮之上，色光白而薄，成点成片，如冰上之瑕。

并病 【bìng bìng】伤寒一经的病变未愈又出现另一经的病变，两经的病变先后并见。如太阳与阳明并病，太阳与少阳并病等。

病传 【bìng chuán】指疾病的传变。

病机 【bìng jī】指病因、病位、证候、脏腑气血虚实变化的机理。

病脉 【bìng mài】病态的脉象，是疾病反映于脉搏的变化。

病能 【bìng néng】既疾病的临床表现及病因、发病机理的统称。

chillness, fever, headache, stuffy nose, cough, thin and whitish fur on the tongue, floating pulse, etc.

Superficies-Syndrome Entering the Interior the development of a superficies-syndrome which tends to become heat and involves the interior; manifested as aversion to heat but not to cold, restlessness, thirst, deep-coloured urine, dry and yellowish fur on the tongue, etc.

Thin Nebula a slight corneal opacity which is thin and transparent.

Complication a condition of seasonal febrile disease in which the disease of another meridian appeaprs when the disease of one meridian is not relieved, and the disorders of both two meridians are found successively, such as taiyang disease complicated with yangming disease, taiyang disease complicated with shaoyang disease.

Development of Disease progress of a disease.

Pathogenesis the mechanism of disease including its etiology, location, manifestations, the changes of deficiency or excess of the zang-fu, qi and blood.

Abnormal Pulse certain changes of the pulse which reflect diseases.

Morbid State a general term for the clinical manifestation, pathogeny and machanism of a disease.

病气标本 【bìng qì biāo běn】从人体与致病因素的的关系来说,人体的正气是本,致病的邪气是标。

病人膏肓 【bìng yù gāo huāng】属疾病由轻转重,发展到了危重的阶段,此时患者往往形体消瘦,神色衰败。

病色 【bìng sè】疾病反映在体表色泽的变化,通常以面部色泽为主。

病㿉 【bìng tuí】指双侧睾丸肿大。多因痰气结于肝经所致。

病温 【bìng wēn】指所患病证属温邪性质。

病因辨证 【bìng yīn biàn zhèng】根据疾病的不同临床表现,了解疾病的原因及其病理变化的一种辨证方法。

病在中旁取之 【bìng zài zhōng páng qǔ zhī】身体内在的脏腑发生病变,可以取分布于四肢经络的穴位来治疗。

剥苔 【bō tāi】舌苔剥脱。若舌苔长期剥脱如地图样,多属虫积。若在热性病中,舌苔在短时间内全部剥脱,且舌质深红或光如镜面,是肝肾真阴亏损,正虚邪内陷的重症。

Branch (Biāo) and Root (Běn) Concerning the Pathongenic Factors and the Body pathogenic factors, the healthy qi is considered as the root, and the pathogenic factors as the branch.

The Disease Has Attacked the Vitals a critical stage of a disease manifested as emaciation and seriously sickly complexion, which is usually not to be cured.

Sickly Complexion the colour change of the skin, which results from various diseases.

Bilateral Enlargement of Testes a condition due to stagnation of phlegm in the liver meridian.

Febrile Diseases a disease in which the syndromes are caused by pathogenic warm factor.

Differential Diagnosis for Detecting the Etiology a diagnostic method by observing the various clinical manifestations of the disease to detect its etiology and pathological changes.

Treating the Diseases of Internal Organs by Managing the Lateral Portion treatment for the diseased internal organs by puncturing the points along the meridians of the extremities.

Exfoliative Fur map-like exfoliation of the tongue fur existing for a long duration is indicative of parasitic infestation. The fur exfoliating completely in a short time during a febrile disease and the tongue appearing smooth as a mirror with bright red colour are indicative of a serious disease due to exhaustion of primary-yin in the liver and kidney or invasion of pathogenic factors in the case of deficiency of healthy-qi.

薄厥 【bó jué】因暴怒等精神刺激,致阳气亢盛,血随气逆郁积头部,而出现卒然头痛、昏厥的重证。

Syncope due to Emotional Upset a serious condition due to overabundance of yang-qi and stagnation of blood in the head, which results from emotional upsets, manifested as sudden onset of headache and syncope.

补法 【bǔ fǎ】(补养) 八法之一。补养人体阴阳气血不足,治疗各种虚证的方法。通常分为补气、补血、补阴、补阳等。

Therapy for Invigoration a therapy for various types of asthenia-syndrome due to insufficiency of yin, yang, qi and blood; which is generally classified into invigoration of qi, tonifying of blood, invigoration of yin and invigoration of yang.

补剂 【bǔ jì】具有补益功用的方剂。

补脾 【bǔ pí】(益脾,健脾)

补脾益肺 【bǔ pí yì fèi】(培土生金) 用补脾的方法,使脾的功能强健,以治疗肺脏亏虚的病变,是五行相生学说在治疗上的具体运用。

Prescription with Tonic Effect

Invigorating the Spleen

Invigorating the Spleen to Benefit the Lung a treatment for the disorder of lung-asthenia by invigorating the spleen and promoting its activity. It is also described as the treatment by building up the "earth" to generate the "metal", which is the application of the theory of five-elements in the medical practice.

补气 【bǔ qì】(益气) 补法之一,是治疗气虚证的方法。适用于气虚证。表现为倦怠乏力,精神不振,呼吸气少,面色㿠白,自汗怕风,大便滑泄,脉弱或虚大无力等。

Invigorating Qi a therapy of invigoration for the treatment of deficiency of qi, which is applicable to the cases manifested as lassitude, listlessness, shortness of breath, pale complexion, spontaneous perspiration, aversion to wind, loose stools or diarrhea, weak pulse or feeble and large pulse, etc.

Replenishing Qi and Strengthening the Superficies 【bǔ qì gú biǎo】治疗气虚致表疏不固的方法。常用于气虚容易出汗的患者。 a treatment for weakness of the superficies due to deficiency of qi, which is applicable to the case manifested as hyperhidrosis.

Hemostasis by Invigorating the Qi 【bǔ qì shè xuà】（补气止血）是治疗由于气虚致出血日久不止的方法。 a treatment for prolonged bleeding due to deficiency of qi.

Invigorating the Kindney 【bǔ shèn】补益肾脏的方法。一般分补肾阴和补肾阳。 a treatment for invigorating the kidney, which is classified into invigoration of kidney-yin and invigoration of kidney yang.

Improving Inspiration by Invigorating the Kidney 【bǔ shèn nà qì】（纳气）是治疗肾虚不能纳气的方法。适用于肾不纳气，症见气短气促、吸气困难、苔淡白、脉细无力等。 a treatment for difficulty in inspiration due to kindney-asthenia, applicable to the case manifested as inspiratory dyspnea, pale tongue, small and weak pulse, etc.

Invigoration and Dispersion 【bǔ tuō】动用补益和消散的药物，扶助正气，托毒外出的方法。 a treatment for strengthening the healthy qi and eliminating the toxic materal by the application of drugs of invigoration and dispersion.

Nourishing the Blood 【bǔ xuè】治疗血虚证的方法。适用于证见面色苍白或萎黄、头晕目眩、心悸气短、唇舌色淡、脉细等血虚证。 a treatment for blood deficiency, which is applicable to the cases manifested as pallor or sallow complexion, dizziness, palpitation, shortness of breath, pale lips and tongue, small pulse, etc.

Invigorating Yang 【bǔ yáng】（助阳）治疗阳虚证的方法，多指补肾阳，适用于证见腰膝酸冷、畏寒乏力、阳萎滑精、小便 a treatment for the syndrome of yang-deficiency, usually referring to the tonification of

频数、舌淡苔白、脉沉细等。

kidney-yang, which is applicable to the cases manifested as soreness and cold feeling in the loins and knees, lassitude, impotance, emission, frequent micturition, pale tongue with whitish fur, sunken and small pulse, etc.

补阴 【bǔ yīn】（滋阴、育阴、养阴、益阴）用甘寒滋养的药物治疗阴虚证的方法。适用于阴虚液亏的各种疾病。

Invigorating Yin a treatment for yin-deficiency with the sweet and cold-natured drugs of nourishing yin, which is applicable to various diseases caused by yin-deficiency and fluid consumption.

不传 【bù chuán】外感病不论病程长短，其主要症状和脉象不变，病邪没有向他经传变的一种病理现象。

Diseased Condition Staying in One Meridian a phenomenon of disease caused by exogenous pathogenic factor in which the factor is kept in one meridian and does not involve the other, and the chief symptoms and pulse condition remain the same no matter how the disease persists.

不寐 【bù mèi】经常性失眠的一种病态，由于阴血亏损、中气不足、心脾两虚或痰多、水饮等使心神不安所致。

Sleeplessness a morbid state with frequent insomnia is caused by mental restlessness resulting from the consumption of yin-blood, insufficiency of middle-energizer qi, and deficiency of both the heart and spleen, and retention of fluid, etc.

不内外因 【bù nèi wài yīn】古代三因分法的一类病因，包括饮食、劳倦、跌扑、虫兽伤等。

Pathogenic Factors neither Endogenous nor Exogenous one of the three kinds of pathogenic factors in accordance with the classification in ancient times, including improper diet, overstrain, trauma, animal bites, insect stings, etc.

不食 【bù shí】由于脾胃虚弱，气滞或

Loss of Appetite a symptom result-

痰湿内阻引起不思饮食的一种病证。ing from asthenia of the spleen and stomach, stagnation of qi or retention of phlegm-damp.

不育 【bù yù】通常指男子无生育能力的一种病证。可因先天性生殖器发育不全或其它疾病引起的肾气亏损、精气虚冷所致。

Sterility in Male a disease in male with lack of reproductive function, which is caused by the congenital malformations of the sexual organs, or the decline of kidney-qi and the asthenia-cold of essence-qi resulting from other diseases.

不孕症 【bù yùn zhèng】由于生殖系统的先天性生理缺陷和畸形或其他各种疾病而致不能受孕的疾病,分原发不孕与继发不孕。辨证分类 1. 肾虚证。2. 痰湿证。3. 肝郁证。4. 血瘀证。

Sterility in Female the inability of production resulting from congenital defect or deformity of the productive system and other diseases, including primary and secondary sterility. Type of differentiation 1. sydrome of the kidney insufficiency 2. syndrome of the pathogenic phlegm-damp 3. syndrome of stagnation of the liver-qi 4. syndrome of the blood stasis.

布指 【bù zhǐ】诊脉时手指布置的方法。为成人切脉,用三指定位。通常沿腕部桡动脉分布,以中指在桡骨茎突处为准,该处为关,然后食指放在其前(寸部),无名指放在其后(尺部)。为三岁以上的小儿诊脉,多用一指(食指或拇指)按脉,不必分三部,对三岁以下的小儿则以望指纹代替脉诊。

Arrangement of the Fingers during Pulse Feeling referring to the pulse feeling with three fingers for the adults, the pulse is palpated over the radial artery proximal to the wrist with styloid process of the radius as a mark where the tip of the middle finger is put over (guan region), the tip of the index finger is placed distal to it (cun region) and that of the ring finger proximal to it (chi region), the pulse feeling for the children over 3 years old with only one finger (index finger or thumb); and observation of the superficial venules of their index fingers is made instead of pulse feel-

仓廪之官 【cāng lǐn zhī guān】指脾和胃,它们是提供脏腑器官和全身营养的"仓库"。

Official of the Granaries referring to the spleen and stomach which serve as the granaries for supplying nutrients to the internal organs and the whole body.

嘈杂 【cáo zá】指自觉胃中空虚,灼热不适的证状。

Gastric Discomfort with Acid Regurgitation feeling of emptiness, burning and uneasiness in the stomach.

草药 【cǎo yào】一般的中药书籍没有记载,而在某一局部地区或民间用以医治疾病的药物。

Herbal Medicine the local medicinal plants which are applied clinically in certain districts by the folk practitioners but not yet recorded in the classical works of Chinese materia medica.

参伍不调 【cēn wǔ bù tiáo】脉搏节律不整,往来不畅的一种脉象。

Irregular Pulse a pulse condition with irregularity in rhythm and interruption in flowing.

插药 【chā yào】将药粉加厚糊制成细药条,插入疮内或瘘管内以去腐生肌,用于一些疮疡或瘘管的治疗。

Insertion of Drugs a traetment for abscess and fistula by inserting the medicinal strip into the lesion which is able to remove the putrid tissues and promote the growth of new tissues.

差经 【chà jīng】(错经)多因嗜食辛辣食品,积热郁久,内扰冲任,迫血妄行所致。症见行经时,大便同时出血。

Supplementary Menstruation menstrual flow from the uterus and meanwhile from the rectum, which is caused by the excessive intake of pungent food, prolonged stagnation of pathogenic heat involving thorough fare and conception vessels leading to the extravasation of blood.

差㿉 【chā tuí】指小儿单侧睾丸肿大。

Unilateral Enlargement of Testis in Children

茶 【chá】指药茶。将药物粗末,制成块状,用沸水泡或煎服以代茶饮。

Medicinal Tea a pharmaceutical preparation made of medicinal gran-

察目 【chá mù】望诊内容之一。眼与五脏六腑的功能活动有密切关系,通过观察眼神、色泽、形态和功能来了解内脏的情况。

Inspection of the Eyes an item of inspection by observing the expression, colour, structure and function of the eyes to understand the condition of internal organs, as the eyes are closely related to the function of the internal organs.

掺药 【chān yào】外用药的一种。把适量的药物放在膏药中心,贴在肿疡上;也可直接掺布于疮面上或粘附于药线上,而插入疮口内,具有消肿、提脓、去腐、生肌、止痛、止血等功用。

Topical application of Medicinal Powder one kind of external application of drugs for subsidence of swelling, pus drainage, clearing of necrotic tissues, promotion of granulation, analgesia, hemostasis, etc.

缠腰火丹 【chán yào huǒ dān】生于腰肋间的泡疹性疾病。由心肝二经火邪湿毒凝结而成。初起患处刺痛发红,继而出现米粒样透明水泡,累累如串珠,呈束带状排列。即带状疱疹。

Herpes Zoster around the Waist groups of deep-seated vesicles on erythematous bases distributed over one side of the waist and hypochondrium following the course of a nerve, associated with neuralgic pain; which is caused by the stagnation of fire and damp in the heart and liver meridians.

产后痹证 【chǎn hòu bì zhèng】产后关节肿痛,多因产后气血大虚,经络、关节受风寒湿邪所致。

Puerperal Arthralgia a condition due to marked deficiency of qi and blood after delivery, and the attack of meridians and joints by the wind-cold-damp factors.

产后遍身疼痛 【chǎn hòu biàn shēn téng tòng】指产后全身肌肉疼痛、乏力、短气等,或伴有头痛、恶寒、发热、多因产后气血虚损,气血运行不畅,瘀血滞于经络、肌肉间;或因外邪侵袭经络、血脉所致。

Puerperal General Aching a condition in puerperium characterized by aching all over the body, fatigue and shortness of breath, probably accompanied with headache, chillness and fever, which is due to retention of

产后病痉 【chǎn hòu bìng jìng】指产后突然出现颈项强直、四肢抽搐、甚至牙关紧闭、角弓反张等症的一种病证,多因产后阴血大亏,复感风邪,引动肝风;或产后亡血伤津,筋脉失养所致。

产后不语 【chǎn hòu bù yǔ】产后失语。多伴有唇舌紫暗、胸闷、喉有痰声、或气短、心悸、自汗等。多因产后痰瘀停滞心下或因心气虚不能通于舌所致。

产后瘈疭 【chǎn hòu chì zòng】产后出现手足交替伸缩,抽动不已,多因产后血虚,筋失濡养所致。

产后疮疡 【chǎn hòu chuàng yáng】产后发生疮疡之病。多因气虚血亏,肌

blood stasis in the meridians and muscles resulting from the consumption of qi and blood during labour with impediment of their circulation, or due to attack of exogenous factors to the meridians and vessels.

Puerpera Convulsion a disorder with sudden onset of stiffness of neck, spasms of extremities or even trismus, opisthotonos, etc. after childbirth, which is due to consumption of yin blood associated with the attack of pathogenic wind leading to hyperactivity of the liver-wind, or due to exhaustion of blood and body fluid resulting in undernourishment of the muscles and vessels.

Puerperal Aphasia a condition in puerperium caused by retention of phlegm and blood stasis in the epigastrium, or deficiency of the heart-qi which fails to flow to the tongue; usually accompanied with dark purplish colouration of the lips and tongue, feeling of oppression over the chest, wheezing sound during respiration, shortness of breath, lassitude, palpitation, spontaneous perspiration, etc.

Puerperal Clonic Convulsion a disorder on puerperium marked by alternating contraction and relaxing of the muscles, resulting from deficiency of blood and failure to nourish the tendons.

Pyogenic Infection of the Skin after Delivery a disorder caused by the

肤受毒邪侵袭而致。 attack of pathogenic factor to the skin in a puerperant with deficiency of qi and blood.

产后大便难 【chǎn hòu dà biàn nán】即产后大便秘结，多因产后血虚津亏，大肠失润或气虚致大肠传送无力。

Puerperal Constipation a condition in puerperium due to dryness of the large intestine resulting from exhaustion of blood and body fluid, or due to hypotonia of the large intestine resulting from deficiency of qi.

产后盗汗 【chǎn hòu dào hàn】妇女分娩后入睡出汗，醒后即止，多因产时耗伤气血，血虚阴亏所致。

Puerperal Nitht Sweat a condition in puerperium caused by consumption of qi and blood during labour leading to deficiency of blood and yin.

产后恶露不绝 【chǎn hòu è lù bù jué】（恶露不下）产后三周以上恶露不绝；引产半月以上或早期流产一周以上，恶露不绝者。多因产后气虚，冲任不固，或败血瘀阻影响冲任，血不归经所致。辨证分类 1. 气虚证。2. 血热证。3. 血瘀证。

Lochiostasis lochina persists in dripping for more than three weeks after labour, or for more than fifteen days after artificial abortion, or for more than seven days after natural abortion in early pregnancy, which is caused by deficiency of qi with impairment of thoroughfare and conception vessels, or the attack of the blockage of stasis to these two vessvels leading to disorder of blood flow. Types of differentiation 1. syndrome of qi deficiency 2. syndrome of blood heat 3. syndrome of blood stasis.

产后腹痛 【chǎn hòu fù tòng】产后小腹痛，多因血虚、血瘀或寒凝所致。

Puerperal Abdominal Pain a condition due to blood-deficiency, blood stasis or retention of pathogenic cold factor.

产后感染发热 【chǎn hòu gǎn rǎn yǎn fā rè】产后十天内，发热不解，连续三天体温在38℃以上，并伴有腹痛及恶露色、质、量、气味等变化。需与血虚、外感、蒸乳发热相鉴别，辨

Pureperal Inflammatory Fever a morbid condition with the temperature above 38℃ lasting more than three days within ten days after labour, which is accompanied with

证分类 1. 邪毒证。2. 血瘀证。

abdominal pain and the changes of the colour, state, amount and smell of the lochio stasis; it should be distinguished from deficiency of blood, exogenous pathogenic factor and the fever due to acute mastitis. Types differentiation 1. syndrome of the pathogenic toxin 2. syndrome of blood stasis.

产后交肠病 【chǎn hòu jiāo cháng bìng】产后大小便从阴道而出，相当于产后伤造成的阴道直肠瘘或阴道尿瘘。

Vaginal Fistula in Puerperium an abnormal passage communicating with the vagina resulting from injuries during labour, similar to rectovaginal fistula, urethrovaginal fistula, etc.

产后惊悸 【chǎn hòu jīng jì】产后易受惊恐而发生心慌、心悸、心中不宁等。多因产后血虚，心气不足所致。

Puerperal Palpitation a disorder in puerperium manifested as timidness, palpitation and restlessness, which is caused by the deficiency of blood and the insufficiency of the heart-qi.

产后拘挛 【chǎn hòu jū luán】指产后感觉肢体牵引不适，活动不能自如，伴头昏目眩、目涩等。多因分娩耗伤气血，阴血不足，筋失所养；亦有因外邪、瘀血留滞筋脉引起。

Puerperal Muscular Spasm a disorder in purperium marked by stiffness and immobility of the limbs, accompained with dizziness, dryness of the eyes, which is caused by the consumption of qi and blood, insufficiency of yin blood and failed to nourish the tendons; or by the attack of exogenous factors or blood stasis in the meridians.

产后口渴 【chǎn hòu kǒu kě】产后渴欲饮水。多因产后失血、多汗、耗伤津液，或阴虚火旺，灼伤津液所致。

Puerperal Thirst a desire for drinking water in puerperium due to consumption of body fluid, which is caused by loss of blood, profuse perspiration, or yin-deficiecy with excessive fire.

产后麻瞀【chǎn hòu mā mào】产妇分娩后感觉四肢麻木,头晕目眩。多因产后气血亏虚,不能濡养周身四肢;或气虚湿停,聚湿成痰,阻滞经络所致。

Puerperal Numbness and Dizziness a morbid condition on puerperium due to deficiecy of qi and the blood failed to nourish the body and the extremities, or due to deficiency of qi and accumulation of pathogenic damp with formation of phlegm leading to the obstruction of meridians.

产后乳汁自出【chǎn hòu rǔ zhī zì chū】(产后乳汁溢)产后不因吸吮而乳汁自动流出,多因脾胃气虚不能固摄,乳汁失约而自溢出;或因肝火亢盛,迫乳外溢所致。

Puerperal Galactorrhea spontaneous flow of milk in puerperium, which is caused by asthenia of the spleen and stomach leading to inability to hold the milk, or by the hyperactivity of the liver-fire which forces the milk to overflow.

产后三冲【chǎn hòu sān chāng】产后出现神志错乱、癫狂、胸闷烦躁、气急咳逆、脘闷呕恶、腹满胀痛等症。多因产后恶露、瘀血不下,或下而不畅,逆而上冲,引起败血冲心、败血冲肺、败血冲胃三种危急证候。

Three Puerperal Lochiostasis-Syndrome three critical conditions resulting from retention of lochia and blood stasis, i.e., that affecting the heart (manifested as alienation, depression and maia), that affecting the lung (manifested as feeling of oppression over the chest, cough, and dyspnea), that affecting the stomach (manifested as nausea, vomiting and abdominal distending pain).

产后三脱【chǎn hòu sān tuō】产后出现气急、喘促不宁、血崩、神志不清等症状。多因产后气、血、神剧损,引起气脱、血脱、神脱所致。

Three Puerperal Exhaustion three syndromes due to over consumption, they are qi-exhaustion syndrome, blood-exhaustion syndrome, and spirit-exhaustion syndrome, manifested as dyspnea, metrorrhagia and unconsciousness.

产后伤食【chǎn hòu shāng shí】产后饮食不节,食积停滞中焦,损伤脾胃所致的病证,症见脘腹满闷、嗳腐吞

Puerperal Dyspepsia a disorder in puerperium due to impairment of the spleen and stomach by retention of

酸、纳呆食少，大便酸臭等。indigested food in the middle-energizer caused by immoderate eating and drinking; marked by abdominal fullness, acid regurgitation, poor appetite, discharge of fetid stools, etc.

产后四肢虚肿 【chǎn hòu sì zhī xū zhǒng】产后出现四肢浮肿，伴有腹痛、恶露不绝。多因瘀血阻滞经络，水湿停留，溢于肌肤所致。

Puerperal Edema of Extremities a disorder caused by retention of blood stasis in the meridians and accumulation of body fluid and damp involving the skin and muscles, usually accompanied with lochiostasis and abdominal pain.

产后头痛 【chǎn hòu tóu tòng】产后出现以头部疼痛为主的病证。多因血虚，脑络失养所致；亦可因外感或血瘀致头部经络受阻引起。

Puerperal Headache headache occurring in puerperium, which is usually due to blood insufficiency of failing to nourish the brain, or due to obstruction of the meridians of the head, resulting from the exogenous pathogenic factors and blood stasis.

产后小便不利 【chǎn hòu xiǎo biàn bù lì】产后出现小便量少或排出困难等症状。多因产后伤肾、肾阳虚衰，气化无力，或情志不舒，肝郁气滞，气化受阻所致。

Puerperal Dysuria difficult urination in puerperium due to hypoactivity of the kindney-yang after impairment of the kidney by childbirth, or due to stagnation of the liver-qi and hypoactivity of qi caused by emotional upsets.

产后虚烦 【chǎn hòu xū fá】产后出现烦热、少气、疲倦、胸膈满闷，不得眠等。多因产后气血亏损，虚火上扰所致。

Puerperal Vexation a condition in puerperium marked by restlessness, fever, short breath, fatigue, fullness over the chest and insomnia, which results from the consumption of qi and blood during labour and the attack of upward asthenic fire.

产后血崩 【chǎn hòu xuè bāng】产后子宫突然大量出血的危证。

Puerperal Metrorrhagia a serious state manifested as profuse uterine bleeding after childbirth.

产后血晕 【chǎn hòu xuè yūn】产后突然发生昏厥,不省人事的证候。因产后气血暴虚,虚阳浮越或恶露不下,败血停瘀,上攻于心所致。

产后腰痛 【chǎn hòu yāo tòng】产后发生腰部隐痛、乏力、耳鸣等,多因分娩伤肾,腰无所主所致;亦有因败血瘀阻滞脉而引起。

产后遗尿 【bhǎn hòu yí niào】产后发生小便不能自制,容易遗出等症状。多因产后肾气虚弱,约束无力;或产时损伤膀胱所致。

产后瘖 【chǎn hòu yīn】1. 产后声音嘶哑,难以发音。多因肺、肾两虚或脾虚气郁所致。2. 指产后失语证,见产后不语。

产后乍寒乍热 【chǎn hòu zhà hán zhà rè】产后出现时寒时热的症状。多因产后气血两虚,阴阳不调或营卫不和所致。

产后中暑 【chǎn hòu zhòng shǔ】盛夏季节,在产褥期出现头晕、恶心、胸闷、口渴、多汗,甚至高热神志不清等症。多因产后气血未复,暑邪乘虚侵袭机体所致。

Puerperal Faintness　a critical condition resulting from sudden deficiency of qi and blood leading to upward attack of the asthenic yang or resulting from the attack of lochiostasis and blood stasis to the heart.

Puerperal Lumbago　a disorder in puerperium accompanied with fatigue and tintus, which is due to impairment of the kindney during labour, or due to the obstruction of blood vessel by blood stasis.

Puerperal Enuresis　involuntary discharge of urine in puerperium, which is due to deficiency of kidney-qi leading to failure of controlling passing urine, or injury of the bladder during labour.

Puerperal Aphonia　difficult speaking in low and hoarse voice in puperium, which is caused by asthenia of both the lung and kindney or stagnation of qi due to deficiency of the spleen.

Puerperal Chills and Fever　a morbid condition due to deficiency of both qi and blood, imbalance of yin and yang, or incoordination between ying and wei after childbirth.

Puerperal Summer-Heat Stroke　a disorder occuring in puerperium during summer time, which is due to attack of summer-heat to the puerperant with deficiency of qi and blood; marked by dizziness, nausea, feeling of oppression over the chest, thirst,

产门 【chǎn mén】即阴道。

Vaginal Orifice

长脉 【cháng mài】脉长超过本位的一种脉象,长而和缓属中气健旺;长而弦硬则属病脉,多因实热内结或热盛所致。

Long Pulse a pulse condition in which the length of pulsation is abnormally long. The long and gentle pulse indicates that the middle-energizer qi is prosperous. The long and wiry pulse is pathogenic and is frequently caused by accumulation of sthenia-heat or domination of excess heat.

长针 【cháng zhèn】一种针体长为20-23厘米或更长的用于深刺的针。

Long Needle a type of acupuncture needle about 20-30 cm long or more, which is used for deep insertion.

肠痹 【cháng bì】指因大小肠的气机痹阻,致小便不利、喘满或飧泄的病证。

Intestinal Bi-Syndrome a syndrome due to dysfunction of the large or small intestine; manifested as dysuria, dyspnea, or lienteric diarrhea.

肠风 【cháng fēng】(肠风便血、肠风下血) 1. 指痔疮出血。2. 泛指因脏腑劳损,气血不调及风冷热毒搏于大肠所致的便血。3. 即风痢。4. 指大便下鲜血,血在粪前。多因外风入客或内风下乘所致。

Fresh Blood in Stool 1. bleeding from the gaemorrhoids. 2. bloody stool caused by the impairment of viscera, disorder of qi and blood, the attack of large intestine by pathogenic wind cold and heat factors. 3. wind-type dysentery. 4. discharge of bright red blood before stool caused by the attack of exogenous wind or downward endogenous wind factors to the large intestine.

肠鸣 【cháng míng】(腹鸣)指肠动作声。因中气虚,或邪在大肠所致。

Borborygmus rumbling noise caused by the propulsion of gas through the intestines, due to deficiency of the middle-energizer qi or the attack of pathogenic factor to the large intestine.

肠痈 【cháng yōng】以右下腹痛,明

Pyoenic Infection of Intestine a dis-

显压痛及反跳痛为特征,伴有发热、恶寒、恶心、便秘或腹泻。相当于急性阑尾炎,辨证分类1.气血瘀滞证。2.瘀滞化热证。3.热毒炽盛证。

order marked by pain in the right lower quadrant of the abdomen with intense local tenderness and rebound tenderness, accompanied with fever, chillness, nausea, etc; corresponding to acute appendicitis. Types of differentiation 1. stagnation of both qi and blood 2. the stagnation transferring to the pathogenic heat factor 3. excess of the pathogenic heat-toxin.

肠痔 【cháng zhì】以肛周出现核肿、疼痛、出血,伴有发热恶寒为主症的一种病证。多由湿热下注所致。

Perianal Abscess abscess located around the anal canal with local pain and bleeding, accompanied by chillness and fever; due to accumulation of pathogenic dampness-heat factors in the lower part of the body.

常毒 【cháng dú】毒性次于大毒的药物,使用时应注意方法和用量,且不宜久用。

Moderate Toxicity referring to drugs with toxicity less than the potent poisons, which should be applied with caution regarding to the usage, dosage, and applied only for a short duration.

潮热 【cháo rè】指发热如潮汛有定时,以阴虚和血虚者为多,常在午后或夜间发热,早晨退热至正常,实证则多为阳明里实证,热退不清,每至下午三至五时热势增高,常伴有大便不通等症。

Hectic Fever a fever recurring daily at regular time most seen in the cases with yin-deficiency and blood-deficiency, the temperature is high in the afternoon or at night, and becomes normal in the morning. In the case of sthenia-syndrome, mostly internal sthenia-syndrome of yang-ming, the temperature is high in the afternoon but could not return to normal and is usually accompanied with constipation.

炒 【chǎo】将药物放入锅内加热,不断拌炒,根据需要可炒至药物爆裂、

Frying a method of processing medicinal herbs by stir-frying the

或炒黄、或炒焦等。

膜胀 【chēn zhàng】指上腹部饱胀不适。多由于脾失健运，气机阻滞所致。

沉脉 【chén mài】脉象之一。脉搏深沉，轻按不应，重按始得。主病在里。沉而有力为里实；沉而无力为里虚。

成方 【chéng fāng】常用的验方，一般药味不变。

迟脉 【chí mài】脉象之一。脉率缓慢，一息不足四至（每分钟搏在六十次以下的一种脉象）。迟脉产寒证，也可因阳气被实邪阻滞所引起。经常锻炼的运动员脉迟缓有力，不属病脉。

尺脉 【chǐ mài】桡动脉搏动的近侧端。右手的称为右尺，候命门；左手的称为左尺，候肾。

齿 【chǐ】又名牙口，为口腔内嚼食物

drug on a heated pan untill it is cracked, or becomes deep coloured or charred as necessary.

Epigastric Fullness a syndrome due to dysfunction of the spleen and sluggishness of qi.

Sunken Pulse a pulse condition in which the beats are located deeply and palpable only by heavy pressure, indicating that the disease involves the interior. The deep and strong pulse indicates an internal sthenia-syndrome, while the deep and weak one indicates an internal asthenia-syndrome.

Formulated Prescription the classical prescription frequently used in clinical practice, generally the medicines of the prescription are unchanged.

Slow Pulse a pulse condition (with less than 60 beats per minute) with less than four beats to a normal cycle of respiration, indicates cold syndrome, also caused by the stagnation of yang-qi by excess pathogenic factor. A slow but vigorous pulse occurring in a well-trained athlete is considered as normal.

Chi Pulse the proximal throbbing of the radial pulse; which of the right hand indicates the state of the gate of life (called right chi), which of left hand indicates the state of the kidney (called left chi).

Teeth a set of small hard structures

的器官，属足少阴肾经，为肾所主。手阳明大肠经与足阳明胃经分别入上、下齿。

in the jaws used for mastication of food, belonging to the kidney meridian of Food-Shaoyin, controlled by the Kidney. The large intestine meridian of Hand-Yangming and the stomach meridian of Foot-Yangming pass through the upper and lower jaw respectively.

齿槁 【chǐ gǎo】牙齿枯槁。由肾阴枯竭，热邪熏蒸所致。

Dryness of Teeth a morbid state caused by exhaustion of kidney-yin or hyperactivity of pathogenic heat factor.

齿痕舌 【chǐ hén shé】舌边缘出现牙齿的痕迹。多属脾虚。

Tongue with Teeth Marks on its Margin a sign which usually indicates the spleen-asthenia.

齿焦 【chǐ jiāo】牙齿焦枯，由于阴液受伤所致。

Dry Teeth a morbid condition resulting from consumption of yin-fluid.

齿衄 【chǐ nǜ】血从齿缝，牙龈处渗出，甚者可流血不止。多因胃腑积热上乘；或肾阴不足，虚火上炎。或脾不统血所致。

Gum Bleeding a disorder due to upward attack of the pathogenic heat which is accumulated in the stomach, or the hyperactivity of asthenia-fire due to insufficiency of kidney-yin or failure of the spleen to control blood flow.

齿龋 【chǐ qǔ】牙齿被蛀空伴有疼痛。多因口腔不洁，或风痰湿热熏蒸手、足阳明二经所致。

Dental Caries localized, progressive decay of the teeth accompanied with toothache, which is caused by the bad oral hygiene, or by the attack of pathogenic wind, phlegm, damp and heat to the Hand and Foot-Yangming meridians.

齿龂 【chǐ xiè】睡觉时牙齿互相摩擦。多由心胃火热或气血两虚所致；小儿则常为肠道寄生虫病所致。

Teeth Grinding involuntary grinding of the teeth while sleeping, which is usually caused by fire-heat retained in the heart and stomach or deficien-

齿龈肿痛 【chǐ yín zhǒng tòng】指牙龈红肿疼痛。多因胃经实火或肾经虚火上炎所致。

赤 【chì】五色之一。即红色，它与五行中的火，五脏中的心及与热邪有密切关系。

赤白带下 【chì bái dài xià】阴道流出赤白夹杂的粘液，连绵不断。多因肝郁犯脾，湿热下注冲、任、带脉所致。

赤白痢 【chì bái lì】指下痢脓血。赤白相杂的病证。多因湿热夹滞，阻于肠道，气分血分均受侵袭所致。

赤白浊 【chì bái zhúo】白浊与赤浊的合称。见白浊及尿血。

赤带 【chì dài】阴道流出血色红似血非血的枯液，淋漓不断。多因忧思伤脾，加之郁怒伤肝，肝郁化火，夹湿热下注所致。

赤面风 【chì miàn fèng】由心胃二经

cy of both qi and blood, it is the indication of parasitosis in children.

Gingivitis inflammation of the gum, which is caused by sthenic fire retained in the stomach meridian or by flaming up of the asthenic fire in the kidney meridian.

Red one of the five colours which matches fire (in the five elements) and heart (in the five zang), and is closely related to pathogenic heat.

Leukorrhagia with Reddish and Whitish Discharge profuse vaginal discharge with reddish and whitish, mucus, which is caused by the stagnation of liver-qi involving the spleen leading to the accumulation of pathogenic damp-heat downward to the TV, CV, and BV.

Desentery with Purulent and Blooby Stools a disease caused by the accumulation of pathogenic damp-heat and indigested food in the stomach and intestines with the involvement of qifen and xuefen.

Reddish and Whitish Turbid Urine

Leukorrhagia with Reddish Discharge profuse reddish, viscid discharge from the vagina resulting from impairment of the spleen by anxiety and impairment of the liver by anger which is transmitted into pathogenic fire attaching the BV with pathogenic damp-heat factors.

Allergic Dermatitis on the Face a

气血壅盛，复感风热、郁阻肌肤而成。初起面部发红作痒，继则灼热肿胀，相当于过敏性皮炎。

赤如衃血 【chì rú pēi xuè】 形容紫黑枯槁的病色。常见于心血瘀阻、胃气衰败的疾病。

赤浊 【chì zhuó】带红色混浊的小便。见尿血。

瘛疭 【chì zòng】指手足伸缩交替，抽动不已的症状。邪热亢盛，引动肝风；津血亏损，虚风内动；或痰火壅滞，上扰心窍等，均可引起本证。

冲服 【chōng fú】将一些散剂，如田七粉先放在碗内，待其余药煎好后，趁热冲入碗内，搅匀，温服下。

冲气 【chōng qì】指在致病因素的作用下，导致冲脉之气上逆的病理。常以患者自觉有气从少腹上冲胸部和咽喉为主症。

冲任不固 【chōng rèn bù gù】指妇女冲任二脉受损，气血两虚的病理。常导致崩漏、流产、阴道分泌物增多等证候。

disease caused by the excess qi and blood in the heart and stomach meridians, the attack of pathogenic wind-heat factors involving the skin and muscles; manifested as erythema, itching, heat and swelling of the face.

Cyanotic Complexion as Coagulated Blood a sickly complexion usually seen in the case of the stagnation of heart-blood and the exhaustion of stomach-qi.

Reddish and Turbid Urine hematuria

Clonic Convulsion a disorder caused by hyperactivity of liver-wind resulting from the overabundance of pathongenic heat; or hyperactivity of asthenic wind resulting from the consumption of body fluid and blood, or the attack of the stagnation of phlegm-fire to the heart.

Be Taken with Decoction a method for oral use of some powdered medicines mixed with the hot decoction for drinking.

Rushing Up of Gas a morbid state of adverse rising of the qi of the chong meridian, resulting from the action of pathogenic factors, manifested as a subjective feeling of rushing up of gas from the lower abdomen to the thorax and throat.

Dysfunction of Thoroughfare and Conception Vessels a morbid condition in female caused by impairment of thoroughfare and conception ves-

冲任损伤　【chōng rèn sǔn shàng】指感染、房室过度或孕育过频,伤及冲、任二脉的病理,症见月经不调、下腹部疼痛、腰酸、崩漏、习惯性流产或不孕等。

Impairment of Thoroughfare and Conception Vessels　a morbid condition, caused by infection, excessive coitus or freqent pregnancy and production, manifested as irregular menstruation, pain over the lower abdomen, lunbago, metrorrhagia, habitual abortion or sterility, etc.

虫积　【chóng jī】多指肠道寄生虫病。由于饮食不洁,生虫聚积所致,症见面黄肌瘦、时吐苦水清水、腹部胀大、腹痛或脐周痛、时痛时止、或可触到积块。

Malnutrition Due to Parasitic Infestation　referring to the intestinal parasitosis due to ingestion of contaminated food, manifested as sallow complexion, emaciation, vomiting of bilious and gastric fluid, tympanites, intermittent abdominal or periumbilical pain, or palpable mass in the abdomen.

虫兽伤　【chóng shòng shāng】虫兽类对人的伤害,如蛇伤、昆虫螫刺伤等。

Injury by Insects and Animals　snake bite, bee sting, etc.

虫痫　【chóng xián】因肠道寄生虫引起的痫证。多见于小儿。

Epilepsy due to parasitic Infestation　convulsive seizures caused by intestinal parasites, mostly seen in children.

重阳　【chóng yóng】两种阳的属性同时出现于一事物上,在病理变化上是阳盛。如身热、脉洪大都属阳,称为重阳。

Double Yang　two matters attributed to yang exist simultaneously, and it appears as excessive yang in pathological changes. For example, fever and full pulse both belonging to yang are considered as double yang.

重阴　【chóng yīn】两种阴的属性同时出现于一事物上,在病理变化上是阴盛,如肢冷、脉微欲绝都属阴,两者

Double Yin　two matters attributed to yin exist simultaneously, and it appears as excessive yin in pathological

同时出现时称为重阴。

抽风 【chōu fēng】(瘛疭、抽搐) 手足伸缩交替,抽动不已的症状。常见于外感热病,热盛伤阴,风火相煽所致;过汗、失血、气血津液损伤,筋脉失养亦可引起,另风痰或热痰也能引起本症。

抽筋痧 【chōu jīn shā】痧证之一。以呕吐、腹泻、两足抽筋、胸闷,体表静脉怒张等主症的一种疾病。

出针 【chū zhēn】针刺完毕后,一手固定穴位,另一手持针,用捻转或直接向外提针将针拨出体外。

初潮 【chū cháo】指女子首次月经。

初持 【chù chí】指诊脉时切按时间较短暂的一种切脉方法。

初生不尿 【chū shēng bù niào】婴儿出生后两天仍无小便。多由于胎热蕴结于膀胱或先天不足,影响膀胱的气化所致。

changes. For example, coldness of limbs and impalpable pulse both belonging to yin are considered as double yin.

Couvulsion a series of involuntary contraction of the voluntary muscles, caused by the attack of pathogenic wind-fire factor resulting from the impairment of yin by the excess heat in the exogenous febrile disease, or by the consumption of qi, blood and body fluid after profuse sweating or bleeding leading to malnutrition of the muscles, by the attack of pathogenic wind-phlegm or heat-phlegm.

Sha-Syndrome with Convulsion a syndrome characterized by vomiting, diarrhea, convulsion, feeling of oppression over the chest, engorgement of the superficial veins.

Withdrawing the Needle the last step of acupuncture manipulation by which the needle is taken off by rotating or dircetly lifting while the skin around the acu-point is pressed downward.

Menophania the first sign of the menses at puberty.

Preliminary Pulse-Feeling pulse feeling for a short time, a method of pulse feeling.

Anuria in Newborns a disorder marked by absence of urination for two days or more after birth, resulting from the stagnation of the fetus-heat in the bladder or congenital de-

初生不乳 【chù shēng bù rǔ】婴儿出生十二小时后,不能正常吮乳。多由于元气不足,胃气上逆所致。

嚏鼻 【chù bí】把药物研成细末,由病人自己吸入或由别人吹入患者的鼻腔内,以治疗鼻部疾患。

触诊 【chù zhěn】诊法之一。医者用手对病人的皮肤、胸腹及疼痛部位进行触摸按压,以了解局部的冷热、弹性、压痛、包块或其他变化。

传变 【chuán biàn】伤寒病发展过程中,病情变化循一定规律或超越规律发展。

传导之官 【chuán dǎo zhī guān】指大肠,因为大肠是传送糟粕的通道。

传经 【chuán jīng】伤寒病发展变化的过程,从一经的病变演变为另一经的病变。通常分循经传、越经传、表里传等。

喘 【chuǎn】指呼吸急促的症状。

fects leading to dysfunction of the bladder.

Inability to Suck in Newborn a disorder of failure to suck for twelve hours after birth, resulting from insufficiency of primodial qi and adverse rising of the stomach-qi.

Nasal Insufflation application of medicinal powder insufflation into the nose for the treatment of nasal diseases.

Palpation a method of physical examination by touching, feeling and pressing the skin, thorax, abdomen and the pain area to understand changes of local temperature, elasticity, tenderness, mass and other condition.

Progress of Disease the development of seasonal febrile disease that follows the ordinary regulation or surpasses the ordinary regulation.

Official of Transportation referring to the large intestine, which is the passage for transporting the residues.

Pathogenic Factor Transmitting from One Meridian to Another development of seasonal febrile diseases in which the meridians are involved by pathogenic factor from one to another, usually as follow ways: transmitting along the meridians, surpass the meridians and transmitting from the superficies to the interior.

Asthma rapid respiration.

喘鸣 【chuǎn míng】指呼吸急促、喉间有痰鸣声的症状。

Bronchial Wheezing a main symptom of asthma, manifested as rapid respiration with wheezing.

喘胀 【chuǎn zhàng】指气喘而见肿胀的病症。多因肺脾气虚；或痰浊内盛，肺气上逆所致。多伴有小便不利。

Dyspnea-Edema Syndrome a morbid state marked by dyspnea and edema, usually accompanied with dysuria; which is caused by deficiency of both the lung and spleen-qi, or overabundance of phlegm in the body and adverse rising of lung-qi, usually accompained with dysuria.

喘证 【chuǎn zhèng】（喘息、喘逆）指以呼吸急促为特征的一种病证。多因风寒痰饮、邪火壅阻于肺，肺失肃降或肺肾虚弱，肺虚气无所主，肾虚摄纳无权所致。

Dyspnea a syndrome characterized by rapid and difficult respiraton, caused by the hypofunction of the lung resulting from the retention of pathogenic wind-cold, phlegm and fire factors, by the inability to control qi by the lung and to acceept qi by the kidney resulting from asthenia of the lung and kidney.

串 【chuàn】民间称药性下行的为串。串药多有泻下作用。

Drugs with Downward Action a term named by folk physicians including drugs which are mostly purgatives.

疮 【chuāng】指皮肤化脓性疾病。

Sore referring to the skin festering diseases.

疮毒攻心 【chuàng dú gōng xīn】毒邪内攻，扰及心营的疮疡，兼见心烦、高热、神昏或恶心呕吐等症。相当于败血症。

Suppurative Inflammation of Skin Complicated with Septicaemia a condition caused by the attack of pathogenic factor to the heart and yingfen, accompanied with irritability, fever, coma, nausea and vomiting.

疮疡 【chuāng yáng】是体表上有形证可见的外科及皮肤疾患的总称。包括所有肿疡及溃疡，如痈、疽、疔疮、痔肿、流注、流痰、瘰疬等，多

Pyogenic Infection and ulceration of Skin a general term, including carbuncle, deep-rooted carbuncle, furuncle, multiple abscess, tuberculosis

由毒邪内侵，邪热灼血，以致气血壅滞而成。 of bone and joint, scrofula, etc, resulting from the attack of pathogenic factors and consumption of blood by pathogenic heat leading to stagnation of qi and blood.

吹药 【chuī yào】将药物研成细粉，用喷药器或细管吹入，是口腔咽喉疾病的一种外治法。 **Insufflation of Drug Powder** a external treatment for oral or throat diseases by insufflating the drug powder into the oral cavity with an insufflator or tube.

春弦 【chūn xián】春季的脉象偏于弦，这是脉象随气候变化而发生相应变化的一种生理现象。 **Taut Wire-Pulse of Spring** a physiological condition that the normal pulse varies with the seasonal changes.

纯阳之体 【chún yáng zhī tǐ】一般指小儿的体质特点，即小儿正在阳气当发，生机蓬勃时期。 **Pure Yang-Body** a term referring to the constitution of infants, which shows the development of yang-qi.

唇 【chún】（飞门）七冲之一。口唇分上、下唇，它与脾有密切关系，常通过诊察口唇来帮助诊脾的疾病。 **Lips** one of the seven important openings, composed of lower and upper lips. The inspection of the lips is helpful to diagnose the spleen disorders because it is closely related to the function of the spleen.

唇疮 【chún chuāng】唇部肿胀疼痛，继则溃烂。多因脾胃蕴热所致。 **Lip Boil** a condition manifested with swelling and pain, furthery ulceration, which is usually caused by the retention of pathogenic factor of heat in the spleen and stomach.

唇疔 【chún dīng】由脾胃火毒上攻，聚于口唇所致。 **Lip Pustule** a disease caused by the attack of pathogenic fire factor in the spleen and stomach to the lips.

唇疽 【chún jū】疽生唇部。多因脾胃积热所致。 **Lip Furuncle** furuncle over the lip caused by the accumulation of pathogenic heat in the spleen and stomach.

唇裂 【chún liè】口唇干燥皲裂。常由 **Cracked Lips** a sign usually seen in

感受燥邪或热病伤津等引起。 the case of attacking to pathogenic dryness factor or a febrile disease in which the boby fluid is consumed.

唇紫 【chún zǐ】口唇紫暗或紫红，属热，多因血分热盛或血瘀所致；口唇青紫则属寒，多因寒邪壅盛，心血瘀阻，缺氧等引起。 **Purplish Lips** dark purple or reddish lips indicating pathogenic heat, resulting from excessive heat in xuefen or blood stasis; and bluish purple indicating cold syndrome, stagnation of heart blood, hypoxidosis, etc.

从外测内 【cóng wài cè nèi】从外表反映出的各种症状和体征，来判断人体内部的病变。 **Estimation of the Disorder inside the Body through the External Manifestation** a method of establishment of the diagnosis of internal diseases through the symptoms and signs reflected to the superficies.

腠理 【còu lǐ】即皮肤，肌肉的纹理及皮肤与肌肉之间的间隙，是气血流通的门户和排泄液体的途径之一，也是防御外邪内侵的屏障。 **Striae** the natural lines of the skin and muscles and the space between them, it works as an entrance and outlet for the flow of qi and blood and one of the way for the excretion of body fluid, and as resistance against the pathogenic exogenous factors.

卒病 【cù bìng】1. 指突发比较急重的疾病。2. 指新得的疾病。3. 指杂病。 **Acute Disease** referring to 1. acute and serious disease 2. new case 3. internal disease.

卒腰痛 【cù yāo tòng】指突然发作的腰痛。多因风邪乘虚侵袭肾经或不慎腰部损伤所致。 **Lumbago with Sudden Onset** a disorder resulting from the pathogenic wind factor attacking the kidney meridian or from sprain.

卒中 【cù zhòng】（中风）常以猝然昏仆，不省人事等为主症。 **Apoplexy** a condition marked by sudden loss of consciousness.

促脉 【cù mài】搏动急促有力，（每分钟脉搏大于 90 次），有不规则间歇，多因阳盛热实所致，也可因气、血、痰、食停滞引起。 **Abrupt and Irregular Pulse** a condition of pulse characterized by short, quick and strong beats with irregular intervals, usually caused by the excess of yang, and sthenia of heat, also by

催乳 【cuī rǔ】（通乳，下乳）治疗产后缺乳的方法。临床上常按病因病机不同，采用补益气血法治疗气血虚弱乳汁全无或乳汁量少；行气通络法治疗气滞所致的乳汁不下。

催吐法 【cuī tù fǎ】治疗八法之一，使用催吐药或物理刺激方法催吐，以祛除病邪。

淬 【cuì】将一些矿物类药物用火烧红后，立刻投入水中或醋中，这样反复多次，淬后不仅容易捣碎，并可缓和药性。

寸白虫病 【cùn bái chóng bìng】（白虫病），因食未熟的猪牛肉而感染绦虫的疾病。

寸、关、尺 【cùn guàn chǐ】是寸口诊脉法所诊三个部位的的名称。穴位是：掌后高骨（桡骨茎突）的内侧定为关，关之前（腕端）为寸，关之后（肘端）为尺，其脉象分别称为寸脉、关脉、尺脉。

寸口 【cùn kǒu】（气口、脉口）两手腕部桡动脉处，是诊脉的主要部位。

寸脉 【cùn mài】桡动脉搏动的远侧端。左手的称左寸脉，该处的脉象候心与膻中；右手的称寸脉，该处的脉象候肺与胸中。

the stagnation of qi, blood, phlegm and food.

Lactogenesis a treatment for lack of lactation in a puerperal woman by invigorating qi and blood in the case of deficiency of both qi and blood, or by activating qi and free the meridians in case of stagnation of qi.

Emisis one of the eight therapeutic methods, eliminating pathogens with emetics or physical irritation.

Tempering a method of processing mineral drug by burning it to a high temperature and then dropping it into water or vinegar immediately. The process is repeated for several times to render it more brittle and to decrease its toxic effect.

Taeniasis an infection of tapeworms of the genus Taenis, resulting from the ingestion of uncooked pork or beef.

Cun, Guan, Chi names of three locations of pulse-feeling, guan is located over the prominent head or the radius at the wrist; as the center the cun, that distal to it; the chi, that proximal to it.

Cunkou the commonly position for pulse feeling, located along the radial artery proximal to the wrist.

Cun Pulse the distal throbbing of the radial pulse; that of the left hand indicates the condition of the heart (the pericardium) the dan zhong while that of the right hand indicates

搓针 【cuō zhēn】一种针刺手法，用右手拇、食指向一个方向捻转刺入穴位，以加强针感。

挫伤 【cuō shàng】多因跌打、挤压、钝挫所致的软组织损伤。患处疼痛、肿胀、青紫、压之痛剧，但皮肤多完整无破伤。

错语 【cuò yǔ】神志清醒而言语错乱，多因心气虚所致。

大便不通 【dà biàn bù tōng】指便秘。

大便干结 【dà biàn gān jié】与便秘不同，指粪便干燥成粒、排便极难的症状。湿热结于大肠，热邪入里，肠中津液耗伤；或肺脾气虚，大肠传送无力；或阴血耗损，肠失滋润等均可引起本症。

大肠 【dà cháng】六腑之一。大肠上接小肠，下通肛门，具有接纳小肠输送下来的食糜并吸收其中的水分和营养物质，把糟粕形成粪便，最后从肛门排出体外的功能。

大肠寒结 【dà cháng hán jié】寒邪结于大肠而引起的病状，表现为便秘、

the condition of the lung and the thorax.

Twisting the Needle an acupuncture manipulation in which the inserted needle is twisted in one direction to strengthen the sensation of acupuncture.

Contusion an injury of soft tissues without a break in the skin with pain, swelling bruise and tenderness, usually resulting from trauma and pressure.

Paraphasia a disturbance of speech marked by substitution of words and disorganized sentence while being in right mind, due to deficiency of the heart-qi.

Retention of Feces referring to constipation.

Dry Stool a morbid condition caused by the retention of dampness-heat in the large intestine, leading to consumption of the intestinal fluid, by the hypofunction of the large intestine resulting from the deficiency of lung-qi and spleen-qi, or by the dehydration of the intestine resulting from the consumption of yin-blood.

Large Intestine one of the six fu organs, extending from the ileum to the anus. It receives the chyme from the small intestine, where the chyme is further absorbed and the residue is discharged from the anus as feces.

Retention of Pathogenic Cold Factor in the Large Intestine a morbid con-

腹部隐痛、口淡、舌白少苔、脉沉弦等。

dition manifested as constipation, dull abdominal pain, flat taste in the mouth, pale and uncoated fur, sunken and wiry pulse, etc.

大肠热结 【dà cháng rè jié】邪热蕴结于大肠引起的病状，多见于温热病阳明腑实阶段，常表现为便秘、腹痛拒按、舌苔黄燥、脉沉实有力等。

Retention of Pathogenic Heat in the Large Intestine a condition seen in the stage of sthenia of yangming fu-organ during seasonal febrile diseases; manifested as constipation, abdominal pain and tenderness, yellow and dry fur on the tongue, sunken and solid pulse, etc.

大肠湿热 【dà cháng shī rè】因饮食不节或不洁，损伤脾胃，湿热之邪侵犯大肠的证候。证见腹痛、下利脓血、里急后重、肛门灼热、小便短赤、舌苔黄腻、脉滑数等。

Pathogenic Dampness-Heat in the Large Intestine a morbid condition caused by immoderate diet or polluted food leading to impairment of the spleen and stomach and accumulation of pathogenic dampness-heat in the large intestine; manifested as abdominal pain, diarrhea with purulent and blood stools, tenesmus, oliguria with deep-coloured urine, yellow and greasy fur, smooth and fast pulse; mostly seen in dysentery, colitis, etc.

大肠虚寒 【dà cháng xū hán】因脾肾阳虚致使大肠虚寒而出现传导功能紊乱的证候。常表现为下利清谷、怕冷纳少、肢冷腰酸、苔薄、脉沉细等，多见于慢性肠炎、慢性痢疾等。

Asthenia-Cold of Large Intestine a morbid condition caused by the deficiency of spleen-yang and kidney-yang leading to the disorder of the large intestine; manifested as watery diarrhea, introlerance of cold, loss of appetite, cold extremities, lumbago, thin fur, sunken and small pulse, etc. mostly seen in chronic enteritis, chronic dysentery.

大肠液亏 【dà cháng yè kuī】因阴血

Insufficiency of Fluid in the large In-

不足或热病伤津引起大肠津液不足的证候。特证为便秘和排便困难,常伴有消瘦、皮肤干燥、咽干、舌红苔少、脉细等症。多见于老年性便秘。习惯性便秘等。

大肠主传导 【dà cháng zhǔ chuáng dǎo】大肠的生理功能之一。大肠具有传化糟粕的作用。

大毒 【dà dú】指毒性剧烈的药物,使用时必须严格掌握适应症、份量和使用方法,以防中毒。

大方 【dà fāng】方剂组成形式之一。特点为药味多、药量重,药力猛,多取一次服完的方法,适用于邪气盛或有兼证或病重者。

大骨枯槁 【dà gǔ kū gǎo】因肾气衰败而见极度消瘦衰弱,全身骨节显露的垂危征象,见于慢性消耗性疾病后期及恶液质病人。

大汗 【dà hàn】汗出过多的一种证候,可伴有伤津的情况,严重时可导致亡阴、亡阳。

testine a syndrome caused by insufficiency of yin-blood or consumption of body fluid during febrile disease; characterizde by constipation or dyschesia, accompanied with emaciation, dry skin, red and uncoated tongue, small pulse; frequently seen in senile constipation and habitual constipation.

Large Intestine Commands Transportation one of the physiological functions of the large intestine to convey and transform waste products.

Strong Toxicity referring to the drugs which are poisonous, and should be used under careful consideration for their indication, dosage and route of application.

Large Prescription a prescription composed of medicines of relatively large number, large dosage and strong potency, generally being taken in one time, suited for the disease due to excessive pathogenic factors, and the disease with complication and serious condition.

Bones Becoming Withered a morbid state marked by muscular wasting and bony appearance caused by failure of kidney-qi seen in the late stage of chronic consumptive diseases and cachexia.

Profuse Perspiration a syndrome which may be accompanied with consumption of body fluid, or may lead to

大 da

大结胸 【dà jié xiōng】《伤寒论》中的一个证型，表现为胸脘少腹硬满疼痛、拒按、口渴舌燥、午后潮热、脉沉紧等。因太阳病表证未愈而误用下法，使热邪内陷所致。

大渴引饮 【dà kě yǐn yǐn】即口渴甚，饮水多的症状。

大脉 【dà mài】脉象之一。脉体阔大，无洪盛汹涌之势。脉大而有力，主邪热实证；大而无力多为正气虚损，气不内守的表现。

大衄 【dà nǜ】口鼻同时出血的病状，严重时可于眼、耳、口、鼻及二阴同时出血。因血热妄行或气不摄血所致。

大头瘟 【dà tóu wēn】感受温毒之邪，以头面红肿或咽喉部痛为特征的温毒证，包括头面丹毒、流行性腮腺炎等多发于春季的急性的传染病。

the exhaustion of yin and yang.

Syndromes due to Accumulation of Pathogenic Factors in the Thorax It recorded in Treatise on Exogenous Febrile Diseases, resulting from the pathogenic heat accumulated in the thorax owing to the erroneous use of purgation when taiyang superficies-syndrome is not yet cured, and manifested as fullness, pain and tenderness of the thorax and abdomen, dry tongue, afternoon fever, tense and sunken pulse, etc.

Extreme Thirst intense dryness of the mouth with polydipsia.

Large Pulse a pulse condition with double width of amplitude as normal one; the large and strong pulse indicates excess-syndrome of pathogenic heat, while the large and weak one indicates deficiency syndrome marked by failure of qi to be kept inside of the body.

Simulataneous Bleeding From the Orifices bleeding from the mouth and nose, and in severe case also from the eyes, ears, rectum and urethra; resulting from the extravasation of blood produced by pathogenic heat or failure to control the blood in the case of deficiency of qi.

Epidemic Disease with Swollen Head acute febrile diseases caused by virulent wind-warm, marked by swelling and redness of face or throat ailment; seen in acute infectious diseases in

大泻 【dà xiè】 针刺手法中泻法的一种，即针插入穴位后用手指紧按针旁的皮肤，同时将针向左右前后大幅度的摇动，使针孔开大，邪气得以从体内透发于外。

Strong Dispersion one of the acupuncture manipulation by press heavily the skin around the needle inserted, and then shaking the needle forward, backward and lateralward to enlarge the puncturing hole so as to dispress the pathogenic factors of the body.

大针 【dà zhèn】 一种针体较粗、针头微圆的针。

Big Needle a type of acupuncture with relativly large caliber and round tip.

大眦漏 【dà zì lòu】（眦漏）症见脓液自大眦部溢出的外眼疾患，多因心火内炽或风热停聚，上攻内眦所致，相当于泪囊炎。

Dacryocystitis inflammation of the lacrimal sac with discharge of pus, caused by hyperactivity of heart fire or attack of pathogenic wind-heat to the inner canthus.

呆病 【dāi bìng】（痴呆）精神病的一种类型，多因肝气郁结，克伐脾胃，致痰湿内生，蒙蔽心窍所致。临床上常见终日不语、精神恍惚、哭笑无常、口中喃喃、行为异常、数日不食而不呼饥等。

Dementia a type of psychosis due to stagnation of the liver-qi impairing the spleen and stomach leading to the production of pathogenic phlegm-dampness involving the heart; manifested as various forms of mental deterioration and abnormal behaviors.

代脉 【dài mài】 脉象之一，搏动缓弱而有规则间歇的一种脉象，主脏气衰弱。常见于心脏病患者。

Intermittent Pulse a pulse condition, characterized by slow and weak beats with regular intervals, indicating deficiency of visceral qi, commonly seen in the patients with heart disease.

代指 【dài zhǐ】 指外伤引起的甲沟化脓性感染。

Paronychia inflammation involving the folds of tissue surrounding the finger nail caused by trauma.

带下 【dài xià】 1. 泛指妇科疾病。2. 指妇女阴道流出一种粘性液体，连绵

Daixia 1. referring commonly to all kinds of gynecopathy. 2. leukorrha-

不断。

带下病 【dài xià bìng】带下有色（白、黄、赤等色）、质（清稀、稠浊）、量（量多、特多）、气味（腥、秽或臭）等改变，可伴有腰酸腿软、小腹坠痛等症状者。辨证分类 1. 脾虚证。2. 肾虚证（肾阴虚、肾阳虚）3. 肝火证。4. 湿热证。

带下医 【dài xià yī】古代专门治疗妇产科疾病的医生。

戴眼 【dài yǎn】指病人眼睛上视，不能转动。多为太阳经气衰竭的危候。亦见于小儿急惊风、厥阴风痰闭阻等。

戴阳 【dài yáng】下真寒、上假热的重危证候。症见两颧色淡红，或口鼻出血，或口燥齿浮，足胫逆冷，大便稀溏，脉浮大无力等。

丹 【dān】药用剂型之一，依方精制，有内服、外用两种。外用的往往用含有汞、硫等矿物药升华提炼而成，如白降丹、红升丹等。内服的丹有各种剂型，如紫雪丹为散，至宝丹为丸。

丹毒 【dān dú】由热毒邪气引起的急

gia.

Morbid Leukorrhea a disease marked by the changes of color, quality, quantity and smell, accompanied with soreness of the low back, lassitude, heavy pain in the low abdomen. Types of differentiation 1. syndrome of spleen deficiency 2. syndrome of kidney deficiency 3. syndrome of liver-fire 4. syndrome of dampness-heat.

Practitioner Specialized in Leukorrhagia an ancient name for the doctors skilled in gynecology and obstetrics.

Hyperphoria permanent upward vision of the eyes; a sign symbolizing the exhaustion of the qi of taiyang meridian; seen in infantile convulsion, stagnation of the pathogenic wind-phlegm in jueying meridian.

Floating Yang a morbid condition caused by deficiency of kidney-yang and hyperactivity of yin-cold in the interior leading to floating of yang; manifested as reddish cheeks, bleeding from the oral cavity and nose, dry nose, swollen gum, cold legs, diarrhea, floating, large, weak pulse, etc.

Dan ready-made medicines prepared according to set prescriptions including sublimated powder of minerals for external application, and medical powder e. g; Zixuedan or pill Zhibodan for oral administration.

Erysipelas acute skin infection

性皮肤感染。患处皮肤红如涂丹,边缘清楚,灼热疼痛,伴有发热恶寒、头痛、全身酸痛、局部淋巴结肿大等证状。辨证分类 1. 风邪热毒证。2. 湿邪热毒证。3. 胎毒蕴热证。

caused by virulent heat, which is manifested as redness of skin with a clear outline and burning pain; accomanied with fever, chillness, headache, general aching and enlargement of local lymphnodes. Type of differentiation 1. syndrome of pathogenic wind and toxic heat 2. syndrome of pathogenic damp-heat 3. syndrome occuring in new-born babies due to internal heat.

丹田　【dān tián】是身体上的重要部位,古代内丹派认为该处是炼丹结丹之处。一般把丹田分为上、中、下三处(腹中线脐下三寸的部位为针灸穴位)。

Dan Tian　certain important regions of the body which include upper, middle and lower Dan Tian. It was regarded by the ancient Nei Dan Pai as the place where the Dan forms.

单按　【dān àn】诊脉方法之一。用一个手指专按某一部位的脉搏。

Feeling the Pulse with a Single Finger　a method of feeling pulse with a single finger putting on a particular locality.

单蛾　【dān é】同单乳蛾,一侧扁桃体肿大。多因肺胃热壅,火毒熏蒸;或因气滞血凝。痰火郁结;或肝肾阴亏津耗,虚火上炎引起。

Unilateral Tonsillitis　a condition due to the attack of fire resulting from the accumulation of pathogenic heat in the lung and stomach, or from the stagnation of qi and blood leading to accumulation of pathogenic phlegm-fire, or from the yin deficiency and the body fluid consumption in the stomach and kidney leading to flaming up of asthenia-fire.

单方　【dān fāng】方剂的一种简单形式。仅用一、二味药,效用专一,取效迅速。往往适应于某个病证。

Single Prescription　a prescription composed of only one or two medicines with specific and prompt effect, commonly applicable to certain syndrome.

单腹胀　【dān fù zhàng】指以腹部胀

Distention of the Abdomen　a mor-

大如鼓为主症的一种疾病。见腹皮青筋暴露，而四肢肿胀不明显。多因肝脾损伤，水湿不运，气血瘀滞所致。

单乳蛾 【dān rǔ é】指发于一侧的扁桃体炎。

单手进针法 【dān shǒu jìn zhēn fǎ】针刺进针法之一。以拇指、食指持针体与针尖之间部分，向下速刺入穴且不加捻转。

单行 【dān xíng】药物配伍七情之一。用一种药物，发挥其专一效能来治疗疾病。如独参汤，取单味人参，用其专一的大补元气之功效。

胆 【dǎn】居六腑之首，又属奇恒之腑，附于肝，内藏胆汁，有助于消化。胆气的盛衰关系决断情志的变化。

胆黄 【dǎn huáng】因受大惊大恐或斗殴受伤，胆气伤败液泄所致的病证，症见身目呈黄绿色、胸中气满、不欲饮食、困倦昏沉。

胆咳 【dǎn ké】指咳嗽而并呕吐胆汁

bid condition characterized by the distention of abdomen accompanied with engorged veins visible over its surface with no significant edema of the limbs; due to accumulation of fluid resulting from the impairment of the liver and spleen, and the stagnation of qi and blood.

Unilateral Tonsillitis referring to the attack only to one side.

Single-Hand Needle Insertion a method of needle insertion by being grasped between the thumb and forefinger and inserting rapidly into the point without twirling.

Single Medicine one of the seven prescriptions, by using only one medicine, exerting its specific effect, e.g., single Ginseng decoction, exerting its effect on tonifying the primordial qi.

Gallbladder the first of the six fu organs and one of the extraordinary fu-organs adhered to the liver, storing bile and aiding in digestion. Its condition affects the ability of its owner to make decisions and control emotion.

Jaundice due to Frigtening or Traumatic Injury a disease due to impairment of gallbladder-qi and extravasation of the bile after being frightened or wounded; manifested as greenish yellow colouration of the skin and eyes, fullness of the chest, loss of appetite, lassitude and sleepiness.

Cough with Vomiting of Bile a syn-

的病证。

胆气 【dǎn qì】指胆的功能。

胆热 【dǎn rè】胆的热证。证见胸胁烦闷、口苦、咽干、寒热往来等。

胆热多睡 【dǎn yè duō shuì】（胆实多卧）由胆腑实热，胸膈有痰，脏腑壅滞所致的病证。症见神思不爽，昏闷如醉，心胸烦闷，口苦而干，头目昏重等。

胆实 【dǎn shí】胆的实证。由于胆气不畅而出现的症状。如胸脘满闷，胁下胀痛等。

胆虚 【dǎn xū】（胆气不足）症见虚烦不眠、心慌、易惊恐等。见于某些神经衰弱、癔病患者。

胆虚不得眠 【dǎn xū bù dé mián】指胆虚受邪，神气不宁所致的失眠。症见心烦失眠、心悸易惊等。

drome of cough with bilious vomiting.

Gallbladder-Qi　　referring to the function of the gallbladder.

Gallbladder-Heat　　heat-syndrome of the gallbladder, manifested as feeling of oppression over the chest and hypochondrium, bitter taste in the mouth, dry throat, alternating episodes of chills and fever, etc.

Somnolence due to Gallbladder-Heat　　a morbid condition caused by sthenic heat in the gallbladder, phlegm accumulated in the thorax; manifested as emotional distress, drowsiness, feeling of oppression over the chest, bitter mouth, dizziness with heaviness of the head.

Gallbladder of Sthenia　　sthenia-syndrome of the gallbladder due to poor flow of gallbladder-qi, manifested as feeling oppression over the chest and epigastrium, distending pain over the hypochondrium, etc.

Asthenia of Gallbladder　　a morbid condition manifested as restlessness, insomnia, palpitation, timidity, etc; seen in some cases with neurasthenia or hysteria.

Insomnia due to Asthenia of Gallbladder-Qi　　a morbid condition caused by irritability due bo the sttack of pathogenic factor to the asthenic gallbladder; manifested as restlessness, insomnia, palpitation, liability to be frightened, etc.

胆胀【dǎn zhàng】胆受寒邪侵袭所致病证。见胁下疼痛胀满、口苦、善太息等症。

Distention of gallbladder a morbid condition caused by the attack of pathogenic cold factor to the gallbladder; manifested as hypochondriac distending pain. bitter in the mouth, frequent deep sighing, etc.

胆主决断【dǎn zhǔ jué duàn】中医学认为,人的勇、怯与胆有关,故中医对易惊胆怯、失眠、善恐、多梦等神态病变,常从胆论治,胆的决断功能有助于防御和消除某些精神刺激的不良影响,以维持人体气血运行的正常和脏腑功能的协调作用。

The Gallbladder Controls the Power of Making decision bravery and timidity are related to the gallbladder; from then on, the diagnosis and treatment of pathological changes in emotion, which is manifested as liabillty to be frightened and scared, insomnia, dreaminess, usually by an overall analysis of signs and symptoms concerned with the gallbladder. This function of the gallbladder is helpful for the avoidance of certain mental upsets and the removal of their harmful effects, so as to maintain the normal circulation of qi and blood and to keep the vicera in coordination.

但欲寐【dàn yù mèi】少阴病主证之一。表现为神志朦胧,似睡非睡的证候。多由邪入少阴,心肾阳气衰竭所致。

Drowsiness the main symptom of shaoying disease, marked by impairment of consciousness appearing as a drowsy state caused by the attack of shaoyin pathogenic factor and collapse of yang-qi of the heart and kidney.

淡渗利湿【dàn shèn lì shī】以味淡利湿药为主,使湿邪从小便排出。适用于偏于湿重者。症见泄泻清稀、小便不利、苔腻、脉濡等。

Eliminating the Pathogenic Dampness With Bland Taste Drugs a treatment for the elimination of pathogenic dampness through the discharge of urine by the application of bland taste drugs, applicable to the

淡味渗泄为阳 【dàn wèi shèn xiè wéi yáng】淡味药多能渗水利湿，其药性属阳。如薏苡仁（味淡能利小便而去湿）性属阳。

刀斧伤 【dāo fǔ shāng】由刀斧锐器所致的损伤。

刀晕 【dāo yūn】因利器创伤后出血、疼痛或精神过度紧张而致的晕厥。

导法 【dǎo fǎ】（导便）将易溶、性润滑的药液灌入直肠或将润滑性的栓剂塞入肛门内，以通下大便。

导气 【dǎo qì】有意识的引导呼吸锻炼。

导引 【dǎo yǐn】古代的一种健身方法。即通过肢体运动，调节呼吸及自我按摩相结合，以达行气活血，强健筋骨，消除疲劳，祛病益寿之目的。

导滞通腑 【dǎo zhì tōng fǔ】下法之一。行气消导药与泻下药并用以治疗积滞内停的方法。

捣针 【dǎo zhēn】一种强刺激针刺手法。针刺于皮下，在皮下一定深度内

case manifested as watery diarrhea, dysuria, whitish fur, soft and floating pulse, etc.

Bland Medicines with Diuretic Effect Belong to Yang for example Semen Coicis with bland taste and diuretic effect belongs to yang.

Incised Wound the injuries by sharp tools such as sword, axe, etc.

Traumatic Syncope syncope due to bleeding, pain and mental stress caused by trauma.

Moving the Bowels by Topical Application a therapy for constipation by applying drugs, made of lubricated and easily fusible medicated mass, into the anus.

The Guiding of Breathing directing respiratory training with will.

Conduction of Qi Flow physical exercise in ancient China, which consists of special ways of the limb exercises, respiratory regulation and automassage, serves to relieve fatigue, cure diseases and prolong one's life, by activating qi flow and blood circulation, and strengthening muscles and bones.

Removing Stagnancy and Obstruction of the Fu-Organs a therapy of purgation, for the retention of indigested food by the complex medicines both qi-activating, digestives and purgatives.

Lifting And Thrusting the Needle Repeatedly an acupuncture manipu-

将针反复上下捣动。

倒睫拳毛【dào jié quán máo】症见睫毛内倒、触刺眼珠、涩痛流泪, 羞明难睁。

盗汗【dào hàn】指入睡汗出, 醒后汗止。多属阴虚火旺之证。

得气【dé qì】针刺入穴位后, 经过手法操作或留针, 病人感觉酸、麻、胀、重, 行针者觉针下沉紧, 这种反应称为得气。得气的程度和持续时间的长短, 往往与疗效有密切关系。

得神【dé shén】具有旺盛的生命活动功能。表现为神志清醒, 机体各脏腑器官功能正常。

涤痰【dí tán】使用作用峻烈的祛痰药, 以荡涤顽痰的疗法。适用于久而不愈的痰证, 但本法作用比较剧烈, 虚人慎用, 孕妇忌用。

巅【diān】即头顶部。

巅疾【diān jí】1、指婴儿癫痫。2、泛指头部痛证。

lation for strong stimulation by which the needle is lifted and thrusted repeatedly after inserting the needle into a definite depth.

Trichiasis a morbid state manifested as ingrowing eyelashes offending to the eye-balls, pain, lacrimation, photophobia, etc.

Night Sweat a morbid condition of sweating during sleep and stopping sweating after waking up, commonly seen in the caes of yin-deficiency and consumption.

Getting Sensation of Acupuncture sensation of soreness, numbness, distension and heaviness, felt by the patient and the tight feeling of the needle felt by the acupuncturist. Its severity and duration are closely related to the curative effect.

Spiritedness a healthy state in which the vital functions of the human body are active, such as full consciousness and normal activities of all organs.

Clearing away Pathogenic Phlegm a treatment for intractable phlegm-syndrome with potent medicines of eliminating phelgm. It should be used carefully in the case of general deficiency and contraindicated in pregnant women.

Vertex the uppermost part of the head.

Dian Diseases referring to infantile epilepsy, headache, etc.

癫 【diān】（失心风）1、精神病的一种类型。多由痰气郁结所致。症见精神抑郁、表情淡漠、言语错乱、不思饮食、舌苔薄腻、脉弦滑等。2、古代的癫即痫病。

癫狂 【diān kuáng】指精神错乱的一类疾病。癫属阴，多属虚证，患者多静默；狂属阳，多属实证，患者多躁动。

癫痫发作 【diān xián fā zuò】指痫证突然发作而出现各种症状。

点刺 【diǎn cì】即速刺法。用左手捏紧皮肤，右手持针疾速刺入皮下浅层静脉，迅速出针，然后挤出数滴血液。通常使用三棱针或短毫针，刺手指、足趾端、耳尖、太阳穴、委中等穴。

电针疗法 【diàn zhēn liáo fǎ】在刺入人体一定穴位后的毫针上，通以适当强度的电流，以加强或维持针刺作用，达到治疗目的的一种方法。

吊脚痧 【diào jiǎo shā】为霍乱吐泻之后，因津液耗失，伤及气阴，筋脉失养所致之病证。症见两腿挛缩，甚则腹部拘急、囊缩舌卷。

Depressive State 1. a psychiatric syndrome caused by stagnation of pathogenic phlegm and qi, manifested as dejected mood, apathy, paraphasia, poor appetite, thin and greasy fur, wiry and smooth pulse. 2. referring to epilepsy in ancient times.

Mania-Depressive Syndrome referring to psychosis, in which the depressive state belongs to yin, as asthenia-syndrome; while the manic state belongs to yang, as sthenia-syndrome.

Epilepsy Seizure

Pricking Acupuncture an acupuncture manipulation by which a short filiform needle or three-edged needle is inserted into the skin of finger (toe) tip, earlobe, or taiyang point and weizhong point, then withdrawn quickly to let out a few drops of blood.

Electro-Acupuncture a method of acupuncture by which the needle is attached to a direct current of optimal intensity after it is inserted into the selected point; by which the effect can be strengthened persistently.

Sha-Syndrome with Cramps of the Calves a morbid condition due to failure of nourishing the muscles and tendons resulting from sudden loss of body fluid and impairment of both qi and yin after severe vomiting and diarrhea caused by cholera; manifested as cramps of the calves, even abdominal cramps, scrotal shrinkage and curled-up of the tongue seen in severe case.

掉弦 【diào xuán】多因肝风内动所致，表现为头昏眼花，肢体震颤的症候。

Dizziness with Trembling Extremities a morbid state marked by dizziness, dim-sightedness and tremor of the limbs resulting from the stirring of liver-wind inside the body.

跌打损伤 【diē dǎ sǔn shāng】包括刀枪、殴打、跌扑、闪压、擦伤及运动伤损等。伤处多见疼痛、肿胀、破损、出血、伤筋、骨折、脱臼等情况。

Wound a body injury caused by physical means, such as incision, contusion, pressure, abrasion, violent motion, etc.; manifested as local pain, swelling, rupture of skin, bleeding, sprain, fracture, dislocation, etc.

跌仆伤胎 【diē pū shāng tāi】孕妇因跌仆闪挫，损伤胎元，气血逆乱，以致胎动不安。症见腰腹坠痛或阴道出血。

Damage of the Fetus due to Trauma a state due to disorders of qi and blood after trauma; manifested as hypermotility of the fetus, bearing-down pain over the loins and abdomen, or bleeding from the vagina.

疔疮 【dīng chuāng】（疔毒）指形小、根深、坚硬的疮疡。多由饮食不节，外感四时不正之气，火热毒邪阻于肌肤所致。初起如粟，坚硬根深，继则迅速发红、疼痛、肿胀、化脓、溃烂等，若疔根随脓排出，则肿消痛止而愈。

Furuncle a painful nodule formed in the skin by circumscribed inflammation of the corium and subcutaneous tissue, enclosing a central slough, with a tendency of healing after the discharge of pus; caused by the attack of irregular meals, exogenous pathogenic factors leading to stagnation of fire-heat to the skin.

聤耳 【dīng ěr】指内耳红肿灼痛，鼓膜破溃，耳道流出黄色脓液的病证。肝胆郁火，三焦湿热所致属实证；肾阴亏损，虚火上炎所致，则属虚证。

Chronic Suppurative Otitis Media chronic inflammation of the middle ear with rupture of the tympanic membrane and purulent discharge. The sthenic type is caused by the retention of fire in the liver and gall-

耵聍 【dīng níng】(耳垢)即外耳道的分泌物,若大量堵塞耳道可影响听力。

Cerumen   the waxlike secretion found in the external meatus of the ear, the accumulation of it may impair hearing.

顶 【dǐng】称药性上行的为顶。顶药多具催吐作用,常用以治疗风痰上涌,突然昏倒等病证。

Drug with Upward Action   a term including a kind of drugs which are mostly emetics and usually applied in fainting due to uprising pathogenic wind-phlegm.

定风 【dìng fēng】治疗因津血亏损或肝肾阴虚筋脉失养或肝风内动的方法。常用于温热病后期。

Calming the Wind-Syndrome   a treatment for the malnutrition of tendon and vessels or hyperactivity of liver-wind due to consumption of fluid and blood or deficiency of liver-yin and kidney-yin; usually applied in the late stage of seasonal febrile disease.

锭 【dìng】将极细的药末加入适当赋形剂,制成如纺锤、圆锥等不同形状的固体制剂,供内服或外用。

Troche   a small circular or oblong tablet consisting of fine medical powder mixed with proper excipient, for oral or topical use.

冬石 【dōng shí】因冬季寒冷,阳气潜藏,所以脉象偏于沉紧,这是脉象随气候改变的生理现象。

Stone-Like Pulse of Winter   a physiological phenomenon that the pulse condition varies with the seasonal change. The yang-qi is deeply stored within the human body due to the cold weather in winter, so the condition of the pulse tends to be sunken and tense.

冬温 【dōng wēn】冬季感受非时之温热之邪而发生的温病。

Winter-Febrile Syndrome   the febrile disease occuring in winter due to exposure to the unseasonable warm

动脉 【dòng mài】脉象之一。脉体较短，滑数有力，应指跳突如豆。

Tremulous Pulse a pulse that feels short, slippery, quick and forceful like a bouncing pea, with irregular beats over a narrow region; resulting from incoordination between yin and yang, and disorder of both qi and blood.

动功 【dòng gōng】（外功）是气功中的一大类功法。它是采取与意念、呼吸相结合的肢体动作或自我按摩等方法，以锻炼内脏，凝静心神，活跃气血，是一种动中求静的功法。

Dynamic Qi Gong also called external qi gong, it is one of the categories in qi gong, which aims at training internal organs, calming spirit of heart, activating qi and blood circulation by certain motions of limbs, combined with will and breath, or by self-massage. In practice, the principle "quiescence in motion" should be adhered to.

冻伤 【dòng shāng】寒冷严重损伤皮肉，气血凝滞而成。多发于手足、面部、耳廓等处。患处先呈苍白色，渐成紫红、肿胀、灼痛、瘙痒。辨证分类：1、阴盛阳衰证。2、血虚寒凝证。3、气血两虚证。4、热结血瘀证。

Chilblain a morbid condition manifested as localized itching, swelling, painess on the fingers, toes, face and ears, which is caused by frost bite with damage of the skin and the stagnation of qi and blood. Types of differentiation 1. syndrome of excessive yin due to hypoactivity of yang 2. syndrome of cold stagnation due to blood deficiency 3. syndrome of deficiency of both blood and qi 4. syndrome of stagnation of heat leading to blood stasis.

独阳 【dú yáng】喻阳的过于偏盛。

Single Yang referring to the excess of yang.

独语 【dú yǔ】患者神志清醒，喃喃自语，属虚证。多由心气不足，神失所养引起。

Soliloquy a morbid state of muttering to oneself under a conscious condition, a deficiency-syndrome, resulting from the insufficiency of heart-qi

毒痢　【dú lì】因热毒所致的痢疾。症见痢下五色脓血而无粪质、心烦、腹痛如绞等。

Fulminant Dysentery　dysentery due to virulent heat factor, manifested as discharge of blood and mucus without fecal material, restlessness and abdominal colic.

毒蛇咬伤　【dú shé yǎo shāng】有毒蛇咬伤史，咬伤处有牙痕，周围可出现血疱、水疱、疼痛；或局部麻木，伤肢肿胀。全身有发热、头昏、嗜睡、复视。严重者出现视觉、听觉障碍，流涎，瞳孔散大；或全身皮下、内脏出血。脉细或沉伏。辨证分类 1、风毒证（神经毒）2、火毒证（血循毒）。3、风火毒证（混合毒）。

Viper Biting　bitten by a viper with the appearance of ophidism, marked by hematic abscess, blister, pain, local numbness, edema of the bitten region as well as fever, dizziness, lethargy, ambiopia, and even disturbances in vision and hearing, salivation, platycoria, or general subcutaneous hemorrhage and visceral hemorrhege. Types of differentiation 1. syndrome of wind-toxin (neurotoxin) 2. syndrome of fire-toxin (toxin flowing along the blood circulation) 3. syndrome of wind-fire-toxin (mixed toxin).

毒药攻邪　【dú yào gōng xié】（以毒攻毒）为达治病目的，使用有一定毒性的药物克除病邪的方法。

Expelling Pathogenic Factors by Poisonous Medicine　applying certain poisonous medicines to cure some pathogenic factors.

妒乳　【dù rǔ】产妇乳汁积蓄过多，而致乳房胀硬掣痛，手不得近；或乳头生细小之疮，痛或痒。

Galactostasis　a condition of excess of accumulated breast milk leading to induration and distending pain of breast, or painful, or itchy nodules over the breast.

短脉　【duǎn mài】脉象之一。脉体首尾俱短，不满寸、关、尺三部。脉短而有力主气郁；短而无力则主气虚。

Short Pulse　one of the pulse conditions, it is only palpable at the guan site but indistinct at cun and chi sites. A short and forceful beat indicates the stagnation of qi, while a short and weak pulse suggests consumption and deficiency of qi.

短气 【duǎn qì】指呼吸短促且不能接续。由体弱久病、元气耗损所致，属虚证。由痰饮瘀阻、气滞所致，多属实证。

煅 【duàn】把药物直接放在火内烧红；或放在耐火容器中间接煅烧，使药物质地松脆，易于煎煮以利发挥效用。

对口疮 【duì kǒu chuāng】(脑疽)生于脑后枕骨之下，大椎穴之上。多由湿热毒邪上壅；或肾水亏损，阴虚火炽所致。

顿服 【dun fú】将汤剂一次服完。一般适用于病在下部。

顿咳 【dùn ké】因时行疫毒犯肺，使肺气不宜，气郁化热，酿液成痰，阻于气道，气机上逆而引起的症状。症见典型阵发性痉咳伴有回声，舌系带溃疡，目胞浮肿。分为1、初咳期；2、痉咳期；3、恢复期，包括脾气虚和肺阴伤。多见于百日咳。

Shortness of Breathing a morbid state resulting from the consumption of primordial qi due to general debility or chronic illness mostly seen in the case of asthenia-syndrome, or from retention of pathogenic phlegm, stasis and stagnation of qi seen in the case of sthenia-syndrome.

Charring a method of processing crude medicine by burning it directly or indirectly to render it more brittle so as to get the effect of the medicine.

Boil on the Nape pyogenic infection over the back part of the neck, resulting from the attack of pathogenic dampness-heat or deficiency of kidney-fluid and hyperactivity of fire factor due to yin-deficiency.

Be Taken Totally at One Time a method of oral use of decoction, it is suited for the case with the disease in the lower part of the body.

Paroxysmal Cough a type of cough due to invasion of the lung by epidemic seasonal noxious agent, leading to obstruction of the lung-qi, and the stagnated qi turning into heat, causing phlegm retention obstructing the qi passage and resulting in abnormal ascending of the lung-qi, with accompanying manifestations such as wheezing sound, ulcer of the frenulum of the tongue, edema of the eyelids. Types of differentiation: 1. incipient stage   2. paroxysmal stage

燉 【dùn】将药物与辅料密封于同一容器内,放入锅内加热煮沸一定时间。

多汗 【duō hàn】指不是由于炎热、运动、药物等因素引起的汗出过多。

多梦 【duō mèng】睡眠不熟多梦扰。常因情志郁结,肝阳偏亢或气血虚少,心神不安所致。也有因肝胃阴虚而致。常见于神经衰弱的患者。

多忘 【duō wàng】指记忆力减退。多因思虑过度,心肾不足所致。

夺汗者无血 【duó hàn zhě wú xuè】治则。血汗同源,故汗液耗伤过度的人,不能再伤其血。

夺精 【duó jīng】指精气严重耗损。症见精神萎靡、耳聋、视物不清。

夺血者无汗 【duó xuè zhě wú hàn】治则。血汗同源,故血液耗伤过度的人,

3. rehabiliating stage, including deficiency of spleen-qi and impairment of lung-yin.

Cooked by Putting the Container in Boiling Water a method of preparation of medicine by putting them in a covered container with water, then cooking in boiling water.

Hyperhidrosis excessive sweating which is not induced by hot weather, physical exercise or drugs.

Dreaminess a morbid condition due to irritability resulting from sorrow, hyperactivity of liver-yang or deficiency of both qi and blood; as well as deficiency of liver yin and kidney yin; usually seen in the case with neurasthenia.

Amnesia lack or loss of memory usually caused by over-anxiety and asthenia of the heart and kidney.

Consumption of Blood Is Contraindicated in the Case with Excessive Sweating a treating principle in which consumption of blood should be avoided in the case of excessive sweating, since the blood and the sweat fluid originate from the same source.

Exhaustion of Vital Essence a morbid state due to excessive consumption of essence and qi; manifested as dispiritedness, deafness, blurring of vision.

Diaphoresis Is Contraindicated in the Case with Consumption of Blood

不能再发其汗。 a treating principle in which sweating should be avoided in the case with over consumption of blood, since the blood and the sweat originate from the same source.

鹅口疮 【é kǒu chuāng】多见于新生儿,因久病体弱或长期使用广谱抗生素之后引起的口腔疾病。症见舌上、颊内、牙龈或上唇、上腭散布白屑,可融合成片,重者可向咽喉等外蔓延,影响吮奶及呼吸。辨证分类:1、心脾积热 2、虚火上浮。

Thrush fungus infection of the mucous membranes of the mouth of infants, which is caused by weak constitution due to protracted illness and long-time use of the broad-spectrum antibiotics, marked by scattered white flakes on the tongue, inner surface of the cheeks, gum or upper lip and palate, which may then form into groups, or even extending to the throat and causes difficulty in feeding and breathing. Types of differentiation 1. accumulation of heat in the heart and spleen. 2. flaming up of the asthenic fire.

鹅掌风 【é zhǎng fēng】即手癣生于手掌部。因风湿聚集,气血失养所致;或由接触传染而得。

Tinea Manuum a fungus infection of the hand skin, resulting from the local accumulation of pathogenic wind-damp interfering the local supply of qi and blood; or by direct contact with the etiologic agent.

额疽 【é jū】(赤疽)即头疽生于前额正中者。多由火毒所致。

Carbuncle on Forehead a disorder frequently due to pathogenic fire toxin.

恶心 【ě xīn】指欲吐不吐的症状。多由胃虚或邪气犯胃所致。

Nausea a symptom due to asthenia of the stomach, or attack of pathogenic factors to the stomach.

恶疮 【ě chuāng】指疮疡由风热挟湿毒之气所致。表现为焮肿痛痒、溃烂后浸淫不休、经久不愈等。

Obstinate Sore a term for the lesion of skin caused by pathogenic wind-heat and damp-toxic, manifested as redness, swelling, pain and itching

恶露 【è lù】指产妇分娩后，由阴道排出的胞宫内残留的余血和浊液。一般在产后三周内完全排尽。

恶色 【è sè】面部颜色的变化，其色显露枯槁晦暗，一般表示病情较重，预后不良。

恶血 【è xuè】是指溢于经脉之外，滞于组织间，且不具有正常生理功能的血液。

恶念 【è niàn】是指练功中胡思乱想，想到一些使人气愤、懊丧、恐惧、恼怒之类的事情，以致情绪激动，心神不宁。

呃逆 【è nì】指胃气冲逆而上，呃呃有声的一种症候。多因脾胃虚寒所致。

儿枕痛 【ér zhěn tòng】（儿枕、血母块）产后恶露未尽或风寒侵袭胞脉，致使瘀血内停所致病证。表现为下腹硬痛拒按或可触及硬块。

耳 【ěr】五官之一。为听觉器官。它的功能靠精、髓、气、血的充盈濡养，赖肾脏功能的正常。耳的疾病常与肾

over the involving area, rupture with profuse watery discharge, and difficulty in healing.

Lochia the vaginal discharge that eliminates during the first three weeks after labor.

Unfavourable Complexion a colour change of the face with dry and lusterless appearance, indicating a severe condition and an unfavourable prognosis.

Extravasated Blood the blood flowing in the interstitial space outside the vessel, which is unable to carry on its normal physiological function.

Virulent Will referring to thinking of things which makes himself angry, frightened, etc. and leads to excitement and mind disturbed in the process of training qi gong.

Hiccup a syndrome caused by the adverse rising of stomach-qi, causing the characteristic sounds; mostly due to asthenia-cold factor of the spleen and stomach.

Lower Abdominal Pain in Puerperium Caused By Blood Stasis a morbid condition of retention of blood stasis as a result of postpartum lochiorrhea, or attack of pathogenic wind-cold to the uterine meridian; manifested as pain, tenderness or palpable mass of the lower abdomen.

Ear one of the five sense organs, the organ of hearing. The function of the ear depends on the nourishment

有关，此外小肠、膀胱、三焦、胆、胃等经脉均循行于耳。所以，它与脏腑经络都有密切关系。全身脏器及肢体常可在耳廓找到反应点。这些反应点用以帮助诊断和治疗多种疾病。

from the vital essense, marrow, qi and blood, as well as the normal activity of the kidney. The disorder of the ear is closely related to the dysfunction of the kidney and also the heart, spleen and liver. The meridians of the small intestine, bladder, triple energizer gallbladder and stomach pass through the ear. Corresponding reflecting points of the viscera and extremities are found on the auricle and are applied to the diagnosis and treatment of various diseases.

耳疔 【ěr dīng】（肾疔）生于耳窍的疔疮，因肾经火毒或过服丹石热药，积毒而成。

Pustule at the External Auditory Meatus a morbid condition caused by the attack of pathogenic fire to the kidney meridian or overtaking of prepared mineral medicines of hot nature.

耳定 【ěr dìng】外耳道肿瘤。伸出于耳外，形如梅子，由肝胆积热所致。

Tumour of the External Auditory Meatus a new growth extending out of the ear, like a plum, resulting from the stagnation of pathogenic heat of the liver and gallbladder.

耳防风 【ěr fáng fēng】多由肝、胆、三焦火盛所致的耳部疾患。症见耳内肿痛流脓，痛甚则耳外周围和面部也肿，不能张口。

Infection of Ear an ear disease marked by swelling and pain of the ear, with purulent discharge, due to the overabundance of fire in the liver, gallbladder and triple energizer. In the serious case, the swelling extends to the area around the auricle and the face, and the opening of the mouth is affected.

耳根毒 【ěr gēn dú】（耳根痈）因少阳胆经风热所致的耳后肿疡，局部红热疼痛。多发于一侧。类似耳后急性淋

Infection Behind the Ear a condition caused by the attack of pathogenic wind-heat to the shaoyang

巴结炎。

耳后疽 【ěr hòu jū】耳后肿痛溃破流脓，伴有发热、恶寒、头痛等全身症状。本病由三焦及肝胆两经火毒引起。类似急性乳突炎。

耳菌 【ěr jūn】外耳道肿瘤，伸出于耳外，形如蘑菇，由肝、肾等经火毒凝聚而成。

耳廓 【ěr kuò】（耳轮）外耳道以外全部耳壳的统称。耳壳内侧面有脏腑和肢体的反应点，应用于耳针。

耳烂 【ěr làn】皮疹溃破流水，缠绵难愈的一种耳壳皮肤病。多由肝胆湿热所致，类似湿疹。

耳聋 【ěr lóng】（耳闭）听力有不同程度障碍的一种症状，可由先天或外感、外伤、内伤所致。急性耳聋多属实证；慢性耳聋多属虚证。

gallbladder meridian, marked by unilateral, local redness, heat and pain; similar to acute retroauricular lymphadenitis.

Acute Mastoiditis a condition caused by the attack of pathogenic fire to the triple energizer and the liver and gallbladder meridians, manifested as swelling, pain and purulent discharge, usually accompanied with fever, chills, headache, etc.

Ear Tumour a new growth like a mushroom extending out of the auditory meatus, caused by the stagnation of pathogenic fire and toxin in the meridians of the liver and kidney.

Auricle corresponding reflecting points of the viscera and extremities are found on the lateral surface of the auricle and have been applied in ear acupuncture.

Erosion of the Auricle a lingering skin disease of the auricle with exfoliation and discharge, resulting from the retention of pathogenic damp-heat factor in the liver and gallbladder; similar to eczema.

Deafness lack or loss of the sense of hearing, congenital or acquired from the attack of exogenous factor, trauma and the impairment of viscera; deafness with sudden oneset usually indicates sthenia-syndrome, while deafness with insidious onset and lasting for a long duration indicates asthenia-syndrome.

耳泌 【ěr mì】小儿因外耳道流出分泌物引起耳部疼痛的一种病证。见于急性中耳炎。

耳鸣 【ěr míng】耳内鸣响,其声如蝉鸣,或如水击,或如钟声等听觉异常的自觉症状。肝胆火气上逆,脾胃痰火上升,或肾精不足,中气下陷均可引起,前者属于实证,后者属虚证。

耳膜 【ěr mó】是一种半透明的薄膜,将耳道分为中耳道和外耳道。

耳内异物 【ěr nèi yì wù】异物留于外耳道的一种病证。多伴有耳痛、听力障碍等症状。

耳衄 【ěr nǜ】血从耳中溢出的病证。多由少阴肾火或厥阴肝火所致。

耳挺 【ěr tǐng】外耳道肿瘤。伸于耳外,形如枣核。

耳痛 【ěr tòng】耳部疾患的一种常见症状。可由肝胆风热,三焦火盛或虚火等引起。

耳痒 【ěr yǎng】因肝风内动,肾火上扰所致的耳内奇痒难忍的一种病证。

Ear Discharge a morbid condition in infants manifested as earache with serous or purulent discharge; seen in acute otitis media.

Tinnitus a noise in the ears, as chirping, roaring, ringing, etc.; resulting from the adverse rising of liver-fire and gallbladder-fire leading to hyperactivity of phlegm-fire in the spleen and stomach; or resulting from deficiency of kidney essence leading to the collapse of middle energizer qi (in the case of asthenia-syndrome).

Tympanic Medbrane a thin, semi-transparent membrane separating the middle from the external ear.

Foreign Body in the Ear a condition with foreign body in the external auditory meatus, marked by earache, auditory disorder, etc.

Bleeding of the Ear a morbid condition caused by the pathogenic fire in shaoyin kidney meridian and jueyin liver meridian.

Tumour of the External Auditory Canal a new growth like a seed of Chinese date, extending out of the auditory meatus.

Earache a common symptom of ear diseases caused by the pathogenic wind-heat in the liver and gallbladder, the hyperactivity of fire in the triple energizer, and feeble fire.

Itching in the Ear a symptom of intolerable itching in the ear caused by the attack of liver-wind or the flam-

耳痛 【ěr yōng】耳部灼热胀痛，有浓液流出。类似外耳道疖肿。

耳针 【ěr zhēn】耳针疗法用的毫针，长约0.7～1.0毫米。

耳针疗法 【ěr zhēn liáo fǎ】在耳壳上按照不同疾病选用特定穴位进行针刺的一种治疗方法。

二十八脉 【èr shí bā mài】1、常见的二十八种脉象，即浮、沉、迟、数、滑、涩、虚、实、长、短、洪、微、紧、缓、弦、芤、革、牢、濡、弱、散、细、伏、动、促、结、代、大等。2、指二十八条经脉，即手足三阴及三阳经、督、任、左右跷脉等。

二阳并病 【èr yáng bìng bìng】《伤寒论》中指太阳、阳明两个阳经先后发

ing up of kidney-fire.

Furuncle of External Auditory Meatus an infection of the external auditory meatus with local heat, swelling, pain and purulent discharge.

Auriculo-Acupuncture Needle the needle of auriculo-acupuncture which is filiform-shaped with 0.7mm to 1.0mm in length.

Otopuncture therapy acupuncture therapy applied to the special points of the auricles selected according to different diseases.

1. **Twenty-Eight Kinds of Pulse Condition** common condition of the pulse, including: floating pulse, sunken pulse, slow pulse, fast pulse, smooth pulse, unsmooth pulse, feeble pulse, force pulse, long pulse, short pulse, bounding pulse, indistinct pulse, tense pulse, even and soft pulse, wiry pulse, hollow pulse, wiry and hollow pulse, sunken and sturdy pulse, soft and floating pulse, weak pulse, scattered pulse, thready pulse, hidden pulse, strong and fast pulse, abrupt and irregular pulse, slow pulse with irregular intervals, slow and weak pulse with regular intervals, and large pulse. 2. **Twenty-Eight Meridians** the three yin meridians and the three yang meridians of the hand and feet, GV, CV and the left and right Heel Vessels.

Disease Involving Two Yang Meridians in Succession a morbid state in

生病变。两经的症状先后出现，但一般是指太阳、阳明先后发生病变。which two yang meridians are involved successively, meridians of tai yang and yang ming; written in **Treatise on Exogenous Febrile Diseases**.

二阴 【èr yīn】即前后阴。前阴指尿道口及外生殖器，后阴指肛门。
Two Yin the anterior yin (external genitals and urethral orifice) and the posterior yin (anus).

发背 【fā bèi】位于背部的有头疽。
Carbuncle on the back of human body

发表不远热 【fā biǎo bù yuǎn rè】风寒表证，须用辛温药以解表散寒，称为发表不回避热药。
Medicines of Hot Nature are not contraindicated in Dispelling the Superficial Factors a medical principle for the superficies-syndrome due to wind-cold factors, in which medicines of acrid taste and warm nature should be applied to disperse the pathogenic cold and to dispell the superfical factor.

发汗禁例 【fā hàn jìn lì】禁用汗法的病例，如无表证的发热、体虚、津亏、失血等。
Case for which Disphoretic Therapy Is Contraindicated referring to the case such as fever not accompanied with superficies-syndrome, general debility of body fluid, bleeding, etc.

发黄 【fā huáng】 1、因火盛血燥或久病气血亏损所致的发色变黄的一种症状。2、肤色黄染的一种病状。见黄疸。
1. **Colour of the Hair Turning to Yellow** a condition due to hyperactivity of fire, blood-dryness, or consumption of qi and blood after long illness. 2. Jaundice

发脑 【fā nǎo】位于玉枕、风池等穴处的有头疽。
Carbuncle at the Occiput carbuncle located over the region around the yuzhen and fengchi points.

发泡 【fā pào】（起泡）用对皮肤有刺激性的药物，捣烂或研末敷在一定部位的皮肤上，使局部起水泡而治疗某些疾病。
Vesiculation a treatment by the application of certain irritative drugs over the skin in order to raise vesicles.

发泡灸 【fā pào jiǔ】用艾炷直接烧灼，
Moxibustion a therapy by applying

或用刺激性药物贴敷穴位,使局部皮肤起泡的一种治疗方法。

发热 【fā rè】体温高于正常标准的一种常见症状。外感六淫之邪或疫疠之气所致的发热称为外感发热,多属实证;脏腑气血损伤或功能失调所致的发热称为内伤发热,多属虚证。有部分内伤发热的病人仅自觉发热,而体温并不升高。

发热恶寒 【fā rè wù hán】 外感热病的症状,常见于感冒、流感、温病等。

发颐 【fā yí】面颊部的化脓性感染,如疖肿、化脓性腮腺炎等。

伐肝 【fá gān】(抑肝)治疗方法之一。是抑制肝气过旺的一种治法。

发 【fà】1、头发。是肾之外华。其生长状况是肾气盛衰的反映。2、病情严重的体表痈疽。

发白 【fà bái】多因肝肾亏损,阴血不

irritant drugs to the acu-point or directly cauterizing the skin over an acu-point with moxa cone to produce visiculation.

Fever a symptom with the body temperature above the normal standard; the fever caused by the six exogenous factors or pestilent factors is termed exogenous febrile disease, categorized as sthenia-type, while the fever caused by the impairment or dysfunction of the internal organs, qi and blood is termed endogenous febrile disease, categorized as asthenia-type. Some cases of the latter have a fever subjectively but the body temperature is not actually increased.

Fever and Chillness symptoms occurring in various kinds of exogenous febrile diseases, commonly seen in common cold, seasonal febrile diseases, etc.

Pyogenic Infection of the Cheek suppurative inflammation over the cheek, including suppurative parotitis.

Suppressing the Sthenic Liver-Qi a therapy to disperse the stagnation of liver-qi.

Hair 1. the external manifestation of the kidney as its condition reflects the sufficiency or deficiency of kidney-qi 2. Suppurative Inflammation referring to the serious case of carbuncle or abscess.

Poliosis the impairment of the liver

足，发失濡养，过早地出现头发花白的一种症状。

发迟 【fà chí】初生儿因禀赋不足，气血不能上荣于发，故头发迟迟不长或头发稀疏萎黄。

发际疮 【fà jì chuāng】在项后发际外的毛囊炎。初起如粟米大，坚硬丘疹，顶白根赤，痛痒，穿破后流出脓液。

发枯 【fà kū】毛发干枯，失去正常光泽的一种症状。多因肾虚血热，阴血不能濡养毛发所致。

发落 【fà luò】头发脱落稀疏，枯燥无光泽的一种症状，多因肾阴虚或血虚，不能荣养毛发所致。多见于大病之后，失血及营养不良的患者。

发为血之余 【fà wéi xuè zhī yú】头发赖于血液营养。所以，头发的生长及分布情况可以部分地反映机体气血的情况。

翻花痔 【fān huā zhì】患痔复感热毒，气血壅滞，肛门四边翻出，形如翻花、

and kidney and the insufficiency of yin-blood leading to the undernourishment of the hair.

Tardiness of Hair Growth in Infancy because of weak constitution with insufficiency of qi and blood which fail to nourish the hair, the newborn has no hair and the hair grows tardily, or the hair is thin and looks sallow.

Folliculitis on the Hair Margin of the Nape inflammation of hair follicles appearing as indurated papules of millet size with white head and red base, and with purulent discharge after ruptured, accompanied with pain and itching.

Dry Hair a morbid state with the hair becoming dry and lusterless, mostly resulting from the kidney-asthenia and blood-heat, and the yin-blood failing to nourish the hair.

Loss of Hair a condition with the hair becoming thin, dry and lusterless, resulting from the kidney-asthenia or blood-deficiency and failure to nourish the hair; usually seen in the patient with long-stage illness, malnutrition after loss of blood.

The Sign of Blood Condition the hair is nourished by the blood, so the growth and distribution of the hair reflects partially the condition of qi and blood.

Hemorrhoids hemorrhoids characterized by flower-like protrusion out-

肉色紫黑、痛流血水。side the anal sphincter, dark purplish colour, pain and discharge of bloody fluid resulting from the repeated attack of heat and the stagnation of qi and blood.

烦渴 【fán kě】指烦热口渴。多由于热盛伤津所致，属实证。

Restlessness and Thirst an excess syndrome usually due to fluid consumption which is caused by the attack of pathogenic heat.

烦热 【fán rè】心烦、体感闷热。在外感热病，见于表邪不得外泄，或里实热盛；在内伤杂病，见于肝火旺盛，阴虚火旺等。

Fever Accompanied with Restlessness a morbid state occurring in exogenous febrile disease while superficial factors fails to be expelled or the sthenic heat is hyperactive in the interior, and also occuring in the syndrome with impairment of the viscera such as an excessive liver-fire, hyperactivity of fire due to deficiency of yin.

烦躁 【fán zào】指胸中热郁不安、手足扰动不宁的症象。常因阴虚火旺或外感经汗下后伤津所致。

Irritability a symptom manifested as being easily annoyed due to hyperactivity of fire caused by deficiency of yin, or consumption of body fluid after sweating in seasonal febrile disease.

反关脉 【fǎn guān mài】桡动脉位于腕关节的背侧，是一种胚胎发育变异的脉位。

Ectopic Radial Pulse the radial pulse palpable at the dorsum of the wrist joint resulting from the radial artery located away from its normal location. This is a condition of variation of embryo development.

反治 【fǎn zhì】（从治）是顺从疾病假象而治的一种治疗方法。如病属真寒假热，在治疗时要在温药中加入少许寒药将温药煎好后冷服。

Treatment Contrary to the Routine treatment applied when the false signs of a disease appear and the routine treatment is not suitable. For example, in the treatment of false heat-

犯本 【fàn běn】治病的时候，由于没有精确地分析正与邪的关系，运用不恰当祛邪法，以致损伤正气，特别是脾胃的功能。

饭后服 【fàn hòu fú】饭后服药。根据病变部位确定，如病在上焦，多数药物可在饭后服用。

饭前服 【fàn qián fú】饭前服药，如补养肝肾的药。

泛恶 【fàn ě】（恶心）多因痰浊、湿邪、食滞等停积于胃所致。

方 【fāng】通常指方剂。是按照治疗原则，由一定的药物配伍组成，用于治疗和预防疾病。

方剂配伍 【fāng jì pèi wǔ】在辨证的基础上，根据君、臣、佐、使的组方原则，选用适当药物组成方剂。

芳香化浊 【fāng xiāng huà zhuó】用气味芳香化湿浊的药物治疗湿浊内阻的方法。适用于症见腹胀、恶心、吞酸、大便稀薄、体倦乏力者。

syndrome in appearance but real cold-syndrome in nature; some drugs of cold nature should be added or the decoction should be taken after cooled.

Weakening the Healthy Qi an improper treatment affecting the healthy qi of the patient, mostly the function of the spleen and stomach because of the erroneous diagnosis.

Be Taken after Meal the time of taking decoction, according to the diseased location, mostly suited for the case with upper energizer disease.

Be Taken before Meal the time of taking decoction, esp. that for nourishing the liver and kidney.

Nausea a symptom caused by the retention of phlegm, damp or stagnation of indigested food in the stomach.

Recipe a formular with the combination of certain medicine in accordance with various therapeutic principles applied for the treatment and prevention.

Composition of Prescription the particular combination of medicines, based on the differentiation of syndromes, in a recipe representing their actions, designated as monarch, minister, assistant and guide.

Eliminating Pathogenic Damp with Drugs of Fragrant Flavour a treatment for the accumulation of dampness in the body by the application of fragrant drugs for eliminating dampness, applicable to the case marked by abdominal flatulence, nausea, acid regurgitation, discharge of loose stools, lassitude.

房劳 【fáng láo】指性生活过度，耗损肾精，成为虚劳病的病因之一。

Sexual Excess a cause of the asthenia-syndrome of viscera which consumes the kidney-essence.

飞痘 【fēi dòu】接种牛痘后，发生在接种部位以外的痘泡。亦称泛发性牛痘。

Vacciniola generalized vaccine after smallpox vaccination.

飞扬喉 【fēi yáng hóu】咽部疾患。心肺二经炽热，上扰喉关所致。表现为血泡发生于悬壅垂上引起的咽部阻塞症状。

Hematoma of Uvula a disease of pharynx caused by the attack of pathogenic heat accumulated in the heart and lung meridians to the oropharngeal isthmus, manifested as hematoma of the uvula and obstruction of the pharynx.

非风 【fēi fēng】类似中风的症状，而非外风所致的中风。

Apoplectoid Stroke a morbid state with apoplectoid attack but not actually apoplexy resulting from exogenous factors.

肥粘疮 【féi niān chuāng】头皮化脓感染，多发于小儿，属感受风热或热毒上攻所致。症见头皮起丘疹，继而成脓疮，破后糜烂流脓。

Pyogenic Infection of Scalp mostly occurring in children, manifested as papules over the scalp, followed by formation of pustules, erosion and discharge of pus; resulting from the attack of the pathogenic wind-heat or heat-poison factors.

肺 【fèi】五脏之一。主要功能是主气司呼吸，主肃降，通调水道。协助心脏维持正常的血液循环，以供给身体各器官生理活动所必需的物质；协助肾脏调节水液代谢。此外，肺与肌表的抗病能力亦有密切的关系。

Lung one of the five zang organs. Its main functions are to regulate qi of whole body, control of respiration, and to keep pure and descendant and to help the heart in regulating blood circulation, so as to provide the substances necessary for the physiological

肺痹 【fèi bì】皮痹日久不愈，复感外邪，损害肺气所致的痹证。症见心胸烦闷、胸背痛、咳嗽气急，或见呕恶。

肺病 【fèi bìng】指肺脏发生的多种病证。通常分为虚实两类。虚证又有阴虚、气虚之别。

肺朝百脉 【fèi cháo bǎi mài】人体全身的血液经脉管循环，都要流经肺脏。故谓肺朝百脉。

肺疳 【fèi gān】（气疳）五疳之一，多因郁热伤肺，出现咳嗽气逆、多涕、咽喉不利、寒热等症。

肺合大肠 【fèi hé dà cháng】指肺和大肠之间通过脉络的联系互为表里，在生理上互相协调，在病理上互相影响。如肺热下注大肠引起大便秘结，往往用通大便来清泄肺热。

activities of the organs of the body. Furthermore, the lung is closely related to the body resistance.

Lung-Bi-Syndrome a type of bi-syndrome caused by intractable skin bi-syndrome complicated by the attack of exogenous factors leading to the impairment of lung-qi; marked by feeling of oppression over the chest, chest pain, backache, cough, shortness of breath, or nausea.

Lung Disorder a general term referring to all kinds of diseases involving the lung, classified into asthenic and sthenic types; the former is further classified into deficiency of lung-yin and lung-qi.

Blood Flow of the Whole Body Converges in the Lung one of the functions of the lung, by which the blood circulation flows through the lung.

Infantile Malnutrition Involving the Lung a morbid state of infantile malnutrition associated with impairment of the lung by the retention of heat, marked by cough, dyspnea, running nose, uneasiness of the throat, fever and chills.

Lung is Connected with the Large Intestine the lungs and the large intestine are exterior-interiorly related due to interconnecting-interpertaining of the meridians. They cooperate in functioning and involve each other when diseased. For instance, lung-heat syndrome may result in constipation, and it can be relieved by relaxing the bowels.

肺和皮毛 【fèi hé pí máo】肺能宣发卫气于皮肤,使皮肤润泽,肌腠致密,抵御外邪的能力增强,肺气虚体表不固,则易于感冒。皮肤汗孔对体温的调节作用也影响着肺的呼吸功能。因此生理上两者互相协调,增强功能;病理上互相影响,导致疾病。

Skin and Hair are Connected with the Lung the lung has the function of dispersing outward defensive qi to the skin, of sending the essence to the skin and vellus hairs, the skin becomes compact and body resistance enhanced, while the resistance aganist foreign pathogens becomes weakened due to the deficiency of lung-qi leading to easy attacks by commom cold. The regulating function of the body temperature of the skin and the hair also affect the respiratory function of the lung. They are coorderated each other physiologically and are affected pathologically.

肺火 【fèi huǒ】指肺热火旺。有实火和虚火两种。实火症见咳剧痰少、咳声有力或咯黄稠痰、痰中带血、舌红苔黄、脉滑数等;虚火多属久咳阴虚、咳声无力,伴有潮热、盗汗、脉细数等。

Lung-Fire a disorder due to accumulation of pathogenic fire in the lung, classified into two types of sthenic-fire and asthenic-fire, manifested as severe and sounding cough with scanty amount of yellowish, thick or bloody sputum, reddish tongue with yellowish fur and smooth, fast pulse in the case of sthenia-fire syndrome, and as feeble cough, hectic fever, night sweat, and small, fast pulse in the case of asthenia-fire syndrome due to deficiency of yin.

肺开窍于鼻 【fèi kāi qiào yú bí】肺主气,司呼吸,鼻为气体出入的门户。另方面,鼻的正常功能也有赖于肺功能

Nose is the Orifice to the Lung the close relationship between the lung and the nose, the lung control breath

的正常。

肺咳 【fèi ké】即肺经病所致的咳嗽。症见咳嗽气喘,甚至咳吐血痰。

肺痨 【fèi láo】因肺脏虚损,并常与肺痨患者接触所引起的病证。症见疲劳乏力、干咳、食欲不振、形体消瘦、咳嗽、咳血、潮热、颧红、盗汗等。辨证分类:1、肺阴亏损证,2、阴虚火旺证,3、气阴两虚证;4、阴阳两虚证。常指肺结核。

肺络损伤 【fèi luò sǔn shāng】指因久咳或剧烈咳嗽,损伤肺脏血络,引起咳血、咯血的病变。常见于支气管扩张和肺结核等疾患。

肺,其华在毛,其充在皮 【fèi, qí huá zài máo, qí chōng zài pí】肺合皮毛,因此,通过望皮肤和毛发的情况来帮助了解肺的功能状况。

and the nose serves as the entrance and outlet of the air to the lung, and the lung is responsible for the normal function of the nose.

Cough due to Disorder of the Lung Meridian cough due to involvement of the lung meridian, manifested as dyspneic cough or even hemoptysis.

Impairment of the Lung Caused by Overstrain a morbid condition due to deficiency of the lung and frequent contact with such patients, marked by lassitude, dry cough, anorexia, emaciation, cough, hemptysis, flushed face, flushing of zygomatic region and night sweating. Types of differentiation 1. syndrome of deficiency of the lung-yin 2. syndrome of yin deficiency and excessive fire 3. syndrome of deficiency of both qi and yin 4. syndrome of deficiency of both yin and yang, usually referring to pulmonary tuberculosis.

Impairment of the Lung-Collaterals a morbid state of hemoptysis caused by chronic cough or severe paroxysmal cough, mostly seen in bronchiectasis, pulmonary tuberculosis, etc.

The Hair and Skin Reflect the Condition of the Lung the lung dominates skin and hair, so the observation of condition of the skin and the hair aids in understanding the state of the pulmonary function.

肺气 【fèi qì】指肺的功能活动。

Lung-Qi referrring to the functional activities of the lung.

肺气不利 【fèi qì bù lì】肺有清肃下降、通调水道的功能。如因某些原因引起功能障碍，则出现咳嗽、鼻塞、小便不利、浮肿等。

Inaction of Lung-Qi a disorder resulting from the failure to keep the lung-qi pure and descendant and to regulate the metabolism of body fluid; manifested as cough, stuffy nose, dysuria, edema, etc.

肺气不宣 【fèi qì bù xuān】因感受风寒邪气，皮毛闭塞，致肺气不能宣通的病变。症见发热、恶寒、鼻塞流涕、咳嗽等。

Sluggishness of Lung-Qi a disorder due to attack of the lung by pathogenic wind-cold factors; manifested as chillness, fever, stuffy nose and running nose, cough, etc.

肺气不足 【fèi qì bù zú】指肺的功能低下。症见气短、语声低微、面色淡白、畏风、自汗等。

Insufficiency of the Lung-Qi hypofunction of the lung, manifested as shortness of breath, pallor, aversion to wind, spontaneous perspiration, etc.

肺气上逆 【fèi qì shàng nì】因病邪犯肺，影响肺之肃降功能所致。症见喘咳气逆、痰多、胸闷等。

Adverse Rising of Lung-Qi a disorder caused by the attack of pathogenic factors to the lung affecting the purifying and descendant functions of lung-qi; manifested as productive cough, dyspnea, feeling of oppression over the chest, etc.

肺气虚 【fèi qì xū】指肺的功能低下的病变。症见面色㿠白、短气、声音低弱、怕风、自汗等。

Deficiency of the Lung-Qi a morbid state of hypofunction of the lung; manifested as pallor, shortness of breath, low voice, intolerance of wind, spontaneous perspiration, etc.

肺热咳嗽 【fèi rè ké sòu】指热邪犯肺，肺失肃降所致的咳嗽。症见咳吐黄痰、咳而不爽、口渴而干或发热等、舌红、苔黄、脉数。

Couhg due to Lung-Heat a disorder due to the lung-qi unable to keep pure and descendant resulting from the heat factor attacking the lung; manifested as cough with yellow thick sputum, thirst, discharge of yellowish urine, red tongue with yellow-

肺热病 【fèi rè bìng】因风热犯肺，蕴热成痰，肺气不宣所致的热性病证。临床以身热、咳嗽、烦渴、或伴气急、胸痛为症。辨证分类：1、邪袭肺卫 2、邪热壅肺 3、肺胃热盛 4、热闭心包 5、阴伤气耗 6、邪陷正脱。多见于急性肺部炎性病变。

Disease due to the Lung-Heat a morbid condition due to invasion of the lung by pathogenic wind and the formation of phlegm because of the heat, resulting in obstruction of the lung-qi, marked by fever, cough, thirst, or accompanied by shortness of breath, and chest pain. Types of differentiation 1. invasion of the lung wei by pathogenic factors 2. accumulation of pathogenic heat in the lung 3. excessive heat in the lung and stomach 4. heat-blockage of the pericardium 5. impairment of yin and exhaustion of qi 6. interior invasion of the pathogen and consumption of the body resistance; usually seen in the acute pneumonia.

肺肾两虚 【fèi shèn liǎng xū】泛指肺肾两脏同时出现虚证。多由于久病耗伤肺肾两脏所致，通常分肺肾阴虚和肺肾气虚两类。

Deficiency of both the Lung and the Kidney a disorder resulting from the damage of both the lung and the kidney during a chronic disease; classified as two types, i.e., yin-deficiency and qi-deficiency of both the lung and the kidney.

肺肾同治 【fèi shèn tóng zhì】用补肺滋肾药物，同时治疗肺肾阴虚。症见咳嗽、气逆、咯血、音哑、潮热盗汗、腰腿酸软、消瘦、遗精、舌红少苔、脉细数等。

Treatment of the Disorders of both the Lung and Kidney Simultaneously treating for deficiency of yin of both the lung and kidney with the drugs of invigorating the lung and the kidney and nourishing yin, applicable to the case manifested or hemoptysis, husky voice, hectic fever, night sweat, nocturnal emission, soreness, and weakness of loins and legs, ema-

肺肾相生 【fèi shèn xiāng shēng】五行学说认为：肺属金，肾属水，金生水。两者是母子关系，在生理上互相滋生，病变时互相影响。

肺失清肃 【fèi shī qīng sù】肺失去清肃下降功能引起的病理变化。症见咳嗽、痰多、气喘、胸隔胀闷等。

肺为娇脏 【fèi wéi jiāo zàng】形容肺是一个娇嫩的脏器，开窍于鼻，直接与外界相通，容易受六淫邪气的侵袭，故称娇脏。

肺痿 【fèi wěi】1、多由燥热熏灼，疾病误治后出现，以咳嗽、吐稠痰白沫为主症的一种病证，并伴消瘦、潮热、口干、气喘、脉虚数等。2、见皮毛痿。

肺系 【fèi xì】即呼吸道，包括鼻腔、咽、气管和支气管等。

肺痫 【fèi xián】 1、指因受惊而得的痫证。2、指小儿惊风。

ciation, reddish and uncoated tongue, thready and fast pulse, etc.

Generation between the Lung and the Kidney the close relationship between the lung and the kidney in accordance with five-element theory, in which the lung belongs to metal and the kidney belongs to water, and metal produces water, analogous to the relation between a mother and her child. They coordinate in functioning each other physiologically and involve each other pathologically.

Failure to Keep the Lung-Qi Pure and Descendant a disorder of pulmonary dysfunction manifested as cough, sputum, dyspnea, feeling of oppression over the chest, etc.

Lung is a Tender Organ the nose is the external orifice of the lung, so the lung is easily attacked by the exogenous pathogenic factors.

Pulmonary Flaccidity-Sydrome
1. a morbid condition due to consumption of body fluid and erroneous treatment; manifested as cough with thick and frothy sputum, accompanied by emaciation, thirst, dyspnea, feeble and fast pulse, etc. 2. Flaccidity-syndrome involving the skin.

Pulmonary System referring to the respiratory tract, including the nasal cavity, larynx, trachea, bronchi, etc.

Lung Epilepsy 1. epilepsy caused by being frightened. 2. referring to infantile convulsion.

肺邪胁痛 【fèi xié xié tòng】指肺受病邪所引起的胁痛。多因寒邪袭肺，水饮内停或邪热灼肺，肺络受伤所致。症见恶寒发热、咳嗽气喘多痰、胁肋刺痛。

肺虚 【fèi xū】指肺的虚证，包括肺气不足和肺阴虚。

肺虚喘急 【fèi xū chuǎn jí】久咳或病久致肺虚，肺气不能肃降引起的喘息。表现为喘急气短不能平卧，言语无力、喘急低弱、自汗畏风等。

肺虚咳嗽 【fèi xū ké sòu】 因肺阴不足所致的咳嗽。症见咳嗽少痰或痰中带血、形体消瘦、心烦失眠、午后潮热、面红颧赤等；也有肺气虚者，症见咳嗽气喘、咳声低微、易出汗、脉软无力。

肺炎喘嗽 【fèi yán chuǎn sòu】因体禀不足，又感受外邪引起的急性病证。症见起病较急，有发热、咳嗽、气促、鼻煽、痰鸣，或有轻度发绀，严重时，喘促不安，烦躁不宁，面色灰白，发绀加重，或高热持续不退。辩证分类：

Hypochondriac Pain due to Involvement of the Lung by Pathogenic Factors a morbid state due to retention of fluid in the lung after the attack of cold factor, or damage of lung collaterals by the heat; marked by chillness, fever, productive cough, dyspnea and stabbing pain over the hypochondria.

Lung-Asthenia a condition referring to the deficiency of lung-qi and lung-yin.

Dyspnea due to Lung-Asthenia a morbid condition caused by the failure of lung-qi to keep pure and descendant as a result of the asthenia of the lung during prolonged cough or chronic diseases; marked by dyspnea, shortness of breath, speaking and coughing in low voice, spontaneous perspiration, intolerance of wind, etc.

Cough due to Lung-Asthenia a disease caused by deficiency of lung-yin, manifested as non-productive cough with blood-tinged sputum, emaciation, restlessness, insomnia, afternoon-fever and flushed face; or caused by deficiency of lung-qi, manifested as cough with light sound, dyspnea, perspiration and weak pulse.

Cough of Pneumonia a morbid condition due to weak constitution complicated by invasion of exogenous factors, marked by sudden onset, fever, cough, shortness of breath, nasal flare or slight syanosis; in severe cases,

1、常证。(1)风寒闭肺，(2)风温闭肺(3)痰热闭肺(4)正虚邪恋，包括阴虚肺热和肺脾气虚。2、变证(1)心阳虚衰，(2)内陷厥阴。常见于小儿支气管肺炎，大叶性肺炎，迁延性肺炎。

gasping for breath and restlessness, pale complexion, worsened syanosis, or persistent high fever. Types of differentiation 1. ordinary syndromes (1) obstruction of the lung by wind-cold (2) obstruction of the lung due to wind-warm (3)obstruction of the lung due to phlegm-heat (4) invasion of pathogenic factors due to deficiency of vital qi, including lung-heat due to yin deficiency and deficiency of the lung and spleen. 2. deteroirated syndrome (1) deficiency of the heart-yang (2)interior invasion of jueyin, commonly seen in infantile bronchopneumonia, lobar pneumonia and persisting pneumonia.

肺阴 【fèi yīn】维持肺脏功能所必需的物质。肺既受脾气上输的水谷精气所滋养，又受肾水濡润，合称肺阴。

Lung-Yin referring to the the blood and bloody fluid nourishing the lung, which are necessary for the maintenance of the normal functions of the lung.

肺阴虚 【fèi yīn xū】肺的阴液亏损的病理变化。症见干咳、少痰、潮热盗汗、五心烦热、咽喉干燥、声音嘶哑、舌质红干、脉细数等。

Deficiency of the Lung-Yin a morbid condition of consumption of yin-fluid of the lung; manifested as dry cough, hectic fever, night sweat, feverish sensation of the palms and soles, dry throat, hoarseness of voice, reddish and dry tongue, small and fast pulse, etc.

肺痈 【fèi yōng】肺部发生痈疡而咳吐脓血的病证。多由外感风邪热毒，蕴阻于肺，热壅血瘀，郁结成痈，久则化脓所致。临床发病多急，常突然寒战高热，咳嗽胸痛，呼吸气粗，咯吐

Pulmonary Abscess a morbid condition mostly caused by exogenous pathogenic wind and heat toxin accumulated in the lung, causing blood stasis which brings abscess, forming

多量黄绿色脓痰或脓血痰。可分为：1、初期 2、成痈期 3、溃脓期 4、恢复期。

pus in the long run, manifested by acute onset, sudden chills and high fever, cough, chest pain, stridor, productive cough with yellow-green mucous sputum or mucous blood sputum. Types of differentiation 1. incipient stage 2. abscess-forming stage 3. pus forming stage 4. rehibilitating stage.

肺燥 【fèi zào】指燥邪伤肺，或肺阴不足伤津燥化的证候，症见干咳、咯血、鼻咽干燥、或咽喉疼痛、声嘶、口干口渴、舌红等。

Lung-Dryness a syndrome due to attack of the lung by pathogenic dryness, or consumption of body fluid with the formation of dryness resulting from the insufficiency of lung-yin; manifested as dry cough, hemoptysis, dryness of nasal cavity, sore throat, hoarseness, dry mouth and throat, thirst, red tongue, etc.

肺胀 【fèi zhàng】1、因邪客于肺，肺气胀满所致的病症。症见胸闷、咳嗽气喘等。2、属胀病。指胀病而见虚满咳喘者。

Lung-Distention 1. disorder due to stagnation of lung-qi resulting from the retention of pathogenic factors, manifested as feeling of oppression over the chest, cough, dyspnea and pain over the supraclavicular region. 2. a type of distention-syndrome with fullness in the chest, cough and dyspnea.

肺主气 【fèi zhǔ qì】肺的主要功能之一。一是指肺具有通过呼吸进行气体交换的功能；二是指肺对其他脏腑的气体活动、气的形成和盛衰均有密切关系，对机体各部生理活动有重要影响。

Lung Controls the Qi one of the main functions of the lung, referring to the gaseous exchange through respiration and the significant influence on the functions of other viscera by the lung.

肺主声 【fèi zhǔ shēng】指人体发声与肺的功能有关。中医学认为人体能正常发出声音，是肺气鼓动声带而发。

Lung is Responsible for the Normal Voice one of the functions of the lung, by which the voice is kept nor-

临床上声音的异常多与肺病相关。

肺主肃降 【fèi zhǔ sù jiàng】肺的生理特点之一。肺气宜清肃下降,才能保持其正常功能活动,否则就会出现喘逆、咳嗽、小便不利等症状。

肺主行水 【fèi zhǔ xíng shuǐ】肺具有调节机体水液代谢的作用,它与脾、肾相互配合以维持体液代谢的平衡。

肺主治节 【fèi zhǔ zhì jié】肺具有协助心进行正常血液循环的功能,只有肺和心的功能互相协调,才能保持其他脏腑的正常活动。

痱疮 【fèi chuāng】(痱子、汗疹、痱疮)由于暑湿蕴蒸,汗泄不畅所致。多见于炎夏。皮肤汗孔发生密集如粟米样的红色丘疹,很快变为小水泡,有瘙痒及灼热感。即红色粟粒疹。

分娩 【fēn miǎn】足月胎儿产出的过程。

粉刺 【fěn cì】(痤疮)皮疹如粟,或见黑头,挤破出白粉汁,感染形成脓泡或疖肿,颜面部较多见。多由肺胃

mal. Clinically, the abnormality of voice is usually imputable to the disorder of the lung.

Lung-Qi Should Keep Pure and Descendant　one of the physiological characteristics of the lung necessary for the maintenance of its normal functional activities, otherwise, symptoms as asthma, cough and dysuria will occur.

Lung Regulates the Metabolism of Body Fluids　one of the functions of the lung, by which the metabolism of body fluid is regulated in cooperation with the spleen and kidney.

Lung is Responsible for the Coordination of Visceral Activities　one of the functions of the lung, by which the lung aids the heart in maintaining the normal blood circulation. Only the lung and heart coordinate each other, can the normal activities of other viscera carry on.

Miliaria　an erpution of puritic papules and vesicles at the mouths of the sweat glands, accompanied with redness and inflammatory reaction of the skin; which is resulted from the obstruction of the ducts of sweat glands due to retention of summer-heat and dampness factors.

Delivery　the process of expulsion of the mature fetus.

Acne　an inflammation of skin mostly seen over the face; manifested as miliary papule or with a black head,

蕴热，血热郁滞而成，亦与过食厚味膏粱有关。

粉瘤 【fěn liù】（脂瘤）多因痰气凝结而成。症见：瘤体形圆质软大小不等，溃后溢出豆腐渣样物。多发于头面背部。

风 【fēng】1、风邪，六淫之一，外感证的常见致病因素，往往挟其他致病因素合而致病。致病特点：发病快且多变，呈游走性。常见症状畏风寒、发热。2、风证，见内风。

风秘 【fēng bì】因风邪侵肺，传于大肠，津液干燥引起以便秘为主症的病证，多伴有头晕、腹胀等症状。

风痹 【fēng bì】（走注）痹证的一种。由于风寒湿邪侵袭肢体、经络、以风邪为主的痹证。特征是关节疼痛游走不定。

风搐 【fēng chù】1、因火盛肝旺，风

whitish discharge when pressed; due to accumulation of heat in the lung and stomach, and stagnation of blood-heat, and also caused by overeating of rich and greasy food.

Lipoma a round, soft tumor usually occurring on the head, face and back, characterized by discharge of bean-curd-like material after rupture; caused by the stagnation of phlegm and qi.

Wind 1. referring to the pathogenic wind factor, one of the six factors which is the common pathogenic factor of the exogenous diseases and usually blends with other factors to attack the human body. The characteristics are sudden onset, changeability and tendency of wandering, manifested as chill and fever. 2. referring to wind-syndrome.

Constipation Caused by Wind Factor a morbid state with constipation as the major symptom due to dryness of the body fluid resulting from the attack of wind to the lung involving large intestine; usually attended by dizziness, flatulence, etc.

Arthralgia Caused by Pathogenic Wind Factor one kind of bi-syndrome, a morbid state characterized by migratory arthralgia, caused by attack of wind, cold and damp factors, predominantly wind factor, to the extremities and meridians.

Tetany 1. a morbid condition with

动痰壅引起的以手足不自主地摇动为主症的疾患。2、见脐风。 involuntary movements of the extremities as the major sign, caused by the domination of pathogenic fire and hyperactivity of liver-qi leading to the agitation of wind and overabundance of phlegm.　　2. neonatal tetanus.

风痱　【fēng fèi】中风后出现的偏瘫。症见肢体瘫痪，身无痛，手足痿废而不收引。 **Hemiplegia after Apoplexy**　a condition marked by paralysis of one side of the body, and limitation of the involved limb movement.

风关　【fēng guān】1、小儿指纹的诊断部位之一。指纹见食指第一指节为风关。观察掌面外侧浅表小静脉的变化，表示病情较轻。2、经外穴名，3、推拿部位名。 **Feng Guan**　one region of diagnosis of infantile finger print which is on the lateral ventral surface of the proximal segment of the index finger, indicating a mild condition of the sick infant.　　2. name of an acupuncture point.　　3. name of Chinese tuina region.

风寒喘急　【fēng hán chuǎn jí】因感受风寒，内郁于肺而致的喘急为主症的病证，伴有发热恶寒而无汗出。 **Dyspnea Due to Pathogenic Wind-Cold Factors**　a disease with dyspnea as the major symptom, caused by the wind-cold factors accumulated in the lung, usually accompanied with fever, chillness, but no sweating.

风寒耳聋　【fēng hán ěr lóng】因风寒束表，经脉凝滞，阻闭清窍引起耳聋为主证的病变，并伴有头痛身疼、发热恶寒、无汗、鼻塞、耳鸣等。 **Deafness Caused by Pathogenic Wind-Cold Factors**　a disorder with deafness as the major symptom, caused by attack of wind-cold, stagnation of meridians involving the superficies and facial orifices, accompanied with headache, body aching, fever, chillness, anhidrosis, stuffy nose, tinnitus, etc.

风寒感冒　【fēng hán gǎn mào】因感受风寒邪气引起的一种感冒。症见发热恶寒、头痛、无汗、鼻塞流清涕、关 **Common Cold of Pathogenic Wind-Cold Type**　a type of common cold caused by exogenous wind-cold fac-

节酸痛、口不渴、苔薄白、脉浮紧等。

风寒咳嗽 【fēng hán ké sòu】因风寒犯肺引起以咳嗽为主症的病证。表现为恶寒、咳嗽、痰稀白、鼻塞流清涕、舌苔薄白、脉浮紧等。

风寒湿痹 【fēng hán shī bì】即风寒湿三邪合而侵袭机体,导致肢体经脉阻闭关节疼痛、运动障碍的一种疾病。

风寒束肺 【fēng hán shù fèi】风寒邪气侵袭肺脏的病理变化。症见鼻塞、喷嚏、流清涕、咳嗽、头痛、恶寒、无汗、或有轻度发热、舌苔白、脉浮等。

风寒头痛 【fēng hán tóu tòng】由于风寒之邪外袭所致以头痛为主症的病证。表现为头痛或连及项背、恶寒、关节酸痛、鼻流清涕、舌苔薄白、脉浮

tors; manifested as fever, chillness, headache, anhidrosis, stuffy nose with watery discharge, sneezing, cough with irritation of throat, arthralgia, thirstlessness, thin and whitish fur on the tongue, floating and wiry pulse, etc.

Cough due to Pathogenic Wind-Cold Factors a condition with cough as the major symptom, in consequence of wind-cold factors attacking the lung; manifested as chillness, general aching, productive cough with thin sputum, stuffy nose with watery discharge, thin and whitish fur on the tongue, floating pulse, etc.

Arthralgia due to Pathogenic Wind-Cold-Dampness Factors a disease marked by arthralgia and limitation of joint movement, resulting from wind-cold-dampness factors involving the body and blocking the meridians of the limbs.

Pathogenic Wind-Cold Factors Tightening the Lung a morbid condition due to the attack of the lung by exogenous wind-cold factors; manifested as stuffy nose, hoarseness of voice, sneezing with thin nasal discharge, cough, headache, chillness, mild fever without sweating, floating pulse, etc.

Headache Caused by Pathogenic Wind-Cold Factors a disorder with headache as the major symptom, in consequence of wind-cold factors at-

紧等。

tacking the head; manifested as headache involving the nape and back, chillness, general aching, stuffy nose with watery discharge, thin and whitish fur on the tongue, floating and wiry pulse, etc.

风寒胁痛 【fēng hán xié tòng】亦称感冒胁痛。因风寒病邪留着胁下所致的胁痛。常伴有寒热、口苦、干呕、脉弦等症。

Hypochondriac Pain Caused by Pathogenic Wind-Cold Factors　a morbid state resulting from the retention of wind-cold factors in the hypochondrium, usually accompanied with fever, chills, bitter taste in the mouth, retching, wiry pulse; also named hypochondriac cold.

风火疬 【fēng huǒ lì】多因外感风热或挟肝胆火邪聚结而成的瘰疬。多发生于耳下，或颈项部，局部有红肿热，甚至破溃。即现代医学的急性淋巴结炎。

Scrofula due to Pathogenic Wind-Fire Factors　scrofula caused by the attack of wind-heat or accumulation of fire in the liver and gallbladder, usually involving the retroauricular and cervical lymphnodes with local redness, swelling, heat and pain; corresponding to acute cervical lymphadenitis.

风火眼痛 【fēng huǒ yǎn tòng】（风热眼）多因感受风热，风热攻目而起病。证见两眼急剧红肿疼痛、羞明、眵多泪热、常伴有发热头痛等。相当于急性结膜炎。

Acute Conjunctivitis　inflammation of the conjunctivitis due to attack of wind-heat factors; marked by sudden onset of redness, swelling and pain of the eyelid, photophobia, profuse secretion and lacrimation, accompanied with fever and headache.

风火相煽 【fēng huǒ xiāng shàn】热病过程中出现的一种症象。由于热邪过盛，火热燔灼肝经，内动肝风而致。症见高热、神志昏迷、惊厥等。

Pathogenic Fire and Wind Factors Stir Up Each Other　a morbid state occurring in the course of febrile diseases resulting from the attack of excessive fire to liver meridian leading to liver-wind stirring inside the body;

风 feng

风家 【fēng jiā】指平时容易伤风感冒的人。

风痉 【fēng jìng】由于感受风寒湿邪引起的一种痉病。症见突然跌倒，身背强直、口噤不开。

风疽 【fēng jū】因湿热阻滞于肌肤、或滞留于血脉引起的一种病变。发生于胫部或足踝处，病变处溃烂流黄水、痒痛相兼。感染后局部红肿，常伴有恶寒发热、腹股沟淋巴结肿大等。即现代医学的慢性湿疹。

风疬 【fēng lì】由风火邪毒引起的一种瘰疬，其形小而痒，数目不等。

风轮 【fēng lún】即黑睛，属于肝胆。病变与肝胆有关。

风疟 【fēng nüè】多因夏凉受风，又感疟邪所致的疟疾。症见先寒后热、寒少热多、头痛烦躁等。

风起㖞斜 【fēng qǐ wāi xié】由于风中经络引起的面神经瘫痪。表现为眼睑

marked by high fever associated with coma, convulsion, etc.

Person Liable to Catch Cold patients suffering from the diseases caused by pathogenic wind factor, such as common cold or apoplex.

Wind-Type Convulsion a type of convulsion due to attack of pathogenic wind, cold and dampness factors; manifested as sudden fall, rigidity, etc.

Chronic Eczema an eczematous dermatitis caused by the accumulation of pathogenic dampness-heat in the skin or in the blood, mostly seen on the leg and ankle; manifested as itching, painful erosion with yellowish discharge, and local redness and swelling after infected; probably accompanied with chillness, fever, and enlarged inguinal lymphnodes.

Scrofula due to Wind small and itching scrofula caused by the attack of pathogenic wind factor.

Wind Wheel referring to the black of the eye, which is linked with the liver and gallbladder. Its disorders usually indicate the involvement of the liver and gallbladder.

Wind-Type Malaria malaria caused by the attack of wind as well as cold in summer; manifested as chills followed by fever, headache, restlessness, etc.

Facial Paralysis Caused By Pathogenic Wind Factor paralysis of the fa-

不能闭合、口眼歪斜,面颊口唇不自主颤动等。

cial nerve caused by wind attacking the meridians, manifested as failure of the eyelid to close, and the eye, cheek and mouth tend to be drawn to the sound side, and may be accompanied with hemiplegia.

风气内动 【fēng qì nèi dòng】由于脏腑功能失调,气血功能障碍,筋脉失养,出现眩晕、抽搐、甚至神志昏迷等神经系统症状时的病理。

Pathogenic Wind Factor Stirring in the Interior a morbid condition due to the dysfunction of the viscera, qi and blood leading to malnutrition of muscles and tendons; manifested as neurological symptoms, such as dizziness, convulsion, or even coma.

风热 【fēng rè】即风和热相结合而致病,症见发热重、恶寒轻、或有咳嗽、口渴、咽喉疼痛、舌质红、舌苔微黄及脉浮数等。

Wind-Heat the pathogenic factor blended with wind heat factors, which may cause symptoms as high fever, mild chillness, cough, thirst, sore throat, reddish tongue with yellow fur, floating and fast pulse, etc.

风热耳聋 【fēng rè ěr lóng】因风热上扰清窍引起的以耳聋为主症状的病证,同时伴有耳鸣、耳痛、头痛、鼻塞等症状。

Deafness Caused by Pathogenic Wind-Heat Factors a disorder with deafness as the major symptom, resulting from the attack of wind-heat involving the facial orifices, accompanied with tinnitus, earache, headache, stuffy nose, etc.

风热感冒 【fēng rè gǎn mào】因外感风热邪气引起的一种类型的感冒。症见发热头痛、恶风自汗、鼻塞涕浊、喉痛、咳嗽、吐黄痰、口渴、舌质红、苔薄微黄、脉浮等。

Commom Cold of Pathogenic Wind-Heat Type a type of common cold due to the attck of exogenous wind-heat; manifested as fever, headache, aversion to wind, spontaneous perspiration, stuffy nose without discharge, sore throat, cough with yellowish and thick sputum, thirst, reddish tongue with thin, white and yellowish fur, floating and fast pulse, etc.

风热喉痹 【fēng rè hóu bì】因风热邪气侵袭咽喉部所引起以咽喉疼痛为主症的病证。表现为咽喉部红肿疼痛、吞咽不利,常伴有头痛、发热、恶寒等。相当于急性咽喉炎。

Sore Throat Caused by Pathogenic Wind-Heat Factors   a disorder with sore throat as the major symptom, caused by the wind-heat attacking the pharynx; manifested as local redness, swelling and pain of the throat, and dysphagia, accompanied with headache, fever and chill; corresponding to acute pharyngitis.

风热惊悸 【fēng rè jīng jì】因风热之邪相搏于心所致的惊悸。多见小儿,以多惊不安为主症。

Infantile Convulsion Caused by Pathogenic Wind-Heat Factors   a syndrome in infant consisting of convulsion and palpitation, caused by the wind and heat blending in the heart.

风热咳嗽 【fēng rè ké sòu】因风热犯肺,肺失肃降引起的以咳嗽为主的病证。症见发热出汗、恶风、咳嗽痰稠、咽痛、苔薄及脉浮数等。

Cough Caused by Pathogenic Wind-Heat Factors   a morbid condition with cough as the major symptom, caused by wind-heat attacking the lung; manifested as fever, perspiration, aversion to wind, cough with thick sputum, dry mouth, sore throat, yellowish and thick nasal discharge, thin fur on the tongue, floating and fast pulse.

风热头痛 【fēng rè tóu tòng】由风热上扰经脉引起的病证。表现为头部胀痛、发热怕风、鼻塞流黄涕、口渴喜饮、溺赤、舌苔薄黄、脉浮数等。

Headache Caused by Pathogenic Wind-Heat Factors   a morbid condition resulting from wind-heat attacking upward the meridians, manifested as distending headache, fever, aversion to wind, stuffy nose with discharge, thirst with desire for drinking, deep-coloured urine, thin and yellowish fur on the tongue, floating and fast pulse, etc.

风热眩晕 【fēng rè xuàn yūn】因风热上壅头部引起以晕为主症的病证。症

Vertigo Caused by Pathogenic Wind-Heat Factors   a morbid condition

见头晕眼花、甚至晕眩欲倒、胸闷呕吐等。

风热牙疳 【fēng rè yá gān】由于阳明蕴热与风热之邪相搏，邪热上冲牙龈所致的病证。症见齿龈红肿疼痛、糜烂、易出血、或伴有发热恶寒、便秘、呕吐等。

风热腰痛 【fēng rè yāo tòng】由风热之邪侵袭肾经所致。主要表现：腰痛牵连脚膝，口干而渴、脉数等。

风痧 【fēng shā】（风疹）为一种较轻的出疹性传染病，流行于冬春季节。多见于五岁以下的婴幼儿。由外感风热，郁于肌表而发，症见初起类似感冒，发热 1——2 天后，皮肤出现淡红色斑丘疹，从头面开始，一日后布满全身，出疹一、二日后发热渐退，疹点逐渐隐退、疹退后脱屑细小或无，无色素沉着。辨证分类：1、邪郁肺卫 2、邪热炽盛。

with vertigo as the major symptom, caused by wind-heat attacking the head; manifested as dizziness, or even fainting, feeling of oppression over the chest, vomiting, etc.

Ulcerative Gingivitis due to Pathogenic Wind-Heat Factors a morbid condition caused by the stagnation of heat in yangming and the attack of wind-heat upward to the gum; manifested as erosion and bleeding of the gum with local redness, swelling and pain, accompanied with fever, chillness, constipation, vomiting, etc.

Lumbago Caused by Pathogenic Wind-Heat Factors a condition with lumbago as the major symptom, caused by wind-heat factor attacking the kidney meridian, marked by loin pain involving the foot, thirst with dry mouth, fast pulse.

Rubella a slight infectious disease usually seen in winter and spring among children under 5 years old, which is caused by exposure to wind-heat dormant in the skin portion, marked by symptoms resembling those of common cold. Light red rash appears after 1-2 days of fever, first on the face, then the whole body within a day. It gradually goes as the temperature comes down gradually 1-2 days later. Thin and small scales or even no scales fall off after the disappearance of rash with no pigmentation of the skin. Types of differentiation 1. accumulation of pathogenic factors in the lung-wei 2. excess of pathogenic heat.

风湿 【fēng shī】风和湿两种病邪同时侵入机体所引起的病变。表现为不同类型的痹证。

Wind-Dampness Syndrome　a syndrome caused by the attack of wind and dampness blended together; usually manifested as arthralgia, myalgia, numbness, as various types of bi syndrome.

风湿头痛 【fēng shī tóu tòng】由风邪外袭,湿浊上扰头部引起的以头痛如裹为特征的病证。常伴有肢体沉重、胸闷腹胀、恶心纳差、口干不欲饮、苔腻、脉濡或浮缓。

Headache Caused by Pathogenic Wind-Dampness Factors　a symptom resulting from blended wind and dampness invading the head; usually accompanied with lassitude, feeling of oppression over the chest, flatulence, nausea, poor appetite, dry mouth but disinclination for drinking, greasy fur, soft and floating pulse or floating and slow pulse.

风湿相搏 【fēng shī xiāng bó】指风邪与湿邪侵入机体,相合为患,导致气血运行障碍,引起全身关节肌肉疼痛等症。

Wind and Dampness Blended to Attack the Body　a morbid state resulting from the pathogenic wind-dampness factors involving the body leading to stagnation of qi and blood flow.

风湿腰痛 【fēng shī yāo tòng】因卧湿受风或肾虚而湿邪乘虚而侵袭,滞留经络引起的以腰痛为主症的病证。表现为腰背部疼痛、活动不利或有恶风、浮肿等症状。

Lumbago Caused by Pathogenic Wind-Dampness Factors　a disease with lumbago as the major symptom caused by exposing to dampness and wind or deficiency of the kidney leading to stagnation of wind-dampness in meridians; manifested as pain and immobility of the waist and back, accompanied with aversion to wind, edema, etc.

风水 【fēng shuǐ】由于风邪侵袭,肺气失于宣降,不能通调水道,水湿潴

Edema Caused by Pathogenic Wind Factor　a disease with edema as

留体内，引起水肿为主的病症。表现为起病急、发热恶风、面目四肢浮肿、关节疼痛、小便不利及脉浮等。

the major symptom resulting from the attack of wind leading to failure to keep the lung-qi dispersive and descendant, and the retention of fluid in the body, manifested as sudden onset of fever, intolerance of wind, dropsy of face and four limbs, arthralgia, dysuria, floating pulse, etc.

风痰 【fēng tán】1. 指因感受风邪或风热内郁引起的素有痰疾发作。2. 痰滞肝经所引起的病证。表现为面青、眩晕、胁满、大小便不利、躁怒、脉弦等症状。

Wind-Phlegm Syndrome 1. recurrence of pre-existing phlegm-sydrome provoked by the attack of wind or stagnation of heat interiorly. 2. a syndrome caused by the accumulation of phlegm in the liver meridian, marked by cyanosis, dizziness, headache, fullness of hypochondrium, difficulty in urination and defecation, irritability, cough with greenish, forthy sputum and wiry pulse.

风痰痓 【fēng tán cì】因风痰壅滞经络所致的一种痉病。症见口眼歪斜、手足搐动或搐搦，甚者昏迷不醒。

Wind-Phlegm Convulsion a convulsion caused by the stagnation of wind-phlegm in the meridians; manifested as distortion of the face, involuntary shaking or spasm of the extremities, or even coma.

风痰头痛 【fēng tán tóu tòng】因风痰上扰引起以头痛为主的病证，伴有眩晕、目闭不欲开、懒言、疲乏、胸闷、恶心、呕吐痰涎等症状。

Headache Caused by Pathogenic Wind-Phlegm Factors a disease with headache as the major symptom resulting from wind-phlegm attacking the head accompanied with dizziness, heavy eyes, disinclination for speaking, feeling of oppression over the chest, nausea, vomiting of mucous fluid, etc.

风痰眩晕 【fēng tán xuàn yùn】因风痰壅闭经脉所致。表现为头晕眼花、

Dizziness Caused by Pathogenic Wind-Phlegm Factors a morbid condi-

头痛、肩背活动不灵、身重、胸闷、心悸、呕吐痰涎等症状。tion resulting from the accumulation of wind-phlegm involving the meridians; manifested as dizziness, headache, immobility of the shoulder and back, lassitude, feeling of oppression over the chest, vomiting with sputum or saliva in the vomitus, etc.

风温 【fēng wēn】 1、指感受风温病邪所致的新感温病,多发于春冬二季。主症为发热、咳嗽、烦渴。2、指太阳病发热而渴、不恶寒,汗出而身灼热者。

Wind-Warm Syndrome a seasonal febrile disease due to the attack of exogenous wind-warm, usually seen in spring and winter, marked mainly by fever, cough, and extreme thirst.

风温痉 【fēng wēn jìng】感受风温病邪所致的痉病。多见于小儿。

Wind-Warm Convulsion a convulsion disease resulting from the attack of wind-warm, it mostly seen in infants.

风痫 【fēng xián】因感受外感风邪引起以抽搐为主症的病证。

Epilepsy Induced by Pathogenic Wind Factor a disease with convulsion as the major sign, in consequence of exposure to exogenous wind.

风消 【fēng xiāo】因思虑过度,心神耗散引起日渐消瘦为主症的病证,常见有发热、经闭、血溢或遗精等。

Emaciation due to Emotional Upsets a disease with progressive emaciation as the major sign, in consequence of emotional upsets, usually accompanied with fever, amenorrhea or emission.

风泻 【fēng xiè】因感受风邪引起以腹泻为主症的病证。表现为头痛、发热、泻下清水或含五谷不化之物、脉浮等。

Diarrhea Caused by Pathogenic Wind Factor a disease with diarrhea as the major symptom resulting from the attack of wind; manifested as headache, fever, intolerance of wind, diarrhea with watery stool or undigested food, floating pulse, etc.

风心痛 【fēng xīn tòng】因风寒邪气内侵所致的心前区疼痛,胸闷。

Precordial Pain Caused By Pathogenic Wind-Cold Factors a morbid condition accompanied with feeling of

风眩 【fēng xuàn】由于身体虚弱，风邪犯脑引起以眩晕为主的病证。症见头晕眼花、发作无定时，呕逆、肢体疼痛，严重者出现昏厥。

风懿 【fēng yì】指猝然昏迷不省人事，伴有舌强、不语、喉有痰声等症状。

封藏失职 【fēng cáng shī zhí】 指肾脏功能失调的病变。症见遗精、早泄、小便失禁、夜尿多频、五更泻等。

疯犬咬伤 【fēng quǎn yǎo shāng】（狂犬咬伤）即被感染狂犬病毒的狗咬伤。由狂犬病毒入体累及中枢神经系统的急性传染病。临床上表现高度兴奋、流涎、恐水、吞咽和呼吸困难等症状。

蜂瘘 【fēng lòu】颈部生瘰疬，肿势明显，垒垒相连，此愈彼溃，溃后脓水不断，疮口似痈。相当于颈淋巴结核。

蜂螫伤 【fēng shì shāng】被蜂螫伤后引起局部红肿疼痛等证。

oppression over the chest, shortness of breath.

Dizziness Caused by Pathogenic Wind Factor　　a morbid state with dizziness as the major symptom, resulting from wind invading the brain, and general debility; manifested as irregular paroxysms of dizziness, accompanied with vomiting, pain in the limbs, and even coma.

Wind-Apoplexy　　a disease characterized by sudden loss of consciousness, accompanied with stiff tongue, aphasia and wheezing sound in the throat.

Dysfunction of Essence Storage　　a morbid condition due to dysfunction of the kidney; manifested as emission, precocious ejaculation, incontinence of urine, frequent nocturnal micturition, morning diarrhea, etc.

Rabies　　an acute infections disease of the central nervous system resulting from the bite of rabid dog or animal, marked by hyperexcitability, salivation, paralysis of the muscles of deglution provoked by the drinking of fluid or by the sight of fluid, respiratory paralysis, etc.

Perforated Scrofula　　enlargement of cervical lymphnodes occurring in clusters, marked by perforation and discharge of purulent fluid; usually due to tuberculosis.

Bee Stings.　　a condition of local reddness, swelling and pain caused by bee bites.

肤胀　【fū zhàng】因阳气不足，寒气留滞于皮肤内而出现的全身浮肿，症见腹部膨大、身肿、按之凹陷。见水肿。

跗阳脉　【fū yáng mǎi】（冲阳脉）古代诊脉部位之一。即足背胫前动脉搏动处。该处的脉搏变化与脾胃有关。

跗骨伤　【fū gǔ shāng】即跖骨骨折，以第五跖骨基底部骨折最多见。伤后局部肿痛，压之痛剧，可有骨声，活动受限。

跗肿　【fū zhǒng】即足背浮肿。

敷　【fū】捣烂新鲜的植物药或将干药末加一定量的溶液调和成糊状，敷在躯体表面的某一部位，定期更换。常用于疮疡、肿痛及外伤。

伏虫病　【fú chóng bìng】多因脾胃虚弱，感染寄生虫所致。症见少食、腹痛腹泻，甚则面黄浮肿、消瘦无力、食味异常等。

伏瘕　【fú jiǎ】古病名。由大肠热气郁积所致。症见下腹部有时隆起呈块状，有时可消散，并有腹痛、便秘等症状。

伏梁　【fú liáng】古病名。由气血结聚

Anassarca　generalized edema due to retention of pathogenic cold factor in the skin resulting from the insufficiency of yang-qi, manifested as ascites and general pitted edema.

Fuyang Pulse　also called chongyang pulse; a position for pulse-feeling in ancient times, located over the anterior tibial artery at the dorsum of the foot, reflecting the disorders of the spleen and stomach.

Fracture of Metatarsus　breaking of the metatarsal bone, esp. the base of the fifth metatarsus, marked by local swelling, pain, tenderness, friction sound and limitation of movement.

Edema of Dorsum of the Foot

Topical Application of Drugs　local application of pounded fresh medicinal herbs or moisturized medicinal powder over the affected part, applicable to local infection, ulcer, swelling, pain and injury.

Parasitosis　infection with parasites due to asthenia of the spleen and stomach; marked by poor appetite, abdominal pain and diarrhea, even sallow and puffy face, emaciation, lassitude, anorexia or heterorexia, etc.

Abdominal Mass　a disorder resulting from the accumulation of heat in the large intestine, manifested as recurrent appearance of lumps over the lower abdomen, accompanied with abdominal pain and constipation.

Fuliang　a name in ancient times for

所致脘腹部痞满有肿块的一类疾病。 a disease resulting from the stagnation of qi and blood, marked by epigastric fullness and mass.

伏脉 【fú mài】脉象之一。脉搏隐若，重按着骨才可触及，甚至难以触到。常见于剧痛、厥证等病情严重的患者。

Hidden Pulse a pulse condition which is deeply sited and impalpable until it is pressed to the bone surface, commonly seen in the patient suffering from serious illness such as severe pain, syncope, etc.

伏气 【fú qì】病邪潜伏体内，经过相当时间才发作的温病。

Disease Caused by Latent Pathogenic Factors seasonal febrile disease with a long incubation period.

伏热 【fú rè】指热邪伏于体内而致病。多因感受热邪，伏而不发，在其它因素诱发下致病。发病时无表证，出现烦热、咽干、口渴引饮等内热症状。

Incubated Heat-Syndrome a syndrome due to attack of pathogenic heat factor which incubates in the body, and aroused by other factors; manifested as internal heat syndrome such as fever, dry throat, thirst, desire to drink, but no symptoms of superficies-syndrome.

伏暑 【fú shǔ】由夏季感受暑湿之邪，留伏于体内，至秋后发病的一种温病。其症状与暑温相似。

Delayed Summer-Heat Syndrome a disorder caused by expoure to summer-heat and dampness factors during the late summer, but occurring in late autumn after a long incubation period. Its symptoms are similar to those of the summer-heat warm syndrome.

伏痰 【fú tán】指痰浊潜伏于体内或久留不去者，常导致某些疾病反复发作。除有一般咯痰症状外，癫痫、某些关节疾病及淋巴结肿大等均与此有关。

Latent Phlegm phlegm retained in the body for a long time, which may cause recurrence of certain disease; marked by frequent expectoration, and also related to epilepsy, arthritis, scrofula, etc.

伏饮 【fú yǐn】饮邪潜伏于体内或留饮去而不尽，反复发作为特点的痰饮

Recurrent Phlegm-Retention Disease phlegm-retention disease with ten-

病。症见喘满咳唾；若外感寒邪则症状加剧，且伴有恶寒发热，腰背痛、肌肉眴动等症。

dency to relapse due to retention of pathogenic factors in the body, manifested as dyspnea and productive cough. The symptom may be aggravated by the attack of cold, and chest pain, backache, muscular twitching, etc.

扶正固本 【fú zhèng gù běn】使用调补阴阳气血的药物，以增强人体的抗病能力的治法。

Strengthening the Body Resistance by Supporting the Healthy Qi a treatment for strengthening the body resistance by the application of drugs for the invigoration of yin, yang, qi and blood.

扶正祛邪 【fú zhèng qù xié】用药物扶助正气，提高抗病能力，以利于消除病邪的一种治法。

Supporting Healthy-Qi to Eliminate Pathogenic Factors a treatment with medicines to support the healthy qi and increase the body resistance and to facilitate the elimination of pathogenic factors.

浮脉 【fú mài】脉象之一。脉浮浅，轻按即得。主表证，浮而有力为表实；浮而无力为表虚。

Floating Pulse one kind of the pulse conditions, in which the beats are superficial and palpable by light pressure, indicating that the disease is on the surface of the body. The floating and strong pulse indicates a superficial sthenia-syndrome, while the floating and weak one indicates a superficial asthenia-syndrome.

浮中沉 【fú zhōng chén】诊脉方法之一。指诊脉手指所用力量分为三种。轻按为浮，中按为中，重按为沉。

Light, Morderate and Heavy Pressure a method of feeling pulse by exerting light, moderate and heavy pressure to the palpated site in order to get the information about the pulse conditions in the shallow, middle and deep sites.

釜底抽薪 【fǔ dǐ chōu xīn】用寒性而

**Taking Drastic Medicine to Treat Dis-

有泻下作用的药物，通泄大便以泻去实热的治法。形容如抽去锅底燃烧的柴草，以降低锅内温度而名。

釜沸脉　【fǔ fèi mǎi】搏动极快、浅表无力的脉象。

腑会　【fǔ huì】八会之一。即中脘穴。六腑水谷精气会聚的地方。

腑精　【fǔ jīng】指六腑中的精气，是六腑进行生命活动的物质基础。

腑证　【fǔ zhèng】伤寒病分类方法之一。即三阳经病影响其所属的腑所致的证候。如太阳经病累及膀胱，症见小腹胀、小便不利等。

腐苔　【fǔ tāi】如豆腐渣堆铺舌面。松散而厚，颗粒大，可刮脱的舌苔。多见于食积不消的患者，多属热证。

附骨疽　【fù gǔ jū】（咬骨疽）指常有明显化脓性病灶存在，或有外伤，感受风寒湿邪等诱发因素所致的骨性疾病。症见起病急聚，开始有寒战高热，患肢疼痛彻骨，不能活动，动则

ease　a treatment for the elimination of sthenic heat factor by increasing bowel movement with purgatives of cold nature, acting as a measure of taking away the firewood from under a cauldron to lower the temperature.

"Boiling" Pulse　a pulse condition with very fast, superficial and weak beats.

Convergent Point of Six Fu Organs　one of the eight convergent points i. e. zhong wan point where the essential substances of the six fu organs gather.

Essence of Six Fu Organs　essential substance stored in the six fu organs, serving as the material necessary for their functional activities.

Fu-Organ Syndrome　a type of seasonal febrile disease occurring in the course of three yang meridian disease with the involvement of their corresponding fu organs, e. g., taiyang meridian disease involving the bladder, marked by fullness of lower abdomen and dysuria.

Residue-Like Fur　a soft thick bean-curd-like covering scattering over the surface of the tongue, easily to be scraped off; which is usually seen in cases of dyspepsia.

Suppurative Ostomylitis　referring to the bone disease with supurative focus predisposing factors such as or trauma, invasion of pathogenic wind, cold, and dampness, characterized by

痛剧，肿胀灼热，化脓溃后，如骨质破坏，骨骼粗大高低不平，脓水淋漓，不能愈合，形成窦道，反复发作。辨证分类：1、热毒凝结证 2、火毒炽盛证 3、脓毒蚀骨证。

sudden onset, chills and high fever at first, severe pain of the affected limb, difficulty in movement, more severe pain on moving, swelling, burning hot. If the bone is impaired after it is ulcerated, the skeleton would be thick and not level, the ulcerated spots are hard to recover, and gradually form fistulas with lingering discharge of purulent fluid and repeated attacks. Types of differentiation 1. accumulation of heat toxin 2. excess of fire toxin 3. corrosion of the bone by pus.

复方 【fù fāng】二个或二个以上的方结合起来组成一个新的方剂称复方。一般适用于病情复杂或慢性疾病经久不愈者。

Complex Prescription a prescription composed of more than one formula, suited for the cases of complicated conditions or the intractable chronic diseases.

腹 【fù】位于人体胸部与骨盆之间的部分。

Abdomen the portion of the body which is between the thorax and the pelvis.

腹满 【fù mǎn】指腹部胀满的症状。有虚实之分，虚证多因脾阳失运所致，喜暖喜按；实证多因热结胃肠所致，腹满痛拒按、大便秘结。

Fullness of the Abdomen a disorder classified into asthenia-syndrome and sthenia-syndrome. The former is usually caused by the dysfunction of spleen-yang; characterized by inclination to local pressure and warm, while the latter is usually caused by the retention of heat in the gastrointestinal tract, characterized by fullness and pain in the abdomen, tenderness and constipation.

腹痛 【fù tòng】因外感六淫、饮食不节、七情所伤、气机郁滞、血脉瘀阻及虫积等因素引起的腹部疼痛。

Abdominal Pain a morbid state caused by the attack of six exogenous factors, immoderate diet, emotional

腹痈 【fù yōng】（腹皮痛）指生于腹壁的痈。

腹胀 【fù zhàng】腹部胀满不适的自觉症状。脾阳不足，寒湿内阻，致脾不健运；或实热内结，壅阻肠胃均可引起。

干霍乱 【gān huò luàn】因饮食不节，或感受瘴气后，秽浊闭塞肠胃所致的疾病。症见突然腹中绞痛、欲吐不吐、欲泻不泻、烦闷不宁、面青、肢冷、汗出、脉伏等。

干脚气 【gān jiǎo qì】脚气没有浮肿。因素体阴虚内热，湿热、风毒之邪从热化，伤营血，筋脉失养所致。症见为下肢无力、麻木酸痛、挛急、脚不肿而日见枯瘦、饮食减少、小便热赤、舌红、脉弦数。

upsets, stagnation of qi, obstruction of blood circulation, parasitic infestation, etc.

Carbuncle on the Abdominal Wall.

Abdominal Flatulence distention of the abdomen due to presence of excessive amount of gas in the stomach or intestine; caused by the hypofunction of the spleen resulting from the deficiency of spleen-yang with retention of cold-damp, or by the stagnation of spleen-qi and stomach-qi resulting from the retention of sthenic heat.

Dry-Type Cholera Morbus a disease caused by improper diet or exposure to pestilent due to retention of dampness in the stomach and intestine; marked by sudden onset of abdominal colic, intending to vomit and defecate but failing to do so, restlessness, pallor, cold extremtities, perspiration, hidden pulse.

Dry Beriberi a condition in the patient suffering from yin-deficiency and internal heat-syndrome due to attack of dampness-heat and wind which turn to heat, damage the ying and blood, and lead to the malnutrition of tendons and vessels; manifested as weakness, numbness, pain and spasm of the lower limbs, muscular wasting but no edema, loss of appetite, hot and deep-coloured urine, reddish tongue, wiry and fast pulse, etc.

干咳 【gān ké】（干咳嗽）以咳嗽无痰为特征，因火郁、伤燥或肺阴不足所致的症证。

干呕 【gān ǒu】(哕)即患者有呕吐动作，有声而无物吐出。多由胃虚气逆或胃寒引起本证。

干癣 【gān xuǎn】由风湿病邪侵及皮肤所致的皮肤病。其皮肤损害界限清楚，皮肤肥厚、瘙痒、干燥有裂口、有白屑脱落。类似慢性湿疹、神经性皮炎等疾病。

干血痨 【gān xuè láo】由于五脏虚劳所伤，虚火久蒸，瘀血不通，干血内结所致。表现为经闭、消瘦、不思饮食、骨蒸潮热、肌肤甲错及面目黯黑等症状。

甘 【gān】指味甘的药物。一般有补益和中的作用，如黄芪补气，大枣和中。

甘疳 【gān gān】因脾虚，过食肥甘、积滞化热所致。症见消瘦、困倦神疲、毛发黄枯、脘腹胀满、青筋暴露、耳鼻生疮、眼涩多困或生白膜、大便泄泻青白黄沫等。

Dry Cough a symptom characterized by non-productive cough resulting from retention of fire, impairment of the lung by dry factor or insufficiency of lung-yin.

Retch a strong involuntary effort to vomit but without vomitus, caused by stomach-asthenia with adverse rising of gas or stomach-cold.

Dry Tinea a dermatosis resulting from pathogenic wind-dampness factors manifested as skin lesions with clear thickened outline, itching, dryness, fissures and white desquamation, similar to chronic eczma or neurodermatitis.

Consumptive Disease Caused by Blood Stasis a morbid state caused by asthenia and consumption of the viscera, hyperactivity of asthenic-fire, and stagnation of blood circulation; marked by amenorrhea, emaciation, anorexia, hectic fever due to yin-deficiency, squamous and dry skin, and dimmish blackish complexion.

Sweet Flavour the drugs of sweat taste which possess the action of invigorating qi or normalizing the function of the stomach and spleen.

Chronic Infantile Malnutrition a disease, seen in children due to spleen-asthenia, caused by the greasy and sweet foods leading to indigestion and fromation of heat factor; manifested as emaciation, listlessness, dry hairs, fullness of epigastrium and abdomen, engorged superficial veins over the abdomen, furuncle on the ear and nose, dryness of the conjunctiva and cornea with membranous formation, heterorexia, diarrhea with forthy or bloody and purulent discharge, etc.

甘寒生津 【gān hán shēng jīn】用性味甘寒滋阴生津药,治疗热盛伤津的一种方法。常用于里热盛,津液耗伤患者,症见发热、口中燥渴或吐粘白沫等。

Promoting the Production of Body Fluid with Drugs of Sweet Taste and Cold Nature a treatment for the consumption of body fluid resulting from excessive pathogenic heat, manifested as fever, dry mouth, discharge of tenacious saliva, etc. by the application of drugs with moisturing effect in sweet taste and cold nature.

甘守津还 【gān shǒu jīn huán】用性味甘寒养阴生津的药物,治疗温病热伤胃津的方法。适用于温热病邪传入气分,胃津损伤患者,症见烦热、口渴、舌苔白厚而干燥等。

Regaining Fluid by Applying Sweet Drugs a treatment for the consumption of stomach-fluid druing a seasonal febrile disease by the application of sweet and cold-natured drugs with the action of nourshing yin and increasing the production of body fluid, which is applicable to the seasonal febrile disease with the attack of dampness to qifen, and the stomach-fluid is consumed, manifested as fever, whitish and thick, dry fur on the tongue.

甘寒滋润 【gān hán zī rùn】用性味甘寒有养阴生津作用的药物治疗内脏津液不足,或热病化燥伤阴的方法。适用于肺肾阴亏、虚火上炎,症见咽燥咯血、五心烦热等。

Nourishing and Moisturizing the Viscera with The Drugs of Sweet Taste and Cold Nature a treatment for the insufficiency of visceral fluid or impairment of yin with formation of pathogenic dryness factor in a febrile disease, by the application of sweet

甘温除热 【gān wēn chú rè】用性温味甘的药物治疗因虚而身大热的方法。因气虚而致的发热而常伴有少气懒言，精神疲乏、舌嫩而淡、脉虚大。产后或久劳内伤发热，症见面赤烦渴欲饮，舌淡红、脉洪大而虚。

Defervescence with the Drugs of Sweet Taste and Warm Nature a treatment for the fever due to deficiency of qi with the drugs of sweet taste and warm nature, it is applicable to the febrile case accompanied with shortness of breath, listlessness, pale and tender tongue, large and feeble pulse, also applicable to the case with fever after labor or overstrain, manifested as flushed complexion, listlessness with intention to drink, slight red fur on the tongue, large and feeble pulse.

甘辛无降 【gān xīn wù jiàng】指味甘、辛的药物其功效一般是向外表发散，没有降的作用。

Sweet and Acrid Drugs Possess No Lowering Action the common effect of drugs of sweet and acrid, which generally act outwards and toward the superficies without the action of lowering.

肝 【gān】五脏之一。主要功能是贮藏和调节血液，主疏泄、主筋，维持全身关节的运动功能及调节脾胃的消化吸收功能，同时，人体精神活动亦与之关系密切。

Liver one of the five zang organs. Its main function is to store and regulate the blood, to command ascending and descending and control the tendons, to control the movement of the joints, and adjust the functions of digestion and absorption of the stomach and spleen, it is also related to the e-

...and cold-natured drugs with the activity of producing body fluid and nourishing yin, applicable to the patient with deficiency of lung-yin and kidney-yin with excessive asthenic fire, marked by dry throat, hemoptysis, feverish sensation over the palms and soles, etc.

肝病【gān bìng】泛指肝脏发生的多种证候。多由七情伤肝,疏泄失常,肝络瘀阻;或阴血不足,肝阳偏亢以至肝风内动;或湿热内蕴,寒滞肝脉等所致。症见胁肋胀痛、头痛眩晕、耳鸣、目赤、易怒、或吐血衄血、肢麻、痉厥以及疝气、少腹胀痛、妇女月经不调等。

肝藏血【gān cáng xuè】肝的生理功能之一。指肝有贮藏和调节血液的功能。

肝胆湿热【gān dǎn shī rè】湿热邪气,蕴蒸肝胆所致肝胆功能障碍的病变。症见发热、恶寒、皮肤及巩膜黄染、口苦、恶心、呕吐、腹胀、小便黄、舌苔黄腻、脉弦数等。

肝风内动【gān fēng nēi dòng】指在病变过程中,出现肢体动摇、眩晕、抽搐等症的病理。通常有虚实之分。虚证多因阴液亏损;实证多因阳热亢盛所致。

肝疳【gān gān】(风疳、筋疳)五疳

motional activity.

Liver Diseases referring generally to various diseases of the liver, caused by emotional upsets leading to stagnation of liver-qi and obstruction of liver yang leading to hyperativity of liver-wind, or retention of dampness-heat and stagnation of cold factor in the liver meridian; manifested as hypochondriac distending pain, headache, dizziness, tinnitus, hematemesis, epstaxis, numbness of limbs, convulsion, hernia, distending pain of the lower abdomen, irregular menstruation, etc.

Liver Stores the Blood one of the physiological function of the liver, by which the blood is stored in the liver and the blood volume is regulated.

Dampness-Heat of the Liver and Gallbladder a dysfunction state due to retention of pathogenic dampness-heat in the liver and gallbladder, manifested as icteric sclera and skin, fever, chill, bitter taste in the mouth, nausea, vomiting, flatulence, hypochondriac pain.

Liver-Wind Stirring inside the Body a morbid condition characterized by trembling, dizziness, and convulsion during the course of a disease; those with asthenia-syndrome are caused by the exhaustion of yin-fluid while those with sthenia-syndrome by the hyperactivity of yang and heat.

Infantile Malnutrition due to Disorder

之一。因乳食不节，肝经受热所致，症见眼睛涩痒、摇头揉目、面色青黄、多汗、下痢频多等。

肝寒 【gān hán】指肝阳不足，功能减退，而出现忧郁胆怯、倦怠、易疲劳、四肢不温等寒性的症状。

肝合胆 【gān hé dǎn】指肝和胆之间通过经络联系构成表里关系。临床上肝气热则胆泄口苦；胆火旺则急躁易怒。

肝火 【gān huǒ】指肝气亢盛而有热象，多因七情所伤。常见有头晕、眼红、口苦、急躁易怒、舌尖红、脉弦数等症状，甚至昏厥发狂。

肝火不得卧 【gān huǒ bù dé wò】指肝火侵扰，神失所守所致的失眠。多由情志失调，肝气郁结，气郁化火；或肝阴素虚，肝阳偏盛，上扰心神所致。症见夜卧不宁、善惊、心烦易怒、口渴多饮、胸胁胀满，或小腹引痛，痛连阴器、脉弦数等。

of the Liver　　a type of malnutrition caused by improper feeding and the involvement of liver meridian by pathogenic heat; marked by dryness and itching of the eyes, involuntary head shaking, greenish yellow complexion, profuse sweating, frequent diarrhea, etc.

Liver-Cold　　hypofunction of the liver due to deficiency of liver-yang; manifested with symptoms of cold nature such as emotional depression, listlessness, fatigue and cold extremities.

Liver is Connected with Gallbladder　　the paired relation between the liver and the gallbladder through the connection of the meridians, both of the liver and gallbladder are cooperated physiologically and affected pathologically.

Liver-Fire　　a condition caused by the hyperactivity of liver-qi with heat-syndrome usually caused by the seven mode of emotions, manifested as dizziness, conjunctival hyperemia, bitter taste in the mouth, wiry and fast pulse, even syncope.

Insomnia Caused by Liver-Fire　　a disorder due to emotional upsets resulting from stagnation of liver-qi, and excessive fire factor caused by the stagnation; or due to deficiency of liver-yin and hyperactivity of liver-yang disturbing the heart, manifested as restlessness at night, frightenedness, irritability, thirst, frequent drinking of water, feeling of fullness in the chest, lower abdominal pain radiating to the external genitals, wiry and fast pulse, etc.

肝火耳聋 【gān huǒ ěr lóng】因肝火上攻所致的耳聋。常有耳鸣善怒、面赤、口苦胁痛、耳窍胀塞、脉弦等症。

Deafness due to Liver-Fire a type of deafness accompanied with tinnitus, irritability, flushed face, bitter taste in the mouth, hypochondriac pain, distending and obstructive feeling of the ear, wiry pulse, etc.

肝火耳鸣 【gān huǒ ěr míng】因肝火上攻所致的耳鸣。常伴有头痛目赤、口苦咽干、烦躁易怒、便秘、苔黄、脉弦数等。

Tinnitus due to Liver-Fire a type of tinnitus accompanied with headache, red eyes, bitter taste in the mouth, dry throat, irritability, restlessness, constipation, yellowish fur on the tongue, wiry and fast pulse.

肝火上炎 【gān huǒ shàng yán】指肝气亢盛的热象。多因五志过极、肝阳化火，表现为上部热象特点者。症见头痛、眩晕、耳鸣、眼红目痛、鼻出血等。

Flaming-Up of Liver-Fire a morbid condition of hyperactivity of the liver-qi, involving the upper part of the body; manifested as headache, dizziness, deafness, tinnitus, congested conjunctiva, hematemesis, etc.

肝火眩晕 【gān huǒ xuàn yūn】因肾水亏少，肝胆相火上炎所致的眩晕，症见头晕头痛、面红、口苦目赤、舌质红、脉弦数等。

Dizziness due to Liver-Fire a disorder resulting from the consumption of the kidney-water and the flaming up of both liver and gallbladder fire, manifested as dizziness, headache, flushed face, bitter taste in the mouth, red eyes, red tongue, wiry and fast pulse.

肝经湿热带下 【gān jīng shī rè dài xià】因肝经郁热与中焦湿邪相互蕴结，注入下焦，损伤任带之脉所致。症见妇女白带增多、淋漓不断、色黄而稠、有臭味、伴胸胁胀痛、口苦咽干、

Leukorrhagia due to Damp-Heat Factor Attacking the Liver Meridian profuse discharge of yellowish, viscid and foul fluid from the vagina, accompained with distending pain over

目眩等。the chest and hypochondrium, bitter taste in the mouth, dry throat, dizziness, etc., which is due to the damage of CV and BV resulting from the pathogenic heat stagnated in the liver meridian which blends with the damp from the middle energizer and attacks the lower energizer.

肝厥 【gān jué】指由肝气厥逆上冲所致。以手足厥冷、呕吐昏晕、状如癫痫、不省人事等为主症的一种病证。

Liver-Syncope a syndrome marked by cold extremities, vomiting, dizziness, epileptiform attack, unconsciousness, etc., usually resulting from the adverse rising of liver-qi.

肝咳 【gān ké】咳嗽伴两胁下痛满,甚至不可转侧的病证。

Cough due to Disorder of the Liver Meridian a syndrome marked by cough with severe pain and fullness in the hypochondria and sometimes the pain is so severe that the patient is unable to turn from one side to the other.

肝劳 【gān láo】见视力疲劳。

Eyestrain

肝脾不和 【gān pí bù hé】由于肝失疏泄,致脾的运化功能障碍的病理。症见精神抑郁、胸胁胀满、腹胀腹痛、泻泄便溏、嗳气、厌食、脉弦等。

Incoordination between the Liver and the Spleen a disorder caused by the failure of the liver in dispersing the stagnant liver-qi, leading to dysfunction of the spleen in digestion and transportation, manifested as emotional depression, distension and fullness in the chest and hypochondria, abdominal distension and pain, loose stool, eructation, anorexia, wiry and fast pulse, etc.

肝,其华在爪 【gān, qí huá zài zhǎo】爪的营养赖于肝血濡养,望爪甲可以判断肝血的盛衰。

Nails Reflects the Condition of the Liver nails depend on the nourishment of the liver-blood, observation of the nails may be helpful in judging

肝气 【gān qì】指肝的功能活动,包括血液调节、神经系统、消化系统和内分泌系统的部分功能。

肝气犯胃（脾）【gān qì fàn wèi (pí)】肝气横逆,疏泄太过,影响脾胃,导致消化功能紊乱的病理。症见头晕、易怒、胸闷、胁肋胀痛、泛酸、食欲不振、泄泻、脉弦等。

肝气胁痛 【gān qì xié tòng】指因情志不舒,肝气失于疏泄,气机郁滞所致的胁痛。症见胁肋胀痛、疼痛部位走窜不定,时痛时歇,嗳气则痛减,情绪波动则疼痛加剧及脉弦。

肝气虚 【gān qì xū】肝功能活动减弱的病理,常伴有肝血不足。症见面白、唇淡、耳鸣失聪、易惊等。

肝气郁结不孕 【gān qì yù jié bú yùn】由于肝气郁结所致的不孕证。多因肝

the condition of the liver-blood.

Liver-Qi referring to the functional activities of the liver, including regulation of the blood, nervous system, digestive system and certain function of the endocrine system.

Hyperactivity of the Liver-Qi Attacking the Stomach (Spleen) a disorder of involvement of the spleen and stomach due to excessive dispersing activity of the liver and up-rising of the liver qi, resulting in dysfunction of digestion, manifested as dizziness, irritability, feeling of oppression over the chest, distending pain over the hypochondrium, acid regurgitation, loss of appetite, diarrhea, wiry pulse, etc.

Hypochondriac Pain due to Stagnation of the Liver-Qi a disorder caused by emotional upsets, failure of the liver in dispersing and the stagnation of the liver-qi, manifested as distending pain over the hypochondrium occurring at intervals and relieved by eructation and aggravated by mental depression and wiry pulse.

Deficiency of the Liver-Qi a morbid condition manifested as pale complexion and lips, tinnitus, deafness, timidness, resulting from the deficiency of the functional activities of the liver and accompanied with the insufficiency of the liver-blood.

Sterility due to Stagnation of the Liver-Qi inability to conceive caused by

郁气血不和，冲任胞脉失于资助，难以摄精成孕。多伴有情志抑郁、胸闷胁胀、乳房胀痛、月经失调等证。

incoordination between qi and blood due to stagnation of the liver-qi, leading to dysfunction of thoroughfare vessel, conception vessel and bao vessel, usually accompanied with emotional depression, feeling of fullness and oppression over the chest, distending pain over the breasts and menoxenia.

肝热恶阻 【gān rè wú zǔ】指妊娠期由于冲脉气盛，冲气挟肝气上逆犯胃，吐苦水或食入即吐、纳差、头晕、心烦易怒等症。

Morning Sickness due to the Liver-Heat a disorder of the attack of the stomach by the up-rising liver-qi resulting from excessive qi of TV, marked by vomiting with bitter fluid, or vomiting after eating, poor appetite, dizziness, irritability, etc.

肝热自汗 【gān rè zì hàn】因肝经热盛所致的自汗。常兼有口苦多涎。

Spontaneous Perspiration due to the Liver-Heat a condition marked by spontaneous perspiration due to the excessive heat involving the liver meridian, usually accompanied with bitter taste and spleepiness.

肝肾亏损痛经 【gān shèn kuī sǔn tòng jīng】指由于肝肾精血亏损，胞脉失养所致的痛经。症见月经量少、经期腹痛绵绵，喜按，伴头晕耳鸣、腰膝酸软等。

Dysmenorrhea due to Impairment of the Liver and Kindney a disorder caused by impairment of the liver and kidney and consumption of the essence and blood, leading to the failure of norishing the uterus; marked by scanty menstruation with continuous abdominal pain, accompanied with dizziness, tinnitus, soreness and weakness of the loins and knees, etc.

肝肾同源 【gān shèn tóng yuán】（肝肾相生）指肝肾之间关系极为密切。肝藏血、肾藏精。而血的化生，有赖于肾中精气的气化；肾中精气的充

The Liver and Kidney Originate from the Same Source referring to closest relationship between the liver and kidney, because the liver stores

盛，亦有赖于血液的滋养。所以精能生血，血能化精，称之为精血同源，即肝肾同源。

肝肾亏损 【gān shèn kuī sǔn】即肝肾阴虚。

肝肾阴虚 【gān shèn yīn xū】（肝肾亏损）指肝阴和肾阴耗损的病理。症见眩晕、头胀、耳鸣、视物不明、咽干口燥、五心烦热、遗精、失眠、腰膝酸痛、舌红少津、脉弦细无力等。

肝肾阴虚崩漏 【gān shèn yīn xū bēng lòu】由于体质因素或因病致肝肾阴虚，阴虚生内热，热扰冲任，损伤脉络，迫血妄行，引起阴道出血，时多时少，淋漓不断，伴头晕耳鸣、腰膝酸软、脉沉细等。

肝生于左 【gān shēng yú zuǒ】指肝气的循行通道。肝位于右，升发，行气在左。

the blood and the kidney stores the essence. The production of the blood depends on the activity of the kidney essence and the activity of the kidney essence depends on the nourishment of the blood; it is also called the essence and blood originate from the same source.

Deficiency of the Liver-Yin and the Kidney-Yin

Deficiency of the Liver-Yin and the Kidney-Yin referring to the condition of consumption of the liver-yin and the kidney-yin, manifested as dizziness, feeling of distention in the head, tinnitus, poor vision, dry mouth and throat, fever sensation in the palms, soles and chest, nocturnal emission, insomnia, lumbago, pain in the kness, red and dry tongue, wiry, thready and feeble pulse, etc.

Metrorrhagia due to Deficiency of the Liver-Yin and Kidney-Yin a disorder manifested as continuous bleeding from the uterus due to constitutional defect, or deficiency of the liver-yin and kidney-yin leading to the production of pathogenic heat attacking the TV and CV, or damaging the meridians and collaterials; accompanied with dizziness, tinnitus, soreness and weakness of the loins and knees, sunken and thready pulse.

Liver-Qi Moves along the Left Side referring to the circulation path of the liver-qi.

肝,体阴而用阳 【gān, tǐ yīn ér yòng yáng】肝为藏血之脏,属阴;但其功能偏于动和向上,而病变时又易出现热证和阳证。所以说它是体阴而用阳。

The Body of the Liver Belongs to Yin but Its Function to Yang the liver is one of the viscera storing the blood, and belongs to yin, however the function of the liver tends to move actively and upwards, so it is considered to belong to yang. When the liver is involved in disease, heat-syndrome and yang-syndrome ensue commonly.

肝为刚脏 【gān wéi gāng zàng】是肝的生理功能特性。肝喜舒畅,恶抑郁,忌过于亢进。如受到情志刺激时,使人易怒、急躁,称为肝气太过;相反,如肝气不足,就会使人产生易惊胆怯的症状。

Liver Is a Rigid Organ one of the physiological characteristics of the liver. It is that the liver-qi inclines to grow freely and is averse to be depressed and stagnated. The hyperactivity of liver-qi is marked by easy to get angry and irritability, however the deficiency of the liver-qi is marked by experiencing fearness and timidity.

肝胃气痛 【gān wèi qì tòng】指因情志不舒、肝郁气滞,横逆犯胃所致的胃脘痛。

Stomachache due to Stagnation of the Liver-Qi a morbid condition marked by stomachache due to emotional upsets leading to stagnation of the liver-qi which attacks the stomach.

肝恶风 【gān wù fēng】当内外致病因素影响累及肝时,常出现眩晕、麻木、抽搐、惊厥等。此证候,中医归属于风,故称肝恶风。

Liver Is Adverse to Wind when the liver is affected by endogenous or exogenous pathogenic factors, symptoms attributed to the wind such as vertigo, numbness, spasm and convulsion may occur.

肝血 【gān xuè】指肝藏的血液。

Liver-Blood the blood stored in the liver.

肝血虚 【gān xuè xū】肝藏血不足的证候。症见心烦失眠、多梦易惊、月

Deficiency of the Liver-Blood a condition of insufficient storage of

经不调等。

肝阳化火 【gān yáng huà huó】肝阳亢盛的进一步发展，出现化热化火的病变。症见目赤面红，易怒，头晕等。

肝阳上亢 【gān yáng shàng kàng】由于肾水不足不能滋养肝木或肝阴虚，阴不潜阳导致肝阳偏亢的病理。症见头晕、头痛、目眩、面赤、口苦、舌红、脉弦细或弦数等。

肝阳头痛 【gān yáng tóu tòng】肝阳上扰髓海所致的头痛。症见头顶痛、眩晕、烦燥易怒、睡眠不宁、脉弦等。

肝阳眩晕 【gān yáng xuàn yūn】因情志不舒，肝阴耗损，肝阳上扰所致的以眩晕为主的病证。常伴有时时头痛，失眠多梦，易怒、脉弦等。

肝阴 【gān yīn】指肝的血和阴液。其与肝阳保持相对的平衡，以维持肝的正常生理功能。

blood in the liver; manifested as restlessness, insomnia, dreaminess, timidness, irregular menstruation, etc.

Fire-Syndrome Derived from Excessive Liver-Yang a condition of significant hyperfunction of the liver due to the further development of the liver-yang hyperactivity; marked by red eyes, flushed cheeks, irritability, dizziness, etc.

Hyperactivity of the Liver-Yang a disorder due to the kidney-water fail to nourish the liver-wood, or deficiency of the liver-yin fail to calm yang; manifested as dizziness, headache, flushed cheeks, bitter taste, red tongue, wiry and thready or fast pulse, etc.

Headache due to Hyperactivity of the Liver-Yang a morbid condition caused by the liver-yang rising up to the brain; manifested as headache, dizziness, restlessness, irritability, sleeplessness, wiry pulse, etc.

Dizziness due to Hyperactivity of the Liver-Yang a morbid condition caused by emotional upsets, resulting in consumption of the liver-yin and up-rising of the liver-yang; accompained with headache, insomnia, dreaminess, irritability, wiry pulse, etc.

Liver-Yin referring to the blood and yin-fluid of the liver. They should keep the relative balance with the liver-yang, so as to maintain the

肝阴虚 【gān yīn xū】又称肝阴不足。指由各种原因所致的肝阴亏虚而不能潜阳的病理。如可因肾精不足而致肝肾阴虚。症见头晕、头痛、视力减退、眼干、夜盲、烦躁失眠、经闭、经少等。

肝痈 【gān yōng】内痈之一。由肝郁化火，气滞血瘀，聚而成痈；或由积湿、虫积，壅结于肝而成。初起右胁部隐痛，拒按，不能右侧卧，常伴有恶寒发热、脉象弦数，继之局部胀痛增剧，身热不退等。

肝郁 【gān yù】（肝气郁结）由于情志不畅，使肝气疏泄受阻而引起的一类病症。可表现为两胁胀痛、嗳气、脉弦等。

肝郁经行先期 【gān yù jīng xíng xiān qī】指因情志所伤，肝郁气滞，郁久化热，热迫血行，冲任失守所致。症见月经期提前，色红或紫，或有瘀块，胸胁小腹胀痛，烦躁易怒等。

normal physiological function of the liver.

Deficiency of the Liver-Yin a morbid condition of failure to calm the yang due to deficeincy of essence and fluid of the liver, and also resulting from the yin deficiency of the liver and kidney due to asthenic essence; marked by dizziness, headache, poor vision, dry eyes, night blindness, restlessness, insommia, amenorrhea, scanty menstruation.

Liver Abscess a morbid condition due to formation of fire from the stagnation of qi and blood in the liver, or due to the retention of dampness or parasitic infestation involving the liver; manifested as dull aching and tenderness of the right hypochondrium, inability to lie on the right side, accompanied with chillness, fever, and wiry and fast pulse, followed by aggravation of local pain and distention, persistent fever, etc.

Stagnation of the Liver-Qi a disorder due to emotional upsets or other factors, marked by bilateral hypochondriac distending pain, eructation, wiry pulse, etc.

Early Menstrual Cycle due to Stagnation of the Liver-Qi a disorder of menstruation resulting from the emotional upsets, or stagnation of the liver-qi generates the pathogenic fire and leading to extravasation of the blood and dysfunction of the TV and

CV; manifested as the menstrual cycle being shifted to an early date, red or purplish menses with blood clots, distending pain over the chest and the lower abdomen, irritability, etc.

肝郁脾虚 【gān yù pí xū】肝气郁结导致脾胃功能减弱的病变。症见胁痛、厌食、腹胀、便溏、四肢倦怠等。

Deficiency of the Spleen due to the Stagnation of the Liver-Qi a morbid condition of hypofunction of the spleen and stomach resulting from the stagnation of the liver-qi, marked by hypochondriac pain, anorexia, flatulence, watery stool and lassitude, etc.

肝郁胁痛 【gān yù xié tòng】指因情志不畅、郁伤肝气、疏泄失调所致的胁痛。症见两胁胀痛，常因情绪变化而增减，伴有胸脘痞闷、食欲不振、烦躁易怒等症。

Hypochondriac Pain due to the Stagnation of the Liver-Qi a morbid condition resulting from emotional depression and anger leading to the disorder of the flow of the liver-qi; manifested as hypochondriac pain varying with emotional changes, accompained with feeling of oppression over the chest, loss of appetite, irritability, etc.

肝主筋 【gān zhǔ jīn】指筋膜有赖于肝血的滋养。肝的血液充盈，才能养筋；筋得其所养，运动才能有力而灵活。若肝的阴血不足，筋膜失养，则表现为筋力不健，运动不利，手足震颤，肢体麻木、屈伸不利、抽搐等症。

The Liver Determines the Tendons the tendons depend on the nutrients from the blood of the liver, the sufficiency of the blood of the liver ensures the strong activity; the deficiency of the liver-blood results in consumption of the tendons, manifested as spasm of the hands and feet, nubmness of the extremities, sluggishness of joint movements, etc.

肝主谋虑 【gān zhǔ móu lù】 肝的生理功能之一。指肝与某些高级神经的功能活动有关，尤其是思维活动。

The Liver Controls Thinking one of the functions of the liver, related to the activity of the higher nerve cen-

肝主疏泄【gān zhǔ shū xiè】肝的生理功能之一。包括以下三个方面：(1)调畅全身气机，推动血的运行和津液的输布代谢；(2)保进脾胃的运化功能，包括对胆汁分泌和排泄；(3)调畅情志的作用。

The Liver Smooths and Regulates the Flow of Qi and Blood one of the functions of the liver, including 1. smoothing and regulating the flow of qi, promoting the blood circulation and the fluid distribution. 2. promoting the digestive function of the spleen and stomach, including the excretion and decretion of the bile. 3. regulating the emotional activity.

肝主血海【gān zhǔ xuè hǎi】指肝具有贮藏和调节血液的功能，故喻为血海。

The Liver is Analogous to a Blood-Sea one of the functions of the liver, serving as a storage of the blood and a regulator of the blood volume.

疳积【gān jī】(疳、疳疾)小儿脾胃受损而虚弱，消化吸收功能长期障碍引起营养不良的一种慢性疾患。症见形体干瘦、懒言少动、毛发焦枯、精神萎靡、腹部胀大、青筋显露、饮食异常等。

Infantile Malnutrition a chronic disease in children due to the impairment of the spleen and stomach and prolonged digestive disorder resulting in malnutrition; manifested as emaciation, lassitude, dry skin, brittle hairs, listlessness, abdominal distention with visible superficial veins, heterorexia, etc.

疳渴【gān kě】疳疾而兼口渴喜饮者。多由于胃热或津液不足所致。

Infantile Malnutrition Accompanied by Thirst a condition caused by the stomach-heat or deficiency of the body fluid.

疳痨【gān láo】属肺疳的重证。由脾肺虚损所致。症见面色㿠白、骨蒸潮热、盗汗、午后两颧发赤、精神疲倦、时有干咳或咽痛等。

Infantile Malnutrition Complicated by Tuberculosis a severe case of infantile malnutrition due to asthenia of the spleen and lung; marked by pale complexion, hectic fever, night sweat, flushed cheeks in the afternoon, lassitude, dry cough or sore throat, etc.

疳痢【gān lì】指疳疾患儿并发痢疾。

**Infantile Malnutrition Complicated by

疳热 【gān rè】指疳疾患儿伴有不同程度发热的症证。

Infantile Malnutrition Complicated by Fever

疳泻 【gān xiè】疳疾患儿的腹泻。

Infantile Malnutrition Complicated by Diarrhea

疳症 【gān zhèng】因长期喂养不当或病后失调，致肚膨腹胀，大便干稀不调等明显脾胃功能失调的病症。伴有形体消瘦，面色不华，毛发稀疏枯黄，或烦躁易怒，或喜揉眉擦眼，吮指磨牙等症。辨证分类：1、疳气证 2、疳积证 3、干疳证。

Infantile Malnutrition a morbid condition due to improper nursing or disturbance after illness, causing abdominal distension, constipation which are the signs of dysfunction of the spleen and stomach, accompanied by emaciation, sallow complexion, sparse dry hair, or restlessness, irritability, or frequent wiping of the eyes, sucking of the fingers and clenching teeth. Types of differentiation 1. type of qi deficiency 2. type of indigested food retention 3. type of deficiency.

感冒 【gǎn mào】指由风邪侵袭人体所致的一种疾病。临床上以发热、头痛、鼻塞、流涕、畏风、脉浮为特征。常分风寒和风热两型。

Common Cold a disease caused by invasion of pathogenic wind, characterized by running nose, sneezing, intching or sore throat, chills, fever, abscence of or less sweat, headache and general aching. Types of differentiation 1. wind-cold type 2. wind-heat type 3. summer-damp type.

感冒头痛 【gǎn mào tóu tòng】因外感风邪所致头痛病证。常伴有鼻塞、自汗恶风、脉浮缓等。

Headache due to Common Cold headache caused by exogenous wind, accompanied by stuffy nose, spontaneous sweating, aversion to wind, floating and slow pulse.

刚痉 【gāng jìng】痉病的一种。由风

Tonic Convulsion one of the con-

热炽盛所致。症见发热、恶寒、无汗、颈项强急、头摇口噤、手足挛急或抽搐，甚则角弓反张、脉弦等。

肛裂 【gāng liè】因血热肠燥，大便干结，排便用力，引起肛门边缘破裂。症见大便秘结、便时肛门灼痛，有时出少量鲜血。

肛漏 【gāng lòu】（肛瘘、牡痔）肛门及周围发生瘘管，常流恶臭脓样物。多因肛门周围痈疽溃后，久治不愈而成瘘管；或因内痔、肛裂等引起。

肛门 【gāng mén】（后阴魄门）消化道最末端，能排泄粪便和控制排便。

肛门痈 【gāng mén yōng】指发生于肛门内外的脓肿。多因过食厚味辛辣煎炒之物；或脾肺不足，肾阴亏损致肠胃受损，湿热下注而成。

高风雀目内障 【gāo fēng què mù nèi zhàng】终年瞳子如金色。由绿风内障恶化而成。

高者抑之 【gāo zhě yì zhī】指应用降逆抑制的方药治疗以向上冲逆为主

vulsive diseases caused by hyperactivity of pathogenic wind-heat, charactized by fever, aversion to cold, abscence of sweat, rigidity of the neck, head tremor, lockjaw, contracture or convulsion of the limbs, or even opisthotons and thready pulse.

Anal Fissure an injury during defecation due to dryness of the intestines and constipation caused by blood-heat, marked by constipation, burning pain in the anus when discharging stool, sometimes with amount of fresh blood.

Anal Fistula fistulas occurring in or around the anus with frequent purulent fetid discharges, mostly caused by the non-healing of boils, or internal hemorrhoid.

Anus the end part of the digestive tract for defecation or controlling defecation.

Perianal Abscess usually referring to internal and external abscess of the anus, mostly caused by eating spicy, oily or fried food, or hypofunction of the spleen and lung, deficiency of the kidney-yin, leading to impairment of the intestines and stomach, and dawnward flowing of damp-heat.

Pigmentary Degeneration of Retina a condition with the pupil golden in color due to the deterioration of glaucoma.

Treating Rush-upward Symptoms with Depressive Therapy a therapeutic

症的疾病的一种治法。如肺气上逆致咳嗽哮喘者用降逆下气的方法。 method to treat diseases characterized by rush-upward symptoms with depressant prescription, e. g., patients with asthma caused by adverse ascending of the lung-qi can be treated by checking upward adverse flow of the lung-qi.

膏 【gāo】分内服、外用膏剂。内服的将药物用水蒸熬,加入冰糖、蜂蜜等调成稠膏,常用于慢性疾病等身体虚弱者;外用的称油膏或药膏。 Soft Extract including extract for oral administration and for external use with the former made by concentrating a decoction to syrupy consistency with addition of sugar or honey, for cases with chronic diseases or those who are weak; extract for external use usually called ointment.

膏肓 【gāo huāng】1、膏,心下之部;肓,心下隔上之部。2、经穴名称,常用来说明病位的隐深,形容病情深重。 Gaohuang 1. "gao" referring to the site below the heart; "huang" referring to the site below the heart and above the diaphragm, mainly used to describe a deep-sited and incurable disease. 2. one of the acupoints on regular meridians.

膏粱厚味 【gāo liáng hòu wèi】指肥腻而味浓的食物。过食这类食物既容易损伤脾胃,又会导致疮疡等多种病证。 Rich Fatty Diet long time feeding or overeating on which will do harm to the spleen and stomach and cause formation of phlegm and heat and development of ulcers and carbuncles.

膏淋 【gāo lìn】(内淋)指以小便混浊如米泔或如脂膏,排尿不畅为主的一种病症。常有虚实之分,虚证多因脾肾虚弱,不能制约脂液引起;实证多因湿热蕴结下焦,气化不利,清浊相混脂液失约所致。 Stranguria Marked by Chyluria a disorder manifested as difficult urination with cloudy rice-water like or oily urine, usually classified as deficiency type and excess type, for deficiency type, mostly caused by hypofunction of the spleen and kidney and failure in controlling the oily urine; for excess type, mostly caused by accumulation of pathogenic damp-heat in the lower energizer, leading to disturbance in qi transformation, the mixing of clear and turbid urine and failure in controlling oily urine.

膏摩 【gāo mó】用膏药涂擦体表的一定部位,以达到治疗目的的一种治法。该治法具有按摩和药物的综合作用。适用于治疗关节或局部肿痛,或某些皮肤病。

Rubbing the Affected Part with Ointment　a maneuver of massage by rubbing the affected part with ointment for the treatment of joint or local swelling and pain, as well as skin disease.

膏药 【gāo yào】(薄贴)敷贴用的膏剂,用时需加热使之柔软。

Adhensive Pulse　a type of soft extract for applying purpose, to be heated to a state of slight melting before use.

革脉 【gé mài】弦大中空,如按鼓皮的一种脉象。多因亡血失精所致。

Tympanic Pulse　an extremely taut and hollow pulse, giving the feeling as if touching the surface of a drum, often seen in patient after loss of blood or spermatorrhea.

隔饼灸 【gé bǐng jiǔ】指施灸时在穴位上隔以用辛温或芳香类药物制成的薄饼的一种灸法。

Cake-Partition Moxibustion　an indirect moxibustion with drug paste, pungent in flavor and warm in property or aromatics, placed between the moxa cone and the acupoint.

隔姜灸 【gé jiāng jiǔ】指把艾炷放在姜片上燃烧灼灸的一种灸法。

Ginger-Partition Moxibustion　an indirect moxibustion by placing a slice of raw ginger upon the acupuncture point and a burning moxa cone over the ginger.

隔蒜灸 【gé suàn jiǔ】指把艾炷放在蒜片上燃烧的一种灸法。

Garlic-Partition Moxibustion　an indirect moxibustion with a thin slice of raw garlic placed over the acupuncture point and a moxa cone then burned on the garlic.

隔盐灸 【gé yán jiǔ】用食盐末将脐窝

Salt-Partition Moxibustion　an indi-

填平，再在盐末上放较大艾炷燃烧的一种灸法。用于治疗腹痛、腹泻、虚脱等症。

瘑疮 【gé chuāng】由风湿热邪客于肌肤所致的一种病证。多见于手掌及足背对称发作粟粒样水疱、自觉瘙痒、破后流黄水，干燥后结成黄褐色痂皮、瘙痒明显、皮肤变厚、粗糙。即慢性湿疹。

膈 【gé】即横膈膜（膈肌）。此膜将体腔分为胸腔和腹腔。

膈痰 【gé tán】因痰水结聚胸膈，气机升降失常，气逆痰壅所致的病证。症见心腹痞满、短气不能平卧、头眩目暗、常欲呕逆等。

膈痫 【gé xián】指风痰阻于胸膈络脉不畅引起的痫证。

更衣 【gēng yī】大便的古称。

攻补兼施 【gōng bǔ jiān shī】攻法和补法同时使用的一种治法，以达到去邪而不伤正的目的。适用于邪气实而正气虚的病人。

rect moxibustion by putting a layer of fine salt on the umbilicus and a large burning moxa cone over the salt, used for treating abdominal pain, diarrhea and prostration.

Chronic Eczema an infected skin disease due to the invasion of pathogenic wind, dampness and heat to the skin, usually appearing symmetrically on the palms and the dorsum of the feet; characterized by itching, oozing and crusting, and later by scaling, thickening and roughening of the skin.

Diaphragm the part which divides the body cavity into thoracic cavity and abdominal cavity.

Diaphragm-Phlegm Syndrome a disease caused by adverse upward flow of qi and accumulation of phlegm due to retention of watery phlegm in the thorax and the disturbance of qi in ascending and descending, characterized by stuffiness of the chest and epigastrium, shortness of breath, inability to lie down, vertigo and nausea.

Epilepsy a disease caused by accumulation of wind-phlegm in the thorax.

An Ancient Name for Defecation

Therapy of the Elimination of Pathogenic Factors and the Restoration of Healthy-Qi a therapeutic method of reinforcement and elimination at the same time for the purpose

攻溃 【gōng kuì】重用消肿排脓药物，使疮疡的脓毒排出后肿痛消退的治法。
Promoting Suppuration a therapy to hasten the rupture of abscess, allowing the pus to evacuate so as to reduce swelling and pain with drugs.

攻里不远寒 【gōng lǐ bù yuǎn hán】热积于内的里证，须用寒性药物来攻下，称为攻里不回避寒药。
The Necessity of Using Drugs in Cold Nature to Treat Internal Heat interior syndrome due to accumulation of heat should be treated with cold nature drugs.

肱 【gōng】上臂。相当肱骨部分。
Upper Arm referring the humerus

孤腑 【gū fǔ】即三焦。
Solitary Fu Organ referring to the triple-energizer.

孤阳上浮 【gū yáng shàng fú】又称虚阳不敛。因精血亏损，致使阴不制阳，虚阳上浮的病变。
Upward Floating of Yang in Deficiency Condition pathogenical changes marked by upward floating of yang due to consumption of esscence and blood and failure of yin to keep yang well.

孤阴 【gū yīn】喻阴的偏盛。
Solitary Yin implying the excess of yin.

孤脏 【gū zàng】指脾脏或肾脏。
Solitary Zang Organs referring to the spleen and kidney.

箍围药 【gū wé yào】（箍药）外治法的一种。在初起的肿疡周围敷一圈湿润的药泥，起消肿、散结止痛或促使脓肿溃破的作用。
Encircling Drugs one of the external therapeutic methods by applying a drug paste around the affected area at its early stage of a suppurative infection, so as to eliminate swelling, remove obstruction and relieve pain as well as to promote the process of suppuration.

谷疸 【gǔ dàn】黄疸的一种类型。因
Jaundice due to Immoderate Eating

饮食不节，湿热食滞阻遏中焦所致。症见寒热、不食、头眩、胸腹胀满、身目发黄、小便不利等。

谷道　【gǔ dào】指肛门。

谷气　【gǔ qì】（水谷之气）指从食物消化吸收的营养物质，即水谷精微。

骨痹　【gǔ bì】指以骨节酸痛、浮肿、运动障碍为主症的痹证。由风寒湿邪乘虚侵袭于骨所致。

骨槽风　【gǔ cáo fēng】（穿腮毒、穿腮发、牙叉发）因手少阳三焦、足阳明胃二经风火邪毒上灼或脾阳虚衰无力托毒外出而成。初起于耳前并连腮项皮下有小结，痛连筋骨，渐大或腐溃流脓，日久排出腐骨，腐臭，甚则牙齿脱落。

骨鲠　【gǔ gěng】因饮食不慎，鸡、鱼等骨梗于咽喉部，咽喉刺痛，吞咽困

a type of jaundices caused by accumulation of dampness and heat as a consequence of food retention in the middle-energizer, characterized by chill or fever, anorexia, dizziness, fullness and distention in the chest and abdomen, yellowish discoloration of the body and eyes, and difficulty in urination.

Anus

Essence Derived from Food　referring to the nutrients from food, i. e. the essence of foodstuff.

Rheumatism Involving the Bone
rheumatism caused by invasion of bone meridians and vessels by pathogenic wind, cold and dampness, characterized by aching pain of the bone joints, and difficulty in movement.

Osteomyelitis of the Maxillary Bone
　a morbid condition caused by the upward wind-fire from the triple energizer meridian of hand-shaoyang and stomach meridian of food-yangming, st. or deficiency of spleen-yang and its inability to expell toxin, first with small subcutaneous nodules appeared in front of the ear and the cheek which are painful, radiating to the bone and ligament, or ulcerated with pus discharge, and much later with the fetid putrefacted bone discharged, or ever loss of teeth.

Bone in the Throat　having a chicken or fish bone or other bone caught

难，甚者唾液和食物中混有鲜血。 in the throat due to carelessness in eating with the manifestations such as irritating pain in the throat, difficulty in swallowing, or even blood seen in the saliva and food.

骨会 【gǔ huì】八会之一，即大杼穴。骨的精气会聚的地方。

Influential Point of the Bone Dazhui point, one of the eight strategic or influential points, where essence of bone assembles.

骨瘤 【gǔ liú】因肾气不足，寒湿挟痰，侵袭骨骼，以致气血凝聚于骨所致的骨骼肿瘤（现代医学指骨细胞的异常增生）。好发于长骨的干骺端。恶性者生长迅速痛甚，肿块与骨相连、推之不移，常伴低热、消瘦、神疲等。良性生长缓慢症状较轻。

Osteoma a disease caused by deficiency of kidney-qi and invasion of the bone by pathogenic cold and dampness as well as accumulation of phlegm, all of these result in stagnancy of qi and blood, in modern term, it is considered as abnormal proliferation of bone cells which usually occurs on the metaphysis of long bones. If malignant, it grows rapidly with the mass adhensive to the bone, unmovable when pushed, usually charaterized by low fever, emaciation, and lassitude; for benign one, it usually grows slowly with less serious symptoms.

骨痛 【gǔ tòng】指肢体某部疼痛彻骨的症状。见于痹证、骨伤、虚劳等。

Osteodynia a symptom of the limbs, seen in bi syndrome, bone traume and consumptive disease.

骨痿 【gǔ wěi】（肾痿）因邪热伤肾，阴精耗损，骨枯髓虚所致的痿症。症见腰脊酸软、不能伸举、下肢痿缩、运动障碍、伴有面色暗黑、牙齿干枯等。

Atrophic Debility of the Bone a type of flaccidity due to impairment of kidney by pathogenic heat, leading to severe exhaustion of kidney-essence and sthenia of the bones, characterized by inability to stand upright due to soreness and weakness of the lower back, atrophic and flaccid muscles or limited movements of the lower limbs, dusty complexion and lusterless teeth.

骨折 【gǔ zhé】因外伤或骨病变造成的骨骼的折断或碎裂。症见:局部肿痛、瘀血、拒按、错位、畸形或有骨声,活动受限及叩击痛等。

Fracture fracture or fragmentation caused by trauma or pathological changes of bones, marked by swelling, pain, tenderness, local blood stasis, dislocation, deformity, bone-tapping sound or pain, and limited movements.

骨蒸 【gǔ zhēng】因阴虚内热所致的一种病证,形容发热自骨髓蒸发而出。以潮热盗汗、喘息无力、心烦少寐、手足心热、小便黄赤等为特征。

Hectic Fever due to Yin-deficiency a condition caused by yin-deficiency and internal heat, implying that the fever starts from the bone marrow, characterized by tidal fever, sweating, dyspnea, restlessness, insomnia, hot sensation in the palms and soles, and dark urine.

蛊 【gǔ】1、指臌胀。由虫毒结聚,肝脾受伤,络脉瘀塞所致。2、指少腹热痛而小便白浊的病证,3、指男子房劳病患。

Tympanites due to Parastic Festation 1. referring to tympanites due to accumulation of parasitic toxins 2. diseases characterized by pain with hot sensation in the lower abdomen and cloudy urine 3. male diseases due to sexual indulgence.

蛊毒 【gǔ dú】由于感染因素导致的以腹水为主症的疾病,多指由寄生虫感染所引起,如血吸虫病。

Diseases due to Noxious Agents Produced by Various Parasites a morbid condition chiefly characterized by ascites due to infections, mostly caused by parasites such as schistosomes.

蛊注 【gǔ zhù】(蛊胀)古病名,指以四肢浮肿、肌肤消索、咳逆、腹大如水状为主要临床表现的疾病,可能指现代医学的结核性腹膜炎等。

Tympanites ancient name of a disease similar to tuberculous peritonitis, mainly characterized by edema of the limbs, cough with dyspnea, and distended abdomen.

鼓胀 【gǔ zhàng】（蛊胀、膨胀）1、指腹部胀大，腹壁浅表静脉显露为特证的病证。多因情志郁结，饮食不节，嗜酒过度，虫积日久，使肝脾损伤，气血瘀滞，水湿不运所致。2、指气胀。腹胀坚满，中空似鼓，只气作胀。

Tympanites 1. diseases marked by distended abdomen with the superficial veins exposed, mostly caused by impairment of the liver and spleen, stagnancy of qi and blood, and retention of water within the body due to emotional distress, improper diet, excessive drinking and long period of parasitic infestation; 2. referring to qi distention, distention of the abdomen like a drum due to the presence of gas.

固崩止带 【gù bēng zhǐ dài】收涩法之一。是治疗血崩（阴道大出血）、月经不止，白带多而淋漓不断等病的方法。

Curing Metrorrhagia and Leukorrhagia one of the arresting methods for the treatment of metrorrhagia characterized by consistent dripping of blood or hematorrhea from the uterus and leukorrhea marked by persistent vaginal discharge.

固瘕 【gù jiǎ】1、大便先硬后溏，杂有不消化的食物和水。因肠胃虚寒，功能低下，水谷不分所致。2、指久治不愈的慢性腹泻。

Watery Diarrhea with Fecal Mass 1. a morbid condition due to hypofunciton of the intestines and stomach in cold insufficiency type, leading to the nonseparation of water from food, characterized by watery diarrhea with hard fecal mass discharged at first and then undigested food. 2. referring to chronic diarrhea incurable and lasting for a long period of time.

固肾涩精 【gù shèn sè jīng】收涩法之一。是治疗肾气不固而遗精、早泄或小便失禁的方法。

Strengthening the Kidney and Controlling Nocturnal Emission one of the arresting methods for the treatment of nocturnal emission, prospermia and incontinence of urine caused by unconsolidation of kidney-qi, characterized by nocturnal emission, pros-

痼疾 【gù jí】指久治不愈,比较顽固的疾病。

痼冷 【gù lěng】指元阳不足,阴寒之邪久伏体内所致的病证。以昼夜恶寒,手足厥冷,经久不愈为主证。

刮肠 【guān cháng】1、见直肠泄。2、指泻脓血的病证。

挂线法 【guà xiàn fǎ】用药制丝线或普通线。通过瘘管两端并扎紧,利用线的张力,促使局部气血不通,肌肉坏死,以达到切开瘘管的目的,一般用于治疗在体表的瘘管。

关格 【guān gé】1、呕吐不止与大便和(或)小便不通并见证候,为六腑功能严重障碍所致。2、指人迎与寸口脉皆盛的脉象。3、指阴阳均偏盛,致阴阳失调不能相互营运的严重病理状态。

关脉 【guān mài】寸口脉的一部分。指腕部桡骨茎突内侧称关脉。左关候肝与胆,右关候脾与胃。

关门不利 【guān mén bù lì】因肾的气

permia, night sweating, and incontinence of urine.

Obstinate Illness referring to diseases which usually last long and difficult to cure.

Obstinate Cold-Syndrome a type of cold syndrome due to insufficiency of genuine yang and prolonged retention of pathogenic cold in the body, mainly characterized by aversion to cold day and night, extreme cold limbs with a prolonged course.

1. **Rectal Diarrhea** 2. **Dysenteric Diarrhea** diarrhea complicated by pus and blood.

Ligation Therapy a method to treat fistula, especially the superficial ones, by ligating it with medicated or the ordinary silk thread in order to necrotize and remove it gradually.

Guan Ge 1. dysuria and constipation with incessant vomiting due to severe functional disturbance of six fu organs. 2. a type of pulse forceful both at renying and cun kou. 3. a severe pathogenical status caused by excess of yin and yang, leading to disturbance of ying and yang and their inability to transport mutually.

The Guan Pulse part of the cun pulse, referring to pulse felt at the radial styloid process with the left guan representing the liver and gall bladder and right guan, the spleen and stomach.

Edema with Difficulty in Urination due

化功能障碍而致小便不利，水肿的病理现象。 to Hypofunction of the Kidney

观神色 【guān shén sè】望诊内容之一。医者运用视觉对患者的精神、意识、思维活动及面部色泽等的变化进行观察，从而了解正气的盛衰。

Inspection of Appearance one of the method in observation, i. e. to observe the patient's complexion, facial expression, the condition of thinking and other outward manifestations to get to know the condition of the healthy qi.

鹳口疽 【guàn kǒu jū】指无头疽生于尾骨尖处。因三阴亏损，督脉经之浊湿痰流结而成。

Carbuncle on the Coccyged Region pointless carbuncles on the coocygeal region caused by impairment of three yin meridians and accumulation of turbid fluid and damp-phlegm in the governor vessel.

光剥苔 【guāng bō tāi】指舌苔突然剥脱。为胃阴枯竭，胃气大伤的征象。分舌前半部分和后半部分剥苔。前者是表邪虽减，但胃肠有积滞和痰饮，后者为病邪入里，胃气已伤。

Uncoated and Smooth Tongue sudden disappearance of tongue fur, usually indicating exhaustion of the stomach fluid and stomach-qi, it is usually classified as the disappearance of the front half of the tongue and that of the back half, with the former indicating the accumulation of indigested food and retention of phlegm still in the stomach and intestines, although the pathogenic factor attacking the exterior of the body weakened; while the latter indicating the invasion of the interior of the body by pathogenic factor and the impairment of stomach-qi.

广肠 【guǎng cháng】包括乙状结肠和直肠。

The Sigmoid and Rectum

归经 【guī jīng】药物对某一经络及其相关的脏腑的病变具有一定的治疗作用。如羚羊角归肝经，能治疗手足

Meridian Tropism (of Medicines) a specific effect of medicines for certain meridian and its corresponding

抽搐的肝经病。一种药物有归入二经或数经的，说明它的治疗范围较大。

龟背 【guī bèi】即脊骨弯曲突起，形如龟背。小儿骨质未坚，曲背久坐，没有及时矫正，脊骨受损或发育障碍或因脊骨局部病变以致变形；或患佝偻病，都可形成龟背。

龟背驼 【guī bèi tuó】属龟背痰的范围。见流痰。

龟背痰 【guī bèi tán】生于脊背部的流痰。见流痰。

龟头肿痛 【guī tóu zhǒng tòng】龟头红肿疼痛。多由湿热下注而致。

鬼击 【guǐ jī】指某些原因不明的暴病、重病。症见突然胸胁腹内绞急切痛、或突然吐血、或鼻中出血、或下血等。

鬼胎 【guǐ tāi】1、相当于葡萄胎。2、指妇女患瘕一类的病证。症见腹似怀孕，面色萎黄、肌肉消瘦，多因素体虚弱、七情郁结，气血瘀结不散，冲任壅滞而致。3、指早产或过期难产的婴儿。出生后体质羸弱多病。

viscera, e. g. , Cornu Saigae Tatericae which is effective for the tremors of hand and foot due to the disease of the liver meridian is said to be distributed to the liver meridian. The medicine which distributes to two or more meridians possesses a wider use for treatment.

Curvature of the Spinal Column abnormally increased convexity in the curvature of the thoracic spine due to the deforming of spine formed by prolonged erroneous sitting position in children, or to the developmental malformation and disease of the spine or rickets.

Kyphosis belonging to tuberculous spine.

Tuberculous Spine tuberculosis that occurs on the vertebrae or back.

Swelling and Pain of Glans Penis a morbid state mostly due to downward running of pathogenic dampness-heat.

Suddn Onset a fulminating or serious disease with unknown cause, manifested as sudden onset of colicky over the chest, hypochondrium or abdomen, or of hematemesis, epistaxis, hematochezia, etc.

Diseased Fetus 1. corresponding to hydatidiform mole 2. referring to abdominal mass in female, manifested as large abdomen like pregnancy, sallow complexion, emaciation, caused by weak constitution, emotional

腘 【guó】膝关节的后方。

过经 【guò jīng】指伤寒病程中,由一经的证候转入另一经证候的变化。

过期流产 【guò qī liú chǎn】怀孕后胚胎死亡已超过1—2个月,而仍稽留在子宫腔内。表现为子宫不增大,反而缩小,有时伴有阴道流血或流褐色分泌物。

海底漏 【hǎi dǐ lòu】病名。多因湿热下注或房劳伤肾所致。证见会阴处肿胀疼痛、溃破流脓、形成漏症、日久不收。

鼾声 【hān shēng】呼吸时发出的一种粗糙而低沉的声音。通常见于熟睡后的正常人;病理性者可见于慢性肥厚性鼻病或痰阻心包、神志昏迷的患者。

寒 【hán】1、病因,六淫之一。寒属阴邪,易伤阳气,寒邪外束,与卫气相搏,阳气不得宣泄可见恶寒、发热、无汗等证。寒气侵入、阻滞气血活动,成为痛证原因之一。2、指机能衰退的

changes, stagnation of qi and blood, and impairment of thoroughfare vessel and conception vessel. 3. a premature and weak baby or a baby born with a delayed and difficult delivery.

The Back of the Knee

Transmission from One Meridian to Another the development of a febrile disease when the manifestations of one meridian change to those of the other meridian.

Missed Abortion retention in the uterus of an abortus that has been dead for more than 1-2 months, indicated by the cessation of increase and even decrease in size of the uterus, accompanied by bleeding or brownish discharge from the vagina.

Anoperineal Fistula diseased condition due to attack of pathogenic dampness-heat or damage of the kidney by frequent sexuel intercourse; manifested as swelling and pain over the perineum, with rupture, discharge of pus and formation of fistula.

Snore a rough, rattling, respiratory noise during sound sleep, and also seen in the patients suffering from chronic hypertrophic rhinitis and coma due to stagnation of phlegm in pericardium.

Cold 1. etiology, one of the six exogenous pathogenic factors, which is yin in nature, consumes the yang qi of the body. Invasion of the body surface by cold, the conflict between cold and

病证。

寒包火 【hán bāo huǒ】指外感风寒，内有积热，寒包于外，热郁于内的病证。

寒痹 【hán bì】（痛痹）痹证的一种。指风寒湿邪侵袭肢节、经络，其中又以寒邪为甚的痹证。症见四肢关节疼痛，痛势剧，遇寒更甚，得热则减轻，可兼见手足拘挛。

寒喘 【hán chuǎn】1、指阳虚寒盛所致的气喘。症见气喘而四肢逆冷、脉象沉细等。2、风寒外束喘证的简称，常兼见表寒症状。

寒呃 【hán è】呃逆的一种。由寒邪犯胃或脾胃虚寒所致。症见呃声连续、胃脘不舒、手足清冷、脉迟无力等。

the defensive qi, and hindrance of yang qi from dispersing cause aversion to cold, fever and anhidrosis, etc. Pathogenic cold is also one of pain reasons by obstructing the circulation of qi and blood. 2. diseases characterized by the hypofunction of the body.

Fire Enveloped by Cold a pathological phenomenon caused by the attack of pathogenic wind-cold from the exterior and the accumulation of pathogenic heat in the interior resulting in cold-syndrome in the superficies accompanied by heat-syndrome in the interior.

Cold-Bi Syndrome a type of bi-syndrome due to attack of the joints and meridians by pathogenic wind, cold and dampness, esp. by pathogenic cold; manifested by severe pain in the joints of limbs aggravated by cold and alleviated by warmth, accompanied by cramps of the extremities.

Cold-Type Asthma 1. a disorder due to yang deficiency and pathogenic cold excess, manifested by dyspnea, cold limbs, deep and thready pulse, etc. 2. as an abbreviation of asthma due to invasion of wind-cold, usually accompanied with symptoms of exterior cold.

Cold-Type Hiccup a type of hiccup due to the attack of the stomach by cold, or hypofunction of the yang in the spleen and stomach, manifested as

寒膈 【hán gé】噎膈的一种。症见脘腹胀满、食不消化、呃逆、腹部苦冷、肠鸣、绕脐痛、消瘦等。

Dysphagia Caused by Cold a type of dysphagia manifested as epigastric and abdominal fullness and distension, indigestion, hiccup, feeling of fullness and coldness over the abdomen, borborygmi; periumbilical pain, emaciation, etc.

寒化 【hán huà】热证后期因阳气虚弱而出现的神倦、肢冷、畏寒、腹泻、舌质淡、苔白滑、脉微弱等证。

Trarsformation into Cold a condition caused by the deficiency of yang-qi during the later stage of heat-syndrome; manifested as general lassitude, cold extremities, chillness, diarrhea, pale tongue with white, smooth fur, weak pulse, etc.

寒霍乱 【hán huò luàn】(寒气霍乱)多因阳气素虚，内伤生冷，外感寒湿所致。症见上吐下泻、吐利清水，或如米泔水，不甚秽臭、腹痛轻微、恶寒、四肢清冷、口唇及指甲青紫、脉沉紧或沉伏等。

Cholera Morbus of Cold Type a disease occurring in the patient with yang-deficiency after overeating cold and raw food or being exposed to cold-dampness; manifested as sudden onset of severe vomiting and diarrhea with watery or rice-water stools, mild abdominal pain, chillness, cold limbs, cyanosis, deep and tense pulse, or deep and impalpable pulse, etc.

寒积腹痛 【hán jī fù tòng】寒积凝滞所致的腹痛。多因脾胃阳虚，伤于生冷或身受寒邪引起，症见腹痛绵绵，得热痛减、得寒更甚、痛则腹泻、脉多沉迟或沉紧。

Abdominal Pain due to Accumulation of Cold this disease caused mostly by the deficiency of yang of the spleen and stomach, overeating cold and raw food or the attack of pathogenic cold, manifested as intermittent dull pain which may be relieved by warmth and aggravated by cold, diarrhea, deep and slow pulse or

寒极生热 【hán jí shēng rè】寒证病情发展到寒极阶段，格阳于外，虚火浮动，出现阴盛格阳的假热现象。

Excessive Cold May Bring About False Heat when the cold syndrome develops to a serious cold stage, excessive cold keeps yang externally, and asthenic fire may flame up. This is yang kept externally by excessive yin.

寒剂 【hán jì】具有寒凉作用的方剂，含有苦寒性药物，如黄连、黄芩之类。

Prescription of Cold Nature prescription with cooling effect referring to medicines of bitter, cold nature, such as Rhizoma Coptidis, Radix Scutellariae, etc.

寒结 【hán jié】（冷秘）指寒气袭于肠道而致的大便秘结，并伴有口唇淡白、口淡、小便清长、舌苔白滑等症。

Cold-Type Constipation constipation due to invasion of the intestine by the pathogenic cold, accompanied by pale lips, flat taste in the mouth, discharge of large amount of clear urine, white and smooth coating of the tongue, etc.

寒痉 【hán jìng】外感风寒而致的痉证。多见于小儿。

Convulsion due to Cold a disorder mostly seen in children, caused by the exogenous pathogenic cold.

寒厥 【hán jué】因阳虚阴盛而引起的一类厥证。症见手足厥冷、恶寒踡卧、下利清谷、口不渴；腹痛面赤、指甲青暗甚则昏厥舌质淡苔润、脉微细等。

Cold-Type Syncope a type of syncope due to deficiency of yang and excess of yin, manifested as cold hands and feet, aversion to cold, lying in a curled up position, diarrhea with undigested food, abscess of thirst, abdominal pain, flushed cheeks, cyanosis of finger tip, even loss of consciousness, pale tongue with moist coating, feeble and thready pulse, etc.

寒冷腹痛 【hán lěng fù tòng】（寒气腹痛）因脾胃虚寒或感受寒邪所致的腹痛。症见腹痛绵绵、得寒痛甚、得热

Abdominal Pain of Cold Type abdominal pain due to asthenia-cold of the spleen and stomach or attack of

稍缓、脉沉迟。 pathogenic cold, manifested as intermittent dull pain, aggravated by cold and relieved by warmth, deep and slow pulse.

寒栗鼓颔 【hán lì gǔ hàn】指极度恶寒而出现全身发抖。

Chill shivering of the body due to aversion to coldness.

寒痢 【hán lì】指痢疾属寒者。多由天热贪凉，多食生冷不洁食物，寒气凝滞，脾阳受损所致。症见痢下纯白或白多红少、质稀气腥或如冻胶、脉迟、苔白等。

Cold-Type Dysentery a type of dysentery due to retention of cold and impairment of spleen yang resulting from excessive intake of raw, cold or dirty food, manifested as diarrhea with white mucus or gelatin-like stool, slow pulse, white coating of the tongue, etc.

寒能去热 【hán néng qù rè】用苦寒的药物以治疗热证，如表里火热俱盛，大热烦躁、口干、出血等实热证。

Medicine of Cold Nature Can Expel the Heat medicine of bitter, cold nature may be used for the treatment of heat-syndrome manifested as extreme fever, irritability, dry mouth, hemorrhage due to excessive heat in the exterior and interior.

寒能制热 【hán néng zhì rè】苦寒的药物可以制止热邪，所以常用苦寒的药物以治疗热性的疾病。

Medicine of Cold Nature Can Eliminate Heat-Syndrome as bitter and cold natured drugs can check heat, the bitter and cold nature drugs are usually used to treat febrile disease.

寒凝气滞 【hán níng qì zhì】因寒邪引起气血流通不畅，而产生疼痛、痉挛等症的病理。

Stagnation of Qi Caused by the Pathogenic Cold a morbid state of stagnation of qi and blood due to attack of cold, manifested as pain, spasm, etc.

寒疟 【hán nüè】以先寒后热、寒多热少或但寒不热、腰背头项痛、无汗、脉弦紧等为特征的一种疟疾。多因寒气内伏，秋凉再感疟邪所致。

Cold-Type Malaria a type of malaria marked by chills followed by fever, or severe chills with low fever, or chills without fever, pain over the loins, back, head and neck, and tense pulse, etc. mostly due to retention of cold and attack of malarial evil in autumn.

寒呕 【hán ǒu】（寒气呕吐、寒吐）因胃气虚寒，或复感寒邪所致的呕吐。症见食久呕吐或遇寒即呕，伴手足清冷、脉沉、细、迟等。

Vomiting due to Pathogenic Cold a disorder caused by deficiency of the stomach yang or repeated attacks of pathogenic cold, manifested as vomiting long after meal or provoked by cold, accompanied by cold limbs, deep, thready slow pulse.

寒癖 【hán pǐ】胁助间有弦索状拱起，遇冷即觉疼痛，脉弦而大的病证。多由寒邪水饮相挟停阻而成。

Hypochondriac Protrusion due to Cold a condition charaterized by stringlike protrusion over the hypochondria, accompanied by hypochondriac pain after exposure to cold, wiry and large pulse, caused by the retension of cold and fluid.

寒热 【hán rè】1、是鉴别疾病属性的两个纲领。是阴阳偏盛偏衰的具体表现，通过鉴别疾病属寒属热，对确定治疗有重要的意义。2、是恶寒发热的简称。

Cold and Heat 1. two principal syndromes for differential diagnosis serving as the concrete manifestation of the changes of yin and yang, and considered as a significant reference for the treatment of disease. 2. referring to chillness and fever.

寒热错杂 【hán rè cuò zá】寒证与热证交错在一起同时出现。如表热里寒、上热下寒等。

Complicated Syndromes of Cold and Heat a condition of cold-syndrome and heat-syndrome appearing simultaneously, e. g. cold in the exterior with heat in the interior, heat above with cold below, etc.

寒热往来 【hán rè wǎng lái】（往来寒热）指不规则的恶寒与发热交替出现的症状。本证多因外感时病邪居半里半表，正邪相争所致。

Alternate Chills and Fever a symptom seen in the case of the exogenous pathogenic factors remain between the exterior and interior, and the pathogenic factor contends with an-

寒疝 【hán shàn】1、指腹中拘挛、绕脐疼痛、出冷汗、恶寒肢冷、甚则手足麻木、周身疼痛的病证,其脉沉紧。多因寒邪凝结腹内所致 2、指以阴囊冷痛为主的疝证。由寒湿之邪侵犯肝经所致。其症阴囊寒冷、硬结如石、疼痛,日久可继发不育。类似附睾结核。

寒伤形 【hán shāng xíng】指寒邪能伤人形体,而出现头痛、恶寒、关节酸痛、肢体麻痹、痉挛等症状。

寒胜则浮 【hán shèng zé fú】寒邪偏胜,引起阳气不足,水湿运行不畅,导致浮肿的病理。

寒湿脚气 【hán shī jiǎo qì】脚气病的一种。多因寒湿外侵,经气不行,血脉不和所致。症见足胫肿大、麻木无力、行动不便、小便不利等。

寒湿久痹 【hán shī jiǔ bì】由寒湿侵袭

tipathogenic qi.

1. **Abdominal Pain due to Cold** a condition marked by colicky pain around the umbilcus, cold sweat, chills, cold extremities, and even numbness of limbs and general aching, deep and tense pulse, which is caused by retention of cold in the abdomen. 2. **Cold Hernia** a disease similar to tuberculosis of epididymis, manifested as coldness of the scrotum with painful and indurated mass, and secondary to sterility caused by the attack of cold-dampness to the liver meridian.

Pathogenic Cold Liable to Damage the Body the attack of cold can involve the superficies of the body, manifested as headache, chillness. arthralgia, numbness and spasm of limbs, etc.

Hyperactivity of Pathogenic Cold May Bring About Edema a mobid condition of retention of body fluid due to deficiency of yang qi and a disturbance in distribution of body fluid resulting from the hyperactivity of pathogenic cold.

Beriberi due to Cold-Dampness a type of beriberi which is caused by the disharmony of qi and blood circulation resulting from the attack of cold-dampness, manifested as swelling, numbness and weakness of the lower limbs, dysuria, etc.

Chronic Arthralgia due to Cold-Damp-

所致的慢性痹证。症见肌肤疼痛、关节挛痹,并有痛处固定和病程缠绵的特点。

寒湿痢 【hán shī lì】痢疾证候类型之一。因脾肾阳虚,湿浊内阻所致。表现为下痢稀、脓色白、脘腹虚胀、腹痛绵绵有下坠感、神疲、不发热、不渴、纳呆、舌淡苔白腻等。

寒湿凝滞经闭 【hán shī níng zhì jīng bì】经闭证型之一。指寒湿与血搏结,冲任胞脉闭阻引起的闭经。常兼见小腹冷痛、形寒肢冷、白带量多等证。

寒湿头痛 【hán shī tóu tòng】头痛证型之一。由寒湿上蔽清阳,血行凝涩,脉络挛急所致。症见头痛而重、天阴易发、胸闷、肢体困重、舌苔白腻、脉缓等。

寒湿眩晕 【hán shī xuàn yùn】指暑令感受寒湿之邪所致的眩晕。症见头晕、恶寒、身重且痛、转则不得、脉虚缓。

ness a disorder characterized by localized and long-suffering arthralgia, accompanied by general aching and stiffness of the affected joint.

Cold-Damp Type Dysentery a type of dysentery due to deficiency of spleen-yang and kidney-yang, and retention of cold-dampness, manifested as discharge of thin and white purulent stool, abdominal flatulence and mile tenesmus, listlessness, absence of fever and thirst, poor appetite, pale tongue, etc.

Amenorrhea due to Stagnation of Cold-Dampness a type of amenorrhea which is caused by the obstruction of thoroughfare, conception vessels and bao vessel resulting from the attack of cold-dampness and blood stasis, usually accompanied by cold feeling and pain over the lower abdomen, chilly sensaion of the body, cold limbs and leukorrhagia.

Headache due to Cold-Dampness a disorder due to cold-dampness attacking pure yang and stagnation of blood flow, manifested as pain and heaviness over the head,, usually occuring in cloudy days, suffocating sensation in the chest, heaviness of the body, white, greasy tongue coating, soft pulse, etc.

Dizziness due to Cold-Dampness dizziness occurring in summer after the attack of cold-dampness, accompanied by aversion to cold, pain and

寒湿腰痛 【hán shī yāo tòng】腰痛的一种。多因寒湿阻滞经络，气血运行不畅所致。症见腰部冷痛重着、转则不利、得热则减、遇寒则增、脉沉紧等。

寒实 【hán shí】寒邪结滞于内所致的一种证候。症见四肢冷、口不渴、小便清长、腹痛拒按、便结、舌苔白、脉沉弦等。

寒嗽 【hán sòu】咳嗽的一种。多由外感寒邪伤肺，或过食生冷伤脾所致。症见咳嗽、痰白带泡沫、面白、脉紧或弦细等。

寒痰 【hán tán】 1、指阳虚寒湿相搏所致的痰证。多有足膝酸软、腰背强痛、骨痛、关节冷痛等症状。2、指素有痰疾，又感寒凉而喘咯咳唾者。症见痰色白而清稀。

heavy sensation of the body, limitation of movement, weak, slow pulse.

Lumbago due to Cold-Dampness a type of lumbago caused by retarded circulation of qi and blood due to obstruction of cold-dampness in meridians, manifested as feeling of coldness, pain, heaviness and stiffness over the lumbar region which can be relieved by warmth and aggravated by cold, sunken and tense pulse, etc.

Cold-Excess Syndrome a syndrome caused by the retention of cold in the body, manifested as cold extremities, absence of thirst, polyuria with clear colour, abdominal pain aggravated by pressure, constipation, white tongue coating, deep and wiry pulse.

Cough due to Cold a disorder due to impairment of lung by the exogenous cold, or impairment of the spleen by overeating cold and raw food, manifested as cough with discharge of white, frothy sputum, pale complexion, tense or wiry and thready pulse.

Cold-Phlegm-Syndrome 1. phlegm-syndrome caused by the attack of cold and dampness due to a yang deficiency, manifested as soreness and weakness of the lower limbs, stiffness and pain of the back and loins, osteodynia, coldness and pain of the joints, etc. 2. a disorder caused by the retention of phlegm in the body and the attack of exogenous cold, manifested as asthma, cough with white, thin

寒无犯寒 【hán wú fàn hán】指季节用药的一般规律，即在冬天不要随便用寒药，以免损伤阳气，发生变证。
Medicines of Cold Nature Should Not Be Used in Winter a general principle of treatment in order to prevent the complication of consumption of yang qi.

寒无浮 【hán wú fú】寒性药的作用，一般是向里向下，没有升浮的作用。
Medicines of Cold Nature Possess No Floating Action a common effect of medicines of cold nature which generally act inwards and downwards but not floating.

寒下 【hán xià】使用苦寒有泻下作用的药物，治疗里热实证的方法。本法只适用于在里的实热证，如燥屎、饮食积滞、积水等。久病体虚者及孕妇忌用。
Purgation by Drugs of Cold Nature a treatnemt for excess heat-syndrome in the interior by the application of purgatives of bitter and cold nature, applicable to the case manifested as dry faces, retention of indigested food, fluid retention, etc. contraindicated for people with general debility after a long illness and pregnant woman.

寒痫 【hán xián】指感寒即发的痫证，多由脾胃内伤，外感风寒，结于胸膈。症见忽然仆倒、不省人事、口涌痰涎。本证多见于小儿。
Cold Type Epilepsy epilepsy provoked by exposure to cold, due to impairment of the spleen and stomach, and attack of exogenous wind cold, both combined together and accumulated in the chest, manifested as sudden loss of consciousness and salivation, mostly seen in infants.

寒邪眩晕 【hán xié xuàn yùn】感受寒邪所致的眩晕。症见身热无汗、恶寒拘紧、头痛身痛、时时眩晕。
Dizziness due to Cold dizziness caused by the attack of exogenous pathogenic cold, manifested as fever, anhidrosis, chillness, muscular stiffness, headache and general pain.

寒泄 【hán xiè】（寒泻）因寒邪客于肠胃所致的泄泻。症见肠鸣腹痛、便
Cold Diarrhea a disease caused by the attack of cold in the stomach and

泻稀水清澈或食物不化或便下清黑、四肢冷、口不渴、苔白、脉沉迟等。

the intestines, manifested as abdominal pain with increased borborygmus, diarrhea with watery or greenish dark discharge, or with discharge containing indigested food, cold limbs, absence of thirst, white tongue coating, sunken and slow pulse, etc.

寒夜啼 【hán yè tí】内脏虚寒所致。症见曲腰而啼、面色清白、腹痛、四肢不温等。

Cold-Type Night Crying a disorder due to deficient cold of the viscera, characterized by crying with flexed gesture, purplish and pale complexion, abdominal pain and coldness of the limbs.

寒疫 【hán yì】指时疫而见阴寒证候者,症见腹痛、肢厥、吐泻清冷、脉沉迟等。

Epidemic Disease of Cold Type an epidemic disease characterized by yin and cold syndrome, manifested as abdominal pain, cold extremities, vomiting and diarrhea with cold, watery discharge, sunken and slow pulse, etc.

寒因寒用 【hán yīn hán yòng】反治法之一。即用寒药治疗真热假寒的疾病。

Treating the Pseudo Cold Disease with Drugs of Cold Nature one of the treatments contrary to the routine, i. e., to treat the diseases which are cold in appearance but hot in nature with drugs of cold nature.

寒因热用 【hán yīn rè yòng】反治法之一。治疗热性病用寒凉的药物的同时,反佐少量热性的药物;或寒性的药物热服,则不格拒。

Treating the Heat-Syndrome with Drugs of Hot Nature one of the treatments contrary to routine, i. e., to treat the heat-syndrome with drugs of cold nature and small amount of drugs of hot nature as well, or being taken hot in order to repel drugs of cold nature.

寒则气收 【hán zé qì shōu】寒邪的致病特点,即寒邪入侵,阳气不得宣泄

Pathogenic Cold Renders the Qi Sluggish a main pathogenic character

而引起毛窍收缩,卫阳闭束的病理变化。

of pathogenic cold, an invasion of pathogenic cold may cause the impairment of the dispersing function of yang qi, the closing of sweat pores leading to the sluggishness of defensive yang.

寒则收引 【hán zé shōu yǐn】寒邪入侵,则筋脉收缩,肌肉拘紧。

Pathogenic Cold May Bring About Contraction an invasion of pathogenic cold may result in the rigidity and spasm of muscle due to stagnation of cold in meridians, joints and muscles.

寒胀 【hán zhàng】因脾胃虚寒,或寒湿郁遏所致的腹胀。症见腹部胀满、不欲饮食、呕吐、心烦、四肢厥冷、脉迟弱等。

Flatulence due to Cold flatulence caused by hypofunction of the spleen and stomach or retention of cold dampness, manifested as fullness of the abdomen, poor appetite, vomiting, restlessness, cold extremities, weak and slow pulse, etc.

寒者热之 【hán zhě rè zhī】指寒证要用温热的方药治疗。临床上一般分表寒、里寒,分别采用辛温解表和温中祛寒的方法进行治疗。

Cold Syndrome Should Be Treated with Drugs of Warm Nature a therapeutic principle for treating the cold-syndrome, i. e., therapy of expelling the exogenous pathogenic factors with drugs of acrid taste and warm nature is applied for cold-syndrome of the superficies and that of expelling cold by warming the middle energizer is applied for cold syndrome of the interior.

寒证 【hán zhèng】由于寒邪引起,或阳气不足,阴气过盛而出现的寒性证候。表现为面色苍白、恶寒肢冷、腹中雷鸣、疼痛得热则减、口不渴、喜热饮、大便不稀薄、小便清长、舌淡苔白润、脉迟或紧等。

Cold-Syndrome as syndrome produced by the attack of exogenous pathogenic cold or the deficiency of yang qi and the excess of yin, manifested as pallor, aversion to cold, cold limbs, increased borborygmus, ab-

寒滞肝脉 【hán zhì gān mài】 指寒邪侵袭肝脉的病机。症见下腹胀痛，牵引睾丸坠痛，并见肢冷畏寒、舌苔白滑、脉沉弦或迟等。

汗 【hàn】 1、汗液、五液之一。是津液代谢产物。汗为心液，汗液的分泌与心脏的功能有关。2、出汗。3、汗法。

汗出汲汲然 【hàn chū jí jí rán】 指汗出连绵不断。此多因胃肠热盛，邪热蒸迫汗液外泄所致。

汗出如油 【hàn chū rú yóu】 指汗出不止，且如油样粘腻的症状。此常是病情垂危的表现之一。

汗法 【hàn fǎ】 又称发汗法，八法之一。通过开泄腠理，调和营卫，发汗祛邪，以解除表邪的治法。它有退热、透疹、消水肿、去风湿等作用。

dominal pain which can be relieved by warmth, absence of thirst, or thirst with a desire for hot drink, loose stools, polyuria with light-coloured urine, pale tongue with moist and white tongue coating, slow or tense pulse, etc.

Retention of Cold in the Liver Meridian a morbid condition due to pathogenic cold attacking the liver meridian, manifested as distending pain over the lower abdomen radiating to testis, aversion to cold, cold limbs, whitish smooth coating of the tongue, sunken and tense or slow pulse etc.

Sweat 1. one of the five kinds of secretion, waste product formed during the process of body fluid metabolism. It's a fluid of heart, which means sweat secretion is related to the function of the heart. 2. perspiration or sweating 3. diaphoresis

Continuous Sweating a sign usually caused by the retention of pathogenic heat in the stomach and intestnes, the pathogenic heat may force sweat to let out.

Oily Sweat profuse perspiration with viscous sweat, usually indicating a critical condition.

Diaphoresis or Sweating one of the eight methods of treatment, which is for expelling superficial pathogenic factors by opening the pores of the skin, regulating the function of ying

汗空 【hàn kōng】即毛孔。其口开于皮肤表面，是汗液排泄的门户。

汗孔 【hàn kǒng】即毛孔。

汗证 【hàn zhèng】指小儿在安静的状态下，全身或局部汗出很多，有盗汗和自汗之分。辩证分类：1、卫表不固 2、营卫不和 3、气阴不足。

毫针 【háo zhēn】古代九针之一。是现代最常用的针刺工具，有多种不同的长度及粗细。

合病 【hé bìng】伤寒病二经和三经同时受病邪侵袭，起病即出现各经主症的一种病变。如太阳与阳明合病等。

合剂 【hé jì】为中药复方的水煎浓缩液，或中药提取物以水为溶媒配制而成的内服液体制剂，如止咳合剂。

和 【hé】1、同和法。2、用功效温和的药物治疗疾病的方法。目的在于调

and wei, and inducing perspiration. It possesses the actions of antipyretic, promoting eruption, reducing edema and antirheumatism, etc.

Sweat Pore　the small opening of a sweat gland in the skin, through which the sweat is discharged.

Sweat Pores　the hair follicle.

Perspiration Syndrome　a condition marked by general or local profuse sweating seen in the infant in calming state, including night sweating and spontaneous perspiration. Types of differentiation 1. deficiency of wei-qi 2. incoordination between ying and wei 3. insufficiency of qi and yin.

Filiform Needles　one of the nine forms of needles in ancient times, used most commonly in acupuncture treatment nowdays, with various length and diameter.

Complicated Disease　a condition of the febrile disease in which two or three meridians are attacked by the pathogenic factor simultaneously with the main symptoms of the affected meridians appearing at the onset, e. g., the disease involving taiyang and yangming meridians, etc.

Mixture　condensed compound decoction or aqueous solution of the extract of drugs on combination, such as mixture pectoral, etc.

Demulcent Therapy　1. same with regulating therapy 2. a treatment

和气血阴阳，使微邪自去，如小寒之病以温药和之。 for mild illness by demulcents to eliminate mild pathogenic factors through the regulation of qi and blood, yin and yang, e. g., to treat mild cold-syndrome by drugs of warm nature.

和法 【hé fǎ】（和解法）即用疏通调和的药物，和解少阳病邪或调和脏腑气血的方法，包括疏肝解郁、和解少阳、调和肝脾、调和肝胃等治法。

Regulating Therapy a treatment for the elimination of pathogenic factors in shao yang meridian or the coordination of functions of viscera, qi and blood by the application of drugs with actions of dispersion and regulation, including various treatments, such as soothing the liver to relieve the depressed liver, relieve symptoms in shaoyang meridian and coordinating the functions of the liver and spleen or of the liver and stomach, etc.

和肝 【hé gān】即滋阴疏肝。以滋阴药与疏肝药合用，使肝气调和通畅。适用于肝虚之郁者，症见胁肋部胀痛、腹胀、舌上无津、咽喉干燥、脉细弱或虚弦等。

Regulating the Liver-Qi nourishing yin and soothing the liver, treating the disorder of liver-qi by the application of drugs for nourishing yin and soothing the liver, applicable to the case with deficiency of liver-yin and stagnation of qi, manifested as distending pain over the hypochondrium, abdominal distension, dry tongue and throat, thready and weak pulse or feeble and wiry pulse, etc.

和缓 【hé huǎn】1、治法，对慢性病的治疗，宜采用从容和缓的方法。2、指医和与医缓两人。他们是春秋时期秦国的医官，医术高明，故后代的医著中将"和缓"并称作为称誉良医的代名词。

Mild Therapy 1. a treatment for chronic diseases by the application of mild therapy. 2. He-Huan, Yi He and Yi Huan, two medical officers of Qin dynasty in the spring and autumn period, because of their skillful medical techniques, the combined na-

和解少阳 【hé jiě shǎo yáng】治疗外感热性病邪在半表半里的方法。适用于邪在少阳,症见寒热往来,胸胁苦满,口苦,咽干,目眩者。

和胃 【hé wèi】(和中)是治疗胃气不和的方法。症见胃脘胀闷、嗳气吐酸、厌食、舌淡苔白等。

和胃理气 【hé wèi lǐ qì】是疏畅胃肠气机,调整胃肠功能的方法、适用于气、食、痰、湿等阻滞中脘,症见脘腹胀闷、吞酸或吐酸水、嗳气等。

和血熄风 【hé xuè xī fēng】治疗肝风内动偏于血虚的方法。适用于热性病后期,阴血耗伤,出现唇焦舌燥、筋脉拘急、手足有轻微不自主的抽动,或头晕目眩,脉细数等症。

me, He-Huan was applied as the representative of skillful doctors in the medical works there after.

Harmonizing ShaoYang one kind of harmonizing therapies, which is used for treating the exogenous febrile disease remaining between the exterior and interior, applicable to the case manifested as alternate chills and fever, fullness in the costal and hypochondriac regions, a bitter taste in the mouth, dryness of the throat, blurring of vision, etc.

Regulating the Stomach a treatment for the disorder of stomach, applicable to the case manifested as distention in the epigastrium, belching and acid regurgitation, loss of appetite, pale tongue, white coating, etc.

Pacifying the Stomach and Regulating the Flow of Qi a treatment for regulation of the function of gastrointestinal tract, applicable to the case with stagnation of qi, indigested food, phlegm and dampness in the stomach, manifested as epigastric and abdominal distention, acid regurgitation, belching, etc.

Regulating the Blood to Calm the Wind a treatment for the hyperactivity of liver-wind inside the body with deficiency of blood, applicable to the case suffering from the consumption of yin-blood during the late stage of a febrile disease, manifested as dry

颌　【hé】下颌骨角的体表部位。

鹤膝风　【hè xī fēng】因病后膝关节肿大，而股胫肌肉消瘦，形如鹤膝，故名。多由三阴亏损、风邪外袭、阴寒凝滞而成。

黑　【hēi】五色之一。即黑色，它与五行中的水，五脏中的肾以及寒邪、寒证、痛证、血瘀等有密切的关系。

黑带　【hēi dài】阴道经常流出黑豆水样稠粘或稀或腥臭的液体，或赤白带中杂有黑色。多因热熏蒸，伤及任、带二脉，肾水亏虚所致。

黑疸　【hēi dǎn】多因黄疸经久不愈，肝肾虚衰，瘀浊内阻所致。症见身黄不泽、目青、面额色黑、肤燥、搔之不觉、大便黑、膀胱急、足下热、甚则腹胀、面浮、脊痛不能立正。

黑睛　【hēi jīng】包括角膜和虹膜。黑

lips and tongue, muscular stiffness with mild spasms of limbs, or dizziness and vertigo, thready and fast pulse, etc.

Lower Jaw　　corresponding to the region of the mandibular angle.

Crane-Knee Arthritis　　arthritis of the knee joint characterized by local swelling and pain with muscular emaciation of the thigh and leg, attack of pathogenic-wind leading to the stagnation of yin cold.

Black　　one of the five colours, which is matched with water (in the five elements) and kidney (in the five zang), and is closely related to pathogenic-cold, cold-syndrome, pain.

Black Vaginal Discharge　　a black vaginal discharge looks like a thick water of black soybean, or thin with fetid odour, or red-white leukorrhea with black colour, resulting from the hyperactivity of heat in the interior, due to impairment of the conception vessel and belt vessel, and consumption of the kidney-fluid.

Black Jaundice　　a disease resulting from prolonged jaundice leading to deficiency of the liver and kidney and retention of blood stasis, manifested as lusterless yellow skin, blue sclera, blackish complexion, dry skin with diminished sensation, urgency for micturition, hot feeling over the feet, abdominal distention and backache.

The Black of Eye　　the dark part of

睛内应于肝，为五轮中之风轮。

黑如炱 【hēi rú tái】指灰黑枯槁的颜色，是肾的真脏色。见于久病肾气将绝、胃气衰败的疾患。

黑苔 【hēi tāi】舌苔色黑。多属里证、重证。若舌苔黑而干燥，属热盛津液枯竭；若黑而湿润，则属阳虚寒盛。

黑子 【hēi zǐ】（黑痣）多发于面部，呈黑褐色扁平隆起，有时表面可生硬毛。

胻骨伤 【héng gǔ shāng】胫骨、腓骨骨折。

横痃 【héng xuán】梅毒发于两腿合缝间，形成核块。

烘 【hōng】把药物放在烘房或烘柜内，用微火加热，使药物干燥而不焦黑。

红丝疔 【hóng sī dīng】因火毒凝聚，或破伤感染所致的疔疮。多发于手脚，初起局部红肿热痛，继而红线由上臂前侧或小脚内侧向上起窜，重者可伴有恶寒发热、头痛、乏力、脉数等证，相当于急性淋巴管炎。辩证分类：1、热毒入络证 2、火毒入营证。

the eye including the cornea and iris, it is related with the liver and is also the wind wheel of five wheel.

Black as Soot Black, Dry and Lusterless Colour referring to the kidney colour of the five colours, indicating the exhaustion of kidney-qi and stomach-qi in prolonged illness.

Blackish Coating it indicates interior syndromes and the severe stage of an illness, a black and dry coating signifies overabundance of heat and exhaustion of body fluid; while a black and moist coating signifies deficiency of yang and overabundance of cold.

Black Nerus a dark brownish, elevated skin lesion, sometimes covered with firm hair, commonly seen on the face.

Fracture of Tibia and Fibula

Bubo an enlarged lymph node in the groin due to syphilis.

Baking a method of processing medicinal herb by drying it in a stove without altering its appearance.

Acute Lymphangitis acute inflammation of lymphatic vessel due to accumulation of fire or injury complicated by infection, usually occurring on the hands and feet with local redness, swelling, heat, pain and a red line extending upward along the anterior side of the upper arm or the medial side of the leg, and accompanied with chilliness, headache, weakness

红臀 【hóng tún】 即尿布皮炎。多因尿布潮湿浸渍，湿毒浸入所致。症见臀部皮肤燉红、粗糙，重则有丘疹、疱疹、甚至形成脓疮。多见于新生儿。

洪脉 【hóng mài】 脉象之一。脉来如波涛汹涌，来盛去衰，一般属热邪亢盛的表现。

齁喘 【hōu chuǎn】 属哮证范畴。多因过食鱼虾盐食，内有积痰寒饮所致的一种病证。症见喘息有声、胸闷气短、坐卧不宁、常随气候变化而发病。

喉痹 【hóu bì】 为咽候肿痛病证的统称。常伴有不同程度的咽喉阻塞、吞咽不利等症。

喉疔 【hóu dīng】 发于喉关两旁或喉关里之疔疮。多因肺胃火燔，痰热内侵，久郁化火，火毒上冲结于咽喉所致。

喉风 【hóu fēng】 咽喉部多种急性感

and fast pulse in sever cases. Types of differentiation 1. syndrome of heat-toxin involving the meridians 2. syndrome of fire-toxin involving ying system.

Diaper Dermatitis inflammation of the skin localized to the area in contact with the diaper in infants, which results from invastion of damp and toxin, marked by local erythema, thickening or even papules, vesicles and pustules formation.

Full Pulse one kind of pulse conditions which come on powerfully and fade away, indicating excessive heat.

Asthma with Wheezing Sound a disease due to over intake of fishes, shrimps and salty food, and accumulation of cold fluid and phlegm provoked by the climatic variation, manifested as paroxysmal ayspnea with wheezing sound, sensation of chest stuffiness, restlessness, etc.

Sore Throat a general term for the various kinds of painful throat, often accompanied by obstruction of the throat and dysphagia, etc.

Abscess of the Throat a pharyngeal lesion occurring on either side of the fauces, which is usually caused by hyperactivity of lung-fire and stomach-fire, invasion of phlegm-heat and fire resulted from prolonged accumulation of phlegm which goes upward to the throat.

Acute Inflammation of the Throat

染性疾病的总称。以咽喉部肿痛连及项颊，痰涎壅盛、语声难出、吞咽及呼吸困难为特征。严重者可致窒息。多由于热毒内蕴，外感风邪所致。

a general term for acute pyogenic infection of pharynx characterized by swelling and pain of the throat, excessive salivation, dysphasia, discomfort in swallowing, difficult breathing, or suffocation in severe case, caused by the accumulateion of heat and toxin in the body and the attack of exogenous pathogenic wind.

喉疳 【hóu gān】（走马喉疳）因风热灼伤肺阴，咽喉失养；或胃经蕴热，火热上攻咽喉；或肾阴亏损，相火上炎所致。喉部有不规则的溃烂，上覆灰白色腐衣，四周围以红晕，伴有剧痛、口臭、吞咽困难、发热等症。

Ulceration of the Throat　a condition due to consumption of lung-yin by wind-heat which leads to poor nourishment of throat, or wind-heat from stomach meridian attacking throat, up-going of prime-minister fire resulting from yin deficiency of the kidney, marked by painful irregular ulcer over the pharyngeal mucosa; covered with whitish grey membrane and surrounded by erythematous induration accompanied by foul odor, dysphagia, fever, etc.

喉关 【hóu guān】位于口咽部，由扁桃体、悬雍垂、舌根等组成。相当于咽峡部，该部是呼吸和饮食的通道，又是抵御外邪入侵的关隘。

Isthmus of Fauces　composed of the tonsils, uvula and the root of tongue, it is the passage for the air and food and also serves as a barrier against the invasion of exogenous factors.

喉核 【hóu hé】即扁桃体。在咽喉部前后腭弓之间，呈长卵圆形。

Palatine Tonsil　a small, oval mass situated between the palatoglossal and palatopharyngeal arches on either sides.

喉间溃烂 【hóu jiān kuì làn】咽喉溃烂。多由阴虚于下，火炎于上，虚火上冲咽喉；肺胃热蕴，毒火上冲咽喉所致。

Ulceration of Pharynx　a disorder due to attack of the pharynx by asthenic fire resulting from yin-deficiency of the lower body and hyperactivity of fire at the upper or up-going

喉癣 【hóu xuǎn】咽喉部粘膜溃腐凹陷,形似苔藓,初觉咽喉部干燥、疼痛,久则声嘶咳嗽、甚至失音、呼吸困难。多因肝肾虚亏、相火上亢、肺阴受伤或胃中积热,胃火熏肺所致。

Erosion of the Throat lichenoid lesion of mucous membrane of the throat, manifested as dryness and pain of the throat, hoarseness, cough, or even aphonia and dyspnea; mostly caused by damage of lung-yin by attacking of prime-minister fire resulting from deficiency of the liver and kidney, or accumulation of stomach-heat, stomach-fire burning the lung.

喉痒 【hóu yǎng】多因阴虚火灼、咽喉失养;或胃火熏肺所致。常为其它咽喉疾病(如喉癣、喉疳等)之兼证。

Itching of the Throat a symptom resulting from poor nourishment of the throat due to yin-deficiency and hyperactivity of pathogenic-fire or from stomach-fire attacking the lung, usually appearing as symptom of other throat disease (such as membranous pharyngitis, ulceration of the pharynx, etc.).

喉音 【hóu yīn】由喉部疾患所致的失音。

Aphonia due to Laryngeal Disease

喉痈 【hóu yōng】痈疡发于咽喉部位。多因六腑不和、血气不调、热毒壅盛所致。局部红肿热痛,伴有恶寒高热或咽喉阻塞痰涎壅盛等症。类似扁桃体周围脓肿、咽后壁脓肿等病。

Pharyngeal Abscess abscess forming on the wall of the pharynx, due to disfunction of six fu organs, disharmony of qi and blood, accumulation of toxic fire, marked by redness, swelling, hot and pain accompanied by chilliness, high fever, obstruction of throat, accumulation of phlegm, including peritonsillar abscess, retropharyngeal abscess, etc.

喉中水鸡声 【hóu zhōng shuǐ jī shēng】形容哮喘病发作时,发出的较高声调的痰鸣音,多因邪阻气道引

Wheezing Sound in the Throat a high-pitched sound produced by the gas passing through the sputum dur-

起。

后阴　【hòu yīn】指肛门。

候气　【hòu qì】针刺入穴位后，用较长时间的留针，使之得气的一种方法。此法多用于身体虚弱的患者。

呼吸补泻　【hū xī bǔ xiè】针刺手法之一。1、患者吸气时进针，呼气时出针，为泻法；反之，呼气时进针，吸气时出针，为补法。2、针刺得气后进行捻转手法，停针时吸气为补法，停针时呼气为泻法。

狐臭　【hú chòu】（腋气、腋臭）腋下汗有特殊臭味，其他如乳晕、脐部、外阴、肛周亦可发生。为湿热内郁或遗传所致。

狐惑　【hú huò】以咽喉及前后阴蚀烂

ing the paroxym of asthma, usually due to the obstruction of trachea by pathogenic factor.

Posterior Yin　referring to the anus.

Waiting for Acupuncture Feeling　a method of retaining the needle in the acupuncture point for a longer duration to wait for the occurrence of acupuncture feeling, usually applied in the debilitated patient.

Tonifying and Dispersing by Manipulating the Needle in Cooperation with the Patient's Respiration
the acupuncture manipulation in which (1) the tonifying effect is attained by inserting the needle while the patient inspires and withdrawing the needle while the patient expires, and the dispersing effect is attained just in the opposite way; (2) during the rotating manipulation of the needle after getting acupuncture feeling, the tonifying effect is attained by stopping the rotation of the needle during inspiration, and the dispersing effect is attained by stopping the rotation of the needle during expiration.

Bromihidrosis Foul　smelling of perspiration commonly occurring over the oxilla, and also over areola, umbilicus, external genitals and around the anus; caused by the stagnation of pathogenic dampnes-heat or hereditary factor.

Throat-Anus-Genitals Syndrome　a

为主症，伴有精神恍惚，惑乱狐疑等一种疾病。多由湿邪浸淫，热毒遏郁所致。

syndrome characterized by erosions in the throat, anus and external genitalia, accompanied with mental confusion and misgiving, mostly caused by attack of pathogenic-dampness and retention of virulent pathogenic-heat.

狐尿刺【hú niào cì】（狐狸刺）因接触昆虫分泌物后引起的皮肤病。患处皮肤起红紫斑点，肿胀焮痛；甚则溃烂成疮，脓水淋漓。即接触性皮炎之类。

Contact Dermatitis an acute inflammation of the skin caused by direct contact with the secretions of insects, marked by purplish red rash with local swelling and burning pain, or even rupture with profuse purulent discharge.

狐疝【hū shàn】多因肝气失于疏泄而发。病发时腹内部分肠段滑入阴囊、阴囊时大时小，胀痛俱作。

Inguinal Hernia herniation of intestine into the inguinal canal, or down to scrotum, accompanied by distending pain, irregular scrotum swelling, caused by the dysfunction of the liver-qi.

猢狲疳【hú sūn gān】由胎中感受遗毒所致。初生儿臀部焮肿溃烂，红赤无皮。即胎传梅毒。

"**Monkey Buttock**" redness, swelling and exfoliation of the buttock in newborns, seen in congenital syphilis.

虎口疔【hǔ kǒu dīng】（虎口毒、虎口疽、虎丫毒）是指疔疮生于手大指、次指岐骨间合谷穴之处。多由阳明经湿热凝结而成。

Pyogenic Infection in Hegu Point a pustule in the part betweeen the thumb and the index finger caused by the accumulation of pathogenic dampness-heat in yangming meridian.

花癫【huā diān】指妇女相火过旺，欲火妄炽而出现情绪激动、语无论次，或沉默痴呆、痴笑无常等精神失常状态。多因情志所伤。

Mania-Depressive Syndrome in Puberty a psychiatric syndrome due to hyperactivity of prime-minister fire which makes female have a stong desire for sexual course consisting of expansive emotional state and dejected mood caused by emotional upset, or

花癣 【huā xuǎn】即颜面单纯糠疹，多因风热郁肺，随阳气上升而成。多发于面部或眉间，呈不规则圆形或椭圆形褪色的丘疹，表面有细屑，时痛时痒，春季易发。

滑剂 【huá jì】用润滑药物组成，具有除去留着作用的方剂。

滑精 【huá jīng】多因肾元亏损，精关不固所致，少数则因下焦湿热而起。

滑可去着 【huá kě qù zhuó】用滑利通淋的药物，去掉凝结在体内的一些病理产物。

滑脉 【huá mài】脉搏流利，应指圆滑的脉象。一般主痰饮、食积、实热。滑数无力者则属虚热。

滑胎 【huá tāi】1、病名。指连续发生三次以上的自然流产者，即习惯性流产。多因气虚、肾虚、血热、外伤等

phlegm-fire attacking the heart.

Pityriasis Alba　　a skin disease due to wind-fire accumulating in the lung and rising up with yang-qi, mostly seen on the face or between eye-brow and usually occurring in spring, appearing as uneven round or oval discoloured papules covered with fine, branny scales, with intermittent itching and pain.

Prescription with Lubricant Effect
　　prescription composed of drugs with lubricant properties, which has an effect of expelling.

Spermatorrhea　　involuntary and frequent discharge of semen without copulation, mostly caused by the inability to control ejaculation resulting from the over consumption of qi of the kidney or by the attack of damp-heat to the lower energizer in a few cases.

Prescription with Emollient Effect May Eliminate a Stagnated Mass
　　the prescription with emollient effect is used for the treatment of elimination of pathological products.

Slippery Pulse　　a pulse condition with fluent and smooth pulsation, indicating phlegm retention, indigestion and excessive heat, that associated with fast and weak beats suggests asthenia-heat syndrome.

Habitual Abortion　　1. name of disease, the spontaneous expulsion deficiency of qi, kidney asthenia, blood-

以致如期而坠或屡孕屡坠。2、使分娩顺利进行的一种治法。heat, trauma, etc. 2. promoting the delivery of a fetus, a therapy for shortening the course of labour.

滑泄 【huá xiè】泄泻不禁，日夜无度，常伴有四肢厥冷或肿胀、形寒短气、消瘦等为主要临床表现的一种病证。多因久泻气陷下脱所致。

Involuntary Diarrhea diarrhea without control of fecal discharge, accompanied by edema, coldness of limbs, chills, shortness of breath and emaciation, which is usually due to collapse of qi resulting from obstinate diarrhea.

化斑 【huà bān】用清热、凉血、解毒的治法，以防热毒继续深陷。适用于温病热入营血致皮肤出现斑点及出血者。

Dissipating Rashes a treatment for skin rashes and subcutaneous hemorrhage, in the case of seasonal febrile disease when the heat involves yin-system and blood system, by the therapies for clearing away heat, cooling blood and eliminating toxic materials to avoid the deterioration of the disease.

化风 【huà fēng】疾病变化过程中出现风证的现象，如眩晕、抽搐、震颤强直等神经症状。

Transformation into Wind-Syndorme wind-syndrome appears during the course of disease, which is marked by neurological symptoms such as dizziness, convulsion, tremor, etc.

化火 【huà huǒ】外感六淫，内伤七情或阴液的亏损，或气血痰食的阻滞，均可在一定条件下，化火而出现病理性功能亢进的现象。

Transformation into Fire-Syndrome a state of pathogenical hyperfunction due to transformation into fire resulting from attacking of six exogenous pathogens, seven emotional upsets, over consumption of yin fluid, or retention of qi, blood, phelgm and food.

化脓灸 【huà nóng jiǔ】引起局部皮肤化脓的一种直接灸法。用艾炷直接置于穴位上，灸至皮肤起疱，并致局部化脓。适用于哮喘 肺结核、瘰疬等

Pustulated Moxibustion a kind of direct moxibustion method by burning a moxa cone directly on the skin over an acupoint to produce local

慢性疾患。

vesiculation, and the suppuration, applicable to chronic disease such as asthma, pulmonary tuberculosis, scrofula, etc.

化热 【huà rè】外感表证传里所表现的内热性病变。症见不恶寒反而恶热、口渴唇干、心烦、便秘、尿黄、舌质红、苔黄、脉数等。

Transformation into Heat-Syndrome a condition of interior heat syndrome resulting from the exogenous pathogenic factors invading the interior from the superficies; manifested as aversion to heat but not to cold, thirst, dry lips, restlessness, constipation, yellowish urine, red tongue with yellowish coating, fast pulse, etc.

化湿 【huà shī】用芳香去湿的药物以宣化上焦湿邪的方法。常分为疏表化湿和清热化湿。

Eliminating Damp a treatment for the retention of dampness in upper energizer by the application of fragrant drugs for eliminating damp, usually accomplished by dispersing the expathogens and clearing away heat-dampness.

化痰 【huà tán】消解痰涎的方法。依据生痰的原因，化痰法通常分为六种，即宣肺化痰、清热化痰、润肺化痰、燥湿化痰、祛寒化痰及治风化痰。

Eliminating Phlegm a treatment for the accumulation of phlegm in the body, it is classified into six kinds: dispersing the depressed lung-qi, clearing away heat, moistening the lung, drying damp, eliminating cold or wind.

化痰开窍 【huà tán kāi qiào】（豁痰醒脑）是治疗痰证神昏的方法。临床上常分为清热化痰开窍和逐寒开窍。

Waking Up the Patient from Unconsciousness by Dissipating Phlegm a treatment for coma due to phlegm, clinically applied by clearing away heat and dissipating phlegm or by dispelling the cold.

化饮解表 【huà yǐn jiě biǎo】运用温化水饮与辛温解表药组成的方剂，治疗素有水饮内停，表有风寒之证，以达

Relieving the Fluid-Retention and Expelling Superficial Coldness a treatment for the case with fluid-re

到既化内饮，又外解表邪的目的。

tention inside the body and wind-cold on the superficies by the application of the warm-natured drugs of promoting fluid excretion and the acrid, warm-natured drugs of expelling superficial coldness.

化燥 【huà zào】因津液消耗而出现燥证的病理。症见口干口渴、唇焦、咽燥便秘、尿少、干咳或咯血等。

Transformation into Dryness-Syndrome a morbid condition resulting from over consumption of fluid in the body, marked by dry mouth, thirst, dry lips and throat, constipation, oliguria, dry cough, or haemoptysis, etc.

怀孕 【huái yùn】（妊娠、妊子、重身、怀娠）指受精卵植入子宫体，并在其中发育的生理现象。

Pregnancy the condition of having a developing embryo in the uterus after union of an ovum and spermatozoon.

坏病 【huài bìng】指疾病发展，是病情恶化的表现。多因一再误治所致。

Disease Deteriorated deterioration of a disease usually due to improper treatment.

环肛漏 【huán gāng lòu】多由结核病引起。症见漏管环绕肛门，偶可见双层漏管。

Anal Fishtula a condition frequently caused by tuberculosis, manifested as fistule surrounding anus or double fistula in a few cases.

环跳疽 【huán tiào jū】生于环跳穴的附骨疽。见附骨疽。

Osteomyelitis with Perforation around the Site of Huan Tiao Point

环跳流痰 【huán tiào liú tán】生于环跳部的流痰。见流痰。

Cold Abscess under Huantiao Point

缓方 【huǎn fāng】即方剂之和缓者。缓方药味虽多，但互相制约，药性和缓；或加甘缓药物以减弱猛烈药的作用；也可制成丸药，以缓缓攻邪，扶助正气或用药治本。适用于体虚而患慢性疾患者。

Prescription with Mild Effect a recipe composed of demulcent medicines, or added with sweet drugs to neutralize the toxicity of the potent drugs, or prepared in pills, which is applicable to the debilitated patient and that suffering from chronic disease, for the purpose of eliminating the pathogenic factors gradually and

缓疽 【huǎn jū】1、因寒凝气滞，瘀于膝关节。生于膝上或膝的两旁，局部肿硬日增，长期不溃。2、腹痈之一种。

缓脉 【huǎn mài】脉率正常，来去舒缓的一种脉象。若和缓、均匀，为平脉；若脉来驰缓松懈为病脉，常见于湿邪致病和脾胃虚弱。

缓下 【huǎn xià】使用性质缓和的药物，通导大便的方法。

缓则治本 【huǎn zé zhì běn】在病情缓慢、病势和缓的情况下，针对疾病的病因进行治疗的方法。

肓 【huāng】即心下隔上的部位。

黄带 【huáng dài】指妇人带下色黄，粘稠而腥臭。多因湿郁化热，伤及任带二脉所致。

黄疸 【huán dǎn】（黄瘅）以身黄、目黄、小便黄为主症的疾病。多由感受

supporting the healthy qi or treating the primary symptom.

Long-Standing Abscess 1. an abscess around the knee joint with progressive swelling and induration, due to accumulation of cold and stagnation of qi in the knee joint. 2. an abscess of abdomen.

Even and Soft Pulse a pulse condition characterized by coming and going insidiously with normal rate, that beating gently and regularly is considered as normal pulse, while that with weak and slow beats is indicative of syndrome of dampness and asthenia of the spleen and stomach.

Purgation by Demulcents a treating method which is for the treatment of constipation by moistening intestine with mild-effect prescription.

Relieving the Primary Symptom in a Chronic Disease a treatment for basic etiology when the temporary secondary symptom has been relieved.

Huang the region below the heart and above the disphragm.

Leukorrhagia with Yellowish Discharge a yellowish viscid and foul discharge from the vagina, which is due to impairment of conception vessel and belt vessel resulting form the stagnation of damp which turns into fire.

Jaundice a disease characterized by yellow appearance of the skin, sclerae

黄   huang

时邪，或饮食不节，湿热或寒湿内阻中焦，迫使胆汁不循常道所致。一般分为阴黄、阳黄两大类。

and urine due to accumulation of damp-heat or cold-damp in the middle energizer which leads to extravasation of the bile; resulting form the attack of seasonal factors or improper diet, it is classified into yin-type jaundice and yang-type jaundice.

黄风内障 【huáng fēng nèi zhàng】由绿风内障恶化而成。瞳神大而黄色昏浊，多致失明。

Absolute Glaucoma an eye disease developed from simple glaucoma, marked by dilatation, yellow coloration and turbid appearance of the pupil, and usually resulting in blindness.

黄干苔 【huáng gān tāi】舌苔黄而干燥。若苔黄干而薄，多为外感化热，初入里而热伤津液；若黄厚而干则属内有实热。

Dry and Yellowish Tongue Coating that with thin coating indicates the attack of heat from outside or just invading interiorly to consume the body fluid, that with thick coating indicates presence of interior heat.

黄瓜痈 【huáng guā yōng】指生于背部两旁的痈疽。由脾经火毒郁结而成。其症色红或不红、疼痛引心，肿高寸许，长则数寸甚至过尺，状如黄瓜。

Cucumber-Like Carbuncle carbuncle appearing on either side of the back, due to accumulation of toxic fire in the spleen meridian. The carbuncle is elevated like a cucumber, several inches or even more than one foot long, red or not red, associated with excruciating pain.

黄汗 【huáng hàn】多因汗出入水，壅遏荣卫或湿热内盛与风、水交蒸溢渗所致。症见头面四肢肿、身热不恶风、汗出粘衣黄色如柏汁、腰髋驰痛、两胫冷、身疼重、小便不利、脉沉迟等。

Yellowish Perspiration a condition resulting from swimming during sweating leading to the disorder of ying system and wei system, or from hyperactivity of damp-heat in the interior complicated by wind and water, manifested by edema of face and limbs, fever but no aversion to wind, yellowish and viscous sweat, dull

黄家 【huáng jiā】指黄疸久不退,已转阴黄的患者。

Patients Suffering from Yin Jaundice Because of Long-Standing Jaundice
aching over the back and hip, cold legs, general heavy pain of the body, dysuria, sunken and slow pulse.

黄腻苔 【huáng nì tāi】舌苔黄厚,表面有一层浑浊粘液覆盖,不易拭去。多因湿热结于中焦或热邪与痰湿互结所致。

Yellowish and Greasy Coating a sign usually indicating the accumulation of damp-fire in the middle energizer or combination of heat with phlegm.

黄胖 【huáng pàng】(黄肿、脱力黄)以全身肌肉萎黄,面浮足肿,神疲乏力为主症的疾病,或兼恶心、呕吐黄水、毛发稀疏、好食生米、茶叶、土炭等。多见于钩虫病。

General Edema with Sallow Skin a disease with puffy face, edematous limbs and lassitude as the major manifestations, or accompanied by nausea, bilious vomiting, dropping of hair, heterorexia, etc. mostly seen in hookwarm disease.

黄如枳实 【huáng rú zhǐ shí】喻脾的真正脏色。枯黄失泽的颜色,多是脾气将绝,胃气衰败的反映。

Yellow as Fructus Aurantii Immaturus the sickly complexion as yellow clay, with red and lusterless, indicating the exhaustion of spleen-qi and stomach-qi.

黄水疮 【huáng shuǐ chuāng】由脾胃湿热过盛,兼受风邪相搏而成。由红斑而变为粟米样水疮,随即变成脓疱痒痛流黄水。多发于小儿头面、耳、项等处,可蔓延至全身。

Pustulosis a skin disease caused by excessive dampness-heat in the spleen and stomach, complicated by attack of wind, manifested as red macules at onset, later with the formation of vesicles and pustules, itching pain and discharge of yellowish fluid; commonly seen in children with it all over the body.

黄苔 【huáng tāi】黄色舌苔。主里热证。根据其厚薄干湿度及颜色的深浅反映不同的病理变化。如黄厚干燥,为胃热伤津。

Yellowish Tongue Coating a sign generally signifying interior heat-syndrome. Different pathological changes are indicated and vary with the thick-

黄液上冲 【huáng yè shàng chōng】多由火热毒邪炽盛所致。常见于凝脂翳瞳孔缩小及外伤。症见风轮内黄色脓液积聚于下部，甚至掩过瞳神。

灰苔 【huī tāi】舌苔色灰白。若灰白而滑润，为三阴寒证；若灰黄而干燥，为里热实证。

恢刺 【huī cì】古代针刺手法之一。在疼痛拘急的筋肉附近斜针刺入，并提插针体以缓解拘挛。用于治疗筋痹。

回肠 【huí cháng】指小肠下端，上接空肠，下连大肠。

回旋灸 【huí xuán jiǔ】将艾卷点燃的一端在施灸部位的皮肤上进行前、后、左、右回旋移动的一种灸法。

回阳救逆 【huí yáng jiù nì】温法之一，救治阳气将脱的方法。适用于汗出不止、四肢厥冷、呼吸微弱、脉微欲绝

ness and moisture of the coating and the degree of its coloration, e. g. thick, dry and yellowish coating indicates impairment of the stomach fluid by heat.

Hypopyon a condition resulting from hyperactivity of toxic fire, manifested as yellow pus accumulating in the lower part of the anterior chamber of the eye, or even over the level of the pupil, usually secondary to purulent keratitis, contraction of pupils and trauma.

Grey Tongue Coating a grey and moist fur on the tongue signifies cold-syndrome of three-yin, while a grey yellowish and dry one indicates sthenia-heat syndrome of the interior.

Soothing Puncture one of the ancient acupuncture manipulation, by inserting the needle slantingly into the painful and cramping muscle and then lifting and thrusting the needle for the purpose of relieving spasm, usually applied for myalgia, arthralgia, etc.

Ileum the distal proprotion of the small intestine extending from the jejunum to the cecum.

Moving Moxibustion a method of moxibustion by which the burning moxa roll is moved over the affected part.

Recuperating the Depleted Yang and Rescuing the Patient from Danger a warming method for the exhaus-

等。

蛔动脘痛 【huí dòng wǎn tòng】蛔虫引起的上腹部痛。症见阵发性上腹部疼痛，发作时疼痛剧烈，伴厥冷或呕吐蛔虫，平时面黄饥瘦，或面有白斑。

蛔厥 【huí jué】指因蛔虫而引起的发作性腹痛、烦躁、手足厥冷等症。

蛔虫 【huí chóng】(蚘虫)寄生于小肠内的大形圆虫，呈白色或淡红色，长15—45厘米。人吞食感染性蛔虫卵而致病。男女老幼均可感染本病，以儿童感染率为最高。

蛔虫病 【huí chóng bìng】(蚘虫病)指蛔虫寄生于人体中。多因脾胃虚弱，杂食生冷甘肥油腻或不洁瓜果蔬菜所致。症见腹痛、痛有休止、亦可有肿块聚起，面色㿠白或黄白相间、或有虫斑、消瘦、呕吐清水或蛔虫等。

蛔疳 【huí gān】因生蛔虫日久而成的疳疾。患儿形体羸瘦、精神不安、腹中作痛、皱眉多啼、呕吐清水、夜间磨牙、易饥、嗜食异物。

蛔厥 【huí jué】见蚘厥。右上腹有钻

tion of yang qi, applicable to the case manifested as profuse perspiration, cold limbs, shallow respiration, small and weak pulse.

Epigastric Pain Due to Irritability of Ascaris a disorder characterized by severe paroxysmal pain over the epigastric region, vomiting of ascaris, pale or sallow complexion with white patches on the face, cold limbs and emaciation.

Colic due to Ascariasis paroxysmal abdominal pain accompanied by irritability, cold limbs, etc.

Ascaris an intestinal nematode parasite, whitish or pink in color, 15-45cm in length, Human of all races, especially children, may be infected by ingeation of its ovum.

Ascariasis infection with worms of the genus ascarus, due to asthenia of the spleen and stomach and ingestion of the indigestable food and contaminated vegetable, characterized by intermittent abdominal pain with visible mass, pale or yellowish complexion, whitish patches on the face, emaciation, vomiting of thin fluid or even of roundworm, etc.

Infantile Malnutrition Caused by Ascariasis a disorder manifested as emaciation, restlessness, abdominal pain, frequent crying, vomiting of thin fluid, teeth grinding at night, liability to be hunger and heterorexia.

Colic Caused by Ascaris a mobid

顶样阵发性剧烈疼痛,痛时患儿坐卧不安,甚则翻滚啼叫,面色苍白,手足厥冷,剧疼时伴有恶心、呕吐,可吐出胆汁或蛔虫。辨证分类 1. 偏寒型 2. 偏热症。

state characterized by severe paroxysmal upward drilling pain which makes the patient restlessness or even turn from side to side on the bed and cry, pale complexion, and cold and rigidity of limbs, usually accompanied by nausea, vomiting with bile or ascarid. Types of differentiation 1. predominant cold-type 2. predominant heat-type.

会厌 【huì yàn】七冲门之一。呼吸时会厌开启,吞咽或呕吐时则关闭,中医认为会厌是声音之户。

Epiglottis one of the seven important opening which opens during respiration and closed during swallowing and vomiting, it is considered as the aperture of voice.

会阴 【huì yīn】1、指肛门及外生殖器之间的部位。2、经穴名称。

Perineum 1. the space between the anus and the external genitals. 2. a name of acu-point.

恚膈 【huì gé】噎膈的一种。因思虑气结所致。症见食不消化、中脘实满、嗳气吞酸、大小便不利。

Dysphagia Due to Anxiety a type of dysphagia due to depression of qi resulting from anxiety, manifested as dyspepsia, gastric distention, eructation, acid regurgitation, constipation and disuria.

昏厥 【hūn jué】突然发作仆倒,四肢厥冷,短暂的意识丧失状态。

Syncope sudden and temporary suspension of consciousness accompanied by cold extremities.

昏愦 【hūn kuì】指神识昏乱,不明事理的症状。

Mental Confusion a state of mental derangement and confused mind.

昏迷 【hūn mí】指神识迷糊或人事不省的证候。多为邪阻清窍,神明被蒙所致。

Coma confused mind or loss of consciousness mainly due to attack of pathogenic factors to the heart orifices resulting in the deterioration of the mind.

昏睡 【hūn shuì】比昏迷较轻的一种神志不清状态。病人日夜沉睡,但能

A Milder State Than Coma a morbid state in which the patient in deep

唤醒。多由邪入营血或心包，神明被扰引起；亦见于中风患者。通常是病情危重的反映。

混合痔 【hùn hé zhì】即内外痔。

混睛障 【hùn jīng zhàng】由肝经风热或湿热，郁久伤阴，瘀血凝滞所致。症见一片灰白混浊翳障，似磨砂玻璃样漫掩黑睛。类似间质性角膜炎。

活血化瘀 【huó xuè huà yū】疏通血脉，消散瘀滞的一种治疗方法。适用于血液瘀滞所致的瘀血症。

火 【huǒ】五行之一。指一类阳性、热性的事物或亢进的状态。1、六淫之一。温热、暑热均属火邪，其性属阳。2、病理性的各种机能亢进的表现。3、生理性的火，为阳气所化，生命的动力，如命门之火等。

火不生土 【huǒ bù shēng tǔ】肾阳虚弱，命门火不足，不能温煦脾胃而出现脾肾阳虚的病理。常见畏寒、四肢不温、消化不良、大便泄泻等症。

火毒 【huǒ dú】1、火热病邪郁结成毒；在各种病证中，尤以外科疮疡肿毒为

sleeping can be aroused, usually caused by the evils invading ying or blood system or pericardium and disturbing mind, also seen in apoplexy.

Mixed Hemorrhoids

Interstital Keratitis a disease usually due to blood stasis and impairment of yin fluid resulting from the prolonged retention of wind-heat cornea with deep deposits in its substance which became hazy throughout and has a ground-glass appearance.

Activating Blood Circulation to Dissipate Blood Stasis a treatment for dredging blood vessel and dispersing blood stagnatition, which is applicable to the blood-stasis syndrome.

Fire 1. one of the five elements, which is yang in nature; one of the six pathogenic factors, which is yang in nature, including the warm-heat and summer-heat. 2. a pathological state of hyperactivity of the body. 3. physiologically referring to the motive force of life which is transformed from yang qi, such as the fire of the gate of life.

Fire Fails to Generate Earth a morbid condition of deficiency of spleen and stomach-yang due to insufficiency of kidney-yang and the fire of the gate of life, manifested as aversion to cold, coldness of extremities, indigestion, diarrhea, etc.

Virulent Fire 1. a pathogenic factor formed by the stagnation of fire, usu-

多见。2、烫火伤感染。

火疳【huǒ gān】（火疡）因火邪上犯白睛的一种急性眼病。症见白睛深部向外凸起，表面覆以暗红色颗粒，逐渐增大，疼痛、羞明流泪、视物不清，严重者可致黑睛溃破以致失明。

火罐【huǒ guàn】拔罐疗法所用的一种杯形工具，多用玻璃、金属、陶土或竹节制成。

火咳【huǒ ké】（火嗽）因火邪伤肺所致。表现为久咳少痰或痰中带血、烦渴面赤、胸胁痛、便秘等。

火逆【huǒ nì】误用烧针、熏、熨、灸等火法，由此导致引起的变证。

火盛刑金【huǒ shèng xíng jīn】1、火同肝火，见木火刑金。2、指火热之邪引起肺阴耗伤的病理，常出现喘咳、咯血痰等症。

火头痛【huǒ tóu tòng】（火邪头痛、火热头痛）因阳明胃火上冲引起头痛为主症的病证。症见头部跳痛或胀痛，痛连颊齿，或自耳前后痛连耳内，伴

ally responsible for the formation of swelling. 2. burn complicated by infection.

Acute Cleritis an acute oculopathy caused by the attack of fire to sclera, marked by bulging of the sclera covering with dark red granules, accompanied by pain, photophobia and blurring of vision, followed by perforation of the cornea and blindness in serious cases.

Cupping Jar a jar used for cupping-therapy which is made of glass, metal, mud or bamboo.

Cough Caused by Fire a disease with cough as the major symptom, which is due to fire impairing the lung, manifested as chronic cough with scanty phlegm or blood-tinged sputum, excessive thirst, flushed face, chest pain, constipation, etc.

Deterioration of Disease by Warming-therapy the condition of a patient who is becoming worse after erroneous application of heat needle, fuming, hot compress, and moxibustion.

Hyperactivity of Fire Impairs Metal 1. fire referring to the liver fire. 2. a morbid condition of over consumption of lung yin resulting from fire or heat, manifestied as asthma, cough with blood, sputum, etc.

Headache due to Fire a disorder with headache as the major symptom, resulting from up-going of stomach fire, manifested as throbbing or

烦热、口渴、便秘、脉洪大等。

火陷 【huǒ xiàn】疮疡邪毒陷入营血时出现的一种逆证。表现为疮色紫暗、疮口干枯、无脓疼痛、底部散漫、局部灼热剧痛。并有高热、口渴、便秘尿赤、烦躁谵语、舌绛、脉数等。

火性炎上 【huǒ xìng yán shàng】比喻火邪致病时病变有向上的特点。如面红、咽痛耳鸣、鼻衄、咯血等症均属火性炎上的病变。

火郁喘 【huǒ yù chuǎn】因火邪郁阻于肺所致的气喘。神情闷乱、四肢厥冷、脉沉伏等。

火针 【huǒ zhēn】针刺疗法用的一种金属针,长三至四寸,针体粗圆,针尖锐利,针柄用角质或竹木包裹,用时先将针尖烧红才入针。

火针疗法 【huǒ zhēn liáo fǎ】将针尖烧红后插入患部的一种治疗方法。操作时,对准患部速入速出,适用于痈疡、瘰疬、顽癣、痹痛等证。

distending pain over the head, involving cheek, teeth, ear, accompanied by fever, thirst, constipation, full and large pulse.

Fire Invading Interior a disorder with bad prognosis resulting from toxic material of carbuncle invading ying and blood system, appearing as dark-purplish lesion without distinct border, opening without drainage, local hotness and severe pain; accompanied by high fever, thirst, constipation, dark-colored urine, irritability, delirium, crimson tongue, fast pulse.

The Nature of Fire is Up-Flaring the character of fire is upward-going, manifested as flushed face, sore throat, tinitus, epistaxis, haemoptysis, etc.

Dyspnea due to Fire Retention a disorder caused by the retention of fire in the lung, manifested as dyspnea, irritability, cold extremities, sunken and hidden pulse, etc.

Heated Needle a metallic needle used for acupuncture therapy, 3-4 inches in legth, with round body and sharp tip, the handle of the needle is made of horn or wood, and the tip is burnt to red before inserting into the skin.

Acupuncture with Heat Needle a therapeutical method by inserting a heated needle into the affected part and withdrawing quickly, applicable to the disease such as abscess, scrofu-

火珠疮 【huǒ zhū chuāng】因心肝二经热毒炽盛所致的皮疹。多见于头部，初起时皮肤红赤、继而出现小泡疹，并有剧痛。类似头部带状疱疹。

Red-Pearl Boils skin eruption caused by hyperactivity of toxic fire in the heart and liver meridians, usually seen over the head. At onset the rashes appear red and then vesiculated, accompanied by severe pain, similar to herpes zoster over head.

霍乱 【huò luàn】以起病突然，大吐大泻为特征的疾病。常因饮食生冷不洁或感受寒邪、暑湿、疫疠之气所致。

Cholera Morbus a disease characterized by sudden onset, frequent vomiting and diarrhea, usually resulting from the intake of comtaminated food, or by the exposure to cold, summer dampness or pestilent factors.

霍乱转筋 【huò luàn zhuǎn jīn】因霍乱吐泻之后，津液暴失，气阴两伤，筋脉失养所致的病证。症见两腿挛缩。重则腹部拘急，囊缩舌卷。

Muscular Cramps Resulting from Acute Diarrhea and Vomiting a morbid condition caused by sudden loss of body fluid and impairment of qi and yin which leading to disnourishment of tendons; manifested as muscular cramps of legs, or even abdominal pain, shinkage of the scrotum and curling up of the tongue.

击仆 【jī pū】1、指击仆损伤而言，是外伤性的致病因素之一。2、见卒中。

Strike 1. injury due to strike, one of the traumatic pathogens. 2. see stroke.

饥不欲食 【jī bù yù shí】指感觉饥饿而又不想进食，因胃虚有热或肾阴虚，虚火乘胃所致的一种症状。

Hunger with Disinclination to Eat feeling hungry with no desire to eat, a symptom due to deficiency of stomach with retention of heat pathogen or deficiency of the kidney-yin with production of asthenia-fire attacking the stomach.

肌 【jī】即肌肉。

Muscle

肌痹 【jī bì】（肉痹）指以肌肤证候为

Myalgia a disease of muscles and

突出表现的痹证。多因伤于寒湿，除肌肤尽痛外，或见汗出、四肢痿弱、皮肤麻木不仁等。skin mostly caused by the attack of cold-dampness, marked by general aching, sweating, weakness of the extremities, numbness of the skin, etc.

肌腠　【jī còu】即肌肉的纹理。肌肉的组织间隙以及其中的结缔组织。**Muscular Striae**　the spaces and connective tissues between the strips of muscle.

肌肤甲错　【jī fū jiǎ cuò】皮肤粗糙、干燥、角化、外观皮肤呈褐色、如鳞甲状，且常兼有身体消瘦、腹满不能饮食等症状。多因内有瘀血，肌肤失养所致。**Squamous and Dry Skin**　skin becomes rough, squamous with brownish, scaling appearance and is often complicated with emaciation, abdominal fullness, loss of appetite, etc.; mostly due to blood stasis in the body which caused disnourishment of skin.

肌衄　【jī nù】（汗衄）指血从毛孔而出的病证。因阴虚火旺，肝胃火炽盛，或气血虚衰致使血不循经引起。**Hematohidrosis**　bleeding from the sweat pores, due to extravasation of the blood resulting from yin-deficiency with hyperactivity of fire, or overactivity of liver-fire and stomach-fire, or deficiency of qi and blood.

肌肉不仁　【jī ròu bù rén】指肌肉麻木不知痛痒冷热，本证可见于痿痹、中风、麻风等病。**Numbness**　lack or diminution of sensation of the skin, commonly seen in case of flaccidity-syndrome, apoplexy, leprosy, etc.

肌肉软　【jī ròu ruǎn】五软之一。指骨肉松软不坚，形体瘦弱。多因脾胃虚弱所致。**Muscular Flaccidity in Infant**　a condition of flabby muscles, emaciation and general debility, caused by deficiency of the spleen and stomach.

鸡胸　【jī xiōng】即胸骨突出形如鸡胸的胸廓畸形。多因佝偻病所致。**Pigeon Breast**　a deformity of the chest in which the sternum is prominent, as a chick, mostly due to rickets.

奇方　【jī fāng】药味是单数或单味药的方。**Prescription Composed of Medicines in Single or Odd Number**

积聚　【jī jù】指腹内结块，或胀或痛的病证。多由七情郁结气滞血瘀，或**Mass**　formation of mass in the abdomen accompanied with distention

饮食内伤,痰滞交阻,或寒热失调,正虚邪结而成。结块明显,固定不移为积;结块陷现,攻窜作胀为聚。

激经 【jī jīng】指孕后仍按月行经并无其他症状,又无损于胎儿,随胎儿渐长,其经自停。

急方 【jí fāng】用气味都很浓厚的药物,组成作用快捷的方剂,大多用汤剂的方式以求速效。急方适用于急性病、病情危重等。

急喉痹 【jí hóu bì】急性咽喉红肿热痛,伴吞咽不利、痰涎涌盛、胸闷气促、恶寒发热、面红赤头痛身疼,甚而牙关紧闭,汤水不下等。多因肺胃积热,邪毒内侵,风痰上涌所致。

急喉风 【jí hóu fēng】喉风之发病急骤,迅即咽喉肿塞者。见喉风。

急黄 【jí huáng】1、黄疸中的一种危重病证,多因湿热毒邪熻灼营血所致。症见发病急骤、突然发黄、黄疸迅急加深,伴有心满气喘、甚者高热神昏、吐衄便血、腹水等。2、即瘟黄。

or pain, caused by emotional upsets, stagnation of qi and blood, or improper diet, phelgm accumulating or disorder of cold and heat, pathogens accumulating due to deficiency of healthy qi.

Regular Menstruation during Pregnancy a condition in pregnancy during which menstruation occurs regularly without interference to the growth of the fetus and stops spontaneously as the fetus grows gradually.

Prescription with Prompt Effect a recipe composed of drugs of heavy flavour and acting promptly, usually prepared as decoction, applicable to acute disease or critical case.

Acute Pharyngitis inflammation of the pharynx marked by local redness, swelling and pain, accompanied with dysphagia, salivation, chocking sensation in the chest, rapid respiration, chilliness, fever, flush face with red eyes, general aching, lockjaw, etc., caused by the accumulation of heat in the lung and stomach, and attack of toxic pathogen leading to up-going of wind-phlegm.

Acute Pyogenic Infection of Pharynx a disease marked by rapid swelling of the throat.

Acute Jaundice a critical condition in jaundice due to involvement of yin-blood by virulent damp-heat, characterized by sudden onset and rapid hematemesis, epistaxia, hema-

急惊风 【jí jīng fēng】多因内热炽盛,外为风邪郁闭,热极生风所致。发病急,突然高热惊厥、牙关噤急、痰壅气促,继而四肢抽搐、神志昏迷、头项强硬,甚则角弓反张。

急劳 【jí láo】指劳瘵病势急暴者。症见憎寒体热、颊赤盗汗、心烦口干、咳嗽咯血、食欲不振,久则形体消瘦等。

急乳蛾 【jí rǔ é】(急蛾)即急性扁桃体炎。多因肺胃热壅,火毒之邪上冲咽喉所致。

急下存阴 【jí xià cún yīn】用泻下作用较强的方药,迅速通便泄热清除燥结,以保存津液,防止痉厥变证的方法。适用于急性热病高热,烦渴、大便秘结、舌苔黄燥、脉沉实有力等实热证。

急者缓之 【jí zhě huǎn zhī】对筋脉拘急强直的病证,宜用平息缓解的方法进行治疗,如因寒邪侵袭筋脉拘急的患者,须用温经散寒法以缓之。

tochezia, ascites in severe case.

Acute Infantile Convulsion a disease caused by the hyperactivity of heat interiorly or stagnation of wind from outside which leads to production of endogenous wind characterized by sudden onset of high fever, convultion and syncope, lockjaw, dyspnea, abundant sputum and followed by convultion, coma, stiff neck, or even opisthotonose.

Acute Tuberculosis an infectious disease manifested as chilliness, fever, flush of cheek, night sweat, restlessness, dry mouth, cough, hemoptysis, anorexia and gradual emaciation.

Acute Tonsillitis acute inflammation of the tonsils due to attack of toxic heat accumulated in the lung and stomach to the pharynx.

Retaining Yin by Emergent Application of Purgatives a treatment for the preservation of body fluid and the prevention of convultion by eliminating the heat and discharging the dry feces with sthenia-heat syndrome manifested as high fever, extreme thirst, constipation, yellowish and dry tongue coating, sunken, solid, strong pulse, etc.

The Spasmodic Disease Should be Relaxed a therapeutic principle for treating muscular spasms, e. g., such case caused by the attack of cold is usually treated with the threapy of

急者治标 【jí zhě zhì biāo】在临床上有的症状虽属于标症，但由于它的起病急、发展快、给病人造成痛苦甚至危险，则应先予以治疗。
Relieving the Secondary Symptom in an Acute Case a principle of treatment applied when the secondary symptom (biao) occurs abruptly with a rapid progress and is harmful to the patient.

疾徐补泻 【jí xú bǔ xiè】缓慢进针，疾速出针为补法；疾速进针，缓缓出针为泻法。
Tonifying and Reducing by Adjusting the Velocity of Manipulation the manipulation of acupuncture in which the tonifying effect is obtained by inserting the needle slowly and withdrawing quickly; the reducing effect is obtained by inserting the needle quickly and withdrawing slowly.

疾医 【jí yī】周代官方卫生机构分科医生的一种，相当于内科医生。
Doctor Specialized in Internal Medicine the medical specialist serving in the official health institute of Zhou Dynasty.

脊 【jǐ】即椎骨。它有支撑人体躯干及脏腑的作用，为督脉所过之处。
Spine vertebrae with the function of supporting the trunk and organs, along which the GV passes.

脊疳 【jǐ gān】是指疳疾患者背部肌肉消瘦，脊骨显露之证。
Infantile Malnutrition with Prominent Spine the infantile malnutrition characterized by emaciation of the back muscles and prominent spine.

忌口 【jì kǒu】由于治疗的需要，要求病人忌食某些食物，如水肿忌食盐，黄疸腹泻忌食油腻等。
Dietetic Restraint certain foods should be avoided for the treatment of diseases, e. g., salty food should be limited for edematous patients, greasy diet should be avoided for diarrheic patients.

剂型 【jì xíng】(剂) 药物制剂的形式，如汤、丸、散、膏、丹等。
Pharmaceutical Forms forms in which medicines are prepared, such as decoction, pill, powder, plaster, pellet,

季肋部 【jì lèi bù】胸部前下侧部位。

Hypochondrium the lower anterolateral region of the chest.

季胁痛 【jì xié tòng】指软肋部疼痛。多属肝虚。兼见胆怯善惊、视物昏糊、耳鸣者，属肝气虚；兼见烦热口干、头眩眼花者，舌质红属肝血不足。

Hypochondriac Pain a symptom belonging to deficiency of liver, that accompanied with timidness, blurring of vision, tinnitus is attributive to the deficiency of liver qi, while that with feverish sensation, dry mouth and dizziness to the insufficiency of liver blood.

悸心痛 【jì xīn tòng】多因心脾不足所致。症见心痛而悸、痛有休止、喜按、得食减缓、饥则更痛、脉虚弱等。

Epigastric Pain with Palpitation a disorder due to insufficiency of the heart and spleen, manifested as intermittent epigastric pain with palpitation which can be relieved by pressure and intake of food, and aggravated by hunger, weak pulse.

夹板 【jiā bǎn】医疗器械、主要用于骨折复位后局部外固定，过去用树皮、竹片制作，现在用塑料制作。

Splint a medical appliance for keeping a broken bone in the right position, made of strips of bark or bamboo in the past and now of plastics in someplace.

颊 【jiá】面部两侧的突起部。

Cheek fleshy protuberance on either side of the face.

甲疽 【jiǎ jū】因外伤所致的甲沟旁组织的炎症，多发生于足大趾。

Paronychia inflammation involving the tissue at the groove of the nail after injury mostly occurring in the big toes.

假寒 【jiǎ hán】热证表现出寒的假象。

Pseudo-Cold Syndrome heat syndrome but appearing as some cold symptoms.

假热 【jiǎ rè】寒证反而表现假热症状的一种病象。

Pseudo-Heat Syndrome cold syndrome but appearing as some heat symptoms.

坚阴 【jiān yīn】固肾精，平相火的治

Fortifying Yin a treatment by

坚肩　jian

法。用于相火妄动，肾气不固致梦遗等证。

strengthening the kidney-essence and calming prime-minister fire, indicated in the case of nocturnal emission due to hyperfunction of prime-minister fire and deficiency of the kidney qi.

坚者削之　【jiān zhě xiāo zhī】病邪积聚形成有坚实包块的疾病，一般采用攻削的方法进行治疗。

A Mass Should Be Eliminiated　a therapeutic principle for treating the indurated mass caused by accumulating of pathogenic factors.

肩　【jiān】上臂和躯干连接的部位。

Shoulder　the juncture between the upper limb and the trunk.

肩背痛　【jiān bèi tòng】肩背部疼痛。因劳伤，或风寒、风湿等外邪侵袭足太阳经或肺经所致。

Pain over the Shoulder and Back　a condition due to over load, or attack of wind-damp or wind-cold to the foot-taiyang meridian or lung meridian.

肩毒　【jiān dú】泛指肩部的痈疽。

Carbuncle of the Shoulder

肩关节脱臼　【jiān guān jié tuō jiù】（肩骱落下）指肱骨头冲破关节囊，致肩关节面的正常关系发生改变。常有局部肿痛、呈方肩、肘部不能贴胸、肩部活动受限等。多因跌闪等外力所致。

Dislocation of Shoulder Joint　displacement of the head of humerus out of the articular bursa due to trauma, marked by local swelling and pain, square-shaped shoulder, inability of abduction of the upper arm, limitation of movement of the shoulder joints, etc.

肩胛　【jiān jiǎ】1、肩胛骨的部位。2、即肩胛骨。

Shoulder Blade　1. scapular region 2. scapula

肩胛疽　【jiān jiǎ jū】即有头疽发生于肩胛部者。多因太阴肺经积热而致。

Carbuncle with Spot on Scapular Region　a condition caused by the accumulation of heat in the lung meridian of hand-taiyang.

肩痛　【jiān tòng】指肩关节、肩胛周围筋骨肌肉疼痛。多因外感风湿或因强力举重、跌仆损伤等所致。

Shoulder Pain　referring to pain of shoulder joint and tissue over scapular region due to attack of wind-damp or over load, or trauma, etc.

肩息　【jiān xī】呼吸时张口抬肩以助

Breathing with Elevation of Shoulders

呼吸的状态。多见于严重呼吸困难的患者,如哮喘病发作、严重肺气肿、心力衰竭等。

肩髃 【jiān yú】1、肩关节上方。2、穴位名称。

兼方 【jiān fāng】用主治不同的药物组合而成的方剂。多用于病情复杂者,如寒热、虚实错杂等。以兼收疗效。

兼证 【jiān zhèng】指主证的伴发症状和体征,与主证相对而言。

煎 【jiān】是汤剂的另一名称。见汤液。

煎药法 【jiān yào fǎ】煎药的方法。煎药时所加水量的多少、火力的大小及煎药时间的长短,应根据药物的性质、药味的多少、病人年龄大小及病的轻重等条件来决定。

茧唇 【jiǎn chún】(唇癌)多由思虑伤脾,心火内炽,脾胃积热;或水亏火旺,火毒蕴结唇部所致。初起在口唇部出现豆粒大小硬结,逐渐增大,白皮皱裂,形如蚕茧,溃破后时流血水,溃疡面高低不平,常覆有痂皮。后期常伴口干咽燥,形体消瘦。

a condition seen in the case of profound dyspnea in order to make breathing easy, as asthmatic attacks, serious case of pulmonary emphysema, cardiac failure, etc.

Jian Yu 1. the upper portion of the shoulder 2. a name of acupoint.

Prescription Composed of Drugs with Different Properties a recipe applied in the complicated cases, such as cold syndrome complicated by heat syndrome, deficient syndrome complicated by excess syndrome.

Associated Symptom and Sign less important symptoms accompanied with principal ones, they are in contrast with principal ones.

Decoction

Method of Decocting Medicine the preparation of decoction in which the amount of water added, the temperature and the time for boiling are adjusted according to the character and number of the medicines, the age of the patient and the severity of the disease.

Lip Carcinoma a morbid condition due to impairment of the spleen by anxiety, hyperactivity of the heart-fire and retention of pathogenic heat in the spleen and stomach, or due to consumption of the body fluid and hyperactivity of fire involving the lips; manifested as a small indurated nodule at onset with gradual enlargement like cocoon, followed by rupture

..., with bloody discharge, and uneven surface covered with scabs; in the later stage, usually accompanied with dry mouth and throat, and hectic marasmus.

间接灸 【jiàn jiē jiǔ】指艾炷与穴位皮肤之间衬隔物品的灸法，如隔姜灸、隔蒜灸、隔饼灸、隔盐灸等。

Indirect Moxibustion a method of moxibustion in which the ignited moxa cone is separated from the skin by a slice of ginger, garlic, herbal cake or a layer of salt.

间日疟 【jiàn rì nüè】指隔日发用一次的疟疾。

Tertian Malaria the malaria in which the febrile paroxysms occur every third day counting the day of accurrence as the first day of the cycle.

间者并行 【jiàn zhě bìng xíng】对于某些慢性病采取标本同治的方法。

A Chronic Case Should Be Dealt with the Treatment Aiming at both the Primary and Secondary Symptoms

健脾 【jiàn pí】治疗脾虚，运化功能减弱的方法。常用于脾气虚弱，症见面色萎黄、疲倦乏力、饮食减少、食后腹胀、大便稀薄、舌淡苔白、脉缓弱者。

Invigorating the Spleen a treatment for the dysfunction in transformation resulting from deficiency of spleen-qi applicable to the case manifested as sallow complexion, lassitude, poor appetite, stomachache which is relieved by pressure, loose stools, pale tongue with whitish coating, slow and weak pulse.

健脾疏肝 【jiàn pí shū gān】治疗肝气郁结，引起脾不健运的方法。临床用于肝郁脾虚，症见两胁胀痛、不思饮食、腹胀肠鸣、大便稀薄、苔白腻、脉弦者。

Invigorating the Spleen and Dispersing the Stagnated Liver-Qi a treatment for the disturbance of transformation and transportation due to the spleen-asthenia caused by stagnated liver qi, which is applicable to the case manifested as distending pain over the hypochondrium, anorexia, abdominal flatulence, increased borygmus,

健忘 【jiàn wàng】指记忆力的严重衰退。多因忧思，用脑过度，心失所养，心肾不交所致。

健胃 【jiàn wèi】加强胃的消化功能的方法。适用于胃消化功能低下，食欲减退等。

降剂 【jiàng jì】用降抑药物组成，具有降逆作用的方剂，常用药物如苏子、旋覆花等。

降可去升 【jiàng kě qù shēng】用沉降的药物，以治疗邪气上逆的病证。

降逆下气 【jiàng nì xià qì】(顺气) 治疗肺胃之气上逆的方法。适用于肺气上逆致哮喘咳嗽、痰多气急和胃气上逆致呃逆不止、胸中不舒、脉迟等。

降气 【jiàng qì】(下气) 治疗气上逆的方法。适用于呃逆等病证。

交通心肾 【jiāo tōng xīn shèn】治疗心肾不交的方法。心肾不交，症见心烦

loose stool, whitish and greasy tongue fur, wiry pulse, etc.

Amnesia lack or loss of memory, usually due to over anxiety, overstrain of brain, disnourishment of heart, disharmony of heart and kidney.

Strengthening the Stomach a treatment for promoting the digestive function of the stomach, indicated in the cases with debility of digestive function of the stomach and poor appetite.

Prescription with Lowering Effect prescription composed of drugs with the action of lowering the adverse qi, such as Fructus Perillae, Flos Inulae, etc.

Prescription with Lowering Effect Can Treat the Adverse-Rising-Qi Syndrome a treatment for the adverse-rising of qi, by using the depressant prescription.

Keeping the Adverse Qi Downwards a treatment for the adverse rising of lung and stomach qi, in that of lung qi manifested as asthma, productive cough and dyspnea, and in that of stomach qi manifested as incessant hiccup, uneasiness in the chest, slow pulse, etc.

Keeping the Adverse Qi Downwards a treatment for adverse rising of qi, such as cough, dyspnea, hiccup, etc.

Restoring the Equilibrium between the Heart and Kidney a treatment

失眠、遗精、头晕、健忘、耳鸣耳聋、腰酸腿软、小便短赤、脉细数等。

for the inequlibrium between heart-yang and kidney-yin, applicable to the case manifested as restlessness, insomnia, nocturnal emission, dizziness, amnesia, tinnitus, deafness, soreness of the loin, weakness of the legs, scanty and dark urine, red tongue, small and fast pulse, etc.

胶 【jiāo】用动物的皮、骨、角等加水反复煎煮,浓缩后制成的干燥固体状物质。如阿胶、鹿角胶等。

Gelatin a product derived from the long-time cooking of the skin, bone, horn of animals, such as gelatin, deer-bone gelatin, etc.

椒疮 【jiāo chuāng】即沙眼。多因眼部受风热毒邪侵染,加之脾胃素有积热而发。症见眼睑内面发生红色细小微粒、自觉眼部沙涩痒痛、羞明流泪。

Trachoma a disease of eye caused by the attack of wind-heat and the accumulation of heat in the spleen and stomach; marked by red granules over the conjunctiva, itching, pain, photophobia and lacrimation.

焦原 【jiāo yuán】即命门。中医学认为命门的功能活动是三焦功能活动的原动力。

Origin of the Triple Energizer the gate of life, which is considered as the motive force for the functional activity of triple energizer.

角弓反张 【jiǎo gōng fǎn zhāng】项背高度强直,使身体仰曲如弓状的症状。多因津血受伤或邪阻筋脉,致筋失濡养引起。常见于痉病、破伤风等。

Opisthotonos a form of spasm in which the head and heels are bent backward and the body bowed, usually seen in convulsive disease and tetanus; it is caused by the failure to nourish the muscles due to the over consumption of fluid and blood and the obstruction of tendons and vessels by pathogenic factors.

脚跟骨伤 【jiǎo gēn gǔ shāng】多因坠跌、压砸所伤,跟部肿痛、压痛明显、不能站立和行走。

Fracture of Os Calcis breaking of the heel bone due to trauma, marked by local swelling, pain, tenderness, and inability to stand and walk.

脚盘出臼 【jiǎo pàn chū jiù】即踝关节

Dislocation of Ankle Joint dis-

脱臼。因跌扑、扭伤所致。局部严重肿胀，明显畸形，疼痛剧烈，皮下瘀血，不能活动。

脚气 【jiǎo qì】（脚弱）。其症先起于腿脚麻木、软弱无力甚者脚气攻心出现神恍。本病多由湿邪壅滞，流注于脚所致。临床上分干、湿脚气两种。

脚气疮 【jiǎo qì chuāng】（脚湿气）脚趾间出现小水泡，瘙痒流水，反复发作，致趾间糜烂或干痒为主，皮肤粗糙脱屑、皲裂。多由脾胃二经湿热下注或接触毒邪所致。即脚癣。

脚心痛 【jiǎo xīn tòng】足底中心肾经涌泉穴处疼痛。多因肾虚湿着，命门之火失于温煦敷布所致。

脚趾骱失 【jiǎo zhǐ jiè shī】即趾关节脱臼。

脚肿 【jiǎo zhǒng】指脚浮肿。多因水湿下注于肾所致。

疖 【jiē】由内蕴热毒或外触暑热引起毛囊和皮脂腺的急性炎症。肿势局限，色红、热疼，脓出即愈。临床分有头疖和无头疖。辩证分类：1、热毒

placement of the ankle joint due to trauma or sprain, marked by local swelling, distending, obvious deformity, intense pain, bruise and immobility.

Beriberi a disease resulting from local retention of damp factor manifested as numbness and weakness of foot and legs or even mental disorder in some cases if damp attacking heart; clinically classified as dry and damp beriberi.

Tinea Pedis a chronic superficial fungal infection of the skin of the foot, esp, betweem the toes, marked by small vesicles, maceration, erosion, scaling and fissures, caused by the attack of damp-heat from the spleen and stomach meridians, or by direct contact with the etiologic agent.

Pain at the Center of the Sole pain at the site corresponding to yongquan acupoint in the kidney meridian, caused by the inability of warming by the life-gate fire resulting from the kidney deficiency and attack of damp factor.

Interphalangeal Dislocation of Foot

Edema of Lower Extremities a sign usually due to attck of the dampness to the kidney.

Furuncle a pyogenic infection of hair follicle or sweat gland due to retention of heat-toxin or attack of summer heat, manifested as superfi-

蕴结证 2、暑热浸淫证 3、正虚毒恋证。

icial circumscribed swelling, redness, heat and pain, and healing after discharge of pus. Types of differentiation 1. stagnation of heat and toxin 2. syndrome of summer-heat attack 3. syndrome of retention of toxin due to deficiency of healthy qi.

节气 【jié qì】农历推算四季气候的单位。一般以十五日为一个节气。一年共有二十四个节气。如立春、雨水……等。

Solar Term a climatic period approximately equivalent to 15 days. There are 24 solar terms in a year, i. e., "the beginning of spring", "rain water", etc.

洁净腑 【jié jìng fǔ】即利小便。

Clearing the Bladder a treatment for promoting diuresis.

结核 【jié hé】多因风火或湿痰气郁凝滞所致。肿块生于皮里膜外，形如果核，坚而不痛。

Subcutaneous Node indurated and painless lumps beneath the skin due to stagnation of qi, accumulation of wind-fire or damp-phlegm.

结脉 【jié mài】脉来缓而时一止，止无定数。主阴盛气结之证，由气壅痰滞，气滞血凝而致。

Slow and Irregular Pulse a pulse condition characterized by slow beating less than 90 beats per minute with irregular intervals; signifies qi stagnation due to sufficiency of yin, the pulse is caused by the obstruction or aggregation of qi and blood or accumulation of phlegm.

结胸 【jié xiōng】指邪气结于胸中，而出现心下痛，按之硬满的病证。多因太阳病攻下太早，以致表热内陷与胸中原有水饮结聚或由太阳内传阳明，阳明实热与腹中原有水饮互结而成。

Syndrome due to Retention of Pathogenic Factor in the Thorax a syndrome with epigastric pain, fullness and rigidity, resulting from early administration of purgative for taiyang disease, leading to the heat in the superficies attacking the interior and blending with the fluid originally existed in the thorax or from the sthenic heat in yangming meridian

结阴 【jié yīn】便血之一种。多由阴气内结或厥阴肝血内结所致。

结阳 【jié yáng】四肢阳气郁结，不得通达，引起水液停滞不行，出现四肢浮肿的病理。

结扎法 【jié zā fǎ】外治法的一种。是利用线的张力，促使患部气血不通，使所需除去的组织坏死脱落，达到治愈的目的。此法多用于痔核、赘疣等。

结者散之 【jié zhě sàn zhī】对结聚之证要使其散之。如浊痰结聚所致的瘰疬，常用软坚散结的方法进行治疗。

睫毛 【jié máo】上下眼睑边缘的细毛，具有保护眼球的作用。

截疟 【jié nüè】在疟疾发作前的适当时候，使用内服药或针刺等法，以制止疟疾的发作。

解表 【jiě biǎo】解除在表的病邪，通常是指汗法。

which is coming from taiyang meridian blends with the fluid originally existed in the abdomen.

Sluggish Yin one kind of hematochezia, resulting from yin-qi or the liver blood of jueyin accumulated interiorly.

Sluggish Yang-Qi a morbid condition with edema of extremities, caused by the stagnation of yang-qi in the extremities leading to the retention of fluid.

Ligation Method an external treatment for hemorrhoid nevus, etc. by ligating the root of a superficial mass tightly to block the blood circulation and to cause it necrotic and dropping.

Disease Caused by Accumulation of Pathogenic Factor Should Be Treated with Therapy of Dispersion a therapeutic principle, e. g. scrofula due to accumulation of phlegm is usually treated with the therapy of softening and dissipating.

Eyelash the hairs growing on the margin of the eyelids, which play a role in protecting the eye.

Stopping the Paroxysm of Malaria a treatment for stopping the attack of malaria by the application of oral medicines or acupuncture at a proper time before the paroxysm.

Expelling Superficial Pathogenic Factors a treatment usually referring to diaphoresis.

解表法 【jiě biǎo fǎ】通过发汗以解除肌表之病邪的方法，临床常分辛温解表和辛凉解表。

Diaphoretic Therapy a treatment for dispelling exogenous factors through perspiration, including pungent-warming method and pungent-cooling method.

解毒 【jiě dú】泛指解除体内毒素。包括解血分热毒、寒盛成毒、误服或接触毒物、蛇虫犬兽伤所致的中毒，以及按特定的炮制方法减除药物的毒性等。

Removing Toxic Material a treatment for eliminating toxin in body, including the virulent heat in blood system or that produced by the hyperactivity of cold, or by the administration and contact with poisonous material, or the poison secreted by animals or insects, and also for the elimination of toxicity of materia medica by special method of preparation.

解肌 【jiě jī】解除肌表之邪，是对外感初起有汗的治法。一般宜根据病症的寒热而采用辛温或辛凉解肌法。

Expelling the Pathogenic Factor in the Muscles a treatment for expelling superfical factors in the case exposed to exogenous factors with perspiration at once, by the application of pungent-warming method or pungent-cooling method according to the symptoms.

解痉 【jiě jīng】（镇痉）解除震颤、手足抽搐及角弓反张等症的方法。

Relieving the Muscular Spasm a treatment for tremor, tetany, opisthotonos, etc.

解颅 【jiě lú】小儿到一定年龄，囟门应合而不合，头缝开解，以致囟门较正常为大，或可见囟门部稍稍隆起。多由父母精血不足，以致小儿先天肾气虚弱，不能充养脑髓而成。多见于脑积水、佝偻病等疾病。

Non-Closure of the Fontanels in Infants a condition due to congenital deficiency of kidney qi with failure to nourish the spinal marrow resulting from the insufficiency of essence and blood of the parents; seen in hydrocephalas rickets, etc.

解索脉 【jiě suǒ mài】快慢不匀，忽慢忽快、节律紊乱的脉象，如解乱绳之状。此为肾与命门之气皆亡之候。

Untying-Knot Pulse a pulse condition characterized by frequent irregular changes in pulse rate and rhythm,

疥疮 【jiè chuāng】因疥虫引起的传染性皮肤病。皮肤出现针头大的丘疹和水泡，痒甚，以手指缝最为多见。

金创 【jīn chuāng】（金疮）指由金属器刃损伤肢体所致的创伤。

金疳 【jīn gān】在白睛上出现局部隆起的小泡，赤脉绕于周围的眼病，多由肺火炽盛，热灼津液所致。

金破不鸣 【jīn pò bù míng】1、由于肺气损伤而致的声音嘶哑。多见于晚期肺结核。2、见久瘖。

金针拨障法 【jīn zhēn bō zhàng fǎ】即针拨白内障术。方法：在角膜颞下方，距角膜约4毫米处做一约2.5毫米长切口，用一特制的拨障针从切口进入眼内，将白内障拨离瞳孔，下沉在眼内直下方，以达到恢复视力的目的。

津 【jīn】人体体液的组成部份，有营养肌肉和滋润皮肤的功能。中医认为，汗和尿液皆来源于此，出汗或排尿过多皆可伤津。

resembling the untying of a knotted rope, which indicates depletion of both the kidney-qi and qi of the life gate.

Scabiies a skin disease due to itch-mite, manifested as papules and vesicle with intense itching, commonly seen over the skin folds at the roots of the finger.

Incised Wound injury by metallic tool.

Follicular Conjunctivitis an epidemic mucopurulent inflammation of the conjunctiva marked by follicles surrounded by hyperemic arterioles, caused by the hyperactivity of the lung-fire leading to the consumption of body fluid.

Broken Bell-Metal Can't Ring 1. hoarseness due to consumption of lung qi mostly seen in the late stage of tuberculosis. 2. see Lingering Dysphonia

Operation of Cataract removal with a metallic needle, an operation for cataract by performing a 2.5mm incision at the sclera 4mm apart from the inferior temporal margin of the cornea, and pressing down the opaque lens to the lower part of the vitreous with a metallic needle.

Thin Body Fluid a component of body fluid with the function of nourishing the muscles and moistening the skin. The sweat and urine are originated from the thin body fluid, pro-

津血同源 【jīn xuè tóng yuán】津血皆由饮食精微所化,可相互转化,并在体液调节中相互协调,在病理上相互影响。 **Body Fluid and Blood are Derived from the Same Source** both body fluid and blood originate from the nutriments of food and can be transformed from each other. They coordinate in the regulation of fluid metabolism and effect each other pathlogically.

津液 【jīn yè】1、机体的水分包括各脏腑组织器官的内在体液及其正常的分泌物,如胃液、肠液和涕、泪等。2、饮食通过胃、脾、肺、三焦等脏的作用而化成的营养物质。 **Body Fluid** 1. all liquid components of the body. 2. the nutriments transformed from foods by the action of the stomach, spleen, lung, and triple energizer.

筋 【jīn】在中医学的概念中,有时候也包含于肌肉。其功能与肝有密切的关系。 **Tendon** it serves as ageneral term for tendons and muscles in TCM, its function is closely related to the liver.

筋痹 【jīn bì】痹证之一种。指筋脉拘挛,关节疼痛,不能行走的病证,由风寒湿邪侵袭于筋所致。 **Tendinous Bi-Syndrome** a syndrome characterized by convulsion of the muscles, arthralgia, debility to walk, resulting from the attack of wind-cold-damp factors to the tendons and muscles.

筋缓 【jīn huǎn】指筋脉弛缓,不能随意运动之证。多因肝肾虚亏或湿热所伤引起。 **Muscular Flaccidity** a morbid state of flabby muscles with difficulty in movements, mostly due to asthenia of the liver and kidney, or impairment of muscles by damp-heat factors.

筋会 【jīn huì】八会之一。即阳陵泉穴,筋的精气会聚的地方。 **Convergent Point of Tendons** one of the eight convergent points, i.e. yangling quan, where the essence of the tendons gathers.

筋膜 【jīn mó】包于肌腱外的结缔组织。 **Aponeurosis** connective tissue covering the tendons.

筋惕肉瞤 【jīn tì ròu rùn】指筋肉抽掣 **Muscular Twitching and Cramp** a

跳动的症状。多因血虚或津液耗伤或因寒湿伤阴，筋肉失养所致。

sign due to disnourishment of muscles resulting from the blood deficiency, over consumption of body fluid, or the impairment of yin by cold-damp.

筋痿 【jīn wěi】（肝痿）1、痿证的一种。由于肝火而阴血不足，筋膜干枯所致。症见筋急拘挛、渐至痿弱不能运动，伴有口苦、指甲枯痿等。2、见阳痿。

Flaccidity-Syndrome Involving the Muscle 1. a type of flaccidity syndrome due to insufficiency of yin blood and dryness of the aponeurosis resulting from liver-fire, manifested as convulsion, followed by flaccidty and immobility, accompanied with bitter taste, withered nails, etc. 2. Impotence

筋瘿 【jīn yǐng】指瘿块局部静脉曲张，结如蚯蚓。多因怒气伤肝，火旺血燥所致。

Goiter Covered with Varicose Veins a condition due to impairment of the liver by a rage, or hyperactivity of fire and blood-dryness.

紧脉 【jǐn mài】指感紧张有力，切之如按转索，左右弹指的一种脉象，多见于寒证及痛证。

Tense Pulse a pulse condition with tense and vigorous beats, like a stretched twisted cord, frequently seen in cold-syndrome and pain-syndrome.

进针 【jìn zhēn】将针由浅入深地刺入预定的深度。一般在进针前已做了选穴及局部皮肤常规消毒等预备工作。

Inserting the Needle a stip of acupuncture manipulation by which the needle is punctured through the sterilized skin to the expected depth after the point is selected.

近血 【jìn xuè】指便血而先血后便者。出血部位多在广肠或肛门，血色多鲜红。

Bleeding from Lower Intestinal Tract discharge of blood which usually comes from the rectum and is bright red in color.

浸洗剂 【jìn xǐ jì】将药煎汤，浸洗全身或局部。

Bathing Preparation a preparation of medical decoction for general or local bath.

浸淫疮 【jìn yín chuāng】由心火脾湿，凝滞不散，复感风邪，郁于肌肤而致。

Acute Eczema an inflammatory skin disorder caused by the stagna-

形如粟米、瘙痒流水、迅速蔓延、浸淫成片、甚者身热。即急性湿疹。tion of heart fire and spleen-dampness, moreover by the attack of wind with involvement of the skin; marked with skin lesion of miliary size, itching and oozing, followed by rapid spreading and coalescence and even fever in severe case.

禁刺 【jìn cì】即针刺的禁忌。包括禁针部位如重要器官动脉附近, 孕妇的腹、婴幼儿囟门部及禁针穴位等禁刺。酒醉、过饥、过饱、过度疲劳、情绪激烈变化等情况下, 不可立刻进行针刺, 以免发生意外。

Acupuncture Contraindication the location of human body and the condition of the patient to which acupuncture is contraindicated. The former includes important organ and big artery, the abdomen of preagnant women, the fontanelles of infants, certain particular points, the latter includes the patients who are drunken, over hunger, over fed, over fatigue, under emotional upsets, etc.

禁方 【jìn fāng】(秘方) 某些有效的方剂被制方人保密, 不传授给他人。

Secret Recipe an effective recipe kept from the knowledge of others.

噤口痢 【jìn kǒu lì】指痢疾患者饮食不进或呕不能食。多因湿浊热毒蕴结肠中, 邪毒亢盛, 胃阴受劫, 和降失常; 或因久病脾胃两伤, 中气败损所致。症见不思饮食、呕恶不纳、下痢频繁、肌肉瘦削、胸腔痞闷、舌绛、苔黄腻等。

Dysentery with Inability to Take Food a serious dysentery caused by the accumulation of virulent dampness and heat in the intestines, leading to consumption of stomach-yin and dysfunction of stomach, or by the impairment of the spleen and stomach and exhaustion of the middle energizer qi; manifested as anorexia, vomiting, frequent diarrhea, emaciation, feeling of oppression over the chest and upper abdomen, crimson tongue with yellowish and greasy coating, etc.

经闭发肿 【jīng bì fā zhǒng】经闭之后发生肢体肿胀的病证。多因寒湿之

Amenorrhea Accompanied with Edema a condition due to the attack of

邪伤及冲任胞脉，气机不行，水失运化所致。

经刺　【jīng cì】1、指某一经脉有病时，在该经经脉上进行针刺。2、古代针法之一。指针刺与患病局部同一经脉上的阳性反应点。

经断前后诸证　【jīng duàn qián hòu zhū zhèng】指妇女更年期月经将断未断时出现一些综合性病证。症见月经紊乱、烦躁易怒、精神疲乏、头昏耳鸣、手足心发热、心悸失眠等症状。多因肾气渐衰，精血不足，导致脏腑经络失于濡养和温煦。

经方　【jīng fāng】一般指汉代以前医著中所记载的方剂。以张仲景的方剂为代表。

经后吐衄　【jīng hòu tù nǜ】月经后，从口或鼻中出血，量少、色鲜红。多因肺胃虚热未尽，血热不得归经所致。

经尽　【jīng jìn】指病邪在某经传变至尽，而趋向自愈。

经绝　【jīng jué】指妇女到五十岁左右，由于肾气衰，天癸衰竭，冲任胞脉俱

damp-cold to TV and CV during amenorrhea, leading to the dysfunction of qi and accumulation of body fluid.

Puncture the Corresponding Meridian　1. puncture the point of the diseased meridian. 2. one of the ancient acupuncture techniques, puncture the positive reflecting points along the corresponding meridian of the diseased part.

Menopausal Syndrome　a syndrome occurring during menopause, manifested as irregular menstruation, irritability, fatigue, dizziness, tinnitus, palpitation, insomnia, etc., due to disnourishment of organs and meridians resulting from deficiency of kidney-qi and the insufficiency of essence and blood.

Classical Prescription　the prescriptions recorded in the medical works before Han dynasty, those of Zhang Zhong Jing as the representative.

Epistaxis and Hematemesis after Menstruation　a condtion which is caused by the retention of asthenic heat in the lung and stomach, the blood heat forces the blood circulation out of the vessels.

Transmission to the End of the Meridian　referring to the pathogenic factor is transmitted to the end of a meridian, and the patient tends to recover.

Menopause　cessation of menstruation in the female occurring usually at

虚，致月经停止的生理现象。about the age of fifty, a physiological phenomenon due to deficiency of the kidney qi, exhaustion of Tiangui and debility of TV, CV and Bao vessel.

经来浮肿 【jīng lái fú zhǒng】月经来潮时颜面和下肢出现轻度浮肿。多因脾虚水湿不化，泛溢肌肤而致。 **Edema during Menstruation** edema of face and lower limbs during menstruation caused by retention of fluid in the body resulting from the spleen deficiency.

经来狂言谵语 【jīng lái kuáng yán zhān yǔ】（经行发狂）月经期间出现的精神状态，如烦躁易怒，或者狂言乱语等。多因经来肝气逆乱，血随气逆上攻于心所致。 **Mania during Menstruation** a mental disorder manifested as irritability or mania during menstruation due to up-going of blood along with qi to the heart resulting from disturbance of the liver-qi.

经来呕吐 【jīng lái ǒu tù】月经来潮期间，发生呕吐的症状。多因脾胃虚弱，水饮食积停滞，胃气上逆所致。 **Vomiting during Menstruation** a condition due to deficiency of the spleen and stomach leading to the retention of fluid and indigestion and adverse rising of the stomach-qi.

经络 【jīng luò】人体气血运行的通道，包括经脉和络脉两部分，其中直行干线称为经脉，由经脉分出网络全身各个部位的分支称为络脉。通过经络系统的联系，人体内外、脏腑、肢节联成为一个有机的整体。 **Meridians and Collaterals** a passage along which qi and blood travel including meridians, which is direct route, and collaterals which is branches from direct line to every parts of the body, its function is connecting viscera with extremities, communicating the interior with the exterior, regulating the function of organs, joining the body to build up an organic entity.

经脉 【jīng mài】是联系人体各部分及运行气血的主要干线。 **Meridians and Vessels** the main passage connecting different parts of the body in which qi flows and blood circulates.

经气 【jīng qì】指运行于经脉中的气。 **Meridian-Qi** qi circulating in the

它包括经脉的功能和经脉中流动着的营养物质。是整体生命功能的表现。

经如虾蟆子 【jīng rú xiā má zǐ】(经来下血胞、经来下肉胞)相当于葡萄胎。已婚育龄妇女在停经后二至四个月间,反复发生不规则的阴道出血,往往排出水泡状物如虾蟆子样。

Hydatidiform Mole an abnormal pregnancy resulting from a pathologic ovum of a mass of cysts resembling a bunch of grapes, accompanied with irregular vaginal bleeding.

经行发热 【jīng xíng fā rè】(经来发热)在月经期间表现有发热的症状。多因感受风邪或血虚所致。

Fever during Menstruation a condition usually due to attack of pathogenic wind or blood deficiency.

经行后期 【jīng xíng hòu qī】(经期错后、经期落后)月经来潮比正常周期推迟一周以上者。

Delayed Menstrual Cycle menstruation occurring later for more than one week at every cycle.

经行衄血 【jīng xíng nù xuè】(倒经)指在月经期间合并有鼻中流血、兼见头痛胁疼、口苦、咽干等证。多因肝郁化火犯肺或阴虚肺热、损伤络脉所致。

Retrograd Menstruation epistaxis during menstruation accompanied with hypochondriac pain, headache, bitter taste in the mouth, dry throat, etc, due to attack of fire transmitted from stagnation of qi in the liver, or due to impairment of collaterals by yin-deficiency and lung-heat.

经行吐血 【jīng xíng tù xuè】经行时周期性的吐血或经血量减少。多因积热损伤胃络所致。

Hematemesis during Menstruation a morbid condition accompanied with scanty menstruation, due to impairment of stomach collacterals by the accumulation of heat.

经行先后无定期 【jīng xíng xiān hòu wú dìng qī】指月经来潮或提前或错后,经期表现不规律。多因肝郁、肾虚致气血不和、冲任不调引起。

Irregular Menstruation the menstruation which does not occur at normal regular intervals, due to disharmony of qi and blood, dysfunction of TV anc CV caused by stagnation of the liver-qi or kidney deficiency.

经行先期 【jīng xíng xiān qī】(经期超

Preceded Menstrual Cycle men-

前、月经先期）指月经来潮比正常周期提前一周以上者。

经行泄泻 【jīng xíng xiè xiè】月经来潮期间，大便次数增多，伴神疲食减、腹胀或浮肿。多因脾肾素虚，当经行之时，脾肾更虚，水湿自盛，影响脾胃消化吸收而致。经期过后，常自行恢复正常。

经证 【jīng zhèng】伤寒病分类法之一。指伤寒病邪在其经的证候。如太阳病的恶寒、头痛、发热；阳明病的身壮热、烦渴、自汗；少阳病的寒热往来、心胸烦闷，均属经证。

惊风 【jīng fēng】四肢抽搐和意识不清的病证，一至五岁的幼儿多见。见急惊风及慢惊风。

惊膈嗽 【jīng gé sòu】小儿患惊风，惊止而嗽作。多由风热挟痰，壅逆于肺所致。

惊后瞳斜 【jīng hòu tóng xié】小儿惊风后，眼球斜向一侧。多属肝经阴血受损，目系失养所致。

惊积 【jīng jī】小儿积食化热，热极生风。多由于饮食不节所引起。症见腹

struation occurring earlier for more than one week at every cycle.

Diarrhea during Menstruation a disorder usually accompanied with fatigue, poor appetite, flatulence, or edema, which subsides spontaneously after menstruation; due to impairment of digestive function by the damp resulting from deficiency of the spleen and kidney aggravated by menstruation.

Meridian Syndrome syndrome of an exogenous febrile disease reflecting the meridian involved, e. g., chilliness, headache, and fever in taiyang meridian disease; high fever, severe thirst, spontaneous perspiration in yangming meridian disease; episodes of chill and fever, feeling of oppression over chest in shaoyang meridian disease.

Infantile Convulsion a disease usually seen in infants of 1-5 years of age, marked by sudden onset of convulsion accompanied with loss of consciousness.

Cough after Convulsive Attack a symptom due to retention of wind-heat blending with phlegm in the lung.

Strabismus after Convulsive Seizure a disorder due to disnourishment of eye resulting from impairment of yin-blood in the liver meridian.

Convulsion due to Indigestion a morbid condition due to the produc-

胀肠鸣、低烧潮热而以午后夜间为甚、睡眠不安、烦躁易惊，甚则手足抽搐、大便干燥秘结或稀稠酸臭等。

tion of interior wind factor by the overabundance of heat, usually caused by imporper diet followed by retention of food in the stomach, marked by abdominal fullness, frequent borborymus, lower grade or hectic fever at night, insomnia, irritability, timidness or even convulsion, constipation or loose stool with foul odour.

惊厥 【jīng jué】指发作性肌肉抽搐和意识不清的一种证候。多因感受温热病邪，热盛风动；或热病伤阴，虚风内动所致。多见于小儿。

Convulsion and Syncope a state marked by paroxysm of involuntary muscular spasm accompanied with loss of consciousness, which is caused by the hyperactivity of wind resulting from the attack of virulent heat, or by the attack of asthenia-wind resulting from the over comsumption of yin in febrile disease usually seen in children.

惊痢 【jīng lì】指小儿受惊而致的下利腹泻。症见腹痛、便下青色稠粘、心烦不食。多由外受惊恐、肝气逆乱、阻滞气机、湿浊内停，下注肠道所致。

Diarrhea after being Frightened a disorder occurring in a frightened child due to disturbance of the liver-qi, stagnation of qi, and accumulation of dampness in the intestines, marked by abdominal pain, diarrhea with greenish and viscous stool, restlessness, loss of appetite, etc.

惊热 【jīng rè】小儿遍身发热，但不太高。颜面有时发青、身上有汗，夜间烦躁多惊、心悸不宁。

Fever due to Frightening a disorder in infants marked by moderate fever, cyanosis, sweating, and restlessness or palpitation at night.

惊伤胁痛 【jīng shāng xié tòng】指因受惊伤及肝气所致的胁痛。

Hypochondriac Pain due to Frightening a condition due to impairment of the liver-qi resulting from fright.

惊水 【jīng shuǐ】指小儿受惊后引起的水肿。由于小儿神气怯弱，元气未

Edema Resulting from Frightening edema occurring in frightened in-

充，易于受惊，致脏腑功能失调，水湿停留引起水肿。

惊瘫 【jīng tān】指惊风后四肢瘫痪。因风毒流入经络、骨节而成。

惊啼 【jīng tí】（胎惊夜啼）指小儿啼哭惊惕的病状。由于小儿肝气未充，胆气怯而易惊所致。饮食不节、哺乳不当或感受风寒也可引起。

惊痫 【jīng xián】1、指急惊风发作。2、指小儿痫证的类型之一。3、泛指惊风、痫证等。

惊则气乱 【jīng zé qì luàn】大惊引起心气紊乱，气血失调的病理。症见心悸、失眠、心烦，甚则精神错乱等。

惊者平之 【jīng zhě píng zhī】惊悸怔忡，心神慌乱的一类病症，可用重镇安神法或用养心安神法以平定之。

惊震内障 【jīng zhèn nèi zhàng】（惊震翳）因眼受到剧烈震击、穿刺，或热、电等损伤，致使睛珠变混而成内障。相当于外伤性白内障。

睛，【jīng】1、指眼球。2、指视觉功

fants due to dysfunction of viscera and retention of body fluid. The infants are liable to be frightened since the spirit and qi are relatively weak, and their primordial qi is not strong.

Paralysis of Extremities Occurring after Convulsive Seizure a disorder due to virulent wind attacking meridians and joints.

Night Cry due to Frightening a condition seen in infants whose liver-qi is immature and gallbladder qi is insufficient, caused by improper diet or exposure to wind-cold factors.

Convulsive Disease 1. acute onset of infantile convulsion. 2. a type of infantile epilepsy 3. generally referring to convulsion, epilepsy, etc.

Terror may Lead to Disorder of Qi a morbid condition of disorder of heart-qi and disharmony of qi and blood, caused by terror; manifested as palpitation, insomnia, restlessness, or even mental confusion, etc.

Frightened Patient should be Calmed a therapeutic principle. The case manifested as mental comfusion and restlessness after being frightened should be treated by the means of sedatives of heavy weight or sedatives of nourishing heart.

Traumatic Cataract cataratic following an injury, such as blow, piercing, heat, electricity, etc.

Jing 1. eyeball 2. visual function.

能。

精 【jīng】 是构成和维持人体生命活动的基本物质,包括先天之精和后天之精。

精巢 【jīng cháo】 即眼。因为机体五脏六腑的精华皆上注于眼,从而使眼保持正常的功能。所以说,眼为精之巢。

精气夺则虚 【jīng qì duó zé xū】 在疾病过程中,正气过分消耗,则表现为虚证。症见面色苍白、神疲体倦、心悸、气短、脉细弱无力等。

精窍 【jīng qiào】 男性尿道口。

精明之府 【jīng míng zhī fǔ】 指头部。五脏六腑的精华都上会于头部,诸髓之精也上聚于头部,所以,头部是精髓神明之府。

精神内守 【jīng shén nèi shǒu】 指精气内存,神不妄动,以保持充沛的正气,从而可以抗拒病邪的伤害。

精微 【jīng wēi】 指精华微细的富有营养价值的物质。与水谷之精涵义相同。

精血同源 【jīng xuě tóng yuán】 见肝肾同源。

精汁 【jīng zhī】 (胆汁) 因胆汁具有帮助消化的作用,属于精华物质,故

Essence of Life fundamental substances constituting the body and maintaining the life activity, including both the congenital and aquired essence.

Essence Nest referring to the eyes. The essence of the internal organs all ascend to the eye so as to keep its normal function.

The Consumption of Healthy-Qi Brings about Asthenia a deficient syndrome due to overconsumption of healthy qi during the process of disease, manifested as pale complexion, lassitude, palpitation, shortness of breath, small and weak pulse, etc.

Orifice of Semen Discharge external orifice of male urethra.

The House of Essential Substance referring to the head. The essence of the viscera and marrows all gather in the head.

Keeping the Spirit in the Interior a state capable of protecting the body from the damage of pathogens, which is accomplished by keeping the peace of mind.

Refined Substance the fine and nutritious substance, the same with essenital substance derived from food.

Essence and Blood are Derived from the Same Source see the liver and kidney originate the same source.

Refined Juice bile, so called because it aids in digestion and is attributed to

称。

井疽 【jīng jū】位于腹上角处（鸠尾穴与中庭穴之间）的无头疽。

颈痈 【jǐng yōng】指痈生于颈部两侧，小儿较为常见。由外感风温，三焦郁火上攻所致，症见恶寒发热，头痛项强，颈部结块形如鸡卵，漫肿热痛。化脓时皮色较红，疼痛加重，核块变软，有应指感。辨证分类：1、风热痰毒证 2、肝郁痰火证 3、湿热蕴结证 4、热胜酿脓证 5、余毒凝滞证。

净腑 【jìng fǔ】指膀胱。因其通过排尿而清除废物，故称净腑。

静功 【jìng gōng】（内功）是气功中的一大类功法，它是采取坐、卧、站等外表上静的姿势，通过放松、入静、意守、调息等炼意、炼气等方法，着重锻炼人体内部的精、气、神，以至脏腑经络，气血津液，是一种静中有动的功法。

essential substance.

Cold Abscess on the Lumber Region a deep abscess under the infrasternal notch (between the Jiuwei and Zhongting point).

Neck Carbuncle carbuncles seen on the two sides of the neck, mostly among infants, caused by exposure to wind and damp leading to the upward attack of the accumulated fire in the triple energizer; marked by chills, fever, headache, rigidity of the neck with carbuncles which are as large as an egg and swelling. The skin of the affected area turns into red and the mass becomes soft with more severe pain and finger-resisting sensation. Types of differentiation 1. type of toxicant of wind, heat and phlegm 2. accumulated phlegm-fire in the liver 3. accumulation of damp and heat 4. formation of pus due to excessive heat 5. accumulation of surplus toxin.

Fu Organ for Clearing referring to the bladder. It is so called because the bladder eliminates the wastes through urination.

Static Qi Gong it, also called inner qigong, is one of the categories in qigong, which aims at training essence, qi, spirit of the body, meridians and organs, blood and fluid in the body by means of training mind and training qi, such as relaxation, staticness, concentration of mind, regula-

痉 【jìng】以项背强急、口噤、四肢抽搐、角弓反张为主症的病证。因风、寒、湿、痰、火邪壅滞经络或因过汗、失血、素体虚弱、气虚血少、津液不足、筋失濡养、虚风内动所致。

炅药 【jiǒng yào】指热性的药。

炅则气泄 【jiǒng zé qì xiè】（热则气泄）指由于热则汗出，阳气随汗外泄的现象。

䐃【jiǒng】肌肉的突起部分。如肱二头肌、腓肠肌等。

九窍 【jiǔ qiào】1. 指眼、鼻、耳、口、尿道（或阴道）肛门。2. 指眼、耳、鼻、口、舌、喉。

九脏 【jiǔ zàng】即心、肝、脾、肺、肾、胃、大肠、小肠及膀胱。

九针 【jiǔ zhēn】古代医学使用的九种不同形状和用法的针，即镵针、员针、鍉针、锋针、铍针、员利针、毫针、长针及大针。

tion of breathing, static qi gong can be practised in sitting, lying, standing position and the principle of motion in quiescence should be adhered to.

Convulsive Disease   a disease marked by rigidity of the neck and back, lockjaw, cramps of the limbs and opisthotonos; caused by stagnation of wind, cold, damp, phlegm and fire in the meridians, or due to oversweating, loss of blood, general debility, deficiency of qi, blood or body fluid resulting in muscular malnutrition and asthenia-wind stirring inside.

Medicines of Hot Nature

Fever Leading to Consumption of Qi
  a condition of letting out of Yang-qi along with sweating during fever.

Muscular Prominence   muscles with prominent appearance, such as the biceps, gastrocnemius, etc.

Nine Orifices   1. referring to the eyes, nares, ears, mouth, urethra (or vegina) and anus 2. referring to the eyes, nares, ears, mouth, tongue and pharynx

Nine Viscera   referring to the heart, liver, spleen, lung, kidney, stomach, large intestine, small intestine and bladder.

Nine Forms of Needles   the needles with various shape for different uses in ancient times, i. e., sharp-tip (chan) needle, ovoid-tip needle, blunt-tip needle, three-edged needle, sword-shaped needle, horse-tail-shaped needle, filiform needle, long needle and big needle.

久咳 【jiǔ ké】经久不愈的咳嗽。久咳多痰者,多属于脾虚生痰之症;久咳无痰者,多属肺阴不足之症。

Protracted Cough chronic and obstinate cough; the productive type is considered as the spleen-asthenia, and the non-productive type as insufficiency of the lung-yin.

久痢 【jiǔ lì】指痢疾日久不愈的病证。多因脾胃虚弱,中气不足所致。

Protracted Dysentery chronic and obstinate dysentery resulting from asthenia of the spleen and kidney and insufficiency of qi in the middle-energizer.

久疟 【jiǔ nüè】经久不愈的疟疾。为气血两亏,脾胃虚寒所致。

Protracted Malaria chronic malaria with recurrent attacks, caused by deficiency of both qi and blood, and asthenia-cold of the spleen and stomach.

久热伤阴 【jiǔ rè shāng yīn】热邪稽留不退,灼烁津液,致阴津耗损的病理。症见皮肤干燥、心烦口渴、干咳无痰、舌红干及脉细数等。

Impairment of Yin due to Prolonged Fever a morbid condition of consumption of yin-fluid due to prolonged attack of the heat; marked by dry skin, restlessness, thirst, dry cough, red and dry tongue, thready and fast pulse, etc.

久泻不止 【jiǔ xiè bù zhǐ】即大便泄泻日久不止。多因脾肾阳虚而致。

Protracted Diarrhea a disease caused by the deficiency of spleen-yang and kidney-yang.

久瘖 【jiǔ yīn】慢性进行性发音困难,多属虚症。

Lingering Dysphonia a chronic progressive difficulty in enunciation, usually manifested as an asthenia-syndrome.

灸法 【jiǔ fǎ】针灸疗法的一大类。指用艾柱或艾条在体表穴位上烧灼,熏熨防治疾病的方法。

Moxibustion Therapy a type of acupuncture and moxibustion therapy by employing moxa cone or moxa-stick to stimulate selected acupoints

酒悖 【jiǔ bèi】指酗酒后胡言乱语,行为妄动的状态。

Irritability after Immoderate Drinking a condition of paraphasia with loss of control over one's act after being drunk.

酒疸 【jiǔ dǎn】(酒黄疸)因饮酒过度,湿热郁蒸,胆热液泄所致的黄疸。症见身目发黄、心中懊侬热痛、鼻燥、腹满不欲食、时时欲吐等。

Jaundice due to Immoderate Drinking a disease caused by retention of dampness-heat in the body with extravasation of the bile resulting from immoderate drinking; manifested as icterus of the eyes and the skin, feeling of oppression and burning pain in the chest, dryness of the nasal cavity, flatulence, poor appetite and frequent nausea, etc.

酒剂 【jiǔ jì】药物剂型之一。把药物浸入酒内,经过一定时间浸泡或隔汤蒸煮,滤去药渣,取液服。多用于祛风活血、通络止痛等。

Medicated Wine a form of medicament, a pharmaceutical preparation made by immersion of medicines in wine for a period of time, ususlly applied for expelling wind, promoting blood circulation, dredging meridian and relieving pain, etc.

酒客 【jiǔ kè】平素嗜酒的人。

Drinker a person who has an addiction for drinking.

酒癖 【jiǔ pǐ】1.嗜酒成性。2.指因长期嗜酒致腹部发生肿块的慢性疾病,常伴有消瘦、腹水。类似酒精中毒所致的肝硬化。

1. Alcoholic Addiction 2. Abdominal Mass due to Alcoholism a chronic disease characterized by abdominal mass, emaciation and ascites; similar to alcoholic hepatic cirrhosis.

酒齇(渣)鼻 【jiǔ zhā bí】病名。由脾胃湿热上熏于肺所致,症见鼻准发红,久则呈紫黑色,老者鼻准皮肤变厚,鼻头大。

Acne Rosacea a chronic skin disease caused by the attack of dampness-heat in the spleen and stomach to the lung; marked by red apex nasi or purple one after lasting for a long time even thickened skin of nose and hypertrophic apex nasi

酒胀【jiǔ zhàng】由于经常饮酒，湿热蕴结肝脾，损伤脾胃所致。症见腹胀、尿少、便血等。

Flatulence due to Immoderate Drinking　a disorder caused by alcoholic addiction causing the accumulation of dampness-heat in the liver and spleen leading to impairment of the spleen and stomach; manifested as abdominal flatulence, oliguria and hematochezia, etc.

救里【jiù lǐ】治疗在里的病变。

救脱【jiù tuō】治疗虚脱的方法。分救阳、救阴两种：(1)救阳，见回阳救逆；(2)救阴，常用益气养阴及收敛的药物，治疗亡阴的方法。

Treating the Disorder in the Interior

Treatment for Collapse　a treatment including 1. recuperating the depleted yang 2. recuperating the depleted yin by applying the drugs of supplementing qi and nourishing yin, or astringents

拘急【jū jí】(挛急)四肢、两胁或少腹等处牵引不适或自觉紧缩感，以致影响活动的证候。多因六淫外邪伤及筋脉或血虚不能养筋；或肝气失于疏泄，经络不得通利所致。

Muscular Stiffness　a disorder frequently occurring in the extremitis, hypochondrium and lower abdomen, caused by the attack of six pathogens on muscle, insufficiency of blood failing to nourish the muscles, or the obstruction of meridians resulting from the hypofunction of the liver-qi.

疽【ju】指疮面深而恶者，是气血为毒邪所阻滞，发于肌肉筋骨间的疮肿。可分为有头疽和无头疽两类。

Deep-Rooted Carbuncle　a kind of infection occurring between the muscle and bone, resulting from the stagnation of qi and blood caused by toxic material; classified into carbuncle and deep abscess.

焗服【jú fú】(泡服)对含有挥发油容易出味，用量较少，久煎失效的药物，如肉桂可泡服。泡时用平杯开水或将煮好的一部分药液趁热浸泡。

Infusing　taking drug after soaking it in hot water or decoction, some drugs with essential oil whose effective ingredients being easily decocted out such as Rougui should be taken in this way, for their dosage is small and they will lose their effect if being de-

举按【jǔ àn】诊脉时不同的指力上下测检脉搏的变化的一种方法。

举、按、寻【jǔ àn xún】切脉时用不同的指力和手法侯测脉象的方法。轻指力浮取为举；重指力沉取者为按；中度指力或适当移动手指寻找者为寻。

巨分【jù fēn】鼻唇沟。

拒按【jù àn】疼痛部位因按压而疼痛增剧，患者往往不愿进行按压检查。多属实证。

聚散障【jù sàn zhàng】（聚开障）因肝肾阴虚，虚火上炎所致的一种眼病。症见黑睛生翳、或圆或缺、或厚或薄、痛则见之、不痛则隐、聚散不一，来去无时。

聚星障【jù xīng zhàng】由肝火内炽，风热外侵，风火相搏上，攻于目或肝肾阴虚，虚火上炎所致。黑睛生翳，呈细颗粒状，聚散如星、抱轮红赤，羞明流泪。

cocted for a long time.

Releasing and Pressing by Fingers (for pulse feeling) a method of pulse feeling by exerting light and heavy pressure alternately by the fingers.

Touching、Pressing and Searching by Fingers (for pulse feeling) a method of pulse feeling by exerting different pressure to the pulse. That with light pressure is said to be touching, that with heavy pressure, pressing; and that with moderate pressure or shifting of the finger, searching.

Nasolabial Groove

Tenderness the pain is aggravated when pressing over the afftected part. It is a sign belonging to sthenia-syndrome.

Interstitial Keratitis a type of keratitis resulting from deficiency of the liver-yin and kidney-yin which leads to flaming-up of asthenic fire; manifested as deep deposits in the substance of the cornea, which becomes hazy throughout, varies in size and thickness and appears more apparent during pain.

Punctate Keratitis a condition due to hyperactivity of the liver-fire and attack of wind-heat pathogen involving the eyes, or resulting from insufficiency of the liver-yin and kidney-yin with involvement of the eyes by asthenic fire; manifested as cellular and fibrinous deposits on the posterior

决渎之官 【jué dú zhī guān】指三焦，由于三焦具有决渎（疏通水道）的功能，故名。

The Organ in charge of Water Circulation referring to triple energizer. It is so named because the triple energizer promotes fluid metabolism of the body.

绝汗 【jué hàn】（脱汗）多因气绝、气散或虚极致汗出如珠、如油或冷汗不止的症状。是病危时阴阳离决的见症之一。

Sweating in Critical Stage a condition in danger of death indicating the separation of yin and yang, caused by the exhaustion of qi or extremely asthenic state, marked by profuse stick or cold sweat.

厥逆 【jué nì】1. 四肢厥冷。2. 指胸腹剧痛、两足暴冷、烦而不能食、脉涩的一种疾病。3. 因寒邪犯脑所致的慢性头痛。症见头痛连及齿痛，日久不愈。

Extreme Coldness and Painess 1. coldness of limbs 2. a disease marked by severe pain in abdomen and chest, dead coldness of feet, restlessness resulting in loss of appetite, uneven pulse. 3. prolonged headache radiating to the teeth, caused by cold factor attacking the brain.

厥逆头痛 【jué nì tóu tòng】（脑逆头痛）即寒邪犯脑所致的头痛。症见头痛连及齿痛。

Headache due to Attack of Cold Factor a disease caused by the cold attacking the brain, marked by headache associated with teethache.

厥气 【jué qì】逆乱之气。多因阴阳气血逆乱。或痰浊、食积、剧烈疼痛所致，引起四肢厥冷或突然昏仆等证。

Chaotic Qi a morbid condition caused by the disorders of yin, yang, qi and blood or phlegm, indigestion, severe pain; marked by cold limbs, sudden syncope, etc.

厥心痛 【jué xīn tòng】属阴寒类型的心痛。症见心痛彻骨，背如锥刺，休息时减轻，活动则加剧。并可见手足逆冷汗出、面色青黑无神、善叹息胸腹胀满、两目直视等症。

Precordial Pain of Yin-Cold Type a syndrome marked by stabbing precordial pain radiating to the back, relieved by rest and aggravated by exertion; accompanied with coldness

厥阳 【jué yǎng】 1. 即狐阳。阳气偏盛,阳失阴的涵养所致。2. 飞阳穴别名。

厥阳独行 【jué yáng dú xíng】指阴阳平衡失调,阳气偏胜,阴分不能维系而孤阳上越的病理,是阴阳平衡失调的严重阶段。

厥阴 【jué yīn】经脉名称之一。包括足厥阴肝经和手厥阴心包经。是阴气发展的最后阶段。

厥阴病 【jué yīn bìng】病邪侵入厥阴,累及肝及心包所致的一种病证。临床主要有上热下寒与厥热胜复两类情况。

厥阴头痛 【jué yīn tóu tòng】1. 指伤寒厥阴病头痛。主症为头痛、干呕、吐涎沫、四肢厥冷等。2. 指头痛表现在厥阴经脉循行部位者,常为头顶痛。

厥证 【jué zhèng】(厥) 1. 泛指突然昏倒,不省人事,但大多能逐渐甦醒的一类病证。2. 指四肢寒冷。3. 指癃证之危重者。

of the hands and feet, sweating, dark complexion, susceptible to sigh, fullness of the chest and abdomen, staring eyes, etc.

Jueyang 1. a morbid state of overabundance of yang-qi, with failure of nourishing yang by yin; also named solitary yang. 2. Acupoint Feiyang.

Solitary Existence of Jueyang a severe stage of failure of yin yang equilibrium in which the yang-qi is overabundant, yin can't restrain yang and the solitary yang floats up.

Jueyin yin meridians including the liver meridian of foot-jueyin and the pericardium meridian of hand-jueyin where the yin-qi develops to its final stage.

Jueyin Disease a disease caused by the pathogen attacking Jueyin meridian and involving the liver and pericardium; marked by heat-syndrome in the upper part but cold in the lower or alternative occurence of chill and fever, etc.

Jueyin Headache headache occurring in jueyin sydrome of exogenous febrile disease accompanied with retching, salivation, cold limbs, etc. 2. pain along the jueyin meridian over the head, i, e., headache at the vertex.

Jue-Syndrome 1. a temporary suspension of consciousness 2. cold limbs 3. the severe stage of dysuria.

君臣佐使 【jūn chén zuǒ shǐ】方剂组成的基本原则,是按君臣佐使的规律配合组成。君是指方剂中治疗主证,起主要作用的药物,按照需要可用一味和几味。臣是加强主药疗效的药物。佐是协助主药治疗兼证或抑制主药的毒性和峻烈之性的药物。使是引导各药直达病变部位或调和各药作用的药物。

Monarch、Minister、Assistant and Guide the terms signifying the different effects of the drugs composed of a prescription. The monarch acts as the chief drug for treating the disease and is composed of one or more drugs; the minister serves to intensify the effect of the monarch; the assistant helps to deal with the secondary symptoms or inhibits the potent effect or toxicity of the monarch; and the guide leads the other drugs to the diseased part and balances the effects of the drugs.

君火 【jūn huǒ】(心火)与相火配合,有推动脏腑功能活动的作用。

Monarch-Fire the heart-fire, cooperation with the prime-minister fire to promote the functional activities of the viscera.

皲裂疮 【jūn liè chuāng】因肌肤骤被寒冷风燥所逼,致血脉阻滞,肤失濡养而成,并与经常磨擦、压力、浸渍等有关。多发于手掌、手指尖或足跟、足底两侧,患部皮肤干燥、增厚发硬,有长短深浅不一的裂口,甚者可疼痛、出血。

Chapped Skin a condition resulting from the sudden attack of the cold, wind or dryness leading to the stagnation of blood vessels and the failure of nourishing the skin, and also related to frequent friction, pressure and wetting; commonly seen over the hands and feet. The skin becomes dry, thickened, indurated, cracked and fissured, and may be painful and bleeding in severe cases.

峻下 【jùn xià】使用有强烈泻下作用的药物,攻逐里实的方法。本法适用于邪实而正气未衰的患者。

Drastic Purgation a treatment for the elimination of sthenic factor in the interior by the application of potent cathartics, suitable to the condition when factor is hyperactive and healthy qi of the patient is not exhausted.

咯血 【kǎ xuè】指喉中觉有血腥，一咯即出血块或鲜血。多因阴虚火旺或肺有燥热，血络受伤所致。

开阖补泻 【kāi hé bǔ xiè】针刺补泻手法之一。出针后揉按针孔，使针孔闭阖，不令经气外泄者属补法。出针时摇大针孔，不加揉按，使邪气外出者属泻法。

开噤通关 【kāi jìn tōng guān】治疗中风牙关紧闭，昏迷不省人事的方法。通常是用辛温芳香通窍的药物制成散剂吹鼻。适用于寒闭证。

开痞 【kāi pǐ】理气法之一。用辛香行气的药物，以开散痞结的治法。适用于胸、胁、脘、腹等处胀闷。

开窍 【kāi qiào】（宣窍、醒脑、开闭）开窍通神治疗邪阻心窍神志昏迷的方法。适用于邪盛气实的闭证。通常有凉开、温开之别。

开胃 【kāi wèi】用行气和助消化的药物，增进食欲的治法。

Hemoptysis bleeding from the respiratory tract resulting from the attack of excessive heat pathogen due to yin-deficiency or the dry-heat in the lung to damage the blood collaterals.

Reinforcing-Reducing Methods by means of Open-Close the acupuncture manipulation in which the tonifying effect is attained by pressing the puretnced hole after the needle is withdrawn, in case of letting meridian qi out and the dispersing effects is attained by enlarging the punctured hole during the withdrawal of the needle to let pathogen out.

Relieving Lockjaw and Causing Resuscitation a treatment for apoplexy with trismus and coma by insufflation of the powder made of acrid, fragrant and warm-natured drugs to the nose, applicable to coma of cold type.

Relieving Fullness a treatment for the feeling of fullness in the chest and abdomen with acrid and fragrant drugs for activating qi.

Inducing Resuscitation a treatment for coma caused by obstruction of the heart-orifice by the pathogens, applicable to the sthenia-syndrom of coma when the pathogen is excessive and qi is deficient, usually accomplished by using cool-natured or warm-natured drugs.

Increasing Appetite using drugs of activating qi and digestives to en-

亢害承制 【kàng hài chéng zhì】五行学说内容之一。五行有生化的一面，也有克制的一面。若有生而无克，亢必盛之极而为害。因此，必须抵御亢盛令其克制，才能维持五行的正常运动。临床上常运用这一观点来指导对脏腑病变的治疗。

亢阳 【kàng yáng】即阳气亢盛，多指阴不足，阳气独亢的病理现象。如肝阴虚而致肝阳上亢。

尻 【kāo】骶尾骨的通称。

颏 【kē】下颚的前中部凹隐处。

咳喘 【ké chuǎn】指肺气上逆引起的喘咳。

咳逆上气 【ké nì shàng qì】指咳嗽气喘的证候。因外感六淫或痰饮内停，肺失宣肃所致；或由于肺气虚耗，脾失健运，肾不纳气引起。

hance appetite.

Excess Will Bring Harm if not Restrained one of the principles of the theory of the five elements, which indicates that the five elements have the funtions of promotion and inhibition one another. If they only have the former and lack of the latter, disease may ensue. Therefore the excess should be suppressed to maintain the normal activities of the five elements, clinically, the treatment of disease of the viscera is under the direction of this principle.

Hyperactivity of Yang a pathological phenomenon of excess of yang while yin is deficient, such as insufficiency of the liver-yin leading to hyperactivity of liver-yang.

Sacrococcygeal Region the region overlying the sacrum and coccyx.

Chain the anterior prominence of the lower jaw.

Dyspneic Cough cough or dyspnea caused by the adverse rising of the lung qi.

Cough and Dyspnea Caused by the Adverse Ascending of the Lung-qi a disorder resulting from dysfunction of the lung caused by the attack of the six pathogenic factors or retention of phlegm, or from consumption of the lung-qi leading to failure of descending the qi, and dysfunction of the spleen, or from failure of the kidney in controlling qi.

咳嗽 【ké sòu】以咳逆有声，或伴咽痒咳痰为主症的病证。多因外邪犯肺，或因脏腑内伤涉及于肺引起。辨证分类：1. 风寒袭肺证；2. 风热犯肺证；3. 燥邪伤肺证；4. 痰热郁肺证；5. 痰湿蕴肺证；6. 肝火犯肺证；7. 肺虚证。

咳嗽失音 【ké sòu shī yīn】指咳嗽伴有发音困难的症状。此多因肺阴不足，肺失肃降，音门受累所致。常见咳嗽无痰、痰中带血或咯血、声音嘶哑、舌干而光、脉细数等症状。

咳嗽痰盛 【ké sòu tán shèng】指咳嗽痰多的症状。由于暑湿之邪犯肺或脾虚湿聚及肺失肃降引起。前者咳嗽痰多而稠，后者咳嗽痰质白而粘。

咳（咯）血 【ké (ka) xuè】（嗽血）指

Cough a condition marked by cough with sound or accompanied by itching throat with sputum, mostly caused by invasion of the lung by exopathic factors, or the involvement of the lung due to impairment of zang-fu organs. Types of differentiation 1. syndrome of attacking the lung by pathogenic wind and cold 2. syndrome of invasion of the lung by pathogenic wind and heat 3. syndrome of impairment of the lung due to dryness 4. syndrome of accumulation of phlegm in the lung 5. syndrome of accumulation of phlegm-damp in the lung 6. syndrome invasion of the lung by the liver-fire 7. syndrome of deficiency of the lung.

Cough with Aphonia a disorder caused by the insufficiency of lung-yin and the dysfunction of the lung with the involvement of the vocal cord; marked by none-productive cough or with blood-tinged sputum or hemoptysis, hoarseness, dry and uncoated tongue, thready and fast pulse.

Productive Cough a symptom due to attack of the lung by summer-heat and dampness, in which the sputum is copious and thick; or caused by hypofunction of the lung resulting from the asthenia of the spleen and the retention of dampness, in which the sputum is whitish and viscid.

Hemoptysis a condition manifested

咳或咯唾鲜红血色呈泡沫状，常混有痰液的病证。多因外感风邪不解，化热化燥，损伤肺络，或肝火犯肺所致。辨证分类：1.肝火犯肺证；2.阴虚火旺证；3.痰热壅肺证；4.气虚络损证。

by cough with blood or with fresh blood involving foams, mostly caused by repeated attacks of exogenous pathogenic wind causing into heat and dryness which impair the lung collaterals, or flaring-up of the lung by the liver-fire. Types of differentiation 1. syndrome of liver-fire attacking the lung 2. syndrome of yin deficiency and excess of fire 3. syndrome of phlegm-fire attacking the lung 4. syndrome of deficency of qi and impairment of the lung collaterals.

客者除之 【kè zhě chú zhī】治则。凡外来邪气客于人体，应当驱除。如疏风、散寒、清暑、祛湿、消导等法。

Exogenous Pathogens Attacking the Body Should Be Eliminated a principle of treatment for the diseases caused by exogenous pathogens by the application of varies therapies, such as dispelling wind and coldness, clearing summer heat, eliminating dampness or promoting digestion, etc

空腹服 【kōng fù fú】 在空腹的情况下服药，一般指早晚空腹时，如服用治四肢血脉的疾病的药物及驱虫药等。

(Decoction) to Be Taken on an Empty Stomach referring to the time of taking decoction before breakfast or at bedtime, esp. for that treating vascular disease of the limbs and the antihelmintics.

空窍 【kōng qiào】泛指体表的孔窍。包括九窍、汗窍、精窍等。

Hollow Orifice generally referring to the orifice on the surface of the body including the nine orifices, sweat pores, orifice for semen discharge, etc.

恐伤肾 【kǒng shāng shèn】突然或过度的惊恐，可损伤肾气而产生惶恐不安、骨酸痿弱、滑精或小便失禁等症。

Terror Impairing the kidney sudden or great terror can disturb the kidney-qi, resulting in such symptoms as irritability, weakness of the limbs,

恐则气下【kǒng zé qì xià】肾藏精，司二便，恐惧过度，则伤肾气，出现二便失禁、遗精、滑泄等正气下陷的病证。

Terror Causing Sinking of Qi the kidney stores essence and is in charge of urination and defecation, great fright can injure the kidney-qi, which leads to some symptoms of sinking vital-qi, such as urinary and fecal incontinence, nocturnal emission, etc.

控脑痧【kòng nǎo shā】1.鼻中流出臭黄水，伴有嗅觉减退，偶有小量鼻出血。相当于萎缩性鼻炎。多因湿热郁结所致。2.指鼻渊重症。

Atrophic Rhinitis 1. a chronic inflammation of the mucous membrane of the nose, manifested as foul, yellowish nasal discharge, accompanied with impairment of smell and occasional bleeding; which is caused by the accumulation of damp-heat. 2. Serious Case of Nasosinusitis

芤脉【kōng mài】脉浅表大而柔软，按之有空虚感的一种脉象。

Hollow Pulse a pulse which is superficial, large and soft, with a hollow feeling while pressing.

口【kǒu】七窍之一。包括唇、舌、齿、腭等部分，通过咽部与食道相连，为脾之外窍。口腔是经脉循行的要冲，大肠、胃、脾、心、肾、三焦、胆、督、任、冲等经脉都循行于此。

Oral Cavity one of the seven orifices, including the lips, tongue, teeth and palate. It connects with the esophagus through the pharynx and is closely related to the function of the spleen. The meridians of the large intestine, stomach, spleen, heart, kidney, triple energizer, gallbladder, GV, CV and TV pass through the mouth.

口不仁【kǒu bù rén】表现为口舌麻木、味觉减退的症状。可见于中风、脾胃积滞等病。

Numbness of Mouth a condition marked by numbness of the tongue and mouth and decrease of taste; seen in apoplexy, indigestion, etc.

口疮【kǒu chuāng】指口腔内粘膜发生红肿或散在小疮，或有糜烂、破溃、流涎、疼痛，可伴有发热，颔颐下淋巴结肿大的病证。发病多与饮食失调

Aphtha a morbid state firstly manifested by redness and swelling of the mucous membrane of the mouth, or scattered aphthae, or erosion, ulcera-

或发热疾患有关。辨证分类：1. 脾胃积热 2. 心火上炎 3. 虚火上浮。

口唇险症 【kǒu chún xiǎn zhèng】危重证在口唇的反映。即口唇反卷、口张气微、口如鱼口、颤摇不定、口不能闭等。

口淡 【kǒu dàn】指口内有淡而无味的感觉，多属脾胃虚。

口疳风 【kǒu gān fēng】（舌生泡）即舌体下生白泡，大小不一，数个连绵而发，伴脉虚无力。

口苦 【kǒu kǔ】感觉口中有苦味，多属实热症的表现。多因肝胆有热，胆气蒸腾而致。

口苦咽干 【kǒu kǔ yān gān】指口中有苦味，咽喉干燥。多由肝胆积热，胆火上炎，灼伤津液所致。常见于少阳实热证患者。

tion, salivation pain perhaps accompanied by fever, enlargement of the submaxillary lymph nodes, mostly caused by improper diet, or diseases with fever. Types of differentiation 1. accumulation of heat in the spleen and stomach 2. flaring-up of the heart-fire 3. upward attack of the fire of deficiency type

Critical Condition Reflected by the Lips and Mouth including abnormal crimping of lips, mouth opened with weak breathing, mouth as that of the fish, trembling of the lips, mouth with inability to close, etc.

Flat Taste in the Mouth referring to the feeling of tastlessness in the mouth. It is usually a sign of deficiency of the spleen and stomach.

Blisters of the Tongue recurrent occurence of blisters of various size on the low surface of the tongue accompanied with feeble and weak pulse.

Bitter Taste in the Mouth a condition usually referring to the sthenia heat syndrome caused by the adverse rising of gallbladder-qi resulting from the retention of heat in the liver and gallbladder.

Bitter Taste and Dry Throat a symptom usually caused by consumption of body fluid resulting from the accumulation of heat in the liver and gallbladder and flaring-up of the gallbladder-fire; it is mostly seen in the patients suffering from shaoyang sthenia-heat syndrome

口糜 【kǒu mí】 口腔有白色糜腐，形如苔藓状溃疡的病证，多因阳旺阴虚，膀胱湿热内郁，热气熏蒸而致。

Erosion of Mucous Membrane of the Oral Cavity a disease manifested as white muscus like ulcers in the oral cavity, which is caused by steaming and fuming of heat resulting from damp-heat retention in bladder or steaming by heat pathogen.

口软 【kǒu ruǎn】 五软之一。症见唇淡、咀嚼无力、时流清涎。多由脾胃气虚所致。

Weakness of Oral Muscles in Infant a disease of under development of infants due to deficiency of the spleen qi and stomach qi; marked by pale lips, powerlessness, mastication, salivation, etc.

口酸 【kǒu suān】 病人自觉口有酸味，多因消化不良所致。

Sour Taste in the Mouth a condition usually due to indigestion.

口甜 【kǒu tián】 （口甘）即口内常觉甜味，多因湿热郁积于脾胃所致。

Sweet Taste in the Mouth a condition caused by the accumulation of dampness-heat pathogen in the spleen and stomach.

口咸 【kǒu xián】 病人自觉口中有咸味，多属肾虚，是肾液上乘引起。

Salty Taste in the Mouth a condition resulting from the ascending of kidney-fluid which is ususlly caused by insufficiency of the kidney.

口眼歪斜 【kǒu yǎn wāi xié】 由于经脉空虚，风邪乘袭所致的面部外形特征性改变。表现为口角下垂及眼裂增宽而不闭合。常见于面瘫，中风等。

Distortion of the face characteristic changes of the face due to insufficiency of meridians and attack of wind pathogen, marked by dropping of the corner of the mouth and widening of the palpebral fissure with inability of eye closure, often seen in facial paralysis and apoplexy, etc.

口中和 【kǒu zhōng hé】 口不燥不苦，食而知味，表示胃阴恢复，胃气正常。

Normal Sensation of the Mouth a condition of feeling neither dry nor bitter in the mouth with normal taste, which is the signifying normal

口中无味 【kǒu zhōng wú wèi】口中淡而无味,往往兼有食欲不佳。常见于脾胃寒湿和肾气虚弱的患者。

枯痦 【kū pēi】白痦的一种。即白色晶亮的皮疹失去光泽变成枯白色,常是气阴枯竭的征象。

枯痔法 【kū zhì fǎ】用枯痔药物敷在痔核上;或用枯痔注射剂注射于痔核内,使痔核干枯、坏死、脱落的方法。适用于脱出性的内痔。

苦寒清气 【kǔ hán qīng qì】用苦寒的药清气分热邪的一种治疗方法。常用于热邪侵入气分,症见发热不恶寒、口渴汗少、小便黄、舌质红、苔黄、脉数等。

苦寒清热 【kǔ hán qīng rè】(苦寒泄热)即用苦寒的药物清除里热的方法。常用于里热重者,症见烦躁不安、甚则发狂、小便红或吐血、发斑、干呕、舌苔黄或干黑起刺、脉沉数有力等。

stomach qi and stomach-yin.

Flat Taste in the Mouth a symptom usually accompanied with poor appetite, seen in the case of cold-dampness of the spleen and stomach, and deficiency of the kidney-qi.

Dried Sudamina sudamina with deadly white and lusterless appearance, indicative of exhaustion of qi and yin.

Necrotizing Therapy for Hemorrhoids a treatment for the prolapsing internal hemorrhoids by topical application or local injection of necrotizing drugs to make it dry and necrotic, and dropping finally.

Applying Drugs of Bitter Taste and Cold Nature to Eliminate Heat at Qifen a treatment for eliminating heat at qifen; usually applied in the case marked by fever without chilliness, thirst, scanty sweat, yellowish urine, red tongue with yellowish coating, fast pulse, etc.

Clearing Away Heat Pathogen with Drugs of Bitter Taste and Cold Nature a treatment for the serious case of heat pathogen accumulation in the interior by the application of drugs of bitter taste and cold nature, suitable to the case marked by irritability of mania, reddish urine, hematemesis, skin eruptions, retching, yellowish or dark and rough tongue coating, sunken and fast forceful pulse.

苦寒燥湿 【kǔ hán zào shī】用苦寒的药物，祛除湿热病邪的方法。常用于肠胃湿热者，症见腹痛腹胀、大便稀薄而臭、舌苔黄腻等。

Drying Damp Pathogen with Drugs of Bitter Taste and Cold Nature a treatment for the elimination of damp-heat pathogen in the middle energizer by the application of drugs of bitter taste and cold nature, which is suitable to the case with retention of damp-heat in stomach and intestines, which is manifested as abdominal pain, flatulence, thin and foul stools, yellowish and greasy tongue coating.

苦温平燥 【kǔ wēn píng zào】用苦温宣肺透表的药物，治疗外感凉燥表证的方法。适用于偏寒燥邪在表症见怕冷无汗、头微痛、鼻塞流清涕、咳嗽痰清稀、唇燥咽干、苔薄白等。

Treating Dryness-Syndrome with Drugs of Bitter Taste and Warm Nature a treatment for the superficies-syndrome resulting from cold-dryness pathogen by applying bitter and warm-natured drugs with the action of dispersing the stagnated lung-qi and superficies, applicable to the case marked by chillness, anhidrosis, mild headache, stuffy nose, sniveling, cough with sputum, dry lips and throat, thin white tongue coating, etc.

苦温燥湿 【kǔ wēn zào shī】用苦温的药物，祛除寒湿病邪的方法。常用于寒湿阻于中焦，症见胸闷呕吐、恶心、腹胀、大便清稀、苔白腻等。

Drying the Damp Pathogen with Bitter and Warm-Natured Drugs a treatment for the disease with cold-damp pathogen stagnated in the middle energizer by the application of bitter and warm natured drugs, suitable to the case manifested as feeling of oppression in the chest, vomiting, nausea, flatulence, discharge of loose stool, greasy and white tongue coating, etc.

胯痈 【kuà yōng】指生于腹股沟处的

Acute Inguinal Pyogenic Lymphadeni-

痈。其基本病因，临床表现及辨证分类同颈痈。

狂 【kuáng】因七情郁结，五志化火，痰蒙心窍所致的精神病。症见过度兴奋、狂妄自大，甚至怒骂号叫、胡言乱语、舌红苔黄腻等。

狂言 【kuáng yán】言语粗鲁狂妄，失去理智控制的一种病状。多由心火炽盛引起，属实证。

揆度奇恒 【kuí dù qí héng】在检查和诊断时，要善于观察一般的规律和特殊的变化，才能正确地判断病情。

溃疡 【kuì yáng】指疮疡溃破后的创面，尤其是日久难于愈合者。

溃疡不敛 【kuì yáng bù liǎn】痈疽溃者，毒去而肌肉不生，形成溃疡，长期不愈合。多由气血虚衰或治疗失当所致。

阑门 【lán mén】指大、小肠交界的部位。

烂疔 【làn dīng】由皮肤破损染毒或湿热火毒蕴蒸肌肤而发。多见于手足

tis a morbid condition whose etiology, clinical manifestations and type of differentiation are the same of those with neck carbuncle.

Mania a kind of mental disease resulting from emotional depression and obstruction of the orifice of the heart by phlegm, characterized by hyperirritability, megalomania, irrational rage and shouting, overtalkativeness, red tongue with yellowish and greasy coating, etc.

Ravings a sign of sthenia-syndrom caused by overabundance of heart-fire, marked by wild talking with loss of mental control.

Observing both the General and Special Aspects a general rule of physical examination, by which the patient is examined carefully for the changes concerning both general and special aspects, so as to make correct diagnosis.

Ulcer local defect or excavation of the surface of tissues produced by sloughing of inflammatory necrotic tissue.

Chronic ulcer a superficial ulcer occuring as sequelae of a ruptured, unhealed carbuncle; resulting from deficiency of qi and blood or improper treatment.

Ileocolic Opening juncture of the large intestine and small intestine.

Gas Ganrence a morbid condition due to invasion of exogenous toxins

部，初起患处胀痛，周围呈暗红色，迅速蔓延成片，继则疼痛剧烈，患肢水肿、皮肤出现水泡，溃后流出淡黄色浆水，皮肉腐坏，周围转为紫黑色，疮面略有凹形，可伴有寒战、高热、头痛、神昏。舌质红绛，苔黄焦糙，脉洪滑数，相当于气性坏疽。辨证分类：1. 湿火炽盛证；2. 毒入营血证。

through skin wound, or the steaming of muscles and skin by toxins of damp and heat, mostly seen on feet and hands, firstly swelling of the affected area with the surrounding area dark red in color, which extends rapidly with severe pain and edema of the affected limb and skin blisters which, later, become ulcerated with light yellowish serous discharge. The nearby area turns purplish black as the muscle and skin become petrefacted with a pitting wound surface, accompanied by chills, high fever, headache, coma, bright red tongue with yellowish dry coating, and full, slippery fast pulse. Types of differentiation 1. excess of damp-fire 2. invasion of the ying-blood by toxins.

烂喉风 【làn hóu fēng】喉䏲风之一种。以咽喉部肿痛及腐溃，上附灰白色腐衣，伴有口臭、吞咽困难、发热为特点。多因肺胃热毒炽盛，熏灼咽喉所致。

Infective Ulceration of Pharyux a kind of acute pyogenic infection of pharynx characterized by swelling, pain and irregular ulcers of the pharynx, covered with whitish gray membrane, accompanied with fetid odor, dysphagia and fever; due to attack on the throat by the hyperactivity of fire-heat retended in the lung and stomach.

劳复 【láo fù】指病初愈，气虚尚未平复或余邪未清而过度的操劳，使疾病复发。

Relapse of Disease due to Overstrain referring to the early stage of convalescence when qi and blood are not yet restored or the pathogen not yet expelled entirely. The patients usually return to a worse state of health due to overwork.

劳倦 【láo juàn】（劳伤）因七情内伤，起居不节，劳伤脾气，气衰火旺所致的病证。症见困乏懒言、动则喘乏、表热自汗、心烦不安等。

Overstrain　　a morbid condition due to impairment of the spleen qi, insufficiency of qi and hyperactivity of fire resulting from emotional upsets or irrational life, marked by lassitude, exertion, dyspnea, superficial feverishness, spontaneous perspiration, restlessness, etc.

劳淋 【láo lín】遇劳即发的淋症。

Stranguria Induced by Overstrain

劳热 【láo rè】指虚劳发热。主要由气血亏损，或阳衰阴虚等所致。常见骨蒸潮热、五心烦热等症。

Fever in Chronic Consumptive Disease　　a disorder due to consumption of qi and blood, or insufficiency of yang and yin, usually manifested as hectic fever, feverish sensation in the five centres, etc.

劳嗽 【láo sòu】（劳咳、火郁嗽、虚劳咳嗽）指肺劳咳嗽，以及因劳倦、酒色过度、损伤内脏所致的咳嗽。

Cough due to Asthenia of Viscera　　cough resulting from pulmonary tuberculosis, or impairment of viscera due to overstrain, over drinking or frequent coitus.

劳则气耗 【láo zé qì hào】指疲劳过度，气喘、汗出过多等都会使精气耗损，出现倦怠乏力、精神萎靡等证。

Overexertion May Lead to Consumption of Qi　　a morbid condition of consumption of essence and qi due to overexertion, oversweat, dyspnea, manifested as lassitude, listlessness, etc.

劳瘵 【láo zhài】（痨病、痨瘵、痨疰、瘵殗、瘵疟）指病程缓慢而互相传染的一种疾病。症见恶寒、潮热、咳嗽、咯血、饮食减少、肌肉清瘦、疲乏无力、自汗、盗汗、舌红、脉细数等。又指虚损之重症。

Consumptive Disease　　generally referring to a chronic infectious disease manifested as chillness, hectic fever, cough, hemoptysis, poor appetite, emaciation, fatigue, spontaneous perspiration and night sweat, red tongue, thready and fast pulse, etc., also referring to the serious case of asthenia syndrome.

劳者温之 【láo zhě wēn zhī】由于疲劳

Warming the Over-Exhausted　　a

过度或久病之后而致体虚，表现为阳气虚弱，一般应采用甘温药调补。therapeutic principle for treating general debility, e. g., that due to overstrain or prolonged illness characterized by yang-deficiency, should be treated with warm-natured drugs.

牢脉 【láo mài】深沉而弦长有力的一种脉象。多因阴寒积聚所致。**Sunken and Steady Pulse** a pulse condition with sunken, wiry, long and vigorous beats, mostly caused by the accumulation of yin-cold.

痨疮 【láo chuāng】指结核性的疮疡。**Tuberculous Abscess**

老妇行经 【lǎo fù xíng jīng】指妇女五十仍然行经者。若月经按正常规律来潮，且全身无其他疾病表现者，为气血旺盛；若经来较频，一月二至三次，血量反见增多者，多属气虚、肝肾不足、冲任虚损，使血失统摄所致。**Menstruation Continuing after the Climacteric age** menstruation occurring regularly in a healthy woman over 50 may be a sign indicating the normal condition of qi and blood. Profuse menstruation occurring more frequently than once a mouth after climacteric is due to loss of blood control resulting from the deficiency of qi, the liver and the kidney, and debility of thoroughfare vessel and conception vessel.

老黄苔 【lǎo huáng tāi】苔色黄而暗晦。主阳热亢盛。**Rough and Dark Yellowish Tongue Coating** a sign indicating the excess of heat pathogen.

老淋 【lǎo lìn】老人的淋证。多属虚证。**Stranguria in the Aged** usually belonging to the asthenia-syndrome.

老痰 【lǎo tán】多由火邪上熏于上焦，肺气被郁，津液凝而成痰的一种痰证。表现为痰结成粘块汇滞咽间，兼见咽干口燥、咳嗽喘促、面白无华等证。**Lingering Phlegm-Syndrome** a syndrome caused by formation of thick sputum resulting from the attack of fire pathogen and depression of lung-qi; manifested as tenacious phlegm retained in the throat, accompanied with dry mouth and throat, cough, dyspnea, pallor, etc.

烙法 【lào fǎ】用烧红的铁器烧烙患 **Cauterization** a treatment with lo-

处，一般用于已成熟而未溃的皮肤脓疡，使脓液顺利流出，以达到排脓的目的。

雷头风　【léi tóu fēng】多由风邪外袭，或痰热生风所致。其症头面起核块肿痛，或憎寒壮热，或头痛、头中如雷鸣。

肋疽　【lèi jū】生于肋骨的疽。相当于肋骨髓炎、肋骨结核等。多由肝经火毒结聚，气血为毒邪阻滞引起。症见患处肿块如梅李，皮色紫暗或红肿热痛，或疼痛连及肩肘部。

泪　【lèi】五液之一。具有清洁和滋润眼球的作用。辨证论治多与肝有关。

泪窍　【lèi qiào】即泪小管的开口，又叫泪点。

类经　【lèi jīng】医书，卅卷，明·张介宾撰。刊于1624年，是学习和研究《内经》的一部重要参考书。

类消症　【lèi xiāo zhèng】指类似消渴的证候，由中气虚寒，寒水上泛，浮火上游所致。症渴欲求饮，饮一、二口即厌，面赤烦躁等。

cal application of a hot iron, usually applied in the fully developed abscess for the discharge of pus.

Wind-Syndrome over the Head　a syndrome due to attack of exogenous wind pathogen or to wind pathogen resulting from phlegm heat, which is characterized by swelling and pain over the head with skin eruptions or chill and high fever, or headache with thunder-like sounding in the head.

Infection of the Rib　a disease due to stagnation of blood and qi resulting from the retention of toxic fire in the liver meridian, marked by local dark purplish or red coloration, swelling, heat and pain, which may radiate to the shoulder and elbow; seen in osteomyelitis or tuberculosis of the rib.

Tears　one of the five kinds of secretions for cleaning and moistening the eyeball. Its disorder usually associates with the disease of the liver.

Orifice for Tears　lacrymal puncture, the opening of the lacrymal canaliculus.

Classified Canon　compiled by Zhang Jie Bin (1624), including 32 volumes, an important reference book in the study of The Yellow Emperor's Internal Classic.

Diabetes-like Syndrome　a syndrome caused by asthenia-cold of the middle-energizer qi or the upward attack of the cold-dampness pathogen and asthenia-fire; marked by thirst but

类中风 【lèi zhōng fēng】1. 指风从内生的中风病。多由肾阴不足，心火炽盛，肝阳偏亢，肝风内动或气虚，气逆；或血脉痹阻，或湿痰壅盛，化热生风所致，症见猝然昏仆、口眼㖞斜、半身不遂、言语謇涩等，常见于脑血管意外。2. 指类似中风的八种病证。

冷秘 【lěng bì】因脾肾阳虚，阴寒凝结，温运无力所致的大便秘结。症见大便秘结、唇淡口和、四肢不温、腰腹觉冷、喜热恶寒、小便清长、舌胖苔白、脉细无力等。

冷服 【lěng fú】 汤剂煎好后，待冷却后再服用，一般适用于热证。

冷汗 【lěng hàn】1. 指汗出而冷者。多因阳虚不敛所致；也有因热聚于内，或痰证而致者。2. 见阴汗。

desinclination for much drinking, flushed cheeks, irritability, etc.

Apoplexy 1. referring to the unconscious state induced by the endogenous wind pathogen which is caused by the insufficiency of kidney yin, the excess of heart fire, the hyperactivity of liver-yang, the stirring of liver-wind, or by the deficiency of adverse rising of qi, or by the obstruction of blood vessels, or by the overabundance of damp-phlegm producing heat and wind pathogens, manifested as sudden syncope, deviation of the face, hemiplegia, dysphasia, etc. frequently seen in cerebral vascular accident. 2. Apoplectoid Stroke

Cold-Type Constipation a disorder caused by the deficiency of spleen yang, and the stagnation of yin-cold leading to delayed peristalsis; manifested as constipation, pale lips, flat taste in the mouth, cold limbs, cold sensation over the lumbar region and abdomen, desire for heat and intolerance of cold, large amount of clear urine, enlarged tongue with white coating, thready and weak pulse, etc.

Decoction to Be Taken Cool the temperature of decoction suited for the treatment of heat-syndrome.

Clammy Sweat 1. a sign mostly caused by yang-deficiency with inability to keep the body fluid and occasionally due to accumulation of heat in the interior or occurring in

冷淋 【lěng lìn】 1. 由肾虚而寒气客于下焦所致的淋症。2. 指小便频数、尿色如米泔的一种病证。3. 血淋属于下元虚冷者。

冷热疳 【lěng rè gān】（热疳）指冷疳和热疳。一般初起，证候偏于外，偏于热者，称为热疳；病程较长，证候偏于内、偏于寒者，称为冷疳。

冷痛 【lěng tòng】痛处有冷感，局部喜热的症状。为里寒证的表现。可见于胃脘痛、腹痛、痹证等。

冷哮 【lěng xiāo】由外感风寒、寒饮内停，痰浊壅聚，阻滞气道所致的哮喘病。症见呼吸急促、喉中有哮鸣声、咳吐清稀粘痰、胸膈窒闷、面色灰黯、舌苔白滑、脉浮紧等。

phlegm-syndrome. 2. see Yin Sweat.

Cold-Type Stranguria 1. slow and painful discharge of urine due to asthenia of the kidney and retention of cold-pathogen in the lower energizer. 2. a disorder marked by frequent urination with discharge of rice-water urine. 3. stranguria complicated with hematuria, a disorder due to coldness and insufficiency of the lower energizer.

Cold-Heat Infantile Malnutrition referring to cold-type malnutrition and heat-type malnutrition. That of short duration, involving the superficies and manifested as heat-syndrome, is attributed to heat-type malnutrition; while that of long duration, involving the interior and manifested as cold-syndrome, is cold-type.

Cold-Type Pain a sign of interior cold-syndrome, which is associated with local cold feeling and can be relieved by heat; seen in some cases of stomachache, abdominal pain, arthralgia, etc.

Cold-Type Asthema a type of bronchial asthema due to obstruction of the air passage by the accumulation of cold-pathogen, fluid and phlegm resulting from the attack of wind-cold pathogen; manifested as fast respiration with wheezing sounds, cough with discharge of thin and mucous sputum, oppression feeling in the chest, dimmish complexion,

冷心痛 【lěng xīn tòng】(冷气心痛、寒心痛)因心肾阳虚，阴寒内盛所致的心痛。症见心痛暴发、心痛彻背，或痛势绵绵不休，伴有手足厥逆、通身冷汗出、脉沉细无力等。

冷罨法 【lěng yǎn fǎ】罨法的一种。用棉织物浸冷水或冰水后，稍拧干，掩盖在局部。一般用于高热或出血病人。

黧黑斑 【lí hēi bān】由肾亏火旺，血虚不荣，火燥结滞或肝郁气滞所致。发于面部，女性多见。皮肤呈黄褐或淡黑色斑块，形状大小不一，枯暗无光泽，境界清楚，不高出皮肤。

里寒 【lǐ hán】即脏腑的寒证。多因阳气不足或外寒传里所致。症见畏寒肢冷、面色苍白、腰膝酸冷、大便溏泄、小便清长、舌质淡、苔白润、脉沉迟或微细等。

whitish and smooth tongue coating, floating and tight pulse, etc.

Precordial Pain of Cold Type　a disorder due to deficiency of heart-yang and kidney-yang and overabundance of yin-cold in the interior, manifested as a sudden attack or steady occurrence of precordial pain rediating to the back, accompanied with deadly cold extremities, cold sweating, sunken and thready weak pulse, etc.

Cold Compress　a treatment for the case with high fever or bleeding disorder by the topical application of cold, wet pad.

Blackish Patch on the Face　a patch of skin colouration mostly seen in female caused by kidney-asthenia and fire-hyperactivity, blood deficiency, accumulation of fire-dryness or stagnation of liver-qi, characterized by rashes of yellowish brown or blackish colour varying in shape and size, with lusterless appearance and clear margin, but not elevated above the skin surface.

Cold-Syndrome in the Interior　a disorder due to insufficiency of yang qi in the internal organs or invasion of exogenous cold-pathogen to the interior; marked by intolerance of cold, cold limbs, pale complexion, loose stools or diarrhea, polyaria with watey urine, pale tongue with whitish and moist coating, sunken and slow pulse or weak and thready pulse, etc.

里寒格热 【lǐ hán gé rè】 1. 体内阴阳失调，下寒格拒上热。2. 见阴盛格阳。

Heat Being Kept Externally by the Interior-Cold 1. a morbid condition of cold-syndrome in the lower conflicting with the heat-syndrom in the upper, due to the incoordination of yin and yang. 2. see **Yang is Kept Externally by Yin-Excess in the Interior**.

里急后重 【lǐ jí hòu zhòng】 腹痛窘迫、时时欲泻、肛门重坠、便出不爽的症状。多因湿热气滞所致。多见于痢疾。

Tenesmus an ineffectual and painful straining in defecation due to stagnation of qi resulting from the attack of dampness-heat pathogen usually seen in dysentery.

里热 【lǐ rè】指胃肠、肺胃实热或肝胆郁热的证候。多因外邪传里化热或内郁生热所致。症见发热不恶寒、口渴引饮、烦躁口苦、小便短赤、舌质红、苔黄、脉洪数或弦数等。

Heat-Syndrome of the Interior referring to sthenic heat of the stomach and intestine, of the lung and stomach or retention of heat pathogen in the liver and gallbladder, usually due to formation of heat pathogen by exogenous involving the interior or by stagnation of qi; marked by fever without chillness, thirst with desiring for drinking water, restlessness, bitter taste in the mouth, oliguria with reddish urine, red tongue with yellowish coating, full and fast pulse or wiry and fast pulse, etc.

里实 【lǐ shí】1. 外邪化热入里，结于胃肠而正气不虚，出现壮热、烦渴、腹痛、便秘等腹实证候。2. 泛指人体内部气血郁结、停痰、食滞、虫积等。

Interior-Sthenia Syndrome 1. a syndrome due to attack of the exogenous pathogens with formation of heat pathogen accumulated in the stomach and intestines and sufficiency of vital qi in the body, appearing as the sthenia-syndrome of fu organs, such as high fever, thirst, abdominal pain, constipation, etc. 2. generally

里虚 【lǐ xū】脏腑气血不足，功能衰退的一种证候。症见少气懒言、心悸神疲、头晕、食少肢倦、失眠梦遗、舌质嫩、脉虚弱等。

Interior-Asthenia-Syndrome a syndrome due to insufficiency of qi and blood, hypofunction of organs, marked by lassitude, palpitation, fatigue, dizziness, poor appetite, weak limbs, insomnia, nocturnal emission, tender tongue, empty and weak pulse, etc.

里证 【lǐ zhèng】1. 外感病表邪内传入里，已无恶寒症状而出现高热、神昏、烦燥、腹胀、便秘或泄泻、小便短赤、舌苔黄干、脉沉数等。2. 内脏病变与外感相对而言。

Interior-Syndrome 1. a morbid condition caused by the attack of the exogenous pathogens which enter the interior, manifested as high fever, coma, restlessness, fullness of abdomen, constipation or diarrhea, scanty and dark colored urine, yellowish and dry tongue coating, deep and fast pulse, etc. 2. diseases of internal organs, comparing with superficial syndrome.

理气 【lǐ qì】是运用有行气解郁、降气调中、补中益气作用的药物，治疗气逆、气虚的方法。

Regulating Qi a treatment for stagnation, adverse rising or insufficiency of qi with the medicines of activating qi to relieve stagnation of qi, keeping the adverse qi downwards, and invigorating spleen qi.

理法 【lǐ fǎ】推拿手法。即用手握住肢体，一松一紧，自上而下循序移动，多用于四肢部。

Regulating Manipulation a tuina method of grasping patient's limb and moving downward with the rhythem of loosening and tightening.

理血 【lǐ xuè】治理血分病的方法。包括补血、凉血、温血、祛瘀活血、止血等。

Regulating Blood Condition a treatment for xuefen syndrome, including enriching, cooling and warming the blood, removing blood stasis

referring to morbid conditions, such as stagnation of blood and qi, retention of phlegm, indigestion, parasitic infestation, etc.

and promoting blood circulation, stopping bleeding, etc.

理中 【lǐ zhōng】调理中焦脾胃的方法。运用温中祛寒药治疗脾胃虚寒的一种的方法。

Regulating the Middle Energizer a treatment for asthenia-cold syndrome of the spleen and stomach with drugs of warming middle energizer and expelling cold pathogen.

历节风 【lì jié fēng】以关节红肿剧痛,活动受限制为特点的疾病,因风寒湿邪侵入关节所致。

Acute Arthritis a disorder marked by redness, swelling, pain and limited mobility of the joints; caused by the attack of wind, cold and damp pathogens.

立迟 【lì chí】五迟之一,小儿周岁后,仍迟迟不能站立,由于肝肾虚弱或哺养不当,影响筋骨发育所致。

Tardiness of Standing one type of five kinds of maldevelopment marked by infant's inability to stand after one year old, caused by deficiency of the liver and the kidney or improper feeding, affecting the growth of muscles and bones.

立法处方 【lì fǎ chǔ fāng】通过辨证,确定为某种病证后,根据其病因病机和脏腑所属,订立治疗原则,并拟以适用处方。

Formular is Prescribed after the Establishment of the Principle of Treatment prescribing recipes based on differential diagnosis, making certain the reason of the disease and its pathogenesis and the affected organs, and then establishing the principle of treatment.

利湿 【lì shī】用渗湿利水药物,使湿邪从小便排出的方法。

Promoting Diuresis to Eliminate Dampness a treatment usually applying diuretics to eliminate dampness.

利水通淋 【lì shuǐ tōng lìn】治法之一。治疗下焦湿热所致淋证的方法,症见少腹急满,小便深赤,溺时涩痛,淋沥不畅等。

Relieving Stranguria by Diuresis a treatment for stranguria due to dampness-heat accumulation in the lower energizer with symptoms of cramping and fullness sensation of

利小便，实大便 【lì xiǎo biàn, shí dà biàn】治疗因湿邪所致的泄泻的方法，即通过健脾祛湿，使小便通畅，湿邪从小便排出，使大便恢复正常。

沥浆生 【lì jiāng shēng】（沥浆产、沥胞生）相当于在分娩时早期破水。

沥青疮 【lì qīng chuāng】因体质关系，接触沥青而发，以颜面、颈、手指及前臂等暴露部位多见。初起为光泽红斑、灼痛或瘙痒，继则肿胀，皮肤起丘疹和水泡，糜烂、滋水。

疠 【lì】1.疠气，即具有强烈传染性的致病因子。2.指某些烈性传染病。3.指麻风病。

疠风 【lì fēng】即麻风。因津虚感受暴疠风毒，或接触传染，内侵血脉而成。患处麻木不仁，继成红斑，肿溃无脓，久之可蔓延全身肌肤，出现眉落、目损、鼻崩、唇裂、足底穿等症。

栗子痔 【lì zǐ zhì】痔疮外形如栗子，

lower abdomen, deep coloured urine, stranguria, etc.

Anti-diarrhea with Diuretics a treatment for diarrhea due to damp, by promoting diuresis to eliminate the damp through urination by means of invigorating the spleen and eliminating damp pathogen.

Premature Rupture of Amniotic Membrane

Asphalt Dermatitis an acute allergic inflammation of the skin due to the contact with asphalt, usually seen on the exposed parts of the body, such as the face, neck, finger and forearm; marked by bright erythema with burning pain or itching in the affected part at onset followed by swelling, papulation, vesiculation, erosion and oozing.

Pestilence 1. the pathogenic factor with intense infectivity 2. referring to certain virulent infectious disease 3. referring specially to leprosy.

Leprosy a chronic communicable disease caused by attack of blood vessels by pestilent wind pathogen or by direct contact with the etiologic agent; manifested as localized numbness, anesthesia, erythema and ulceration, and later by involvement of all over the body, such as madarosis, eye trouble, depression of the nose bridge, labial fissure, necrosis of the sole, etc.

Chestnut-like Hemorrhoids hemor-

痢风 【lì fēng】指患痢疾后发生的鹤膝风。

痢疾 【lì jí】（注下赤白）因外受湿热疫毒之气，内伤饮食生冷，积滞于肠中所致的疾病。症见腹痛，里急后重，痢下赤白，脓血粘冻，便次增多等，多见于夏秋季节。辨证分类：1. 湿热痢 2. 寒湿痢 3. 虚寒痢 4. 疫毒痢 5. 休息痢。

莲子发 【lián zǐ fā】发背的一种。疮头多突起，形如莲子。即肩胛疽。

莲子疬 【lián zǐ lì】指瘰疬核块簇聚，一包生数十个，形同莲蓬之子。

臁疮 【lián chuāng】（裙边疮、烂腿）多由湿热下注，瘀血凝滞经络所致。多生于小腿内外侧，初起痒痛红肿，破流脂水，甚则腐烂，皮肉灰暗，久不收口，反复发作。辨证分类：1. 湿热下注证；2. 脾虚湿胜证；3. 气虚血瘀证。

rhoids appearing as chestnut, purplish-red in colour, referring to interal hemorrhoids being strangulated.

Dysenteric Arthritis crane-knee arthritis secondary to dysentery.

Dysentery a morbid condition caused by impairment of the stomach due to invasion of epidemic damp-heat or improper intake of raw, cold food, marked by abdominal pain, tensesmus, frequent stools with pus and mucous or stools, mostly seen in summer and autumn. Types of differentiation 1. damp-heat type dysentery 2. cold-damp type dysentery 3. cold-deficiency type dysentery 4. epidemic toxin type dysentery 5. chronic recurrent dysentery.

Carbuncle with Multiple Opening carbuncle over the scapular region composed of many sinuses like a seed-pot of lotus.

Scrofulae in Cluster a lot of scrofulae growing together like the seeds in the seedpod of the lotus.

Ecthyma a morbid condition due to downward drive of the damp-heat and blood stasis in meridians and collaterals, mostly seen on the inner side of the small leg, firstly manifested by itching, pain, redness, swelling, lipid watery discharge, or even putrefaction with the skin and muscles grey in color, difficulty in healing and repeated attacks. Types of differentiation 1. downward drive of damp-heat

敛肺止咳　【liǎn fèi zhǐ ké】收涩法之一。治疗久咳肺虚的方法。症见久咳痰少、呼吸迫促、自汗、口舌干燥、脉数无力等。

敛汗固表　【liǎn hàn gù biǎo】收涩法之一。是治疗表虚或气阳两虚多汗和自汗的方法。常用于气虚自汗或阴虚盗汗等证，临床上往往采用补益药（补气或补阴）和收敛药同用。

敛阴　【liǎn yīn】用酸涩收敛的药物，收敛阴气的治法。

练功反应　【liàn gōng fǎn yìng】是指练功过程中或练功后的自我感觉和正常效应。也包括因练功中掌握功法，运用意念不当所产生的副反应或异常反应。

练功要令　【liàn gōng yào lǐng】是指锻炼各种功法所必须共同遵循的基本要求。主要有：松静自然，动静结合，练养相兼，意气相依，循序渐进等。

2. spleen deficiency and excess of damp 3. qi deficiency and blood stasis

Astringing the Lung-Qi to Relieve Cough　a therapy for chronic cough caused by lung-asthenia, suitable to the case marked by protracted cough without phlegm, dyspnea, spontaneous perspiration, dry mouth and tougue, weak and fast pulse, etc.

Relieving Excessive Sweat and Strengthening the Superficies　a therapy for excessive or spontaneous perspiration caused by insufficiency of superficies or deficiency of qi and yin, by applying tonics (for qi and for yin) and astrigents, indicated in the case with spontaneous perspiration resulting from deficiency of qi, or night sweat due to yin-deficiency.

Retaining Yin with Astrigents　applying sour and puckery flavoured drugs to retain yin, a therapy for the febrile disease when the yin-fluid is exhausted and the pathogen has been relieved, marked by fever subsided, appetite restored, but night sweat.

The Effect of Practising Qi Gong：referring to the self-feeling or normal reaction during or after practice of qi gong, also including side effect or abnormal reaction due to uncorrect method or unfit use of will.

Principle of Practising Qi Going　referring to the basic regulations which mustbe obeyed in practising qi gong, including, being relaxed and

练功杂念 【liàn gōng zá niàn】是指在练功过程中，各种杂乱的念头，纷至沓来，此伏彼起，以致意念不能集中，思想不能安宁，影响了练功的正常进行。

恋眉疮 【liàn méi chuāng】(链眉疮)婴儿出生后，眉间皮肤糜烂、流水、结痂、脱屑，形状如癣，时轻时重、经久不愈。

炼意 【liàn yì】是指气功中的意念锻炼。即如何掌握运用意念，又称用意。

凉血 【liáng xuě】(凉血散血)清热法之一。即清血分热邪的方法。适用于热性病进入血分，迫血妄行。症见吐血、尿血、便血、神昏谵语、舌紫红等。

凉血解毒 【liáng xuě jiè dú】用清热、凉血、解毒的药物，治疗温疫、温毒等热毒炽盛的方法。

static naturally, being both dynamic and static, combining active exercise with inner health cultivation, coordinating the will and qi, proceeding in an orderly way and step by step.

Distraction during Practising Qi Gong being absent-minded during the period of practising qi gong resulting from other thoughts insuminating mind intermittently so as to affect the progress of training.

Eczema Located between the Eyebrows a lingering skin lesion of newbornes marked first by weeping, oozing and crusting and later by scaling and lichenification.

Training Will also called using will, referring to the training of mental activity, mainly involving with the grasping and application of will.

Cooling Blood a kind of therapy for cleaning away heat pathogen in xuefen, suitable to the febrile disease with bleeding, such as hematemesis, hematuria, hemafecia and accompanied with dilirium, dark red tongue, etc.

Cooling Blood and Clearing Away Toxic Material a treatment for the hyperactivity of intense heat pathogen in the case of pestilence and acute febrile disease caused by virulent heat pathogen by the application of drugs of clearing away heat, cooling blood and removing toxic material.

两感伤寒 【liǎng gǎn shāng hán】指阳经和阴经同时感受寒邪而致病。

Both Yin and Yang Meridians are Attacked by Exogenous Cold Pathogen

两胁拘急 【liǎng xié jū jí】指两胁部牵引不舒的感觉。多因肝气郁结或水饮之邪聚结于两胁所致。

Feeling of Contraction over the Hypochondria a symptom caused by stagnation of the liver qi or retention of fluid in the hypochondria.

两虚相得 【liǎng xū xiāng dé】指人体正气发虚,感受虚邪,两虚相合而发病的病因病理。

Deficiencies of Abnormal Seasonal Change and Deficiency of Healthy-Qi Acting on Each Other stimultaneous occurrence of both irregular seasonal changes and insufficiency of healthy qi in the body can easily result in the disease

临睡前服 【lín shuì qián fú】在睡眠之前服药。一般适用于胸膈有积滞者。

Be Taken at Bedtime the time of taking decoction suited for the case with retention-syndrome in the chest.

淋 【lìn】指小便急迫、短、数、涩、痛的病证。多因湿热结聚流注膀胱或中气下陷,肾虚气化无力所致。

Stranguria a disorder marked by frequent, scanty, slow and painful urination, caused by accumulation of damp and heat pathogens in the bladder, or descending of the middle-energizer qi or insufficiency and hypofunction of the kidney.

淋家 【lìn jiā】平素患有淋证的病人。

Patients Suffering from Frequent Stranguria

淋浊 【lìn zhuó】1. 淋证与浊病的合称。2. 性病的一种。症见排尿时阴茎痛,精浊下滴如败脓,有恶臭。

Stranguria with Turbid Urine 1. a syndrome manifested as difficult, slow and painful urination with discharge of turbid urine. 2. a kind of veneral disease, marked by penial pain during urination and purulent, foul discharge from the urethra.

留饮 【liú yǐn】积饮痰饮病的一种。因饮邪日久不化,留而不去。症状可因

Chronic Fluid-Retention Syndrome a disorder resulting from prolonged

留积部位不同而异。如饮停胸膈，可见短气而喘；如饮结经络，可见四肢历节痛。饮留于脾，则腹肿身重等。

accumulation of excessive fluid, consisting of symptoms with the parts affected, e. g., hypochondriac pain due to fluid retention in the hypochondrium can radiate to the clavicular fossa; shortness of breath and dyspnea caused by accumulated fluid in the chest; arthralgia due to fluid in the meridians, fullness of abdomen and heaviness sensation of the body induced by fluid in the spleen.

留者攻之 【liú zhě gōng zhī】病邪滞留于体内，一般宜用攻逐的方法进行治疗。如水肿属水邪滞留体内者，可用逐水的方法。

Retention of Pathogens in the Body Should be Eliminated a therapeutic principle for treating the retention of pathogens in the body, e. g., accumulation of body fluid should be treated with diuretic therapy.

留针 【liú zhēn】得气后，根据病情的需要将针留置穴内不动，经过一定时间再行出针。留针时间的长短可根据病情需要而定。

Retaining the Needle after having got the acupuncture feeling, keep the needle in the acupoint for certain time based on the condition of the patient, then withdraw the needle.

流产 【liú chǎn】指妊娠妇女在胎儿未成活前妊娠中断，由于气血虚弱或肝肾亏损所致。

Abortion interruption of pregnancy before the fetus has attained a stage of viability, caused by deficiency of qi and blood, or insufficiency of the liver and kidney.

流痰 【liú tán】（龟背痰）指骨关节慢性破坏性疾病。多为先天不足，或久病肾阴亏损，骨髓不充，外邪乘虚而入，痰浊凝聚，或跌扑损伤，气血不和而诱发。好发于儿童及青少年。起病缓慢，初起关节酸痛，皮色不变，活动不利，动则疼痛加剧。数月或数年以后，可有寒性脓肿出现，脓肿溃后，脓水稀薄，不易收口。辨证分类：1.

Tuberculosis of The Bone and Joint a chronic destructive disease of the bone and joint, mostly due to congenital deficiency, or impairment of kidney-yin because of long-standing illness, causing insufficiency of bone marrow and invasion of pathogenic factors which further results in stagnation of phlegm, or trauma and

肾虚寒痰证 2. 阴虚内热证 3. 肝肾亏损证。

流涎 【liú xián】（流涎不收）多由脾热或脾胃虚寒所致。

流注 【liú zhù】肢体深部组织的化脓性疾病。多因疮疖感染，跌仆损伤或感受暑湿引起。症见躯干或四肢有一处或相继数处肌肉酸痛漫肿，初起皮色不变，成脓后肿痛显著，皮色转红，按之应指，溃后脓出稠厚，肿痛渐消，疮口愈合。辨证分类：1. 余毒攻窜证 2. 暑湿交阻证 3. 瘀血凝滞证。

流注疬 【liú zhù lì】为瘰疬生于遍身

sprain, disharmony of qi and blood, mostly seen in children or youngsters, manifested by chronic onset, aching of the joints at first, normal skin color, limited movement, more painful on moving, abscess of cold-nature seen several mouths or years later with watery pus discharge when it becomes ulcerated and difficult to heal. Types of differentiation 1. deficiency of kidney and phlegm of cold nature 2. yin-deficiency and interior heat 3. impairment of the liver and kidney.

Salivation a sign of excessive secretion of saliva resulting from spleen-heat or asthenia-cold of the spleen and stomach.

Multiple Abscess a suppurative disease of the deep layer of tissues of the limbs, mostly caused by carbuncles infection, trauma and sprain or exposure to summer-damp, manifested by aching and swelling of one or more places of the trunk or limbs, normal skin color at first, more severe swelling and pain when pus formed with the skin color turning red and with finger-resistent sensation, thick pus discharged after the ulceration with the pain gradually relieved and the wound healed. Types of differentiation 1. attack of retained virulence 2. complicated attack of summer-damp 3. blood stasis.

Multiple Scrofulae suppurative ab-

者。

瘤 【liú】（瘤赘）多因七情劳欲，复感外邪，脏腑失调，聚瘀生痰，随气留滞凝结而成。症见体表出现肿物，界限分明，有的可破溃化脓，病程漫长。

六腑 【liù fǔ】（传化之腑）指胆、胃、大肠、小肠、膀胱和三焦六个器官的合称。

六经 【liù jīng】太阳经、阳明经、少阳经、太阴经、少阴经、厥阴经的合称。

六极 【liù jí】六种因伤所致极度虚损的病症。即气极、血极、筋极、骨极、肌极及精极。

六经辨证 【liù jīng biàn zhèng】《伤寒论》辩证方法之一。根据外感疾病的临床表现，运用六经病理、生理理论加以分析、归纳，以判断病变的部位、性质、正邪盛衰的情况，进而作出诊断。

scesses of lymphnodes all over the body.

Tumor a new growth of tissue which is superficial and well demarcated; and may be ruptured with pus formation; resulting from the accumulation of blood stasis and the production of phlegm, which is collected to form a mass following the stagnation of qi, due to emotional upsets, exposure to exogenous pathogen and dysfunction of the viscera.

Six Fu Organs referring to the gallbladder, stomach, large intestine, small intestine, urinary bladder and triple energizer.

Six Meridians a general term for taiyang, yangming, shaoyang, taiyin, shao yin and jueyin meridians.

Six Extremes of Consumptions six kinds of serious asthenia-syndrome due to overstrain, i. e., extreme deficiency of qi, of blood, of tendon, of bone, of muscle, of essence.

Differential Diagnosis in Accordance with the Theory of Six Meridians one of the Method of differential diagnosis in the Treatise on Exogenous Febrile Disease. i, e., to determine the nature and site of pathological changes and the confliction between the healthy qi and pathogen, based on the analysis and comprehension of the clinical manifestations of the febrile diseases with the theory of pathology and phsiology of the six

六经病 【liù jīng bìng】《伤寒论》把外感热病按其所犯的经络部位、受邪的轻重、病情的进展,归纳为六个不同的证候群,即太阳病、少阳病、阳明病、太阴病、少阴病及厥阴病。

六气 【liù qì】1. 指人体气、血、津、液、精、脉等六种基本物质。2. 指风、热、湿、火、燥、寒等六种气候。

六神之府 【liù shén zhī fǔ】即脑。因它是控制思维活动的高级中枢,故称。

六阳脉 【liù yáng mài】1. 正常脉象之一。两手寸关尺脉象一向比较洪大,但无病态表现。2. 指手足三阳经脉。

六阴脉 【liù yīn mài】1. 正常脉象之一。两手寸关尺的脉象一向比较沉细,但无病态表现。2. 指手足三阴经脉。

六淫 【liù yín】即风、寒、暑、湿、燥、火六种致病因素的合称。

六郁 【liù yù】六种郁证的总称。即气郁、湿郁、热郁、痰郁、血郁及食郁。

Six-Meridian Disease in the Treatise on Exogenous Febrile Diseae, the exogenous febrile disease is classified as six kinds of syndromes, i. e., taiyang, shaoyang, yangming, taiyin, shaoyin, jueyin syndrome, according to the meridians involved, the degree of involvement and the progess of the illness.

1. **Six Kinds of Body Substance** referring qi, blood, saliva, fluid, essence and vessels. 2. **Six Kind of Weather** referring to wind, heat, dampness, fire, dryness, coldness.

Supreme Mental Palace the brain, it acts as the high center controlling the mental activities.

Six Yang Pulse 1. a normal pulse condition with relatively full and large beats over the cun, guan and chi sites of both hands. 2. referring to three yang meridians of hand and foot.

Six Yin Pulse 1. a normal pulse condition with relative deep-small beat over the cun, guan, chi sites of both hands.

Six Factors a general term for the pathogenic factors, i. e., wind, cold, summer-heat, dampness, dryness, fire.

Six Kinds of Stagnation-Syndromes referring to qi stagnation, dampness stagnation, heat stagnation, phlegm stagnation, blood stagnation,

六脏　【liù zàng】指心、肝、脾、肺、肾、心包络或命门。

聋哑　【lóng yǎ】耳聋并口哑，多由热病后遗或先天缺陷所致。

癃　【lóng】（闭癃）1.指小便不利。2.指小便频数。3.淋的古称。

癃闭　【lóng bì】以小便难出，点滴不畅，或小便闭塞不通，小腹胀满为主症的病症。多见于术后、产后及高年男性患者。因肺气壅滞，气机郁结，或脾肾阳虚所致。辩证分类：1.膀胱湿热证　2.肝郁气滞证　3.浊瘀阻塞证　4.脾肾两虚证。

癃疝　【lóng shàn】指少腹引痛睾丸、小便不通的症候。

偻附　【lóu fù】指行走时曲背弯腰，头向下俯的一种体态。常是肾气衰而筋脉虚疲的表现。

蝼蛄窜　【lóu gū cuàn】是流痰的一种。发于前臂及腕部的骨关节，因其内的溃穿头较多，如蝼蛄窜穴，故名。包括前臂及腕关节骨结核。

dietetic stagnation.

Six Zang Organs　referring to the heart, liver, spleen, lung, kidney, pericardium or the life gate.

Deaf-mutism　a disorder resulting from the sequela of febrile disease or congenital defect.

1. **Dysuria** 2. **Frequent micturition** 3. **Straguria named in ancient China**.

Dysuri　a morbid condition characterized by difficult urination with dripping or obstructed urinary discharge with distending and urgent feeling in the lower abdomen, mostly seen after surgical operation or among senile males, caused by stagnation of the lung-qi and yang deficiency of the spleen and kidney. Types of differentiation 1. damp-heat in the urinary bladder 2. stagnation of the liver-qi 3. urethral obstruction 4. deficiency of both the spleen and kidney.

Disuria-Colic Syndrome　a syndrome consisting of colicky pain over the lower abdomen radiating to the testes, and difficulty in urination.

Humpback　an abnormally increased convexity in the curvature of the thoracic spines as viewed from the side, usually due to deficiency of the kidney-qi and muscular weakness.

Tuberculosis of Bone and Joint with Multiple Fistula　a condition mostly seen in the bone of forearm and the wrist.

漏底伤寒【lòu dǐ shāng hán】指外感症初起，洞泄不因攻下而自利者。

Exogenous Febrile Disease with Diarrhea a disease of exogenous febrile disease marked by diarrhea at onset.

漏汗【lòu hàn】汗液漏出不止的现象。多由表证过汗致阳气受伤，卫气不固所致。常伴有小便短少、排尿困难、四肢微拘、关节屈伸不利等症。

Profuse Spontaneous Perspiration a disorder due to impairment of yangqi and dysfunction of wei-qi, usually resulting from the usage of diaphoretics for the treatment of superfical syndrome, often accompanied with oliguria, dysuria, slight stiffness of the limbs, limited movement of the joints, etc.

漏睛【lòu jīng】（眦漏）由心经郁热或风热上攻内眦所致。症见内眦穴处按之脓出，或内眦近鼻隆处起一核，红肿灼痛拒按，生疮成脓。见于泪囊炎。

Dacryopyorrhea a condition due to retention of heat in the heart meridian or attack of wind-heat to the inner canthus, manifested as local erythema, swelling, burning pain, formation of pus in the lacrimal sac; seen in the case of dacryocystitis.

漏疬【lòu lì】为瘰疬破溃成瘘。
漏项【lòu xiàng】为项部瘰疬破溃者。

Perforated Scrofula with Fistula
Perforated Cervical Scrofula

禄食泻【lù shí xiè】（漏食泄）多因脾胃虚弱所致。症见食毕即肠鸣腹急、尽下所纳食物、泻后宽快、经年不愈。

Lienteric diarrhea a chronic disease due to deficiency of spleen and stomach manifested as increased borborygmus abdominal pain and discharge of indigestive food upon ingestion, which are alleviated after diarrhea.

露【lù】把药物放在容器内加水蒸馏，收集所得的澄清透明蒸馏液，称为露。

Distillate a pharmaceutical preparation obtained by distillation of medical solution.

膂【lǚ】脊椎骨两侧的肌肉群。

Muscles along the Spine

绿风内障【lù fēng nèi zhàng】（青光眼）多因肝胆风火升扰；或阴虚阳亢，气血不和等引起。症见瞳神气色浊而

Glaucoma a disease due to attack of wind-fire factor from the liver and gallbladder, or yin deficiency with

不清、散大呈淡绿色、视力减退、眼珠胀痛。yang hyperactivity, or disharmony of qi and blood; marked by opacity and dilatation of the pupils, light green gleam of the eyes, defects of vision and distending pain of the eyeball.

螺疔 【luó dīng】生于手指螺纹处之疔。

Pustule at the Articular Part of the Finger

瘰疬 【luǒ lì】（老鼠疮、疬子颈）指颈部一侧或两侧有单个或多个核状肿块，推之可移，皮色不变，有轻度疼痛，化脓后皮色暗红，肿块变软，破溃后脓液稀薄，夹有败絮样物，疮口久不愈合。多因肺肾阴虚、肝气久郁，虚火内灼，炼液为痰，或受风火邪毒，结聚而成，辩证分类 1. 肝郁痰凝证 2. 阴虚火旺证 3. 气血两虚证。

Scrofula referring to one or more masses which are movable on pushing with normal color and slight pain in one or both sides of the neck. Ulceration occurs when the masses become soft upon palpating and dark red. The ulcerated areas may appear to have purulent substance of dilute quality like bean curd residue. The ulcerated spots are hard to recover. This condition is mostly caused by the action of pathogenic fire consuming the body fluid, resulting from prolonged stagnation of liver-qi and deficiency of lung-qi and kidney-qi, or exposure to toxins of wind and fire. Types of differentiation 1. stagnation of liver-qi and accumulation of phlegm 2. deficiency of yin and excess of fire 3. deficiency of both qi and blood.

络刺 【luò cì】用三棱针刺破皮下小血管放血，以达到治疗目的的方法。

Collateral Puncture a method of treatment by puncturing the subcutaneous small blood vessels with a three-edged needle to cause bleeding

麻疹 【má zhěn】以发热、咳嗽、眼泪汪汪、口腔颊部粘膜上有粟形白点为特征的出疹性疾病。多见于小儿，发病主要在肺胃二经。辩证分为顺证和逆证两大类。顺证又分疹前期（初热

Measles a morbid condition which mainly involves the spleen and stomach meridians characterized by fever, cough, tears in the eyes, white spots shaped like millets in the mucous

期)、出疹期(见形期)和疹回期(收没期)三期;逆证又分毒热闭肺、毒热攻喉和邪陷心肝三型。

membrane on the inner side of the cheek, mostly seen in infants. Types of differentiation, it is usually classified as favourable case and deteriorating case with the former further classed into three stages, incipient stage of measles, rash-eruption stage, and recovering stage, with the latter further divided into three types, 1. toxic heat blocking the lung 2. attack of the throat by toxin and heat 3. invasion of the heart and liver.

麻疹闭证 【má zhěn bì zhèng】指麻疹不能透发,邪毒内闭的证候。症见疹当出而不出、见点不透,或收没太快。多由外感风寒、内热炽盛、饮食积滞、痰湿过盛等导致肺气受阻,腠理闭塞而影响麻疹透发。

Measles Complicated by Retention of Pathogenic Factors measles characterized by delayed incomplete appearance, or precocious subsidence of the skin eruption usually due to attack of wind-cold, accumulation of interior heat, indigestion, stagnation of phlegm-damp leading to retention of lung qi closing of skin pores which effect the eruption of measles.

麻疹喉痛 【má zhěn hóu tòng】麻毒上攻咽喉的证候。多由表邪郁遏,麻毒不能舒发;或里热炽盛,上攻于喉所致。症见咽喉肿痛,甚至汤水难下。

Measles with Sorethroat measles characterized by swelling and pain over throat, due to retention of pathogen in the superficies or hyperactivity of heat in the interior with involvement of the throat.

麻疹逆证 【má zhěn nì zhèng】麻疹患者正虚邪盛,而在各阶段中,病情逆转的各种表现。患者表现为高热、呼吸困难、口唇青紫、出疹不顺利且疹色紫暗、脉洪大疾数,甚或神志不清、烦燥谵语、惊厥抽搐等。

Case of Measles with an Unfavourable Prognosis deterioration of measles due to deficiency of antipathogenic qi and hyperactivity of pathogenic factors manifested as high fever, dyspnea, cyanosis, interrupted eruption with purplish rashes, bounding and fast pulse, or even coma, irri-

麻疹失音 【má zhěn shī yīn】患麻疹出现声音嘶哑。多由热毒闭塞清窍所致。

麻疹顺证 【má zhěn shùn zhèng】麻疹患者，正气充沛而邪毒较轻的表现，患者表现为神气清爽、身热和缓、咳嗽而无呼吸困难，出疹顺利等。病程较短，恢复较快。

麻证齁齁 【má zhèng hōu hē】麻疹呼吸困难，喉中痰鸣的证候。多因痰火炽盛所致。

麻木 【má mù】证名。以感觉减退为特征。多由气血俱虚，经脉失于营养或气血凝滞或寒湿痰瘀留于脉络所致。

马桶癣 【mǎ tǒng xuǎn】对马桶的新漆过敏所致的臀部接触性皮炎。

马牙 【mǎ yá】胎儿受热毒所致的牙龈疾病。新生儿牙龈起白色小泡，妨碍吮乳。

脉 【mài】1. 指脉管，是气血运行的通道。2. 指脉膊、脉象。3. 脉法，见切脉。4. 指女子无月经或月经不调所致的原发性不孕证。

脉暴出 【mài bào chū】原为微细欲绝难以触及的脉象，突然转为短暂的搏

tability, delirium, convultion.

Measles Complicated by laryngitis a disorder due to damage of the throat by the heat toxic factors.

Case of Measles with a Favourable Prognosis measles that occurred in patients with strong antipathogenic qi and attacked by a mild pathogen manifested as prothymia, slight fever, cough without dyspnea, erupting regularly, short course and rapid recovery.

Measles with Dyspnea and wheezing symptoms in measles due to the overabundance of phlegm.

Numbness a disorder marked by hypoesthesia due to disnourishment of meridian resulting from qi and blood deficiency or stagnation of qi and blood in meridian or damp-cold and phlegm accumulating in the vessels.

Contact Dermatitis of Buttock an acute allergic inflammation of the skin caused by contact with the newly lacquer-painted commode.

Gingivitis of Newborn inflammation of the gingival tissue with blisters formation, due to attack of virulent heat factors.

1. **the Vessels through with Qi and Blood Circulate** 2. **Pulse and its Condition** 3. **Pulse Feeling** 4. **Sterility due to Primary Amenorrhea or other Menstrual Disorder.**

Rebeunding of Very Feeble Pulse a phenomenon usually seen in the criti-

动明显的现象,但临床症状却无改善。常是病情危重的表现。

cal condition of a patient, in which the very feeble and impalpable pulse becomes throbbing for a short time, but without the improvement of his critical condition.

脉痹 【mài bì】因脏腑移热于经脉,复遇外邪客搏经络所致的痹证。症见肌肉热极,感觉异常及颜色改变、唇口反裂等。

Meridian Bi-Syndrome a type of bi syndrome caused by the retention of heat factor in the meridians coming from the viscera, associated with the attack of exogenous pathogen to the meridians; manifested as apparent feverishness of the muscles, abnormal sensation and color change of the skin, fissure of the lips and oral mucosa, etc.

脉管 【mài guǎn】(血之府)气血运行的通道。

Vessels the passage along which the blood and qi circulate.

脉合四时 【mài hé sì shí】(脉应四时)指脉象随着四季气候的变化而相应变化的生理现象。

Pulse Condition Corresponding with Seasonal Variations a physiological variation of the pulse condition.

脉会 【mài huì】八会之一。即太渊穴。脉的精气合聚的地方。

Convergent Point of Vessels one of the eight convergent points, i. e., taiyuan point where the essential substances of vessels gather.

脉静 【mài jìng】指脉搏和缓平静,是病情好转的佳兆。

Pulse Calmed the pulse becoming gentle and calm, indicating the convalescence of disease.

脉口 【mài kǒu】即寸口。

The Site of Cun Pulse

脉逆四时 【mài nì sì shí】脉象不能随四季气候的改变而相应变化的病理现象。出现这种情况,往往是身体不能适应四季气候变化的反映。

Pulse Condition Failing to Correspond with Seasonal Variations a morbid condition indicating that the body fails to accommodate to the seasonal variation.

脉微肢冷 【mài wēi zhī lěng】指脉象沉微,四肢厥冷,为阳气衰微的表现。

Weak Pulse and Cold Extremities a condition indicative of deficiency of yang-qi.

脉痿 【mài wěi】（心痿）由于心火上炎，血气随之上逆，下部血脉空虚所致的痿证。症见四肢关节松驰、不能举动、下肢萎软、不能站立。

脉无胃气 【mài wú wèi qì】脉搏失去从容和缓及正常节律，表现出弦劲绷急，坚硬搏指，或浮散无根、杂乱不均等。出现这种脉象往往是胃气将绝，生命垂危的表现。

脉象 【mài xiàng】脉动应指的形象，包括脉搏的频率、节律、充盈度、强弱、幅度及势态等情况。

脉象主病 【mài xiàng zhǔ bìng】脉象变化所提示的病证。如浮脉主表证，沉脉主里证等。

脉阴阳俱浮 【mài yīn yáng jù fú】寸部和尺部都出现浮脉。多因温热病误治，津液受伤，使热邪充斥内外所致。

脉阴阳俱紧 【mài yīn yáng jù jǐn】即寸部和尺部都出现紧脉，常因外感寒邪所致。多见于表实证。

Vascular Flaccidity-Syndrome a type of flaccidity-syndrome due to vacancy of blood vessels of the lower part resulting from the flaming up of heart-fire with the adverse rising of blood and qi, manifested as weakness and dyskinesia of the limbs, and muscular atrophy of the lower limbs with inability to stand up.

The Pulse Loses its Stomach-Qi the pulse condition indicative of exhaustion of stomach-qi and critical state of the patient, manifested as rigid, abrupt, floating without root pulsation instead of its smooth and calm state with regular.

Pulse Condition the sense of fingers when feeling pulse, which is including its frequency, rhythm, fullness, intensity, range and figure, etc.

Pulse Condition Indicating Disease the change of pulse conditions gives a clue to the differentiation of disease, e. g the floating pulse signifying superficies-syndrome, the sunken pulse indicating interior-syndrome.

Both Yin-Pulse and Yang-Pulse Are Floating a floating pulse at both cun and chi sites due to accumulation of heat factor in interior and exterior, resulting from the uncorrect treatment of febrile disease and impairment of the body fluid.

Both Yin and Yang Pulse Are Tense a tense condition at both cun and chi sites usually due to exposure to

脉有胃气 【mài yǒu wèi qì】脉搏往来从容和缓，节律正常，这种脉象往往是胃气尚存，虽病预后常较好。

脉证合参 【mài zhèng hé cān】指辩证过程中，把脉象和症候互相参照，推断病情的方法。

慢肝风 【màn gān fēng】婴儿一月之内目闭不开，或肿胀羞明，或出血。多因心脾蕴热，复感风邪所致。

慢肝惊风 【màn gān jīng fēng】 小儿抽搐，兼有目如橘黄、上视、不乳食、气虚欲脱等。多因泄泻日久，损伤脾胃、肝失营养、虚阳上犯所致。

慢惊风 【màn jīng fēng】抽搐表现为缓而无力，时发时止。体温不高，面色淡黄或青白相间。神疲懒言，大便

the exogenous cold factor, mostly seen in superficial excess syndrome.

The Pulse Has the Stomach-Qi the pulse condition indicative of the presence of stomach-qi and favourable prognosis of a disease, manifested as smooth, calm beats and regular rhythm.

Comprehensive Analysis of Pulse Condition and other Manifestations a diagnostic rule for the differentiation of syndrome by a comprehensive analysis of both the pulse condition and other symptoms and signs.

Chronic Hepatic Wind-Syndrome a syndrome in infants within one month, marked by inability to open the eyes or swelling of eyelids with photophobia, or subconjunctival bleeding, due to accumulation of heat in the heart and spleen complicated by exposure to the pathogenic wind factor.

Intermittent Infantile Convulsion due to Disorder of the Liver a type of infantile convulsion accompanied with yellow tinged eyes, upward staring, refusing to suck milk, deficiency of qi with tendency to collapse; resulting from the impairment of the spleen and stomach due to prolonged diarrhea, and upward attack of the asthenic yang due to the liver dysfunction.

Intermittent Infantile Convulsion a disorder marked by insidious onset mild degree and occurring at interval-

色青；或下利清谷，脉沉缓或沉迟无力。多由气血不足，肝盛脾虚所致。 s, accompanied with normal body temperature, slight yellowish or bluish-white complexion, lassitude, discharge with loose stool, sunken and slow or weak pulse, which is caused by the insufficiency of qi and blood, and liver-sthenia and spleen-asthenia.

慢脾风 【màn pí fēng】小儿由于吐泻过度，正气虚弱，出现闭目摇头，面唇青暗，神昏、嗜睡、四肢厥冷、抽搐无力等症。多由脾阴虚损，脾阳衰竭所致。 **Chronic Splenic Wind-Syndrome** a syndrome seen in infants with deficiency of qi after frequent vomiting and diarrhea, manifested as colsing eyes, involuntary shaking of head, cyanosis coma, sleepiness, coldness of limbs and atonic spasm, which is caused by the consumption of spleen yin and exhaustion of spleen yang.

猫眼疮 【māo yǎn chuāng】多发于头面手足，起红斑成片，或有水泡，有的形如猫眼。因内蕴血热，外感风热或风寒触发。即多形红斑。 **Erythema Multiforme** lesions usually occurring on the face and extremities, appearing as patches, vesicles or bullae, or as the figure of a cat's eye, due to accumulation of blood-heat in the body and provoked by the attack of wind-heat or wind-cold pathogen.

毛际 【máo jì】耻骨处的毛际部位。 **Pubic Hair Margin**

冒家 【mào jiā】常患眩冒的病人。 **The Patient Suffering from Frequent Dizziness**

瞀瘛 【mào chì】以眼昏花及筋脉拘急为特征的一种病症。多因火热上扰心神，引动肝风所致。 **Dizziness with Muscular Spasm** a disorder due to attack of the heart by fire which provokes the activity of liver-wind.

梅毒 【méi dú】（杨梅疮毒）由梅毒螺旋体引起的传染性性病，通过性交或其他直接接触传染。其原发病灶为下疳，并逐步累及身体各组织和器官。 **Syphilis** a contagious venereal disease caused by the spirochete treponema pallidum, transmitted through sexual intercourse or any direct con-

梅核气 【méi hé qì】患者自觉咽部有异物堵塞感的一种证候。多由肝郁气滞,肝气夹痰凝于咽部所致。

猛疽 【měng jū】(结喉痈)痈疽发于咽喉,肿甚疼痛,影响吞咽、呼吸、寒热大作。多因肺肝热蕴,邪毒痰火上冲咽喉所致。

梦遗 【mèng yí】(梦遗精)指因梦交而精液遗泄的病症,多因感情上的刺激,相火妄动,或心火亢盛所致。

泌别清浊 【mì bié qīng zhuó】小肠在承受胃中饮食以后,进行消化和分清别浊的过程,其饮食精微在小肠吸收后,由脾转输到身体各部,糟粕部分下注大肠或渗入膀胱,经大小便排出的功能。

密煎导法 【mì jiān dǎo fǎ】导法之一。用蜂蜜适量,在锅内煎熬浓缩,趁热

tact, its primary local seat is a hard chancre, whence it extends to all tissues and organs of the body.

Globus Hystericus a symptom characterized by subjective feeling of a foreign body obstructing the throat, caused by the stagnated liver-qi and phlegm accumulating in the throat.

Retropharyngeal Abscess a collection of pus on the posterior wall of the pharynx, characterized by intense pain and marked swelling impeding deglutition and respiration, accompanied with chills and fever, which is due to pathogenic heat accumulating in the lung and liver and attack of phlegm fire to the throat.

Nocturnal Emission involuntary discharge of semen during sleep which is due to hyperactivity of sexual action resulting from emotional irritation or due to hyperactivity of heart-fire resulting from overstrain of the heart.

Separating the Pure Substance from the Turbid One a process of small intestine digesting food, by which the nutrients are absorbed and sent to the all parts of the body by the spleen, while the residues are passed to the body by the spleen, with the residues are passed to the large intestine and the bladder and discharged as feces and urine.

Moving the Bowels with Honey Suppository a treatment of constipation

取出，做成大小适中的栓子，塞入肛门内。一般适用于津液缺而大便干燥难解者。

面部疔疮　【miàn bù dīng chuāng】指生于面部唇、鼻、眉、颧等处的疔疮。多因饮食不节，外感风邪火毒及四时不正之气所致。辩证分类　1. 热毒凝结证　2. 火毒炽盛证。

面尘　【miàn chén】指面色灰暗如蒙尘灰。实证多属燥邪所伤，或伏邪内郁；虚证多属久病，或肝肾阴虚。

面疔　【miàn dīng】生于面部的疔疮。多由热毒蓄结所致。

面垢　【miàn gòu】指面部污秽如蒙尘垢。多因感受暑邪，胃热熏蒸；或积滞内停所致。

面黄肌瘦　【miàn huáng jī shòu】指面色暗黄枯槁，肌肉消瘦，多因脾胃虚弱，气血亏损引起。多见于慢性消耗性疾病。

面目浮肿　【miàn mù fú zhǒng】指虚证引起的面部虚浮作肿。多因脾肺阳虚，输化失常；或肝肾阴虚，阳气上

which is due to insufficiency of fluid by suppository made of concentrated honey.

Pustule on Face　referring to the pustule on the lips, nose, eyebrow and zygomatic arch, mostly caused by improper diet, exogenous pathogenic wind and heat as well as some other epidemic exopathic factors. Types of differentiation 1. accumulation of toxic heat 2. excess of toxic fire.

Dusty Complexion　a face that is dark-grey in color as if covered with dust, which indicates injury by dryness or latent pathogens in excess syndrome, and long-standing disease or yin deficiency of the liver and kidney, which is mostly seen in deficiency syndrome.

Furuncle of Face　a disease which is caused by the accumulation of heat-toxin.

Dirty Complexion　a face appearing as if covered with dirt, mostly caused by stomach-heat due to invasion of summer-heat pathogen, or by retention of food in the stomach.

Emaciation with Sallow Complexion　a face that is thin, sallow and dry, mostly due to deficiency of the spleen and stomach as well as consumption of qi and blood, seen in chronic and consumptive disease.

Edema of the Face　edema of deficiency type, mostly due to yang deficiency of the spleen, lung and distur-

浮所致。

面色苍白 【miàn sè cāng bái】指面部失去红润光泽的病色。常伴有口唇和指甲淡白。多由于气血虚亏所致。

面色苍黑 【miàn sè cāng hēi】指面部泛现晦黑的病色。多因肾气虚耗，血气失荣于面所致。可见于阴黄，黑疸等病。肾上腺皮质功能减退亦多有此症。

面色萎黄 【miàn sè wěi huáng】指面部呈现枯萎晦黄的病色。多因脾胃虚弱，气血不能上荣所致。常见于慢性消耗性疾病。

面色缘缘正赤 【miàn sè yuán yuán zhèng chì】形容面色通红，见于急性热病，是热邪炽盛所致病变的面部反映。

面脱 【miàn tuō】指面部肌肉严重消瘦的危重证候。

面游风 【miàn yóu fēng】因平素血燥，过食辛辣厚味，胃蕴湿热，外受风邪所致的病证。症见面目发红，痒如虫爬，肌肤干燥，时起白屑或破流脂水。相当于脂溢性皮炎或湿疹。

bance in their transportation and transformation; or due to yin deficiency of the liver and kidney, and the upwardness of yang-qi.

Pale Complexion a diseased state with the disappearance of the ruddy complexion, often accompanied by pale lips and nails, indicating blood and qi deficiency.

Darkish Complexion dimmish and blackish complexion usually due to exhaustion of the kidney qi and poor blood supply to the face as seen in yin jaundice and blackish jaundice or mostly seen in hypoadrenocorticism.

Sallow Complexion a condition due to hypofunction of the stomach and spleen and poor supply of qi and blood to the face usually seen in chronic consumptive disease.

Flushed Face bright red facial complexion, often seen in acute febrile disease, which is the representation of pathological changes on the face due to excess of pathogenic heat.

Emaciated Face a sign of critical condition with wasted condition of the body easily seen on the face.

Seborrheic Dermatitis a morbid condition due to constitutional dryness of blood, overeating greasy and spicy food, accumulated damp-heat in the stomach and exopathic factors, characterized by flushed face, insect-crawling, dryness of the skin, sometimes with crusts bulging or broken with

面针疗法 【miàn zhēn liáo fǎ】针刺面部特定穴位的一种治疗方法。

面肿 【miàn zhǒng】面部浮肿，因外感风邪或脏腑虚损，致机体水液转输失常所引起。

明堂 【míng táng】1. 指鼻。2. 针灸模型表明腧穴标志点。

命关 【mìng guān】小儿指纹的诊断部位之一。指食指第三指节掌面外侧浅表小静脉的显露，观察此处小静脉的变化可预测病情严重程度。

膜 【mó】1. 体内形如薄皮的组织，如耳膜、筋膜等。2. 病证名。指眼生片状薄膜，通常有血丝，从白睛发出，侵向黑睛，甚至遮盖瞳神，影响视力。

膜入水轮 【mó rù shuǐ lún】黑睛宿翳掩及瞳神的病证。多因黑睛受损其瘢痕侵入水轮所致。

母病及子 【mǔ bìng jí zǐ】根据五行学说理论，说明在病理情况下脏腑间的互相影响。是指疾病的传变，从母脏传及子脏。如肾属水、肝属木、水能生木，故肾为母脏，肝为子脏，肾病及肝，即是母病及子。

lipid discharge, it is corresponding to seborrgeic dermatitis, exzema.

Face-Acupuncture Therapy a technique in which specific on the face are needled to treat disorders in other parts of the body.

Edema of the Face a condition due to pathogenic wind or deficiency of zang-fu organs, leading to failure of the body to transport fluid.

Ming Tong 1. nose 2. chart with diagram of meridians and acupoints.

Life Pass the distal segment of the index finger of an infant, the superficial venules on the palmar side of which are inspected for the diagnosis of diseases on their severity.

Membrane 1. tissue within the body shaped like thin skin 2. symptom referring to patchy membrane appeared in the eye, usually streaked with blood, involving from the white of the eye to the black part, or even covering the pupil, resulting in poor eyesinght.

Nebula Corering the Pupil a condition mostly caused by invasion of the pupil by the scar from the injury of the black of the eye.

Disorder of the Mother Organ Affecting the Child Organ the principle of the mother-child relation of interpromotion of the five elements is used to explain the mutual pathological influence between five zang organs, eg, the kidney being water, liver being wood, water can produce wood, hence, the kidney being the mother organ, liver being the child organ, kidney disease may affect the liver, ie, disease of the mother organ affecting the child organ.

母气 【mǔ qì】在五行中,具有相生关系的两脏中,生者称为母气。如土(脾)生金(肺),则土(脾)为金(肺)的母气。

Mother Organ Qi in the producing sequence of the five clements, the element that produces the other is known as the mother, correspondingly. the mother organ's qi is called mother-qi eg, the earth (the spleen) produces the metal (the lung), thus, the former is the latter's mother-qi.

牡脏 【mǔ zàng】指心和肝属阳之脏。

Male Organ organs of yang nature, ie, the heart and the liver

木火刑金 【mù huǒ xíng jīn】指肝火过旺耗伤肺阴的病理。症见干咳、胸胁疼痛、口苦、心烦、甚至咯血等。

Wood-Fire Impairs Metal fire of the liver (wood) injures the lung (metal) by the latter's essence and fluid and brings on dry cough, chest pain, bitter taste in the mouth, dysphoria, or even hemoptysis

木克土 【mù kè tǔ】根据五行学说理论,肝属木,脾属土。木克土,即是指肝对脾(胃)的正常制约作用。

Wood Restricts Earth according to the theory of the five elements, liver being wood, spleen being earth; here referring to the normal physiological restriction of the liver to the spleen (stomach)

木舌 【mù shé】(死舌)以舌肿胀坚硬为特征的病证。因心脾积热上冲所致。多见于小儿。

Swollen and Rigid Tongue a morbid condition characterized by rigid swollen tongue like a log, usually caused by the flaming-up of the accumulated heat in the heart and spleen, mostly seen in infants.

木肾 【mù shèn】睾丸肿胀而无疼痛的一种病证。

Swollen and Painless Testicles a morbid condition characterized by swollen and painless testicles.

木喜条达 【mù xǐ tiáo dá】肝主疏泄，具有调节气机的作用，宜调和畅达，而恶抑郁。故用树木的生发以比喻肝的生理特点。
Wood Has a Desire for Freely Growing Activites   the liver governs normal flow of qi, capable of regulating functional activities of qi, desiring for freely growing activity, but harmed if stagnated. Hence, this physiological characteristic of the liver is often likened to that of the tree-growing.

木郁达之 【mù yù dá zhī】对肝气郁结的病证，应采用疏肝理气解郁，使肝气畅达的治疗法则。
Depression of the Liver (wood) Should Be Relieved   a therapeutic principle for the treatment of diseases with stagnancy of the liver-qi to soothing the liver and regulating the circulation of qi.

木郁化风 【mù yù huà fēng】由于肝气郁结久而导致肝风内动的病理，常表现为眩晕、震颤或抽搐等证。
Depression of the Liver Causes Wind-Syndrome   a morbid condition due to long-standing depression of the liver, leading to the appearance of the liver-wind such as dizziness, tremor or convulsion of the extremities.

木郁化火 【mù yù huà huǒ】由于肝气郁结日久化火的病理。常见有头痛、眩晕、烦躁、面红、眼赤、舌红、脉弦等。
Depression of the Liver Causes Fire-Syndrome   a morbid condition caused by long-standing depression of the liver, resulting in fire syndrome, characterized by headache, dizziness, dysphoria, flushed face, blood-shot eyes, reddened tongue and wiry pulse.

目不瞑 【mù bù míng】不能闭目的症状，含有失眠的意思。
Unclosed Eyes   a symptom of difficulty in closing the eyes and in falling asleep.

目飞血 【mù fēi xuè】巩膜血管充血成片状分布的征象。常见于椒疮、火疳等多种眼病。
Hyperemia of Bulbar Conjunctiva   a condition in which congested blood vessels of the eyes appear in patches, usually seen in many eye diseases such as trachoma and acute scleritis.

目封塞 【mù fēng sāi】眼睑重度浮肿
Severe Palpebral Edema   severe ede-

以致不能开睑的症状。

目干涩 【mù gān sè】指眼结膜干涩不适。多由肝阴不足或肝肾阴虚所致。

目纲 【mù gāng】眼睑边缘，该部与脾胃有密切关系。

目昏 【mù hūn】指视物模糊不清。多因脏腑精气虚损，不能注于目或风、火、湿、痰上扰清窍所致。

目窠 【mù kē】眼的凹陷处，容纳眼球的地方。

目窠上微肿 【mù kē shàng wēi zhǒng】指两侧上下眼睑轻微浮肿。多因脾不制水，肾不化气，或外感风邪与水气相搏所致。

目涩 【mù sè】指自觉眼睛干燥涩而不适。多因阴液亏损或脏腑虚热所致。

目沙涩 【mù shā sè】眼结膜涩痛，有异物感的一种症状，多伴有羞明流泪、红痒等。多因风热或阴虚火旺所致。见于多种外障眼病。

ma of the eyelid, resulting in failure of eyes to open.

Dryness and Uneasy Feeling of the Conjunctiva a condition usually caused by insufficience of liver-yin or yin deficiency of the liver and kidney.

Margins of Eyelids a part which is closely related with the spleen and stomach.

Blurred Vision a condition mostly caused by decline of vital qi in zang-fu organs and its inability to ascend to nourish the eyes or the upward disturbance to the eye by wind, fire, dampness and phlegm.

Eye Socket the pitting part of the eyes where eyeballs contained.

Blepharoedema referring to the slight edema of both the upper and lower eyelids, mostly caused by the inability of spleen to manage water and of the kidney to transform qi, or due to retention of fluid in the body complicated by attack of pathogenic wind.

Dryness and Uncomfortable Feeling of the Eye spontaneous feeling of dryness and uncomfort, mostly due to consumption of yin fluid or asthenia-heat in zang-fu organs.

Dryness and Pain of the Conjunctiva a condition as if presence of foreign body exists, mostly accompanied by photophobia and lacrimation, redness and itching of the eyes, mostly caused by pathogenic wind-heat, hyperactivity fire due to yin deficiency, seen in many

目上胞【mù shāng bāo】即上眼睑。

目上纲【mù shàng gāng】(目上弦)上眼睑的边缘部。

目下纲【mù xià gāng】(目下弦)指下眼睑的边缘部。

目疡【mù yáng】因火毒郁结、邪热上攻所致的眼睑疾病。初起时眼睑红肿生疮，继而成脓溃烂，可伴有恶寒发热。

目痒【mù yáng】指眼结膜奇痒。多由风火、湿热或血虚引起。

目晕【mù yūn】1.指黑睛与白睛交界处出现的环状混浊。2.指观灯时有彩环。

目直【mù zhí】指定眼直视。可见于肝风窜动之证，如急惊风、惊痫等。

目中不了了【mù zhōng bù liǎo liǎo】指视物模糊不清。因阳明腑热，灼伤津液，邪热上蒸所致。

目眦【mù zì】即眼角。是上下眼睑连结的部位。

募原【mù yuán】1.指膈肌和胸膜之间的部位。2.人体的半表半里的位置。

of external oculopathy.

Upper Eyelid

Margin of the Upper Eyelid

Margin of the Lower Eyelid

Blepharitis a disease of eyelids caused by accumulation of toxic fire and upward attack of pathogenic heat, at onset characterized by swelling of the eyelid, then with the appearance of abscess, at last, broken and the discharging of pus, or accopanied by chills and fever.

Itching of the Eye mostly referring to the itching of conjunctiva due to pathogenic wind, fire, dampness and heat or deficiency of blood.

Turbidity 1. arcus senilis referring to the circular turbidness between the black and white of the eye 2. halo vision colourful circles appeared around lamps on looking at them.

Staring Blankly a symptom seen in syndromes of up-stiring of liver-wind, such as convulsion and epilepsy.

Blurring of Vision a symptom caused by pathogenic heat in fu organs of yangming meridian, resulting in consumption of body fluid, and the steaming-up of the heat pathogen.

Canthus the connective part of the upper and lower eyelids.

Mu Yuan 1. pleurodiaphragmatic interspace 2. space between the exterior and interior in the human body.

纳呆 【nà dāi】(胃呆)即食欲不振。多因中气虚弱,湿浊内阻所致。

Anorexia a condition caused by deficiency of qi in middle energizer and retention of pathogenic dampness.

奶癣 【nǎi xuǎn】(湿疹、胎癣、乳癣)婴儿湿疹。多因素体过敏,风湿热邪蕴阻肌肤所致。

Infantile Eczema a morbid condition due to allergic constitution, retention of pathogenic wind, dampness and heat at the superficial portion of the skin

难产 【nán chǎn】指分娩过程中,胎儿难于娩出。可因产道狭窄、胎位不正、胎儿过大或宫缩无力等引起。

Dystocia a condition caused by stricture of the parturiet canal, abnormal fetal position postmature infant or uterine inertia.

难乳 【nán rǔ】初生儿,风热从脐而入,流入心脾,以致唇舌的活动受影响,不能吮乳;或因小儿初生,口中秽血咽入腹中,致胸腹痞满,短气急促,不能吮乳。

Difficulty in Suching a condition of newborn due to the invasion of the heart and spleen by pathogenic wind and heat entering from the umbilicus, leading to the inability of the mouth to suck, or due to swallowing the dirty blood in the mouth from the mother, resulting in fullness in the chest and abdomen, shortness of breath and inability to suck.

囊缩 【náng suō】(卵缩)指阴囊上缩,常与舌卷并见。多因阳明热盛,邪传厥阴;或寒邪直中少阴所致。属危重症候之一。

Shrinkage of the Scrotum a sign often seen in critical cases together with curling of the tongue, mostly caused by excessive heat in yangming meridian, invasion of jueyin by pathogenic factors, or direct invasion of shaoyin by pathogenic cold.

囊痈 【náng yōng】(肾囊痈)多由肝肾两经湿热下注或外湿内浸,蕴酿成毒所致的病证。症见身发寒热、口干饮冷、阴囊红肿热痛,甚至囊皮紧张光亮,久则成脓。

Scrotal Carbuncle a disease due to the downward flowing of dampness and heat in the liver and kidney meridians or invasion of exopathic dampness, resulting in the formation of toxins, characterized by chills, fever, dry mouth with preference for

蛲虫病 【náo chóng bìng】(肾虫病) 因蛲虫寄生于肠道所致，小儿患者较多。症见夜晚肛痒，甚者烦惊不安。

脑 【nǎo】奇恒之腑之一。脑居颅内，由髓汇集而成。中医认为脑的生长发育及正常功能与肾精有密切关系，是主管人的高级神经活动的重要器官。

脑风 【nǎo fēng】古病名。指以后枕部痛不可忍、项背怯寒为主症的一种病证。多由风邪入脑所致。见头风。

脑疳 【nǎo gān】指疳疾患儿头部生疮或毛发焦枯等局部症状。多因气血不足，或由于感染所致。

脑骨伤 【nǎo gǔ shāng】多因外伤所致。局部有肿胀，或颅骨凹陷、眼结合膜、耳鼻道出血或流出脑脊液、昏睡不知人事，甚者死亡。

脑疽 【nǎo jū】(脑后发) 生于脑后枕骨、大椎穴之间的痈疽。多因湿热

cold drink, redness, swelling, hotness and pain of the scrotum, or even with its skin rigid and bright, pus formed in the long run.

Enterobiasis a disease caused by the parasitic infestation in the intestinal tract, mostly seen in young children, characterized by night itching of the anus or even restlessness.

The Brain one of the extraordinary organs where the marrow converges, hence also known as the sea of marrow, which is thought to be closely related with kidney essence in its development, responsible for the control of the most important nerves.

Headache Caused by Pathogenic Wind
a morbid condition characterized by unbearable pain in the post-occiptal part, chilly sensation of the nape and upper back, mostly caused by invasion of the brain by pathogenic wind.

Head-Boid of Malnutrient Infant
referring to local symptoms such as head-boils and sparse, dry hair of malnutrint infant, mostly due to deficiency of qi and blood or caused by infection.

Fracture of the Cranial Bone a condition usually caused by trauma, characterized by local swelling or depressed skull, bleeding from conjunctiva, ear and nostrils, or discharging cerebral spinal fluid, lethargy or unconsciousness, or even resulting in death.

Carbuncle of the Nape carbuncles seen in the place between the post-oc-

毒邪上壅，或阴虚火炽所致。症见红肿疼痛，易溃，易敛。cipital bone and dazhui acupoint, mostly caused by upward disturbance of pathogenic dampness and heat, or due to yin deficiency and fire flaming, marked by redness, swelling, hotness and pain with the liability to ulceration and astringency

脑鸣 【nǎo míng】指自觉头内鸣响。伴有耳鸣、目弦等症。多因髓海虚衰或因火郁，湿痰阻遏所致。 Tinnitus Crani　　a condition accompanied by tinnitus of the ear and dizziness, mostly caused by asthenia of sea of marrow, or stagnancy of fire and retention of damp-phlegm.

脑髓 【nǎo suǐ】即脑与脊髓。 Brain and Marrow

臑骨伤 【nào gǔ shāng】指肱骨骨折。 Fracture of Humerus

臑痈 【nào yōng】 即上臂。痈指生于上臂的痈。由风温或风火凝结而成。 Carbuncle of Upper Arm　　carbuncle caused by accumulation of pathogenic wind or wind and fire.

内吹 【nèi chuī】指发生于妊娠期的乳痈。 Acute Mastitis during Pregnancy

内钓 【nèi diào】以抽搐、腹部剧痛为特征的病证。发生于婴幼儿，多由受风或受惊所致。 Infantile Tic　　a morbid condition marked by convulsion and severe abdominal pain, seen in infant, mostly due to pathogenic wind or fright.

内毒 【nèi dú】指热毒蕴伏体内，当抵抗力下降或遇诱发因素时，发生的急性化脓性皮肤或软组织感染。伴有高热头痛、口干咽痛、骨节烦痛、皮肤发斑、神志不清等症。相当于败血症的临床表现。 Endogenous Toxin　　toxin retended in the body. when the resistance of the body weakened or due to some predisposing factors, it can result in acute supurative skin infection or soft tissue infection, accompanied by high fever, headache, dryness in the mouth, sore throat, joint pain, maculation and unconsciousness, the same symptoms as those in septicemia.

内风 【nèi fēng】指疾病发展过程中出现眩晕、抽搐、震颤等一类风证症候，它不同于外感的风，故名。 Endogenous Wind　　a wind syndrome manifested as dizziness, convulsion and tremor, which is different from

内寒 【nèi hán】因阳气虚弱、脏腑功能衰退引起水液潴留的病证。症见呕吐、泄泻、手足逆冷、出冷汗或水肿痰饮、脉沉迟等。

内踝疽 【nèi huái jū】位于内踝上的疽。多因寒湿下注、气滞血凝所致。

内漏 【nèi lòu】指因外伤引起的内出血。

内取 【nèi qǔ】1. 诊察脉象的虚实来判断病情的方法。2. 指用内服药来治疗疾病的方法。

内热 【nèi rè】1. 阴液亏损所致的热性证候。症见潮热、五心烦热、盗汗、心烦口渴、舌红少苔，脉细数等。2. 指热邪入里所致的里热证。症见发热、面红目赤、心烦、口渴、便秘、小便短赤、舌红苔黄燥、脉沉实等。

内伤 【nèi shāng】（内损）1. 泛指内损脏气的致病因素，如七情不节、饮食不调、劳倦、房事过度等。2. 病名，同内损。

syndrome caused by exopathic wind.

Endogenous Cold a morbid condition due to yang deficiency and hypofunction of zagnfu organs, leading to retention of body fluid, manifested by vomiting, diarrhea, cold limbs, cold sweating or edema phlegm retention, sunken and slow pulse.

Carbuncle on the Medial Malleolus
a condition caused by downward flowing of pathogenic cold and dampness, leading to stagnancy of qi and blood.

Internal Hemorrhage due to Trauma

Internal Management 1. a diagnostic method by feeling the pulse 2. a therapeutic method to treat diseases by taking medicine orally.

Interior Heat 1. a morbid condition manifested as hectic fever, feverish sensation in the chest, palms and soles, night sweat, dysphoria, thirst, reddened tongue with little coating, fine and fast pulse. 2. interior heat syndrome characterized by high fever, flushed face, dysphoria, thirst, constipation, scanty deep-colored urine, reddened tongue with dry yellowish coating, sunken and forceful pulse.

Internal Injury 1. impairment of the function of the internal organs, caused by emotional strain, improper diet, strain, or intemperance in sexual life. 2. name of disease, referring to internal injury due to severe trauma.

内伤不得卧 【nèi shāng bù dé wò】指由于肝火、胆火、胃不和、心血虚、心气虚等内伤病引起的失眠病证。

Insomnia due to Internal Injury   referring to insomnia due to disease of internal injury caused by the fire of the liver and gallbladder, disorder of the stomach-qi, deficiency of the heart blood and heart-qi.

内伤发热 【nèi shāng fā rè】由脏腑气血虚损或功能失调引起的发热。

Fever due to Internal Injury   fever caused by deficiency of qi and blood in the fu organs or due to their functional disorder.

内伤头痛 【nèi shāng tóu tòng】指脏腑气血内伤或痰湿壅阻所致的头痛病证。以起病缓慢、时发时止为特征。

Headache Caused by Internal Injury   a morbid condition caused by internal injury of qi and blood in the fu organs or phlegm retention characterized by slow onset with the pain off and on.

内伤胃脘痛 【nèi shāng wèi wǎn tòng】指因积冷、积热、脾胃虚寒、阴虚及食积、痰饮、气滞、瘀血、虫积等所致的胃脘痛。

Stomachache due to Internal Injury   a morbid condition due to accumulation of cold, heat, asthenic cold in the spleen and stomach, yin deficiency as well as retention of food and phlegm, stagnancy of qi, blood stasis and parasition infestation

内伤腰痛 【nèi shāng yāo tòng】由于肝脾肾虚损或痰湿、瘀血、内伤所致的腰痛。一般病程较久,以虚证为多。

Lumbago Caused by Internal Injury   a morbid condition caused by deficiency of the liver, spleen and kidney or phlegm-dampness, blood stasis, and internal injury, generally the course is longer and mostly seen in asthenia-syndrome.

内伤饮食痉 【nèi shāng yǐn shí jìng】因饮食停滞,伤及脾胃而致的痉症。多见于呕吐、泄泻之后。

Convulsion Caused by Improper Diet   a condition due to food retention, leading to the impairment of the spleen and stomach, mostly seen after vomiting and diarrhea.

内湿 【nèi shī】指体内水湿停滞。由脾

Endogenous Dampness   retention of

肾阳虚运化水湿功能障碍所致。临床表现食欲不振、腹胀、腹泻、尿少、浮肿、舌质淡、苔润、脉濡缓等。
water within the body, caused by hypofunction of the spleen and kidney and functionl disturbance in water transport, manifested by poor appetite, abdominal distention, diarrhea, oliguria, edema, pale tongue with moist coating, soft and slow pulse.

内托 【nèi tuō】（托法）用内服药治疗外科疮疡的三大治法之一。即使用补益气血的药物，扶助正气，使毒邪消散，以免毒邪内陷。
Expelling from Within one of the three chief therapeutic methods in treating surgical, skin and external diseases with internal application, ie, administering tonics for invigoration and nourishing qi and blood to eliminate toxins of supurative infections from the body.

内消 【nèi xiāo】1. 以多食、多尿而不渴为特征的消渴病。2. 运用内服药使疮疡消散的一种治疗方法，亦称外科消法。
Diabetes 1. diabetes chararcterized by polyphagia, polyuria but with no thirst. 2. resolution of soft tissue inflammation by internal application of drugs.

内因 【nèi yīn】中医病因之一，即喜、怒、忧、思、悲、恐、惊等致病因素。
Endopathic Factors one of the disease-causing factors in TCM i. e, joy, anger, anxiety, worry, grief, fear and fright.

内痈 【nèi yōng】位于胸腹腔内或内脏的脓肿。
Abscess of Internal Organs abscess occurring in the thoracic and abdominal cavities or viscera.

内燥 【nèi zào】因热病、吐泻、出汗、失血等导致体内津液耗伤所致的燥证。症见潮热、心烦、唇燥、皮肤干燥、舌干无津等。
Endogenous Dryness syndrome of dryness due to consumption of body fluid brought about by febrile diseases, vomiting, diarrhea, sweating or loss of blood, marked by hectic fever, dysphoria, dry lips and skin, and dryness in the mouth.

内治 【nèi zhì】用内服药物，治疗机体发生的病证。
Internal Application treatment of diseases with drugs taken orally.

内痔 【nèi zhì】位于肛门齿线以上的痔疮。

能远怯近症 【nèng yuǎn qiè jìn zhèng】即远视眼。视近物模糊，视远物反清晰。

能近怯远症 【néng jìn qiè yuǎn zhèng】即近视眼。视远物模糊，视近物反清晰。

泥鳅疽 【ní qiū jū】（泥鳅疔，泥鳅痈）一手指通肿，色紫灼热，形如泥鳅，痛连肘臂。即化脓性腱鞘炎。

逆传 【nì chuán】疾病的变化不按一般规律发展。如温热病从卫分迅速发展到心包证候。

逆传心包 【nì chuán xīn bāo】指温病不按一般规律发展。即温邪不由卫分经气分的次序传变而侵入心包的病理现象。症见高热、神昏、谵语、心烦、舌绛、脉数等。

逆流挽舟 【nì liú wǎn zhōu】痢疾初起的一种治法。表现为患者既有大便脓血、里急后重、腹痛等湿热内蕴的症状，又有恶寒发热、身痛头痛的外感表证。治以解表药与清热利湿及消滞药同用，以达到既清在里的湿热又解表邪的目的。

Internal Hemorrhoids hemorrhoids occurring above the anal dentate line.

Hyperopia the condition of seeing near objects dimly but being able to see distant ones clearly.

Myopia the condition of being able to see near objects clearly but not the distant ones.

Acute Purulent Tenosynovitis of the Finger a condition marked by swelling purple finger which is burning hot and shaped like a loach, and pain radiating to the elbow corresponding to purulent tenosynovitis.

Reverse Transmission abnormal transmission of a febrile disease, eg, from the weifen rapidly to pericardium as seen in epidemic febrile disease.

Reverse Transmission of an Epidemic Febrile Disease Directly to the Pericardium pathogenic heat invades the pericardium directly after breaking through the weifen (superficial defensive) instead of trasmitting in an ordinary order to qi fen, with the manifestations such as high fever, coma, delirium, dysphoria, deep-red tongue and fast pulse

Boating Up the Stream metaphorically referring to the treatment of dysentery both interiorly and exteriorly at its initial stage for patients with symptoms due to the interior damp-heat, such as purulent stool, tenesmus and abdominal pain, and those of exterior syndrome, such as chills and

逆腻愿捻尿 ni nian niao

逆证 【nì zhèng】指因正气虚衰，邪气亢盛，病情不按一般规律发展而突然加重，病情恶化的现象。

腻苔 【nì tāi】舌苔浑浊而粘腻。多见于湿浊内阻或消化不良及痰饮内阻的疾病。

愿疮 【nì chuāng】妇人阴户生疮。

捻针 【niǎn zhēn】将针左右反复捻转的一种针刺手法。在进针、出针和运针过程中都可以使用。

尿 【niào】1. 尿液。尿液的生成和排泄与肺、肾、脾、三焦及膀胱等脏腑的功能有密切关系，对津液的代谢有着重要的作用。观察尿量和尿的颜色有助于判断病情。2. 指排尿。

尿血 【niào xuè】（溺血、溲血）指小便中混有血液的病证。因阴虚火旺者，症见尿血鲜红、腰腿酸软、耳鸣目花、心烦口干、舌质红、脉细数；脾肾两亏者，症见尿血淡红、面色萎黄、饮食减少、腰酸肢冷、舌质淡、脉虚弱。

fever, pain over the body and headache by using diaphoretics and damp-heat expelling drugs at the same time.

Deteriorating Case a worsening case in which the body resistance qi is overpowered by the pathogenic factors with an abnormal progress.

Greasy Fur slimy and greasy fur ussually indicating stagnancy of dampness, undigested food or damp-phlegm.

Ulcer of the Female External Genitals usually regerring to ulcers appeared around the vaginal orifice.

Twirling the Acupunctune Needle a manipulation of acupuncture by twirling the needle, a technique which can be applied in needle insertion, withdrawal and manipulation.

Urine 1. the formation and excretion of urine closely related with the functions of zang-fu organs such as the lung, kidney, spleen, triple energizer and urinary bladder, which plays an important role in the metabolism of body fluid. Observations on the quantity and color of urine would aid in the diagnosis of diseases 2. Urination

Hematuria a condition in which there is blood in urine, if caused by yin deficiency and excess of fire, it is marked by bright red blood in urine, weakness and soreness of the loins and legs, tinnitus, dizziness, dysphoria, thirst, reddened tongue, thready and fast pulse; if caused by hypofunction of

尿浊 【niào zhuó】(尿白) 以小便混浊, 乳白如膏为主证, 或伴见血尿、血块的病证。多因疲劳过度, 脾肾气虚, 饮食不节等诱发或加重。辨证分类: 1. 湿热下注证 2. 脾虚气陷证 3. 肾虚不固证。

Turbid Urine a morbid condition marked by milky white turbid urine or accompanied by hematuria, blood clot, mostly caused by overstrain, deficiency of kidney and spleen-qi, as well as improper diet which can induce or worsen the disease. Types of differentiation: 1. downward drive of pathogenic damp-heat 2. deficiency of the spleen resulting in qi collapse 3. deficiency of the kidney both the spleen and kidney, manifested by light red urine, sallow complexion, poor appetite, lumbago, cold limbs, reddened tongue and weak pulse.

捏脊 【niē jǐ】(捏积) 属外治法的一种。方法是让患者俯卧, 操作者从尾骶正中两侧, 两手拇指与食指捏起皮肤, 沿脊柱正中线向上移动, 边提边捏, 直推进到脊柱上端, 如此反复操作三至七次。多用于治疗小儿消化不良等症。

Chiropractic one of the external therapeutic methods, mostly for the treatment of indigestion of infants, in which the manipulator, with the patient in supine position, squeezes the skin of the two sides of the mid-coccyx with the thumb and index finger of both hands, moving upward along the mid-line of the spine, drawing and squeezing alternatively. Repeat it three to seven times.

颞颥 【niè rú】眼眶的外后方颧骨弓上方的部位。

Temple the external posterior part of the orbit above the malar bone arch.

凝脂翳 【níng zhī yì】因风热毒邪外侵, 肝胆实火内炽, 风火毒邪搏结于上所致的眼疾。证见黑睛生翳、色带鹅黄, 状若凝脂、头眼剧痛、目赤羞明、泪热多稠, 发展迅猛, 可溃穿黑睛甚则失明。类似化脓性角膜炎。

Purulent Keratitis an eye disease due to exopathic wind-heat and the upward disturbance of excessive fire retained in the liver and gallbladder, characterized by nebulae on the black of the eye which is light yellow in color and shaped like coagulated oil, severe headache, pain of the eye, hyper-

牛皮癣　【niú pí xuǎn】（摄领疮）因风、湿、热毒蕴郁肌肤或营血不足，血虚风燥，肌肤失养所致的苔藓样皮肤病。皮损初起为大小不等的扁平丘疹，呈淡褐色。逐渐融合成片，呈苔藓样改变，干燥肥厚，有阵发性奇痒。病程呈慢性经过，其发作与精神因素有关，类似神经性皮炎。

扭伤　【niǔ shāng】多因旋转外力超越关节的正常活动范围所致。常见于肩、腕、膝、踝等关节处。伤后局部肿胀、疼痛、活动受限、皮色青紫，但无骨折及关节脱位。

脓耳　【nóng ěr】耳内红肿疼痛，鼓膜溃破，耳道流出脓液，称为脓耳。多由肝经火热引起。

脓窝疮　【nóng wō chuāng】由湿热蕴蒸皮肤，或因湿疹、痱子等感染而成。好发于颜面、手臂、小腿等处。

脓血痢　【nóng xuè lì】痢疾的一种。以

emia of bulbar conjunctiva, photophobia, lacrimation with hot sticky discharge and rapid development, possibly leading to the ulceration of the black of the eye and loss of eyesight

Neurodermatitis　licken-like skin caused by invasion of exogenous wind, dampness and heat at the superficial portion of the skin, first with the appearance of flat papules which are various in size and light brown in color, and then gradually extend in area with the skin appearing as licken, which is dry and thick with paroxysmal intense itching. The course of the disease is chronic with its attacks closely related to emotional changes.

Sprain　a condition caused by rotation of joints beyond their normal limits, usually occurring to the shoulder, wrist, knee, and ankle, characterized by local swelling, pain, limitation in movement, blue skin but with no fracture and dislocation

Otitis Media Suppurativa　a morbid condition marked by redness, swelling and pain in the ear, ulcerated ear drum with purulent discharge, mostly caused by pathogenic fire and heat in the liver.

Impetigo　a condition caused by accumulation of pathogenic dampness and heat in the skin or due to infections of eczema of sudamina, usually seen on the face, arms and small legs.

Dysentery with Pus and Blood in the

排脓血便较多为特征。多因湿热蕴结引起。

弄产 【nòng chǎn】孕妇在妊娠后期，胎动次数增加但无其他分娩征兆的一种临床表现。

弄舌 【nòng shé】（吐舌）指时时把舌头伸出口外之症。因心脾积热或脾肾虚热所致。

胬肉攀睛 【nú ròu pān jīng】多因心肺二经风热壅盛，气滞血瘀所致的病证；也可由阴虚火旺引起。症见淡赤胬肉由眦角发出，似昆虫翼状，横贯白睛，渐侵黑睛，甚至掩及瞳神。

怒伤肝 【nù shāng gān】郁怒不止，可影响肝脏的生理功能，使肝气上逆，血随气逆，出现胁痛、善太息、面赤、头痛、眩晕，甚则吐血或昏厥等症。

怒则气上 【nù zé qì shàng】是指过度愤怒可使肝气横逆上冲，血随气逆，并走于上。症见气逆，面红目赤，或呕血，甚则昏厥卒倒。

Stool a type of dysentery marked by pus and blood in the stool, mostly due to accumulation of dampness and heat.

Hyperactivity of the Fetus in Late Pregnancy a clinical manifestation marked by increased fetal movement but with no other signs of delivery.

Sticking Out the Tongue a morbid condition marked by extending the tongue out and drawing it back frequently, indicating excessive heat in the heart and spleen, or asthenic heat in the spleen and kidney

Pterygium a morbid condition mostly caused by excessive wind and heat in the heart and lung meridians, resulting in stagnance of qi and blood stasis, or caused by yin deficiency and excessive fire, marked by pterygium from the canthal corner like insect's wing, covering the white of the eye and gradually invading the black part, or even covering the pupil

The Liver is Easily Affected by Anger long-lasting anger can affect the physiological function of the liver, resulting in upward adverse flow of liver-qi, together with the blood, marked by pain in the hypochondrium, flushed face, headache, dizziness, or even hematemesis or syncope.

Rage Causes Adverse Flow of Liver-Qi a condition which goes adversely upward and even brings blood up, giving rise to reversed flow of qi, flushed

女劳疸 【nǚ láo dǎn】《金匮要略》描述的一种黄疸病。多因劳累或房劳过度所致。症见身目发黄，额部色暗黑、少腹满急、大便色黑、小便自利、傍晚手足心热而恶寒。

Jaundice due to Sexual Intemperance a type of jaundice described in Synopsis of Prescriptions of the Golden Chamber, mostly caused by tiredness or intemperance in sexual life, marked by yellowish brown pigmentation of the skin and sclera, dark brow, fullness of the lower abdomen, dark brown stool, normal urination, hot sensation on the palms and soles with aversion to cold in the evening.

女劳复 【nǚ láo fù】大病初愈、气血尚未恢复，不注意调养、或房事过度，损伤肾精所出现的一种证候。主要症状有头重、眼花、腰背疼痛或小腹拘急绞痛等。

Relapse of Disease due to Intemperance in Sexual Life a condition caused by poor nourishment at the time when the patient has just recovered from a serious illness, qi and blood still remains unhealthy, or caused by intemperance in sexual life, leading to the impairment of kidney essence mainly characterized by heaviness in the head, dim eyesight, pain in the loin and back, and cramping sensation of the lower abdomen.

女子胞 【nǚ zī bāo】（子脏、胞宫、胞脏）奇恒之腑之一。包括妇女整个生殖系统，主管月经、受孕及胎儿发育，与心、肝、脾、肾等脏有密切关系。

Uterus one of the extraordinary fu organs, including the whole female reproductive system, which performs the function of regulating the menses, falling pregnant and breeding of fetus, and which is closely related with some other organs such as the heart, liver, spleen and kidney.

衄家 【nǜ jiā】平素容易流鼻血的人。

Patient Suffering from Frequent Epistaxis

衄血 【nǜ xuè】 1. 指非外伤所致的某些外部出血证候。如眼衄、耳衄、鼻衄、齿衄、舌衄、肌衄等。 2. 指鼻出血。

疟疾 【nüè jí】（疟、疟病、痎疟）指以间歇性寒战、高热、出汗为特征的一种疾病。多发于夏秋季节和疟疾流行地区，或有输血史。辨证分类：1. 正疟 2. 温疟 3. 寒疟 4. 疫（瘴）疟 5. 久疟。

疟母 【nüè mǔ】 指疟疾日久不愈，顽痰挟瘀，结于胁下，形成的痞块。本病相当于久疟形成的脾脏肿大。

疟邪 【nüè xié】 引起疟疾的病邪。

呕家 【ǒu jiā】 经常患有恶心呕吐的病人。

呕乳 【ǒu rǔ】 吐乳直出而不停留，为胃气上逆所致。

呕吐 【ǒu tù】 饮食、痰涎从胃中上涌自口而出的证候。因胃失和降，胃气上逆所致。

呕吐苦水 【ǒu tù kǔ shuǐ】（呕胆）指呕吐黄色苦味之胆液。多因胆经有病所致。

呕血 【ǒu xuè】 血随呕吐而出。多因恼怒伤肝；或饮食、劳倦伤脾；或饮酒过多，积热动血所致。

Bleeding　　1. referring to non-traumatic bleeding, such as bleeding from the eye, ear, nose, gum, tongue, and subcutaneous tissue. 2. Epistaxis.

Malarial Disease　　malaria and other disease characterized by intermittent rigor, high fever and sweating, mostly occurring in summer and autum, and malaria epidemic area or caused by blood transfusion. Types of differentiation: 1. ordinary malaria 2. warm malaria 3. cold malaria 4. epidemic malaria 5. chronic malaria.

Malaria with Hepato Splenomegaly
　　a morbid condition due to the accumulation of stubborn phlegm in the subhypochondrum, forming a mass in spite of the lingering malaria.

Pathogenic Factor of Malarial Disease

Habitual Vomiter　　patient suffering from repeated nausea and vomiting.

Mild Regurgitaion　　a condition due to the upward adverse flow of the stomach-qi.

Vomiting　　a condition referring to the casting up of food substance or gastric fluid from the stomach through the mouth, caused by derangement and abnormal ascending of stomach-qi.

Bilious Vomiting　　a condition mostly caused by disease of the gallbladder meridian.

Hematemesis　　a condition caused by the impairment of the spleen due to improper diet and over-exertion or by over-drinking and accumulation of pathogenic heat, causing damage to the blood vessels.

偶方【ǒu fāng】药味数目是双数的方剂叫做偶方。
Prescription with Ingredients Even in Number

盘肠产【pán cháng chǎn】分娩时肠随儿下，产后肠仍不收，相当于临产时产妇直肠脱出。多由于产妇平素气虚所致。
Prolapse of Rectum during Delivery a condition in which rectum comes out together with the fetus during delivery and is unable to restore to its normal position, mostly caused by constitutional deficiency of qi.

盘肛痈【pán gāng yōng】指肛门周围的脓肿。多因过食辛甘厚味，日久湿热下注所致。
Perianal Abscess referring to abscess appeared around the anus, mostly caused by downward flowing of pathogenic damp-heat resulted from food which is pungent in flavor and sweet in taste.

盘疝【pán shàn】脐旁疼痛。多由感寒气滞所致。
Periumbilical Colic pain in the area around the umbilicus, mostly due to affection by cold and stagnancy of qi.

蟠蛇疬【pán shé lì】指瘰疬绕项串生，如蛇盘绕。见瘰疬。
Scrofula around the Neck scrofulas appeared around the neck in clusters, like snake twining around.

膀胱【páng guāng】（尿胞、脬、玉海）六腑之一。位于盆腔的前方，具有贮藏和排出尿液的功能。
The Urinary Bladder one of the six fu organs lying in the anterior part of the pelvic cavity, having the function of storing and discharging urine.

膀胱咳【páng guāng ké】指咳而小便自出的证候。
Cough with Incontinence of Urine

膀胱气闭【páng guāng qì bì】膀胱气化功能障碍，引起小便不畅的病理。症见小便困难或尿闭，伴有下腹部胀满等。
Dysuria due to Dysfunction of the Bladder a morbid condition due to dysfunction of the bladder in qi activity, resulting in oliguria, characterized by difficulty in urination or dysuria, accompanied by distention and fullness in the lower abdomen.

膀胱湿热 【páng guāng shī rè】湿热之邪蕴积膀胱的病理。症见尿频、尿少、尿痛或血尿、舌红苔黄、脉数等。

Damp-Heat in the Urinary Bladder a morbid condition caused by accumulation of damp-heat in the bladder marked by frequent urination, dysuria, pain during urination or hematuria, red tongue with yellowish coating, thready and weak pules

膀胱虚寒 【páng guāng xū hán】由于肾阳虚，膀胱气化不利或受寒邪影响而引起的一种病理变化。症见遗尿、尿频而清长或排尿无力、脉细弱等。

Hypofunction of the Bladder with Cold Syndrome a morbid condition caused by deficiency of kidney-yang and hypofunction of the bladder in qi activity or due to pathogenic dampness, characterized by enuresis, frequent urination, clear light colored urine or dribbling of urine, thready and weak pulse.

膀胱胀 【páng guāng zhàng】指小腹胀满、小便不利等症。多因膀胱有寒所致。

Distention of the Urinary Bladder referring to the condition of distention and fullness in the lower abdomen and dysuria, mostly caused by retention of pathogenic cold.

胇气不固 【pāo qì bù gù】指膀胱气虚，气化不利，不能约束小便引起的一种病变。症见小便淋沥不断，或小便失禁，或遗尿。

Hypofunction of the Bladder a morbid condition marked by loss of control of urination such as dribbling or incontinence of urine, or enuresis.

炮 【páo】中药炮制法之一。把药物放在高温的铁锅内急炒，致药物表面焦黄而炸裂。如炮附子，可减少它的毒性。

Stirring-Baking one of the methods in processing Chinese medicine by baking a drug in an iron pot with constant stiring till it becomes dark-brown or cracks, eg, processing Acointe by stirring-baking can reduce its toxic effect.

炮炙 【páo zhì】对药物进行加工与处理，意义同炮制。

Preparation of Drugs with the same meaning as the list of processing drugs

炮制 【páo zhì】（修事、修治）对生药加工处理的过程。其目的主要是加强药效，减除药物的毒性和副作用，

Processing Drugs referring to the whole course of processing drugs, the aim of which is to improve the drug's

改变药物的性能，便于服用和保存等。

泡 【pào】（浸泡）一些药物需放在容器内，用水浸泡。经一定时间后，药物质地变软，便于切片加工。

泡服 【pào fú】有些药物不需煎煮，只要用沸水泡后即可服用，如胖大海、菊花等。

衃血 【pēi xuè】指已凝固呈紫黑色的败血。

培土 【péi tǔ】培补脾土，促使脾的运化功能恢复正常的方法。适用于脾虚运化功能低下的病证。症见饮食减少、大便泄泻等。

披肩 【pī jiān】医疗器械。按要求将熟牛皮剪成一定规格，夹于伤处，以作骨折固定之用。适用于肩部骨折，尤其是肱骨颈骨折。

砒霜中毒 【pī shuāng zhòng dú】因突然吸入或误服大量砒粉引起的急性中毒。症见咳嗽、胸痛、呼吸困难或剧烈腹痛、呕吐、腹泻，可迅速出现休克。

effect, reduce its toxicity and side effects, change its property or for the sake of the convenience on use and storage.

Soaking a processing procedure by soaking crude drugs with water in a container to soften them for further preparation.

(Drug) to Be Taken after Being Infused some Chinese medicine can be taken after infused in hot water or decoction, such as Boat Fruided sterculia Seed, Chrysanthemum Flower.

Darkened Extravasated Blood

Building up the Earth (reinforcing the spleen) therapeutic method of restoring and promoting functioning of the spleen, for cases with spleen deficiency and hypofunction of the spleen in transportation, characterized by poor appetite and diarrhea.

Orthopedic Shawl an appliance used to wrap around the patient's shoulder for fixation with a piece of oxhide which is boiled into a certain size according to the requirement, which is usually applied to cases with bone fracture of the shoulder especially the fractures of humerus and neck bone.

Arsenic Poisoning acute poisoning caused by inhaling or taking large dose of arsneic trioxide by mistake, characterized by cough, chest pain, difficulty in breathing or severe abdominal pain, vomiting, diarrhea, or even sudden

皮痹 【pí bì】因风寒湿侵袭皮肤引起的皮肤瘙痒为主症的一种病证。

Skin-Bi a morbid condition caused by attack of wind, cold and dampness, chiefly marked by itching.

皮腠 【pí còu】即皮肤与肌肉交接间的组织。

Myocutaneous Junction referring to the site where the skin and muscle are joined.

皮肤针 【pí fū zhēn】其头端固定若干枚短针的槌状针具,用以弹刺穴位。

Skin Needle a mallet-shaped needle with several short needles fixed on its top to puncture the skin over the acupoints by flicking.

皮毛 【pí máo】中医认为皮毛与肺脏有密切关系。

Skin and Hair skin and hair are considered to be closely related with the lung in TCM.

皮毛痿 【pí máo wěi】伴有皮毛枯槁失去润泽的痿证,多由肺热引起。常并见咳嗽、气急等症状。

Dermatrophia flaccidity syndrome accompanied by dryness of the skin and hair, mostly due to lung-heat, usually manifested by cough and dyspnea.

皮内针 【pí nèi zhēn】专用于皮下埋藏的一种小毫针。颗粒式皮内针的针头如麦粒,针身长五分或一寸;撒钉式皮内针的针头为扁圆形,针身长一至二分。

Intradermal Needle a small filiform needle embedded beneath the skin. The tip of the pellet-style needle is shaped like wheat grain with a total length of 5 fen or 1 cun, while the tip of the thumb-tack needle is oblate-shaped with a total length of 1—2 fin.

皮水 【pí shuǐ】因脾虚湿盛,水溢肌肤所致的水肿病。症见起病缓慢,全身浮肿,按之没指,无汗、不渴、脉浮。

Severe Edema due to Hypofunction of the Spleen a variety of edema due to effusion of water into the skin due to weakness of the spleen and excessive dampness, marked by insidious onset, which is general and pitting, abscence of sweat, thirst and floating pulse.

罴极之本 【pí jí zhī běn】指肝。因肝主筋,是机体运动的根本。体力活动时,对疲劳的耐受性与肝的功能活动有

Origin of Fatigue referring to the liver which is closely related to the physiological function of the tendons

密切关系。

脾 【pí】五脏之一。位于中焦,在膈之下。其主要生理功能是主运化、升清和统摄血液。某些消化系统疾病、水肿、慢性出血性疾病都可能与脾的功能紊乱有关。

脾痹 【pí bì】内脏痹证之一。因肌痹日久不愈,复感外邪、或饮食不调,脾气受损所致。症见四肢懈惰、呕吐清水、胸闷气窒、腹胀、不欲饮食、咳嗽等。

脾病 【pí bìng】五脏病候之一。泛指脾脏发生的多种病证。多由饮食劳倦所伤,脾失健运,水湿不化;或脾阳虚衰,中气下陷等所致。症见腹胀、肠鸣泄泻、面黄肌瘦、食少难化、肢倦乏力、水肿、脱肛等。

and is the essence of the body in performing its activities. The endurance of the body to fatigue is closely related to the physiological function of the liver.

The Spleen one of the five zang organs which is in the middle energizer below the diaphragm. Its main function is digestion and transformation, sending nutrients upward and keep the blood flowing in vessels. Some digestive diseases, edema and chronic hemorrhagic diseases can be possibly resulted from the functional disturbance of the spleen.

Spleen-Bi one of the Bi syndrome of the visceras caused by long-standing rheumatism with the muscle involved, complicated by exopathic factors or improper diet and the impairment of the spleen-qi, manifested by lassitude of the limbs, watery regurgitation, chest stuffiness, abdominal distention and cough.

Spleen Disease one of the manifestions of the five zang disease, generally referring to all the diseases occurring to the spleen, mostly due to improper diet, over-exertion, dysfunction of the spleen in transport and retention of water in the body, or due to insufficiency of spleen-yang and sinking of qi of middle energizer, marked by abdominal distention, borborygmi, diarrhea, emaciation, poor appetite, dyspepsia, weakness of the limbs and relapse of the rectum.

脾不统血 【pí bù tǒng xuè】脾气虚不能统摄血液，致血不循经所引起多种慢性出血病症的病理。如功能性子宫出血等。
Failure of the Spleen to Keep the Blood Flowing within the Vessels a morbid state due to insufficiency of the spleen-qi, leading to chronic hemorrhagic disease, such as functional uterine bleeding.

脾肺两虚 【pí fèi liǎng xū】指脾气虚弱，不能把营养物质上输于肺，使肺气亦虚，两脏同病的病理。症见面色苍白、食欲减退、便溏、短气、咳嗽痰多、消瘦等。
Deficiency of both the Spleen and Lung a morbid condition in which the spleen fails to transport the nutrients to the lung due to the insufficiency of spleen-qi, leading to the deficiency of lung-qi, marked by pallor of the face, poor appetite, loose stools, dyspnea, productive cough and emaciation.

脾风 【pí fēng】1. 见慢脾风。2. 急性抽搐后，变成疟疾者。
Spleen-Wing 1. see Chronic Wind-syndrome 2. malaria accompanied with tetany.

脾疳 【pí gān】（肥疳、食疳）因脾胃虚损，运化失职所引起的疳积。症见形体消瘦、神疲乏力、乳食懒进、能食易饥、肚腹胀大、大便溏泄、夜睡不宁、易哭易怒等。
Spleen Malnutrition in Infant a morbid condition caused by impairment of the spleen and stomach causing their dysfunction in trasporting and transforming, manifested by emaciation, listlessness, abnormal intake of food with irregular hunger, abdominal distention, loose stools, restless sleep and crying with irritability.

脾和胃 【pí hé wèi】指脾和胃之间的互相关联和影响。它们通过经络的联系，互为表里。胃主受纳，脾主运化，共同完成饮食物的消化吸收及其精微的输布，从而滋养全身，故称脾胃为"后天之本"。
The Spleen Is Connected with the Stomach the spleen and stomach are interior-exteriorly related. The function of the stomach is to receive food while the spleen is in charge of transporting and transforming flood, both of which work together in digesting food, absorbing and distributing nutrients so as to nourish the whole body. Thus, the spleen and stomach provide the mate-

脾精 【pí jīng】脾脏的精气。即脾所具有精华物质，属脾阳，是脾进行功能活动的物质基础。

Essence of the Spleen the vital essence and energy of the spleen, which is part of the spleen-yang and the essential substance of the spleen to perform its functional activities.

脾开窍于口 【pí kāi qiào yú kǒu】指饮食口味等与脾运化功能有密切关系。口味正常与否，全赖于脾胃的运化功能是否正常。如脾运正常，则口味正常，而增进食欲，脾失健运，则出现口淡无味、口甜、口腻等口味异常感，从而影响食欲。

The Mouth is the Body Opening of the Spleen this implies the close relationship between the appetite and function of the spleen in transporting and transforming food. The former depends much on the condition of the latter, ie, when the function of the spleen is normal, there will be a normal and good appetite; otherwise, manifestations of poor appetite such as tastelessness, sweet or greasy taste may occur.

脾咳 【pí ké】由于脾病而导致的咳嗽。症见咳嗽、右胁下痛、痛引肩背，甚则不能动、动则咳剧。

Cough Related to the Spleen Meridian a condition caused by spleen diseases, marked by cough, pain in the right hypochondrium radiating to the shoulder and back, and aggravated by exertion.

脾劳 【pí láo】五劳之一。指由于饥饱失调；或忧思过度，致脾受损伤而引起的一种病证。症见身体消瘦、四肢倦怠、食欲减退、便溏等。

Impairment of the Spleen due to Overstrain syndrome of dysfunction of the spleen due to improper eating or mental distress, marked by muscular wasting, weakness of limbs, anorexia and loose stools.

脾，其华在唇四白 【pí, qí huá zài chún sì bái】脾的生理功能是否正常可以在口唇及其周围的组织反映出来。如脾的生理功能正常，则口唇红润有光泽。

Lips Reflicting the Condition of the Spleen the physiological state of the spleen is reflected on the lips and their surrounding muscles. If the former is normal, the lips would look red, moist and bright.

脾气 【pí qì】指脾的功能，包括消化食物、转输营养与调节水液代谢、统摄血液循行于血管内等功能。

The Spleen-Qi functional activities of the spleen including transformation, transportation, sending nutrients upward, regulating water metabolism and keeping blood flowing within the vessels.

脾气不升 【pí qì bù shēng】指脾气衰弱，不能把营养物质上输到心肺的病理。症见面色不华、眩晕、短气、食欲不振、倦怠或视蒙、耳聋、舌淡、苔白、脉虚缓等。

Failure of Spleen-Qi to Send up Nutrients a morbid condition due to insufficiency of the spleen-qi and inability to send nutrients upward to the heart and lung, marked by dim complexion, dizziness, shortness of breath, poor appetite, lassitude or dim eyesight, deafness, pale tongue with whitish coating, feeble and floating pulse.

脾气不舒 【pí qì bù shū】因肝疏泄功能失常或湿邪内侵，导致脾胃消化吸收功能障碍的病理。症见脘腹胀闷、消化不良、厌食、呃逆等。

Depression of the Spleen-Qi a morbid condition due to impairment of digesting and absorbing function of the spleen resulted from hypofunction of the liver in governing the normal flow of qi and invasion of pathogenic dampness, marked by epigastric stuffiness and distress, dyspepsia, anorexia, and hiccup.

脾热 【pí rè】脾受热邪或过食辛燥食物引起的病证。症见唇红、咽干、腹胀或腹痛、大便秘结、小便少而色黄等。

The Spleen-Heat Syndrome heat syndrome caused by attack of pathogenic heat in the spleen or excessive intake of heat-producing pungent food, marked by reddened tips, dry throat, abdominal distention or pain, constipation, oliguria with the urine yellowish in color.

脾热多涎 【pí rè duō xián】指风热壅结于脾，致脾不能摄所致的多涎证。

Salivation due to Spleen-Heat excessive salivation caused by pathogenic wind-heat attacking the spleen meridi-

脾肾两虚 【pí shèn liǎng xū】由肾阳虚衰，不能温养脾阳或脾阳久虚不能充养肾阳而导致的脾肾阳气俱虚的一种病理变化。症见形寒肢冷、面色㿠白、腰膝或少腹冷痛、泄泻完谷不化、或五更泄泻、或浮肿、小便不利或多尿、舌质淡嫩、苔白润、脉沉弱等。

Insufficiency of both the Spleen and the Kidney a morbid condition caused by failure of the insufficient kidney-yang to warm and nourish the spleen-yang, or failure of the long-standing insufficient spleen-yang to nourish kidney-yang, marked by cold limbs, pale complexion, cold pain in the loin or knees or lower abdomen, loose stools with undigested food, diarrhea at dawn, or edema, difficult urination, or polyuria, pale tongue proper, white moist tongue coating, sunken and weak pulse.

脾失健运 【pí shī jiàn yùn】脾运化功能失常的病理。症见腹胀、食欲减退、泄泻、甚则面黄消瘦、四肢乏力或浮肿等。

Dysfunction of the Spleen in Transport a morbid condition manifested as abdominal distention, poor appetite, diarrhea, or even sallow complexion, emaciation, weakness of the limbs and edema.

脾统血 【pí tǒng xuè】脾的主要功能之一。指脾有统摄血液在经脉中流行，防止溢出脉外的功能。如脾的这一功能障碍，常可发生出血性疾病。

The Spleen Governs Blood the spleen has the function of keeping the blood flowing within the vessls, hemorrhagic diseases may occur if anything wrong with the spleen in performing its function.

脾胃湿热 【pí wèi shī rè】湿热之邪内蕴脾胃的病理。症见皮肤及巩膜黄染、腹胀、食欲减退、恶心、倦怠、尿少而黄、苔黄腻、脉濡数等。

Damp-Heat in the Spleen and Stomach a morbid condition marked by yellow pigmentation of the sclera and skin, abdominal distention, poor appetite, nausea, lassitude, oliguria with the urine yellow in color, greasy yellowish tongue coating, soft and fast pulse.

脾恶湿 【pí wù shī】脾的生理特点之一。脾主运化水湿，湿盛则易伤脾阳，影响健运而产生泄泻、四肢困乏等症，所以说脾恶湿。

The Spleen Being Averse to Dampness one of the physiological characteristic of the spleen which is in charge of transporting and transforming fluid. Excessive dampness is liable to impair spleen-yang and cause diarrhea and weakness of the limbs.

脾消 【pí xiāo】（中消）指以多食易饥、消瘦为主要临床表现的一种疾患。多由胃火炽盛所致。

Diabetes with the Spleen Involved a morbid condition which is also called diabetes with the middle energizer involved, mainly characterized by polyphagia, emaciation, mostly due to excessive stomach-fire.

脾泄 【pí xiè】泄泻因于脾病者。常兼见肢体重著、脘腹不适、面色虚黄。

The Splenic Diarrhea a morbid condition marked by diarrhea accompanied by heaviness of the limbs, discomfort in the abdomen and sallow complexion.

脾虚 【pí xū】通常指脾气虚弱或脾阴不足。表现为食不消化、腹满、肠鸣、泄泻等。

Insufficiency of the Spleen usually referring to insufficiency of the spleen as well as that of spleen-yin marked by dyspepsia, abdominal distention, borborygmi and diarrhea.

脾虚带下 【pí xū dài xià】带下证型之一。由于脾失健运，湿聚下注，伤及任带二脉所致。症见带下量多、色白或淡黄、如涕如唾、连绵不断，兼见面色淡黄、精神疲倦、不思饮食、腰腹酸坠，或有下肢浮肿、大便不实等。

Leukorrhagia due to Deficiency of the Spleen a type of gynecological disease caused by hypofuntion of the spleen leading to downward drive of collected dampness which impairs the conception and governor vessels marked by persistent white or slight yellowish leukorrhea which is accompanied by sallow complexion, general lassitude, anorexia, soreness in the lumbar region and tenesmus in the abdomen or edema of the lower limbs and loose stools.

脾虚多涎 【pí xū duō xián】指脾气虚弱不能摄津所致的多涎。症见神疲，面色萎黄，涎多清稀。
Excessive Salivation Caused by Deficiency of the Spleen a morbid condition characterized by lassitude, sallow complexion and excessive salivation.

脾虚经闭 【pí xū jīng bì】经闭证型之一。因脾胃损伤，纳食减少，生化之源不足，难已生成经血所致。除经闭外，兼见食欲不振、脘腹痞满、大便不实等证。
Amenorrhea due to Deficiency of the Spleen impairment of the spleen and the stomach reduces food intake, so there would be insufficient nutrient essence to produce blood for normal menstruation, which is usually complicated by poor appetite, fullness in the abdomen, and loose stools.

脾虚湿困 【pí xū shī kùn】指脾气虚弱导致内湿阻滞的病理。症见食欲减退、上腹部胀闷、大便泄泻、恶心呕吐、口粘不渴、肢体困倦、甚或浮肿、舌苔厚腻、脉缓等。
Water Retention due to Deficiency of the Spleen a morbid condition marked by anorexia, epigastric distress, abdominal distention, diarrhea, nausea, vomiting, absence of thirst, lassitude and weakness or even edema of the limbs, thick sticky coating of the tongue, slow and sunken pulse.

脾虚泄泻 【pí xū xiè xiè】指因脾虚运化失职，水谷不化引起的泄泻。症见泄泻、食欲减退、面色萎黄、神疲乏力、舌淡、苔薄白、脉弱等。
Diarrhea due to Deficiency of the Spleen a morbid condition marked by diarrhea, anorexia, sallow complexion, lassitude, pale tongue, whitish thin tongue fur, weak pulse.

脾阳 【pí yáng】指脾的运化功能及在运化活动过程中起温煦作用的阳气，是人体阳气在脾脏功能方面的反映。如脾阳虚衰，可出现饮食不化、腹痛腹胀、大便溏泄、四肢不温、水湿停滞、浮肿等。
The Spleen-Yang referring to the transporting and transforming function of the spleen and the yang-qi required to carry on the warming process, which are the yang-qi of the body reflected in the spleen functions. Manifestations such as indigestion, abdominal pain and distention, loose stools, cold limbs, water retention and edema may appear if there is insufficiency of spleen-yang.

脾阳虚　【pí yáng xū】（脾胃虚寒）脾胃功能明显低下而出现虚寒证候的病理。症见上腹部冷痛、腹胀、呃逆、食欲不振、慢性泄泻、倦怠、尿少、浮肿、消瘦、舌淡、脉虚等。

脾阴　【pí yīn】指脾的阴液，包括血液和津液等，是脾进行功能活动的物质基础。

脾阴虚　【pí yīn xū】脾的阴液不足，导致消化吸收功能障碍的病理。症见饥不欲食、消瘦、便秘、体倦乏力等。

脾约　【pí yuē】指脾虚，气不化津，致肠中津液不足引起的大便坚硬难出的病证。

脾主后天　【pí zhǔ hòu tiān】人出生以后生长发育所需的营养物质，主要靠脾胃的消化吸收功能来化生，所以说脾主后天。

脾主肌肉　【pí zhǔ jī ròu】脾的功能之一。因为脾胃为气血生化之源，全身的肌肉，都需要依靠脾胃运化的水谷精微来营养，才能使肌肉发达丰满，臻于健壮，因此，人体肌肉的壮实与否，与脾胃的运化功能相关，运化功能障碍，必致肌肉削瘦，软弱无力，甚

Insufficiency of Spleen-Yang　a morbid condition marked by asthenia-cold syndromes; manifested as cold pain in the upper part of the abdomen, abdominal distention, dyspnea, poor appetite, chronic diarrhea, lassitude, oliguria, edema, emaciation, pale tongue, feeble pulse.

The Spleen-Yin　the yin fluid of the spleen, including blood and saliva, which constitutes the material basis of the functional activities of the spleen.

Deficiency of the Spleen-Yin　deficiency of yin fluid in the stomach and spleen which impedes their normal functioning, marked by hunger but with no appetite, emaciation, constipation, lassitude and fatigue.

The Splenic Constipation　constipation due to lack of fluid in the large intestine leading to dryness of feceds as a conseqence of dysfunction of the spleen in fluid transformation.

The Spleen Determines the Condition of the Required Constitution　this implies that the growth and development of the human body mainly depends on the nutrients digested and absorbed by the spleen and stomach.

The Spleen Dominates the Muscles

the spleen and stomach are the source where qi and blood are transformed and produced, when nourished with the nutrients of the food stuff digested and transported by the spleen and stomach, the muscles can remain

至痿废不用。

strong and healthy. Therefore the conditions of the muscles are closely related to the functions of the spleen and stomach. Thus the former might become thin and weak or even flaccid if any functional disturbances occur with the latter.

脾主升清【pí zhǔ shēng qīng】脾的功能之一。指脾能吸收水谷精微等营养物质，并上输于心、肺、头目，通过心肺的作用化生气血，以营养全身。这种功能以上升为主，故有脾气主升的说法。

The Spleen Dominates Sending up Essential Substances one of the functions of the spleen is to send up essential substances to the heart and lung, head and eyes, there the substances are transformed into qi and blood by the activity of the heart and lung to nourish the whole body.

脾主四肢【pí zhǔ sí zhī】脾的功能之一。脾有为四肢活动提供营养和能量，以维持四肢正常活动的功能。

The Spleen Dominates the Limbs referring to one of the functions of the spleen to supply the limbs with nutrients and energy to maintain their normal functional activities.

脾主为胃行其津液【pí zhǔ wéi wèi xíng qí jīn yè】指脾有把胃所受纳水谷中富含的营养物质输送到其他脏腑和人体各部分的作用。

The Spleen Helps thd Stomach in Digestion and Fluid Transportation referring to the function of the spleen to transport the nutrients of the food stuff received by the stomach to the other zang organs as well as the other parts of the body.

脾主运化【pí zhǔ yùn huà】脾的主要功能之一。是指脾具有把水谷（饮食物）化为精微，并将精微物质转输至全身的生理功能。包括对饮食物的消化和吸收与对水液的吸收、转输和布散作用。

The Spleen Dominates the Transportation and Transformation of Nutrients one of the main functions of the spleen, ie, to transform nutrients and transport the essential substances to the whole boby, including the digestion and absorption of food and the absorption, transport and distribution of water.

脾主中央 【pí zhǔ zhōng yāng】按五行学说的归类，在五脏配五方（东、南、西、北、中央），脾为中央。但主要的是指脾有把营养物质输送到其他脏腑组织器官的作用。

The Spleen Transports Nutrition from the Centre to all Parts of the Body according to the classification in the five-element theory in which the five visceras are matched with the five positions (east, south, west, north, centre), the spleen is the centre, which implies that it has the function to transport nutrients to the other zang-fu organs and tissues.

癖积 【pǐ jī】多由水饮停结，痰瘀凝滞，食积内阻，寒热邪气搏结而成的慢性疾病。症见肋下弦硬有条块状物、胀痛或刺痛或兼见喘息短气。

Hypochondriac Lump a chronic disease caused by retention of water, accumulation of phlegm and food, and the invasion of pathogenic cold and heat, marked by hard strip-like lump in the subcostal area with distending or stabbing pain or even complicated by shortness of breath.

痞块 【pǐ kuài】指腹腔内的积块。

Mass in the Abdomen

痞满 【pǐ mǎn】指胸腹间气机阻滞而引起闷或胀满等不适的感觉。

Feeling of Fullness in the Chest or upper Abdomen a morbid condition caused by stagnancy of qi.

痞气 【pǐ qì】1. 为五积之一，属脾之积。多因脾虚气郁，留滞积结而成。症见胃脘部有肿块突起状如复盘，伴消瘦、四肢无力等。日久可发生黄疸。2. 指胸前痞满不舒的症状。多由伤寒误用攻下，而邪不解所致。

Mass at the Right Hypochondrium (at spleen) 1. one of the five types of accumulation in the abdomen mostly caused by deficiency of the abdomen, accompanied by deficiency of the spleen and qi stagnancy, marked by disc-like mass bulging from the abdomen, accompanied by emaciation, weakness of the limbs, and jaundice appeared in the long run 2. feeling of fullness in the chest and upper abdomen, mostly due to erroneous administration of purgatives in the treatment of exogenous febrile disease and

偏方 【piān fāng】未经医学家记载、流传于民间的一些简单、有效的方剂。

偏沮 【piān jù】即半身出汗、半身无汗的症状。多由气血不能畅流全身所致。可见于中风或某些植物神经功能紊乱的疾患。

偏瘫 【piān tān】(偏枯、偏风)指一侧肢体偏废不用，久则见患肢肌肉枯瘦的病证。多由营卫俱虚，真气不能充于全身；或兼邪气侵袭所致。

偏头风 【piān tóu fēng】(偏头痛、头偏痛)其痛多在一侧颞部或头角，有痛连目或视力受损者，有兼恶心呕吐者。多因风邪侵于少阳，或肝虚痰火郁结所致。

偏坠 【piān zhuì】一侧睾丸肿大、疼痛下坠的病证。多因痰湿、瘀血、肝火亢盛所致。

胼胝 【pián zhī】因患处长期受压、磨擦、局部气血阻滞,皮肤失养所致。多见于常突起部位。患处皮肤增厚，呈黄白或淡黄褐色，触之坚硬或疼痛，边缘不清。

the existing pathogenic factors.

Folk Prescription the simple but effective prescriptions which are not recorded in medical books but used among the people.

Hemihidrosis a symptom seen in apoplexy and some diseases with vegetable nerve functional disturbance, mostly due to the poor circulation of qi and blood.

Hemiplegia a morbid condition in which one-side limbs paralysed and, in the long run, with muscular atrophy, mostly caused by the inability of the genuine qi to circulate over the whole body resulting in deficiency of ying and wei; or complicated by the attack of pathogenic factors.

Migraine a morbid condition usually with the pain localized to the temple and radiating to the eyes or causing dim eyesiggt, or complicated by nausea, vomiting, mostly due to invasion of shaoyang meridian by pathogenic wind, or liver deficiency and stagnancy of phlegm-fire.

Swelling with Bearing-down Pain of One Side of Testis a morbid condition mostly caused by phlegm-dampness, blood stasis, excessive liver-fire.

Callosity a condition caused by persistent rubbing on the affected area or poor nourishment of the skin due to stagnancy of qi and blood, mostly seen on the protruding areas of the palms or soles, characterized by thickened

片 【piàn】中药炮制法之一。把药料细粉加入适量的赋形剂,或将药汁浓缩后再吸附药末或赋形剂,经模压成片剂。

漂 【piǎo】中药炮制法之一。某些药物用流水或经常换水的办法浸漂,以除去毒性、盐份、杂质、腥味等的一种炮制方法。

频服 【pín fú】一般指汤剂。根据病情需要,采取少量多次的分服法,适用于病在上部。

牝疟 【pìn nüè】患者素体阳虚,疟邪伏于少阴所致的疟疾。症见寒战较甚、无热或微热、发有定时、面色淡白、脉沉而迟等。

牝脏 【pìn zàng】指肺、脾、肾等属阴之脏。

牝痔 【pìn zhì】即肛门周围脓肿及部分混合痔。

平旦服 【píng dàn fú】在早晨未进食前空腹服药。

平肝熄风 【píng gān xī fēng】(镇肝熄风)是治疗由于肝肾阴虚,肝阳上亢,引动内风的方法。症见头痛、头晕目

skin, in whitish or light yellowish brown color, hard and pain on pressing with unclear margins.

Tablet one of the methods in drug preparation with which tablets are morulded by adding a certain amount of excipient into the fine drug powder, or by absorbing the powder, with the concentrated drug juice or excipient.

Rinsing Medicinal Herbs process of washing crude drugs with flowing water or with frequent change of water to remove dirt, salty ingredient, bood odor and reduce toxicity.

(Decoction) to Be Taken in Small Doses at Short Intervals a method for taking decoctions, suitable for upper-part diseases.

Malaria of Yin-Type chronic malaria due to constitutional yang deficiency and invasion of shaoyin meridian by pathogenic factor of malarial disease, characterized by severe chill and rigors, slight fever, attacks recurring at a regular time each day, pale complexion, sunken and slow pulse.

Yin Organs (zang-organs) zang-organs of yin nature, ie, the lung, the spleen and the kidney.

Mixed Hemorrhoids and perianal Abscess

Taking Drug in the Morning when the Stomach is Empty

Calming the Liver to Stop the Wind a method to check stiring interior wind due to yin deficiency of the liver

眩、口眼歪斜、肢体发麻或震颤、舌体活动不灵或偏斜、语言不清、甚至突然昏倒、手足抽搐、舌质红、苔薄、脉弦等。

and kidney and hyperactivity of the liver-yang, manifested by headache, dizziness, distortion of the mouth and eyes, numbness and tremor of the limbs difficulty in the movement of the tongue or even deviated, slurred speech, and even falling suddenly in a faint with spasm of the limbs, red tongue, thin tongue coating and wiry pulse.

平脉 【píng mài】正常的脉象。其主要特点是脉搏和缓,不快不慢,脉律整齐。

Normal Pulse a pulse condition of healthy person which is mild, regular rhythm and normal frequency.

平人 【píng rén】指健康的人。

A Healthy person

破气 【pò qì】使用较峻烈的理气药,以散气结,开郁滞的方法。本法作用较剧烈,易伤正气,体虚气弱者慎用。

Dispersing Qi a method of removing stagnation or obstruction of qi circulation with drastic drugs, which should be used cautiously to patients who are constitutionally weak since it is potent and may do harm.

破伤风 【pò shāng fēng】(金疮痉、伤痉)因跌打损伤,产褥破伤,脐带剪伤,手术创伤等引起的疾病。症见恶寒发热,颜面肌肉痉挛,呈哭笑面容,牙关紧闭,舌强口噤,流涎,继则角弓反张,频频发作;后期说话、吞咽、呼吸俱感困难,甚则窒息。辨证分类:1. 风毒在表证 2. 风毒入里证。

Tetanus a morbid condition caused by traumatic injuries, dilivery injuries, cutting injury of the umbilicus, and operational injuries marked by chills, fever, spasms of the facial muscle, sad smile complexion, trismus, stiff tongue, locked jaws, salivation, then, opithotonos, with repeated attacks; at last, difficulty in speading, swallowing and breathing or even suffocation. Types of differentiation 1. wind toxic in the superfice 2. interior invasion of wind toxic.

破头疮 【pò tóu chuāng】患处皮破肉烂,色黑形陷,流出水液,不易生肌,顽固难愈。多因素体虚弱或病久脾

Chronic Ulcer a skin lesion marked by ulceration of the affected area which is pitting and black in color

虚，湿邪浸淫所致。 with fluid discharge, failure of the muscle to grow and difficult to heal, mostly due to constitutional weakness or spleen deficiency caused by long-standing disease, and invasion of pathogenic dampness.

破血 【pò xuè】使用作用剧烈的祛瘀药，如桃仁、穿山甲、红花、䗪虫等，以达到祛瘀的目的。 **Removing Blood Stasis** a method of removing blood stasis by using potent drugs such as Semen Persicae, Squama Manitis, Flos Corthami, Eupolyphagaseu Steleophaga, etc.

破瘀消癥 【pò yū xiāo zhēng】（通瘀破结、逐瘀、散瘀）是治疗腹中瘀血积块的方法。通常以活血祛瘀药和行气药同用，治疗因气滞血瘀引起的腹腔或子宫肿块。 **Removing Blood Stasis and Lumps** a therapeutic method by using both blood-stasis-removing drugs and drugs of relieving stagnation of qi to treat lumps in the abdominal cavity or uterus caused by stagnation of qi and blood stasis.

魄 【pò】以机体的本能行为和各种感觉为特征的精神活动。 **Inferior Spirit** emotional activties characteristic of the instinctive behaviors and feelings.

魄汗 【pò hàn】见汗。肺藏魄，汗液透发于肺，故名。 **Inferior-Spirit Perspiration** so called because the spirit is stored in the lung and sweat comes from the lung.

魄门 【pò mén】即肛门。 **Outlet for Discharging Dregs** referring to the anus.

扑粉 【pū fěn】把药物研成细粉，扑撒在皮肤上，用于敛汗、止痒等。 **Applying Medicinal Powder** grinding the drug into fine powder and applying it to the skin to arrest sweating and stop itching.

葡萄疫 【pú táo yì】多因脾胃积热，热损血络，血热妄行所致。症见身起大小青紫斑点、色若葡萄、压之不褪色，甚则牙根腐烂出血。 **Hemorrhagic Disease with Purpura** a morbid condition due to accumulation of pathogenic heat, leading to the impairment of the blood vessels and bleeding due to blood heat, characterized by pelidnomas which are various

七冲门 【qī chōng mén】即飞门、户门、吸门、贲门、幽门、阑门、及魄门。

七方 【qī fāng】按方剂组成的不同，可分为大方、小方、缓方、急方、奇方、偶方及复方等七种。

七怪脉 【qī guài mài】生命垂危时出现的七种异常脉象，即雀啄脉、屋漏脉、弹石脉、解索脉、虾游脉、鱼翔脉及釜沸脉，出现这些脉象往往是脏气将绝，胃气枯竭的表现。

七窍 【qī qiào】指面部的七个孔窍：眼、耳、鼻、口、五脏的精气通于七窍，故从七窍的变化可帮助诊断五脏的疾病。

七情 【qī qíng】1. 即喜、怒、忧、思、悲、恐、惊等七种情志活动，它是人的精神意识对外界事物的反应。2. 作为致病因素，是过于强烈而持久的情志活动引起脏腑气血功能失调而致病。

in size and in grape color that does not fade when pressed, or even accompanied by putrefacted tooth root and bleeding.

Seven Important Portals denoting the following portions of the alimentary tract, viz, lips teeth, epiglottis, cardia, pylorus, ileocaecal valve and anus.

Seven Kinds of Prescriptions classification of prescriptions by their composition: large, small, insidious effect, prompt effect, with ingredients odd in number, with ingredients even in number and compound prescriptions.

Seven Moribund Pulses pulse conditions seen in critical cases, ie, bird-pecking pulse, roof-leaking pulse, flicking pulse, untying-knot pulse, fish-swimming pulse, shrimp-darting pulse and bubble-rising pulse, the appearance of which usually shows the impending dysfunction of the visceras and stomach-qi.

Seven Orifices seven openings of sense organs of head, ie, the eyes, ears, nose and mouth, with which the primordial energy of the five zang organs is linked, by observing changes of the seven orifices would aid in the diagnosis in the zang organs.

Seven Emotions 1. joy, anger, melancholy, meditation, grief, terror and fright, being the response of the mind to the environment. 2. persistent and violent emotions as pathogenic factors causing functional derangement of qi,

七日风 【qī rì fēng】即新生儿破伤风。

漆疮 【qī chuāng】(漆咬、漆湿疮) 因感受漆气而发的过敏性皮肤病。

奇恒之腑 【qí héng zhī fǔ】包括大脑、髓、骨、脉、胆、子宫等。这些器官结构类似腑，作用又类似脏。

脐 【qí】腹壁中央的陷窝，为出生后的脐带断落结疤所形成。

脐疮 【qí chuāng】患儿常先有脐湿，使皮肤破损，再感毒邪所致的病证。症见脐部红肿，甚至脐部周围蔓延糜烂，脓水外流，伴有发热烦躁，唇红口干等。

脐风 【qí fēng】即新生儿破伤儿。是由于断脐不洁，感染外邪所致。症见全身各部发生强直性痉挛、牙关紧闭、面呈苦笑状。

脐漏 【qí lòu】(脐漏疮) 多由脐痈久治不敛，形成漏管。症见脐中时流脓血臭水、久不收口。

脐疝 【qí shàn】多见于幼儿，为脐中

blood and zang-fu organs.

Tetanus Neonatorium

Dermatitis Rhus an alergic skin disease caused by affection of rhus and its products.

Extraordinary Fu-Organs the brain, marrow, bone, vessels, gallbladder, and uterus are called extraordinary fu organs because of their similarities to the ordinary fu organs but having the function to store essence like the zang organs.

Umbilicus a pitting at the center of the abdomen which formed when the umbilicus cord dropped after being delivered.

Omphalitis a morbid condition of infant first with intertrigo umbilicus then affected by toxins, marked by redness, swelling and erosion around the umbilicus with purulent discharge, accompanied by fever, restlessness, redness of the lips and dryness in the mouth, etc.

Neonatal Tetanus a morbid condition due to invasion of exopathic factors through the infected umbilical wound, marked by generalized tonic spasm, locked jaw and sad smile complexion.

Umbilical Fistula a condition due to long-standing umbilical carbuncle, characterized by intermittent fetid watery discharge with pus and blood, and remaining unhealed for a long period of time.

Umbilical Hernia a disease mostly

有包块突出，可闻及肠鸣音。

脐湿 【qí shī】（脐湿肿）指新生儿脐带脱落后，脐孔湿润不干，甚或有水溢出或脐孔周围稍现红肿。由于断脐后护理不当，为水湿所浸而成。

脐下悸 【qí xià jì】指自觉脐下跳动不宁的症状。多因素有水饮内停或发汗不当，心阳不振，水气上逆引起。

脐血 【qí xuè】断脐后脐部有血渗出，经久不止。大都在出生后第一周，脐带脱落前后出现。

脐痈 【qí yōng】 1. 生于脐部之痈。由心经火毒流入小肠积聚而成或搔抓脐部后继发感染而致。症见脐部肿突，皮色或红或白。即脐部感染。2. 见腹痈。

气 【qì】 1. 指呼吸过程中进出人体的空气。2. 体内流动着的富有营养的精微物质。3. 人体及脏器组织的功能。

气秘 【qì bì】由于气滞或气虚引起以便秘为主症的病证。

seen in infant with protruding mass in the umbilicus with borborygmi being heard.

Oozing from the Umbilicus moist navel of the newborn occurring after the umbilical cord has dropped, sometimes even with fluid oozing out, or slight redness and swelling in the surrounding area, usually caused by improper care, and invasion of water.

Subjective Throbbing in the Lower Abdomen a condition caused by excessive accumulation of fluid in the body or improper use of diaphoresis, insufficiency of the heart-yang, upward flowing of the retained fluid.

Bleeding from the Umbilicus a morbid condition occurring in infant after or before the dropping of umbilical cord mostly in the first week after being delivered.

Umbilical Carbuncle 1. carbuncle around the umbilicus caused by fire-toxin in the heart meridian attacking the small intestine or secondary infection because of scratching, marked by swelling with the skin red or white in color, ie, the umbilical infection 2. see Abdominal Carbuncle.

Air 1. the air breathed in and out 2. refined nutritive substance flowing within the body 3. qi functional activities of the body and of the internal organs and tissues.

Constipation due to Disorder of Qi constipation caused by stagnation of qi or deficiency of qi.

气痹 【qì bì】指由于情志刺激等因素致邪气闭阻引发的痹证。因影响部位的不同，可表现为吞咽困难、语言障碍、腰痛脚重、半身不遂、或排尿困难等。

Qi-Bi　arthralgin due to stagnation of qi due to emotional distress with different manifestations for the different positions involved, such as difficulty in swallowing, aphasis, lumbago, heaviness of the feet, hemiparalysis, or difficulty in micturition.

气喘 【qì chuǎn】1. 各种呼吸困难的证候的通称。2. 由于气机郁结而引起的呼吸急促。

Dyspnea　1. general term for difficulties in breathing 2. a condition due to stagnation of qi.

气短 【qì duǎn】呼吸无力、浅表、急促的症状。常由于气虚所致。

Shortness of Breath　respiration which is weak, superficial and rapid, usually caused by insufficiency of qi.

气呃 【qì è】由于气机郁滞或气虚引起的呃逆。

Hiccup Caused by Disorder of Qi　a morbid condition due to stagnation of qi or insufficiency of qi.

气分证 【qì fēn zhèng】温热病邪由表入里，侵及气分，但未侵及营血的阶段。多由卫分证不解，邪热内传气分所致。症见高热不恶寒、汗多、口渴喜冷饮、舌苔黄燥、脉滑数或洪大等。

Syndrome of Qi Fen　the second stage of an acute febrile disease showing invasion of the interior of the body but not yet the ying blood, mostly caused by the existing weifen syndrome and interior invasion of qifen by pathogenic heat, marked by high fever without chills, profuse sweating, thirst and the preference for cold drink, yellowish dry coating of the tongue, slippery and fast or full pulse.

气膈 【qì gé】由于气机郁结引起以噎膈为主症的病证。

Dysphagia Related to Qi　a morbid condition mainly characterized by dysphagia, due to stagnation of qi.

气功 【qì gōng】是运用意识的引导作用，通过调节呼吸、意守等，对生命活动过程实行自我调节、控制，以达到防治疾病，强身延年的一种自我身心锻炼方法。

Qigong　a kind of psychosomatic regime aimed at disease prevention and treatment, health preservation and longevity through training of mind, breating and posture, and regulation of

气功功能态 【qì gōng gōng néng tài】是指气功锻炼时通过对意念、呼吸和姿势等的锻炼，在入静状态中所表现的人体功能状态。

Functional State of Qi Gong referring to the functional state of body after entering static state by the training of mind, breathing and posture in process of practising qi gong.

气功疗法 【qì gōng liáo fǎ】利用气功以治疗某些疾病的方法。见气功。

Qigong Therapy method to treat some certain diseases by means of qigong.

气功学 【qì gōng xué】是研究气功的历史、现状、锻炼功法、程序、机理及其应用的科学。气功学是中国传统医学的一个组成部分，也是一门涉及人体身心互相作用的，复杂的生命现象和规律的人体科学。

Qi Gong Subject a subject about Qigong's history, presence, training skill, process, mechanism and application. It is an important part of TCM, and also a subject of body concerning the interaction between body and mind, the relation between complex life appearance and essential.

气鼓 【qì gǔ】由于气机郁滞所致的鼓胀病。见鼓胀。

Tympanites due to Stagnation of Qi

气臌 【qì gǔ】即气机郁滞所致的鼓胀。症见腹部胀大、青筋暴露、全身浮肿、肤色苍黄等。

Tympanites due to Stagnation of Qi a morbid condition marked by abdominal distention, visible vein vessels on the abdomen, generalized edema and yellowish skin.

气关 【qì guān】小儿指纹的诊断部位之一。指食指第二指节掌面外侧浅表小静脉的显露，此处浅小静脉的变化通常表示病情较重。

Qi Pass the middle segment of the index of an infant, the superficial venules on the palmar side which are inspected for diagnosis, and changes of which usually means that the status of illness is serious.

气海 【qì hǎi】1. 即膻中。是宗气聚集和发源的地方。是四海之一，又叫上气海。2. 经穴名。

Reservoir (Sea) of Qi 1. referring to danzhong, the confluence and source of (pectoral) zong-qi, the upper reservoir (sea), one of the four reservoirs. 2. acupoint.

气化 【qì huà】1. 气的产生、循行及其功能。2. 指某些器官的生理功能，如三焦对体液的调节、膀胱的排尿功能等。

Functional Activity of Qi 1. the formation, circulation and functions of qi 2. referring to the physiological functions of cartain organs, for instance, regulation of body fluid by triple energizer, micturating functoin of the urinary bladder.

气会 【qì huì】八会之一。即膻中穴，精气会聚的地方。

Qi-Assembling Point a point where qi assembles, ie, point of danzhong.

气积 【qì jī】与精神因素如忧思、恼怒等有关的积病，以腹胀时隐时现，痛处游走不定为特征。

Qi Mass abdominal mass due to emotional factors such as melancholy, anxiety, anger etc, marked by abdominal mass which comes and goes, and wandering pain.

气机 【qì jī】指气的功能活动。

Functional Activities of Qi

气机不利 【qì jī bù lì】泛指脏腑功能活动失调。通常用以说明升清降浊的功能紊乱，常见有呃逆、胸腔痞闷、腹胀、腹痛、大小便失常等症状。

Disorder of Qi generally referring to the functional disorders of zang-fu organs, usually denoting their functional disturbances in ascending and descending, usually manifested by hiccup, fullness and stuffiness in the chest, abdominal distention and pain, difficulty in defecation and urination.

气绝 【qì jué】机体生命活动功能严重衰竭的一种危象。临床上常分为阴气绝、阳气绝、脏气绝和腑气绝等。

Depletion of Qi a critical condition denoting the severe functional failure of the body in performing its life activities, usually classified clinically as depleted yin-qi, yang-qi, zang-qi and fu-qi.

气厥 【qì jué】因气机逆乱所致的昏厥。有气虚、气实之分。

Syncope Resulting from Disorder of Qi a morbid condition usually classified as insufficiency of qi and excess of qi.

气疬 【qì lì】指一种瘰疬，其增大与恼怒有关。

Scrofula Aggravated by Anger

气痢 【qì lì】指由于气虚或气滞引起的

Dysentery due to Disorder of Qi

痢疾。

气淋 【qì lín】（气癃）以下腹至阴囊胀痛、小便不畅或尿后疼痛等为特征的病证。多因膀胱气滞或脾肾虚膀胱热所致。

气瘤 【qì liú】因劳伤肺气，腠理不密，复为外邪所袭而引起的皮下肿瘤。以瘤体质软、色如常、大小随情志变化而改变为特征。

气轮 【qì lún】即白睛部分，配属于肺，其疾患多与肺和大肠有关。

气门 【qì mén】1. 指阳气散泄的门户，即毛孔。2. 穴位名称。

气逆 【qì nì】为气机升降失常，脏腑之气逆上的病理。多由情志所伤，或因饮食寒温不适，或因痰浊壅阻等所致。最常见于肺、胃和肝等脏腑。

气呕 【qì ǒu】由于情志不舒（如盛怒、忧思等）或脾气郁结引起以呕吐为主症的病证。可见于神经性呕吐、慢性胃炎等疾病。

dysentery either due to deficiency of qi or stagnation of qi.

Qi Stranguria a morbid condition caused by qi stagnation in the urinary bladder or deficiency of qi in the spleen and kidney and heat in the bladder, marked by distending pain in the scrotum, dysuria or pain after urination.

Tumour due to Disorder of Qi a subcutaneous tumor brought about by damage of the lung-qi due to overstrain and lower resistance of the superficies with simultaneous attack of pathogenic factors from outside; characterized by soft tumor, covered with normal skin, and varying in size with emotional changes.

Qi Wheel (the white of the eye) referring to the white of the eye which belongs to the lung and whose diseases are mostly related to the lung and the large intestine.

Qi Gate 1. referring to the gate through which yang-qi is dispersed, ie, the sweat pore. 2. acupoint

Reversed Flow of Qi a morbid condition mostly due to emotional distress or intake of cold food, or accumulation of phlegm, mostly seen in the zang-fu organs such as the lung, stomach and liver.

Vomiting due to Disorder of Qi vomiting due to stagnation of the spleen-qi resulting from fury, anxiety or emotional depression, seen in neurogenic vomiting, and chronic gastritis.

气痞 【qì pǐ】由于气滞引起的胸腹胀满症状。多因外感误下，或七情所伤，气机阻塞所致。

Flatulence due to Stagnation of Qi stuffiness, distention and fullness in the chest and epigastrium resulting from stagnation of qi which is usually caused by erroneous downward drive of exopathic factors or the hurt of the seven emotions.

气怯 【qì qiè】由于胆气不足而出现的心慌易惊的症状。

Fright due to Deficiency of Qi a morbid condition resulting from deficiency of the gallbladder-qi manifested by palpitation panic and cowardice.

气疝 【qì shàn】1. 因饮食寒温失调，气机阻滞而致的腹痛。2. 由于气郁诱发的阴囊坠痛。

Colic due to Disorder of Qi 1. abdominal pain due to intake of cold food, and stagnation of qi. 2. bearing-down pain of the scrotum due to stagnation of qi.

气上冲心 【qì shàng chōng xīn】自觉有一股气从下腹部上冲至胸部的一种自觉症状。多由寒邪客于下焦及胃肠或肝胃之气上逆所致。

Reflux of Qi to the Heart a subjective sensation of gas rushing from the lower abdomen up to epigastric region and the chest mostly caused by invasion of the lower engergizer as well as the stomach and intestines by pathogenic cold or adverse upward flowing of the liver and stomach-qi.

气嗽 【qì sòu】1. 指因七情内伤所致的咳嗽。2. 指咳嗽而见气机不利，胸膈满闷之症。

Cougth due to Disorder of Qi 1. cough due to emotional upset 2. cough complicated disorder of qi, fullness and stuffiness in the chest.

气随血脱 【qì suí xuè tuō】指由于失血过多，气失依附，导致阳气虚脱的病理。常见有面色苍白、四肢厥冷、大汗淋漓、脉微欲绝等症。相当于出血性休克。

Exhaustion of Qi Resulting from Hemorrhea pathological changes showing exhaustion of yang-qi caused by massive bleeding, manifested by pale complexion, cold limbs, profuse sweating, thready and barely perceptible pulse as seen in hemorrhagic shock.

气痰 【qì tán】1. 即燥痰。2. 指梅核气。3. 因情志刺激致症状加重的痰证。

Phlegm-Syndrome due to Disorder of Qi 1. dry-phlegm syndrome 2. globus hystericus 3. phlege-syndrome aggravated by meytal strain.

气痛 【qì tòng】由于气机郁滞引起的疼痛。多发于胸腹腰胁等部位。

Pain due to Disorder of Qi a morbid condition mostly seen in the chest, abdomen as well as the lumbocostal region.

气为血帅 【qì wéi xuè shuài】指气对血的推动,统摄和化生的作用。中医学认为血能在经脉中运行,是依靠气作为它的动力。

Qi as the Commander of Blood it is so said because qi transforms blood, activates and gorverns the blood circulation. Qi is regarded as the motive force in activating the blood circulation in vessels.

气味 【qì wèi】(性味) 药物的性味。指药物的寒、热、温、凉四气和辛、甘、酸、苦、咸五味的基本属性。药物气味不同,可产生不同的作用。如黄连苦寒,能清热燥湿;浮萍辛寒,能疏风清热。

The Nature and Taste of a Drug referring to the four natures of drugs such as cold, hot, warm and cool and their five kinds of flavor, acrid, sweet, sour, bitter and salty. Drugs of different natures and tastes have different roles, e. g. , Rhizoma Coptidis which is bitter and cold can be used to clear heat and dry damp, while Herba Spirodelae which is acrid and cold can be used to dispel wind and remove heat.

气味阴阳 【qì wèi yīn yáng】指药物四气五味和升降浮沉的阴阳属性。如四气中热、温属阳;寒、凉属阴。五味中辛、甘属阳;酸、苦、咸属阴。升、浮属阳;沉降属阴。

Yin-Yang Categorization of Natures and Tastes the natures and tastes of drugs may be ategorized according to yin and yang. Hot and warm natures belong to yang while cold and cool natures to yin; of the tastes, pungent and sweet belong to yang while sour, bitter and salty to yin; the ascending and floating effects belong to yang while the descending and sinking effects to

气泻 【qì xiè】由于肝气郁结所致的泄泻。以恼怒后症状加剧为特征。

气心痛 【qì xīn tòng】由情志因素所诱发的胸痛。

气虚 【qì xū】1. 指元气耗损、功能失调、脏腑功能衰退、抗病能力下降的病理。症见精神萎靡、面色㿠白、头眩耳鸣、心悸短气、倦怠乏力、自汗、脉虚弱等。2. 指肺气虚，症见面色淡白、短气、声音低弱、畏风、自汗等。

气虚崩漏 【qì xū bēng lòu】因气虚引起的崩漏。症见突然阴道大量出血或淋漓不断，血色淡红而清稀，伴有乏力气短、不思饮食、面色㿠白、心悸等。

气虚痹 【qì xū bì】因气虚阳弱，寒湿内盛，引起四肢关节活动不利，或兼有肢体寒冷麻木的病证。

气虚便秘 【qì xū biàn bì】指因气虚引

yin.

Diarrhea due to Stagnation of Qi a morbid condition due to stagnation of the liver-qi which is aggravated by anger.

Chest Pain Aroused by Emotional Factors

Deficiency of Qi 1. a morbid condition due to exhaustion of qi, functional disturbance, hypofuction of zang-fu organs and reduced ability to resist diseases, marked by poor spirit, pallor complexion, dizziness, tinnitus, palpitation, shortness of breath, lassitude, listlessness, spontaneous sweating, weak pulse. 2. denoting hypofunction of the lung, a morbid condition characterized by pale complexion, shortness of breath, weak voice, fear of wind and spontaneous sweating.

Metrorrhagia due to Deficiency of Qi a morbid condition marked by profuse vaginal bleeding or persistent dripping, with the blood light red in color and watery, accompanied by lassitude, shortness of breath, poor appetite, pale complexion, and palpitation.

Arthralgia due to Deficiency of Qi a morbid condition due to deficiency of yang-qi and interior excessive pathogenic cold and dampness, resulting in difficulty in the movement of limbs and complicated by coldness and numbness of the limbs.

Constipation due to Deficiency of Qi

起的大便秘结。多由劳倦或饮食不慎，损伤脾气；或肺气素虚，大肠传送无力所致。a morbid condition caused by overstrain or improper diet, leading to the impairment of the spleen-qi, or due to constitutional deficiency of the lung-qi and hypofunction of the large intestine to transport.

气虚不摄【qì xū bù shè】1. 泛指脏气虚，统摄失职而出现自汗、遗精、泄泻、遗尿、崩漏、便血等症的病理。2. 指气虚不能摄血而发生各种出血证的病理。**Failure in Governing due to Deficiency of Qi** 1. generally referring to the morbid conditions in which zang-qi fails to govern, marked by spontaneous sweating, spermatorrhea, enuresis, metrorrhagia, hemafecia. 2. referring to bleeding caused by hypofunction of qi in governing the blood.

气虚喘【qì xū chuǎn】指元气不足或脾肺气虚导致的气喘病证。**Dyspnea due to Deficiency of Qi** dyspnea caused by insufficiency of qi or deficiency of spleen-qi and lung-qi.

气虚耳聋【qì xū ěr lóng】因年老体衰或病后气虚引起的耳聋病证。伴有耳鸣、乏神急倦、心悸气短、口淡纳呆、脉弱无力等症状。**Deafness due to Deficiency of Qi** a morbid condition due to old age, poor health or qi deficiency after just recovering from illness, accompanied by tinnitus, lassitude, listlessness, palpitation, shortness of breath, loss of appetite, and weak pulse.

气虚耳鸣【qì xū ěr míng】因气虚引起的耳鸣病证。其鸣声持续而声小，有如蝉鸣或笛声，并可伴有急倦、食少、便溏等症状。**Tinnitus due to Deficiency of Qi** a morbid condition characterized by long-lasting light ringing sound in the ears like a cicada singing or the sound of flute-playing, accompanied by lassitude, anorexia, and loose stools.

气虚腹痛【qì xū fù tòng】因气虚引起的腹痛病证。表现为腹痛绵绵、按之痛感、劳倦时加重，伴有面色萎黄、气短声微、纳呆、脉细涩或虚大等症状。**Abdominal Pain due to Deficiency of Qi** a morbid condition markde by persist abdominal pain relieved on pressing, and aggravated on overexertion, accompanied by sallow complexion, shortness of breath, low voice,

气虚滑胎 【qì xū huá tāi】由于中气不足而出现先兆流产的证候。多见于习惯性流产的病人。

气虚热 【qì xū rè】泛指脾胃气虚或脾肺气虚所致的虚热证,亦有指暑湿伤气而致的发热。

气虚头痛 【qì xū tóu tòng】由于脾胃不足,气虚而清阳不升引起的头痛病证。

气虚痿 【qì xū wěi】由于劳倦内伤或病后饮食失调导致脾胃气虚,不能充养肢体,肢体痿弱无力的病证。

气虚心悸 【qì xū xīn jì】由于阳气虚弱所致的心悸病证。

气虚眩晕 【qì xū xuàn yūn】因气虚阳衰,清阳不升而引起眩晕。常伴有神疲乏力、食少便溏、脉虚遇劳则发等症。

气虚月经过多 【qì xū yuè jīng guò duō】因身体虚弱,忧思伤脾致中气不足,冲任失固引起的月经过多。症见经行血量过多或行经时间过长。色淡

poor appetite, thready and unsmooth pulse or weak and gigantic.

Threatened Abortion due to Qi Deficiency a morbid condition commonly seen in patients with habitual abortion.

Fever due to Deficiency of Qi generally referring to fever of deficiency type due to the deficiency of spleen and stomach-qi or of spleen-and lung-qi, sometimes referring to fever due to impairment of qi by summer-dampness.

Headache due to Deficiency of Qi headache due to insufficiency of the spleen and stomach and failing of lucid yang to rise.

Flaccidity of Limbs due to Deficiency of Qi a morbid condition caused by orverexertion or improper diet after illness, leading to qi deficiency of the spleen and stomach and inability to nourish the limbs.

Palpitation due to Deficiency of Qi a morbid condition due to deficiency of yang-qi.

Dizziness due to Deficiency of Qi a morbid condition due to hypofunction of qi and failure of lucid yang to rise, usually accompanied by lassitude, anorexia, loose stools, weak pulse and recurring on overstrain.

Profuse Menstruation due to Deficiency of Qi a morbid condition due to general weakness, emotional distress and impairment of the spleen, leading

质稀、面色㿠白、疲倦气短、心悸、纳呆等。

气虚月经先期 【qì xū yuè jīng xiān qī】因身体虚弱，忧思伤脾所致中气不足，冲任失固，引起的月经先期。症见经期提前、经血量多、色淡红质稀，面色㿠白、疲倦气短、心悸、纳呆等。

气虚则寒 【qì xū zé hán】指阳气不足，不能温养脏腑，脏腑功能减弱，而出现阴寒证候的病理。

气虚中满 【qì xū zhōng mǎn】指脾胃气虚，消化吸收功能障碍引起腹部胀满的病理。症见食欲不振、腹胀满而按之不痛或大便溏泄、面白唇淡、舌淡、脉弱等。

气虚自汗 【qì xū zì hàn】由于气虚，表卫不固引起的自汗病证。常伴有汗出身冷、恶风、疲乏无力、脉微而缓或虚大等。

气血辨证 【qì xuè biàn zhèng】根据气

to qi deficiency in the middle energizer and debility of TV and CV, characterized by profuse and persistent menstruation which is light in color and watery, palpitation, loss of appetite.

Preceded Menstrual Cycle due to Deficiency of Qi a morbid condition due to general weakness, emotional distress, and impairment of the spleen, resulting in qi deficiency in the middle energizer and debility of TV and CV, characterized by profuse blood which is light red and watery, pale complexion, lassitude, shortness of breath, palpitaion, poor appetite.

Deficiency of Qi Resulting in Clod-Syndrome a morbid condition due to insufficiency of yang-qi and its inability to nourish zang-fu organs leading to hypofunction of viscera.

Flatulence Resulting from Insufficiency of Qi a morbid condition due to insufficiency of the spleen and stomach-qi, leading to functional disturbance in digestion, marked by poor appetite, distention and fullness of the abdomen which is painful when pressed, loose stools, pale complexion, lips and tongue, weak pules.

Spontaneous Sweating due to Deficiency of Qi sweating due to debility of the superficial defence from deficiency of qi, marked by chilly sweating, aversion to wind, fatigue, weakness, feeble but soft or gigantic pulse.

Differentiation of Syndromes according

血的生理病理特点，以气血的病证为纲的一种辨证方法。它与脏腑病证有密切关系。

气血冲和 【qì xuè chōng hé】（气血调和）指气血功能协调、运行通畅。是保证人体进行正常生命活动的重要条件之一。

气血失调 【qì xuè shī tiáo】指气血之间互不协调的病理。临床上凡是久痛、月经不调、慢性出血等病证多与气血失调有关。

气血痰食辨证 【qì xuè tán shí biàn zhèng】内伤杂病的辨证方法之一。根据气血的生理病理特点及痰食致病的特征，对复杂的临床表现分别以气血痰食的病证为纲进行分析归纳，以判断病情，确定诊断。

气血虚弱痛经 【qì xuè xū ruò tòng jīng】因身体虚弱，气血不足，胞脉失养引起的痛经。症见小腹绵绵作痛、喜温喜按、经血量少、色淡而稀。

气血两虚 【qì xuè liǎng xū】即气虚和血虚同时存在的病理状态。多因久病消耗，气血两伤；或先有失血，气随血耗；或先有气虚，血的生化无源而

to the State of Qi and Blood a method to differentiate syndromes by studying the physiopathological changes of qi and blood, which is closely related to the syndromes of zang-fu organs.

Harmony of Qi and Blood harmony of qi and blood in performing their functions with smooth circulation, which is an important condition to ensure the normal life activities.

Disharmony of QI and Blood a morbid condition to which clinical manifestations such as long-standing pain, irregular menstruation, and chronic bleeding are related.

Differentiation of Syndromes according to the State of Qi and Blood, Phlegm and Diet a method to analyze, sum up and determine the states of illness by studying the physio-pathological changes of qi and blood as well as the disease-causing features of phlegm and diet in making a diagnosis.

Dysmenorrhea due to Deficiency of Qi and Blood a morbid condition caused by general weakness, deficiency of qi and blood, poor nourishment of the uterine vessels, manifested by slight pain in the lower abdomen, alleviated by warming and pressing, scanty menstruation in less red color.

Deficiency of both Qi and Blood a morbid condition mostly due to consumption of both qi and blood because of prolonged illness, or exhaustion of qi

日渐衰少，从而形成气血两虚。症见面色淡白或萎黄，少气懒言，疲乏无力，形体消瘦，心悸失眠，肌肤干燥，肢体麻木等。

resulting from bleeding, or less source of blood, because of deficiency of qi, marked by pale or sallow conplexion, disinclination to talk, listlessness, asthenia, emaciation, palpitation, insomnia, dry skin, numbness of limbs.

气营两燔 【qì yíng liǎng fán】即气分和营分邪热亢盛的病理现象。症见高热、口渴、烦躁、谵妄、斑疹、甚或吐血、衄血、舌绛、苔黄、脉细数等。

Intense Heat in both Qi and Ying Systems a syndrome marked by high fever, thirst, dysphoria, delirium, eruptions, or even haematemesis, epistaxis, deep red tongue with yellowish coating, thready and fast pulse.

气营两清 【qì yīng liǎng qīng】（清气凉营）使用清气分和营分的药物以治疗热性病热邪侵入气分和营分的方法。常用于高热、心烦、口渴、舌质深红、苔黄而干、脉洪数者。

Clearing away the Heat from both Qi and Ying Systems a therapeutic method to clear the pathogenic heat when it invades both the qi and ying systems, for the case marked by high fever, dysphoria, thirst, deep red tongue with yellowish dry coating, and full fast pulse.

气瘿 【qì yīng】由于情志抑郁或水土因素所致的颈部肿块。其边缘不清、质软、皮色如常，一般无痛，可随情志变化而增大或缩小。多见于青年妇女。类似地方性甲状腺肿和青春期甲状腺肿。

Qi Goiter goiter due to emotional depression or geographical factors which is soft with unclear-cut margins and normal skin color, the size of which increases and decreases along with the emotional changes, and which is most commonly seen in young women, pertaining to endemic goiter and puberty goiter.

气由脏发 【qì yóu zàng fā】五脏主藏精气，所以体内流动着的精微物质及机体的功能活动都来于五脏。

Qi Originating from the Five Viscera the five viscera store the vital essence, therefore, all the refined nutritious substances flowing in the body and the functional activities of the body originate from and supported by the five viscera.

气有余便是火【qì yǒu yú biàn shì huǒ】指阳气偏盛，而呈现病理性机能亢进的病理。由阴液不足所致者，属虚火上炎，由情志过极所致者，则属气郁化火。

Hyperfunction of Qi Leading to Fire-Syndrome referring to the pathological hyperfunction because of excessive yang-qi, if caused by insufficiency of yin-fluid, it belongs to flaring-up fire of insufficiency type; if caused by emotional distress, belongs to fire transmission due to stagnation of qi.

气郁【qì yù】由于情志郁结，肝气不舒所致的郁证。表现为胸满胁痛、脉象沉涩。

Stagnation of Qi a pathological change caused by emotional depression which leads to stagnation of the liver-qi, manifested as feeling of distension in the chest, pain in the hypochondrium, sunken and unsmooth pulse.

气郁脘痛【qì yù wǎn tòng】由于情志不舒、肝气郁结，横逆犯胃所致的胃脘痛。表现为上腹部胀痛无定处，痛连两胁，按之痛减并伴有嗳气、泛酸等症。

Stomachache due to Stagnation of Qi epigastric pain due to invasion of the stomach by adverse flow of the liver-qi resulting from emotional depression, marked by unfixed upper abdominal distension pain, and radiating to the two hypochondria, relieved when pressed, accompanied by belching, and acid regurgitation.

气郁胁痛【qì yù xié tòng】由于情志不舒、肝气郁结所致的胁痛病证。

Hypochondriac Pain due to Stagnation of Qi hypochondriac pain due to stagnation of the liver-qi resulting from emotional depression.

气郁眩晕【qì yù xuàn yùn】因情志郁结所致的眩晕病证。表现为眩晕、精神抑郁、心悸、面部发热、眉棱骨痛等。

Dizziness due to Depression of Qi a variety of dizziness accompanied by palpitation, flushed face and pain of the supra-orbital bone.

气郁血崩【qì yù xuè bēng】因暴怒伤肝，气乱血动，冲任失调引起的崩漏证。症见阴道突然大量出血、血色紫红有块、烦躁易怒、胸胁不舒等。

Metorrhagia due to Stagnation of Qi a morbid condition caused by great anger resulting in the impairment of the liver, disturbance in qi and blood circulation and incoordinnation of TV and CV, manifested by a sudden onset of massive bleeding, scanty flow of dark red color with clots, dysphoria, irritability, discomfort in the chest and hypochondrium.

气胀 【qì zhàng】因七情郁结，气机不畅引起的腹部胀满。
Qi Distension abdominal distention and fullness due to emotional depression and poor circulation of qi.

气痔 【qì zhì】每因忧思恼怒而症状加重的痔疮。见于某些内痔合并脱肛的病人。
Internal Hemorrhoid with Prolapse of Rectum a morbid condition aggravated by emotional up-set or anger.

气滞 【qì zhì】即气机郁滞不畅。主要由于情志内郁，或痰、湿、食积、瘀血等阻滞，影响到气的流通，形成局部或全身的气机不畅或阻滞，从而导致某些脏腑、经络的功能障碍。常见胀满和疼痛。
Stagnation of Qi a morbid condition mainly due to emotional depression, or accumulation of phlegm, dampness and food or blood stasis, resulting in impairment of local or general qi circulation or stagnation of qi as well as the functional disturbances of some zang-fu organs and meridians marked by distension, fullness and pain.

气滞腹痛 【qì zhì fù tòng】（气结腹痛）因情志不舒，使气机郁滞引起的腹痛病证。其腹痛每因精神受刺激而诱发或加重，嗳气或矢气后可减轻，常伴有胸闷胁痛。
Abdominal Pain due to Stagnation of Qi a morbid condition due to emotional upset which is induced or aggravated wherever one is irritated emotionally, relieved where there is belching or breaking wind, usually accompanied by stuffiness in the chest and pain in the hypochondrium.

气滞经行后期 【qì zhì jīng xíng hòu qī】因情志不舒，肝气郁结，气机不畅引起的经行后期。常伴有小腹及乳房胀痛、拒按、月经量少、滞涩不畅等。
Delayed Menstrual Cycle due to the Depressed Qi a morbid condition caused by emotional distress and impaired circulation due to stagnation of the liver-qi, usually accompanied by distending pain of the lower abdomen and breast, tenderness, hypomenorrhea and uneven flow.

气滞痛经【qì zhì tòng jīng】因情志抑郁，气机不畅，冲任血行郁滞所致的痛经。症见经前或经行时上腹部胀痛、经行涩滞不畅或伴有胸部、乳房等处胀闷不舒。

Dysmenorrhea due to Stagnation of Qi a morbid condition due to emotional distress, impaired circulation of qi, leading to stagnation of blood in TV and CV, marked by distending pain in the lower abdomen which occurs before or during the menstrual flow and uneven flow or accompanied by distension, stuffiness or discomfort in the chest and breast.

气滞血瘀经闭【qì zhì xuè yū jīng bì】因情志不舒、肝气郁结，瘀血阻滞冲任胞脉而引起的经闭。

Amenorrhea due to Stagnation of Qi and Blood Stasis a morbid condition due to emotional distress, obstruction of the TV, GV and uterine vessel by stagnation of the liver-qi and stasis of blood.

气滞血瘀心悸【qì zhì xuè yū xīn jì】因气滞血瘀引起的心悸病证。伴有心烦不安、胸闷痛、气喘、舌色紫暗、脉涩等。

Palpitation due to Stagnation of Qi and Blood Stasis a morbid condition accompanied by dysphoria, restlessness, stuffiness and pain in the chest, dyspnea, dark red tongue and unsmooth pulse.

气滞腰痛【qì zhì yāo tòng】因情志不舒或跌扑闪挫致经脉气滞，引起的腰痛病证。

Lumbago due to Stagnation of Qi lumbago due to emotional depression or stagnation of qi in the muscles and tendons resulting from sudden sprain and contusion, and trauma.

气肿【qì zhǒng】因气滞湿阻所致的浮肿。其特点是其肿按之觉皮厚，随按随起。

Edema due to Disorder of Qi edema caused by stagnation of qi with the characteristic of thick sensation of the skin when pressed and immediate rebounding afetr being pressed.

泣【qì】即眼泪。

Tears

千日疮【qiān rì chuāng】（疣疮、疣、疣赘）多由风邪搏于肌肤，或肝虚血燥、筋气不荣所致。好发于背、指背、头

Verruca Vulgaris wart mostly caused by invasion of the skin by pathogenic wind or liver deficiency and

皮等处。初起状如粟米，渐增大突出皮肤，色灰白或污黄、蓬松枯槁，数目多少不一，挤压时疼痛，碰撞或摩擦易出血。

dryness of blood leading to poor nourishment of the skin, commonly seen on the back, on the fingers and skin with the newly appeared ones being like rice particles then becoming higher than the skin in pale or slightly yellow skin color. They are soft and dry, and various in number, painful when pressed. Bleeding is liable to be the result of collision or pressing friction.

千岁疮 【qiān suì chuāng】生于遍身的瘰疬。 **Widespread Scrofula** scrofula seen all over the body.

前后不通 【qián hòu bù tōng】指大小便不通。 **Constipation and Dysuria**

前阴 【qián yīn】指外生殖器及尿道口。 **External Genitalia** referring to the genitals and urinary tract.

潜阳 【qián yáng】用质重具有镇静和收敛固脱的药物，以治疗阴虚阳亢或阳虚浮越的方法。本法常与平肝、滋阴等法同用。 **Suppressing the Asthenic Yang** a treatment for debilitating hyperactivity of liver-yang due to deficiency of yin with sedatives and asthenic yang astringents of heavy weight; usually applied together with therapy for calming the liver and nourishing yin.

潜镇 【qián zhèn】（镇潜）镇静安神药和潜阳药合用，以治疗因心神浮越表现惊悸失眠或肝阳上亢所致头痛眩晕。 **Calming and Suppressing the asthenic Yang** a treatment with the application of sedatives and of suppressing the asthenic Yang, for the cases manifested as palpitation, insomnia or as headache, dizziness due to hyperactivity of the liver-yang.

强阴 【qiáng yīn】使用药物补益阴精的方法。适用于肾阴虚而致的腰酸、遗精、盗汗等证。 **Strengthening Yin** a treatment with medicines of restoring the yin-essence, applicable to the case marked by lumbar, nocturnal emission, night sweat caused by deficiency of the kidney-yin.

强中　【qiáng zhōng】指阴茎勃起坚硬，久久不萎而精液自泄的病症。多由肝肾阴虚阳亢或性欲过度所致。

Prolonged Erectness of Penis　a disorder usually accompanied with spontaneous emission, due to deficiency of both the liver and the kidney-yin leading to hyperactivity of yang or excessive libido.

切脉　【qiè mài】（诊脉、按脉、持脉）诊查脉象的方法。目前常用的诊脉部位是两手腕部桡动脉，并从脉的位置、次数、性状、形势等分为多种，以诊察机体的病变。

Pulse Feeling　a method of examining pulse condition usually by palpating the pulse of the radial arteries of both hands proximal to the wrists, to observe the pathological changes in its frequency, nature, state and rhythm.

切诊　【qiè zhěn】四诊之一。是医者运用手和指端的感觉，对病人体表某些部位，进行触摸按压的检查方法，包括按脉和对患者的体表、胸腹及手足等部位的触摸、按压，以掌握脉象和胸腹等部位的变化，帮助了解病情。

Palpation　a method of physical examination by which the practitioner palpates the various parts of the body surface of the patient with the touching sensation of the hands and the ends of fingers, for the purpose of investigating the condition of pulse, chest, abdomen and extremities to establish a diagnosis.

噙化　【qín huà】将丸剂或锭剂含在口腔内，使药物在口中溶化。

Letting the Drug Dissolved in the Mouth　a method for oral use of certain medicines which are prepared as pills or lozenges.

揿针　【qìn zhēn】亦名揿钉或皮内针。针柄扁，针体长约2—3毫米，形似图钉。是一种专用于皮下埋藏的小型针具。

Drawing-Pin-Like Needle　a type of acupuncture needle with flat handle and 2-3mm in length, specially used for intradermal acupuncture or auriculo-acupuncture.

青　【qīng】五色之一。即青色，它与五行的木，五脏的肝及与风邪有密切的关系。

Green　a colour which is matched with the wood (in the five elements) and the liver (in the five viscera), and is closely related to pathogenic wind.

青带　【qīng dài】阴道流出青绿色粘

Leukorrhagia with Greenish Discharge

液，气味臭秽，连绵不断。多因肝经湿热下注，伤及任、带二脉所致。profuse greenish, viscid and foul discharge from the vagina due to the attack of pathogenic damp-heat to the liver meridian with the involvement of conception vessel (CV) and belt vessel (BV).

青风内障 【qīng fēng nèi zhàng】多因肝肾阴虚，风火升扰所致。症见瞳神呈淡青色、略微散大、头眼胀痛不堪，视力渐降。**Simple Glaucoma** a disorder caused by the deficiency of liver-yin and kidney-yin and the attack of pathogenic wind-fire; manifested as greenish coloration and slight dilatation of the pupil, usually accompanied with mild distending, pain over the eye and the head, and gradual diminution of vision.

青盲 【qīng máng】眼外观无异常而逐渐失明。相当于视神经萎缩。多因肝肾亏衰，精血虚损，目窍萎闭所致。**Blindness with Insidious Onset** gradual loss of vision without change of appearance of the eyes, corresponding to advanced optic atrophy; due to consumption of the essence and blood leading to asthenia of the liver and kidney.

青如草兹 【qīng rú cǎo zī】是肝的真脏色，形容青如枯草样的颜色。是风邪盛极，胃气将绝的反映。**Dark Green as Withered Grass** the sick colour symbolizing the exhaustion of essence and energy of the liver, in which the skin appears dark green, dry and lusterless, indicating overabundance of pathogenic wind and exhaustion of stomach-qi.

轻方 【qīng fāng】单用一种方剂，如单用奇或偶方。**A single Prescription** application of only one prescription at a time, e.g., only prescription composed of medicines in odd number or that in even number is used.

轻剂 【qīng jì】用具有轻清疏解作用的药物组成的方剂。用以治疗外感表**Prescription Composed of Light Drugs** a prescription containing aromat-

邪，腠理闭塞无汗之症。ics with the action of expelling the exogenous factors in the superficies, usually applied for the case with exterior syndromes due to exogenous pathogenic factor, and absence of sweat.

轻可去实 【qīng kě qù shí】用轻剂可治疗感受风邪而致的表实症，如发热、恶寒、头痛、无汗、脉浮等。

Treatment of Sthenia-Syndrome with Light Medicine the prescription of comparatively light weight medicines is applied for the case of sthenia-syndrome in the superficies due to attack of wind, seen in fever, chillness, headache, absence of sweating, floating pulse, etc.

轻清疏解 【qīng qīng shū jiě】指用辛凉轻清、疏解表热的方药，治疗风热表症的治法。

Dispelling Superficial Factors with Mild Diaphoretics Medicines a treatment for the syndrome of the pathogenic wind-heat factors attacking the superficies, with the light and mild diaphoretics medicines.

轻清宣肺 【qīng qīng xuān fèi】用轻清上浮泄热的药物，以宣通肺气，清气分热邪的一种治法。多用于感受温燥之邪，症见头痛身热、口渴咽干、干咳无痰等。

Opening the Inhibited Lung-qi with Drugs of Mild Action a treatment for promoting lung qi circulation and clearing pathogenic heat from the qi fen with mild, light, heat-expelling drugs, mostly used for the cases catching pathogenic warm-dryness manifested as headache, fever, thirst, dry throat, cough without sputum.

轻宣润燥 【qīng xuān rùn zào】治疗外感燥热伤肺，肺气不宣的方法。本法既要用轻度发散祛邪的药物，又要用滋润以扶正气的药物。适用于凉燥犯肺和温燥伤肺。

Opening the Inhibited Lung-qi by Moisturizing Dryness-Heat a treatment of lung impairment by dryness-heat due to exopathy and obstruction of the lung-qi with both mild drugs for dispersing expathogens and drugs for moisturizing to strengthen the body resistance for cases with lung invasion due to cool-dryness and lung impairment due to warm-dryness.

清肠润燥 【qīng cháng rùn zào】治疗大肠燥热便秘的方法。适用于大肠燥热,而见大便干结、口臭、面赤、口唇生疮、小便短赤、苔黄燥、脉滑实等症。

Moisturizing Dry-Heat by Clearing the Bowels　a treatment for constipation due to large intestinal dry-heat for cases with dryness of the stool, halitosis, flushed face, lip sores, scanty dark urine, dry, rough and yellowish tongue fur, slippery and forceful pulse.

清法 【qīng fǎ】(清热法)用寒凉药物以清解火热之邪的一种治法。适用于热性病和其他热证。临床上常视邪热的深浅及所在脏腑的不同而采用不同的清法。

Therapy for Clearing Away Heat (Heat-clearing Method)　a treatment for removing pathogenic fire with drugs of cool or cold in nature, for cases with febrile diseases or other heat syndromes. Different clearing methods are clinically used by the different depth and visceras of pathogenic heat.

清络保阴 【qīng luò bǎo yīn】即清肺络之热邪以保肺阴之法。适用于暑温病主要症状已消退,但肺络仍有热邪、肺阴受伤。症见咳嗽无痰或咯血、鼻衄等。

Clearing Away the Lung Heat and Retaining the Lung-Yin　a treatment for clearing away heat from the pulmonary vessels to retain lung-yin for cases with the disappearance of the summer heat symptoms, but still with the existance of pathogenic heat and the damage of lung-yin characterized by dry cough or hemoptysis and epistaxis.

清气 【qīng qì】1、运用苦寒或辛寒的药物,清解里热的一种方法,适用于热在气分。2、指水谷精华的轻清部分。3、秋令清肃之气。

Clearing away the Heat in Qifen　1. a treatment with drugs bitter or pungent in taste and cool in nature to clear up internal heat for cases with

清热化湿 【qīng rè huà shī】用清热药和芳香化湿或辛开苦降的药,以治疗湿热病邪互结于上、中焦的一种治法。症见胸闷腹胀、口苦纳呆、舌苔黄腻、脉濡数等。

清热化痰 【qīng rè huà tán】化痰法之一。是治疗热痰的方法。适用于热邪壅肺炼液成痰。症见咳嗽不利痰黄难咯、面赤烦热、舌红苔黄等。

清热化痰开窍 【qīng rè huà tán kāi qiào】用清热化痰和芳香开窍的药物,以治疗痰热蒙闭清窍致神志昏迷的方法。

清热解表 【qīng rè jiě biǎo】用清热与解表药组成的方剂,治疗里热较重而表证较轻的病证。是表里双解的一种

syndrome of qi fen. 2. the refined essence of food and water conveyed up to the lung and distributed to the internal organs and tissues. 3. cool air in autumn.

Clearing Away Heat and Eliminating Damp a treatment with heat-clearing drugs and drugs for dampness-removing by acromatics or pungent and bitter drugs for dispersion and purgation for cases with diseases caused by dampness in combination with heat as a pathogenic factor in the upper and middle energizer characterized by chest tightness, epigastric distention, bitter taste, anorexia, yellow and greasy coating of the tongue, soft and fast pulse.

Clear Away Heat and Disperse Phlegm one of the therapeutic methods indicated for the treatment of the retention of heat-phlegm in the lung manifested as cough with expectoration of yellowish sputum, flushed face, dysphoria with smothery sensation, red tongue with yellow coating.

Waking Up the Patient from Unconsciouseness by Clearing Heat and Dispersing Phlegm a treatment of coma caused by the accumulation of phlegm and heat with heat-phlegm-removing and resuscitation drugs of aromatics.

Clearing Away Heat and Relieving Exterior Syndrome a prescription of drugs with the actions of removing

方法。

清热解毒 【qīng rè jiě dú】用清热邪解热毒的药物,治疗热性病里热亢盛及痈疮、疔肿、疔毒、斑疹等病证。

清热解暑 【qīng rè jiě shǔ】用清热药结合解暑药,治疗外感暑热的方法。症见发热、头痛、汗出、烦渴、小便黄、苔薄黄、脉浮数等。

清热开窍 【qīng rè kāi qiào】(凉开、清心开窍)以芳香开窍药与清热药合用,治疗温热病神志昏迷的方法。适用于温病高热、神志昏迷、烦躁不安、胡言乱语、四肢抽搐等。

清热利湿 【qīng rè lì shī】使用清热利湿通利小便的药物,治疗湿热之邪蕴结于下焦的一种治法。症见小腹急

exterior syndrome applied for cases with severe internal heat but mild exterior syndrome, which is a therapeutic method for expelling the pathogenic factors from both interior and exterior.

Clearing Away Heat and Toxic Material a treatment with drugs of clearing away toxic heat for cases with febrile diseases characterized by excessive internal heat, or cases with carbuncle, furuncle, furunculosis, and skin eruption.

Clearing Away Summer-Heat a treatment with heat-clearing and summer heat-relieving drugs for cases with heat syndrome due to invasion of pathogenic summer-heat charaterized by fever, headache, sweating, thirst, yellowish urine, thin and yellowish tongue coating, and fast floating pulse.

Waking Up the Patient from Unconsciousness by Clearing Away Heat also called removing heat from the heart to resuscitate, a treatment with resusciation reducing drugs of aromatics taken together with heat-clearing drugs for cases with seasonal febrile disease indicated by high fever, unconsciousness, restlessness, raving and convulsion of the four extremities.

Clearing Away Heat and Promoting Diuresis a treatment with heat-clearing and diuresis-promoting drugs

胀、小便浑赤、涩痛、淋沥不畅、舌苔黄腻等。 for cases with diseases caused by the retention of warm-heat pathogen in the lower energizer indicated by acute epigastric distention, clouding dark urine, painful and dribbing urination, yellowish and greasy tongue fur.

清热止血 【qīng rè zhǐ xuè】止血法之一。是用清热凉血药治疗血热妄行致出血的方法。适用于出血伴有热证表现的患者。 **Clearing Away Heat to Stop Bleeding** one of the therapeutic methods to stop bleeding with which heat-clearing drugs are used to stop bleeding caused by blood heat, for cases with bleeding accompanied by heat syndrome manifestations.

清暑利湿 【qīng shǔ lì shī】用清热解暑药合利湿药,治疗暑病夹湿的方法。症见发热、心烦、口渴、多汗、小便不利等。 **Clearing Away Summer-Heat and Eleminating Dampness** a treatment with summer heat-clearing drugs and drugs of removing dampness by diuresis for cases with summer-heat diseases accompanied by dampness which is indicated by fever, vexation, thirst, hyperhidrosis and difficulty in urination.

清暑益气 【qīng shǔ yì qì】用清热和益气生津的药物,治疗暑热耗伤津液的外感暑热证。 **Clearing Away Summer-Heat and Reinforcing Qi** a treatment with heat-clearing drugs and drugs of supplementing qi and promoting the production of body fluid, for cases with heat syndrome due to invasion of pathogenic summer-heat characterized by the consumption of body fluid.

清肃肺气 【qīng sù fèi qì】(清金降火)治疗肺气上逆的方法。适用于热邪迫肺所致的喘咳气急、咯黄痰、口干、发热、苔黄、脉浮数等。 **Keeping the Lung-Qi Pure and Descendant** a treatment of adverse ascending of the lung-qi characterized by cough, dyspnea, yellowish sputum, thirst, fever, yellowish tongue coating, fast and floating pulse caused by the invasion of the lung by pathogenic heat.

清胃降逆 【qīng wèi jiàng nì】治疗胃热呃逆的方法。适用于胃热所致胃的呃逆的病症。

Clearing Away the Stomach-Heat and Lowering the Adverse Flow of Qi a therapeutic method to treat patients with hiccup caused by the stomach-heat.

清泄少阳 【qīng xiè shào yáng】治疗热性病，邪在半表半里的一种方法。症见往来寒热、口苦咽干，胁肋苦满，心烦欲呕、不欲饮食、目眩、脉弦等。

Clearing Away the Heat Located in Shaoyang Meridian a treatment of a febrile disease with the pathogenic factor half exterior and half interior manifested by alternating chills and fever, fullness of the chest, hypochondriac discomfort, retchig, anorexia, dizziness and thready pulse.

清心 【qīng xīn】（清宫、清心涤热）用清心热、凉血养阴液的药物，治疗热邪侵入心包的方法，适用于热入心包，症见神昏谵语、高热、烦燥不安、舌质绛等。

Clearing Away the Heart-Fire a therapeutic method to treat the cases with diseases caused by the attack of pericardium by heat with drugs to clear heat-fire, remove heat from the blood and nourish the yin-fluid, applicable for the cases manifested as unconsciousness, high fever, restlessness, dark tongre, etc.

清阳 【qīng yáng】阳气的轻清部分，运行于心、肺、头部、肌表与四肢。

Lucid Yang the light and clear yang-qi that circulates in the heart, lung, head, muscle surface and limbs.

清阳不升 【qīng yáng bù shēng】指由水谷精微所化的轻清阳气不能荣养头目、肌表和四肢以维持正常的生理功能,通常是由于脾胃功能障碍所致。

Lucid Yang Failing to Rise the light and clear yang-qi from the food essence fails to nourish the head, eyes, skin and limbs to maintain the normal physiological functions, which is usually caused by the functional disturbances of the spleen and stomach.

清阳出上窍 【qīng yáng chū shàng

Lucid Yang Ascending to the Upper

qiào】阳主气而上升，轻清升发之气（包括呼吸之气）多出于口鼻等上窍。

Orifices the light and clear yang-qi that usually goes upward (including the air breathed) mostly from the upper orifices such as the mouth and nose.

清阳发腠理 【qīng yáng fā còu lǐ】阳主卫外，轻清之气多充于腠理，起到温养肌肤，抗御外邪的作用。

Lucid Yang Acting on the Body Surface the light and clear yang-qi mostly in the striae of skin which plays the role of warming and nourishing the skin and defending the body against exopathogenic factors.

清阳实四肢 【qīng yáng shí sì zhī】四肢为诸阳之本，所以清阳充实四肢，使四肢得以温暖以维持其正常的生理功能。临床上常以触摸四肢的温冷，作为诊断阳气盛衰的依据之一。

Lucid Yang Strengthening the Four Extremities yang dominates the four extremities, when strengthened by lucid yang, they are warm and able to perform their normal physiological functions. Clinically, the warmness or coldness felt by hand is one of the evidences to prove whether yang-qi is sufficient or deficient.

清营 【qīng yíng】（清营泄热）使用具有清热解毒和养阴作用的药物，以清除热邪侵入营分的一种治法。

Clearing up the Yingfen also called clearing up the ying-fen to dispell pathogenic heat; a therapeutic method to dispell pathogenic heat from ying-fen with heat-clearing and detoxifying drug, and drug for nourishing yin.

清营透疹 【qīng yíng tòu zhěn】使用清泄营热、辛凉透疹的方法，治疗热入营分。症见高热烦躁、口不甚渴、睡眠不安、皮肤疹点隐隐、舌绛而干、苔少、脉细数等。

Clearing Away Heat Located at Yingfen and Letting the Eruptions Out a therapeutic method of letting eruptions with drugs of acrid and cool in nature to treat diseases caused by the invasion of pathogenic heat into the yingfen marked by high fever, restlessness, slight thirst, faint skin rashes, dark-red dry tongue, thin

秋毛 【qiū máo】秋天的脉象微细，这是脉象随气候改变而发生相应变化的生理现象。因秋天阳气转向收敛，故脉搏的搏动幅度相对地减弱。

虬脉纵横 【qiú mài zòng héng】球结膜充血。

虬蟠卷曲 【qiú pán juǎn qū】球结膜充血。

鼽 【qiú】（鼻鼽、鼽鼻、鼽水）因肺气亏虚；卫气失固，外感风寒所致的病症。症见鼻中常流清涕、鼻塞、喷嚏。类似过敏性鼻炎。

曲 【qū】把药粉与面粉混合，制成块状，发酵后称为曲剂，如六神曲。

驱虫 【qū chóng】（杀虫）使用具有驱杀寄生虫作用的药物,以治疗人体寄生虫病的治法。

祛风 【qū fēng】疏散风邪的统称。即祛除表里、经络、脏腑间留滞的风邪。祛风法用于外风。通常分为祛风除湿、疏风泄热、祛风养血、搜风逐寒等法。

coating, thready and fast pulse.

Weak and Floating Pulse in Autumn the pulse is usually weak in autumn, which is a physiological phenomenon that the pulse condition changes with climate. The amplitude of the pulsation becomes relatively weak since the yang-qi in autumn weakens.

Hyperemia of Bulbar Conjunctiva congestion of bulbar conjunctiva.

Hyperemia of Bulbar Conjunctiva congestion of bulbar conjunctiva.

Allergic Rhinitis or Rhinallergosis a morbid condition due to insufficiency of the lung-qi, weak defensive energy and wind-cold pathogen marked by running nose, nasal obstruction and sneezing.

Fermented Herb fermented lumps made by mixing medicinal powder and flour together, such as Liu Shen Qiu.

Expelling Worms (Destroying Parasites) a treatment of parasitosis with antiparasitics.

Expelling Pathogenic Wind Factor a general term for expelling pathogenic wind, i. e. expelling the wind from the body surface, meridians, and from the space between the zang and fu-organs. A therapeutic method for exopathic wind which is usually classified as methods of expelling wind and removing dampness, expelling wind and clearing away heat, expelling wind and nouring blood as well as arresting wind and expelling cold.

祛风除湿 【qū fēng chú shī】用祛风除湿的药物，治疗风湿之邪留滞经络、肌肉、关节等部位，出现游走性疼痛症状时的治法。

Expelling Wind and Removing Dampness a treatment with antirheumatics for cases affected by pathogenic wind-dampness in the meridians, muscles and joints marked by wandering pain.

祛风养血 【qū fēng yǎng xuè】用具有祛风湿、补肝肾和营养气血作用的药物，治疗感受风湿日久，血脉不和，肝肾亏虚的方法。适用于腰膝冷痛、关节活动障碍或麻痹不仁等。

Expelling Wind and Nourishing the Blood a treatment with antirheumatics and drugs with the actions of supplementing the liver and kidney, and nourishing the blood for cases suffering from a long-time wind-dampness syndrome, disorder of blood and meridians, deficiency of the liver and kidney marked by cold-pain in the loins and knees, limited movement or numbness of the joints.

祛寒化痰 【qū hán huà tán】采用温性的化痰药物治疗寒痰的方法。适用于脾肾阳虚，寒饮内停。症见吐痰清稀、怕冷、手足不温、舌淡苔滑等。

Eliminating Phlegm by Expelling Coldness a therapeutic method to treat cold syndrome by using phlegm-resolving drugs warm in nature for cases with hypofunction of the kidney and spleen, and retention of cold phlegm marked by thin sputum, aversion to cold, cold limbs, pale tongue with moist and glossy fur.

祛痰 【qū tán】帮助痰浊排出与祛除生痰病因的方法。常分为化痰、消痰、涤痰等。

Eliminating Phlegm a method to aid in the expulsion of sputum and eliminate the factors of phlegm formation, usually classified as resolving phlegm, clearing away phlegm, removing phlegm, etc.

祛邪扶正 【qū xié fú zhèng】是针对邪

Eliminating Pathogonic Factors to Sup-

祛去 qù

实而正稍虚的病情，以祛邪为主，扶正为辅的治则。取邪去则正自安之意。

祛瘀活血 【qū yū huó xuè】（祛瘀生新、活血生新、化瘀行血）使用活血祛瘀的方药，祛除瘀血，流通血脉的治法。适用于气滞血瘀、血脉阻滞引起的疼痛、肿胀等。

祛瘀消肿 【qū yū xiāo zhǒng】治疗因瘀积而引起的肿痛的方法。适用于因外伤或气血阻滞引起的肿痛。

祛瘀止血 【qū yū zhǐ xuè】止血法之一。用于治疗瘀血内阻所引起的出血证，通常采取活血化瘀药与止血药同用。适用于出血伴有瘀血之证者。

去火毒 【qù huǒ dú】中药炮制法之一。指除去新制膏药中的火毒。即将新制的膏药放在阴凉处较长时间，或浸泡在凉水内几天后待用，以减少膏药对皮肤的刺激性。

port the Healthy Qi a principle in the treatment of morbid conditions in which pathogenic factors prevail over the body resistance, i. e. taking the elimination of the former as the key link while making the support of the latter subsidiary with the idea that the healthy-qi can restore automatically as the pathogenic factors eliminated.

Promoting Blood Circulation by Removing Blood Stasis a method to treat blood stasis by using blood-activating and stasis-eliminating drugs for cases with pain and swelling caused by stagnancy of qi and blood stasis, and block of blood vessels.

Removing Blood Stasis and Promoting the Subsidence of Swelling a method to treat pain and swelling due to blood stasis usually applied for those caused by trauma or stagnation of qi and blood.

Hemostasis by Removing the Blood Stasis one of the methods to stop bleeding applied for cases with hemorrhage caused by blood stasis due to blocks, usually with stasis-removing drugs and hemorrhage arresting drugs taken together for blood bleeding complicated by stasis.

Releasing Fire-Toxin one of the methods to prepare Chinese drugs which means to get rid of the fire-toxin from the newly prepared plasters, i. e. to relieve the skin-irritating

去菀陈莝 【qù yù chén cuò】驱除郁结在体内已久的水液废物的一种治法，通常指通便逐水法。

去油 【qù yóu】中药炮制法之一。对油质多的药物通过煨法去油，或放在吸水纸内压榨去油；或研细加水，待油质浮起，倒掉水和油等。药物去油可减低某些药物的烈性和毒性。

全身浮肿 【quán shēn fú zhǒng】指遍体浮肿。多由脾肾虚弱，水液代谢障碍，水湿潴留，外溢肌肤所致。

全身痛 【quán shēn tòng】全身肌肉、关节疼痛。多因外感寒湿邪毒或跌打损伤等引起经络阻滞，气血不和所致。

全身无力 【quán shēn wú lì】即全身疲困乏力。多由气血俱虚或湿邪内阻引起。

quality of newly prepared plasters by placing it in cool shade or cold water for a few days before using it.

Clearing Away the Excessive Fluid from the Intestine with Potent Purgative a therapeutic method to clear away the retained fluid and waste in the body, usually referred to as the hydragogue method by inducing diuresis.

Getting Rid of Oil a process of preparing Chinese drugs in which oil is removed from drugs that are rich in oil to reduce their drastic reaction and toxicity by roasting in ashes or by pressing the drugs that are wrapped in water-absorbing paper, or by grinding the drugs into fine powder, adding water to it, and then getting rid of the water and oil when the oil goes upward.

Anasarca referring to the general dropsy usually caused by hypofunction of the kidney and spleen, disturbance in water metabolism, retention of water within the body and effusion of water into the skin.

Pantalgia generalized pain of the muscles and joints caused by blockage of the meridians and collaterals and disord or of blood and qi due to exopathic cold and damp or traumatic injury.

General Weakness fatigue and weakness over the whole body usually caused by the deficiency of both qi

颧赤 【quán chì】指颧部泛现红色。多由肝肾阴亏，虚阳上浮所致。

Flushing of Zygomatic Region a condition usually caused by deficiency of the liver-yin and kidney-yin, and the upward floating of asthenic yang.

缺盆 【què pén】1、即销骨上窝。2、经穴名。

1. **Supraclavicular Fossa** 2. **an acupoint (st12).**

缺乳 【qué rǔ】产后乳汁甚少或全无。多因产后气血亏虚，乳汁化源不足；或肝郁气滞，气血运行不畅，乳汁壅滞不行所致。

Lack of Lactation little or no milk after child birth chiefly caused by the deficiency of qi and blood, insufficiency of the milk source, or by the stagnation of the liver-qi or by blockage of qi and blood, the resultant blockage of collaterals and milk passages.

雀斑 【què bàn】发于颜面、颈和手背等处，皮肤呈黑褐色或淡黑色散在斑点，小如针尖，大如绿豆，数目多少不一。多由火郁孙络血分，复感风邪凝滞；或肺经血热所致。

Freckle appearing on the face, neck and the back of the hands with the skin dark brown or with pale black spots on the skin among which some are as small as pinpoints, some as large as mung beans and various in number, mostly caused by fire stagnancy in the minute collateral blood and associated infections caused by wind factor; or by blood heat in the lung meridian.

雀啄脉 【què zhuó mài】反复出现的急速而节律不整的脉象。

Bird-Pecking Pulse pulse beating with fast, irregular rhythm.

阙 【què】（阙中）两眉之间的部位。对该部望诊，有助于了解肺部疾患。

Glabella the glabellar region, inspection on which is one of the ways in the diagnosis of pulmorary diseases.

阙上 【què shàng】天庭、阙之间的部位。古人认为可作望诊咽喉病证的参考。

Lower Middle Part of the Forehead region above glabellar, inspection on which would aid in the diagnosis of throat diseases.

染苔 【rǎn tāi】舌苔被食物和药物所染而改变了的舌苔颜色,在观察时必须排除这种假象。

Stained Tongue Fur tongue coating discolored by food or drug taken, called also pseudo-coating which should be distinguished from the true color of coating on inspection.

热 【rè】1、见热邪。2、热证。即八纲之一。指各种原因引致阳气亢盛的病证。(表现出热象如发热、面红、目赤、口渴等)。3、治法之一。即温法或祛寒法。4、药物寒热温凉的四气之一。

Heat (hot) 1. pathogenic heat 2. heat syndrome, one of the eight principal syndromes serving as guidelines in diagnosis, referring to the syndrome due to hyperactivity of yang-qi caused by various factors. 3. one of the therapeutic methods, i. e. therapy by warming or therapy by dispelling cold 4. one of the four natures of Chinese medicine, i. e. cold, hot, warm and cool.

热秘 【rè bì】热结大肠所致的大便秘结。症见身热面赤、恶热喜冷、口舌生疮、小便黄赤、脉数实等。

Constipation due to Heat a condition caused by the accumultion of heat in the large intestine marked by fever, flushed face, aphthae, parched lips, dark brown urine, fast and forceful pulse.

热痹 【rè bì】指热毒流注关节;或内有蕴热,复感风寒湿邪,与热相搏所致的痹证。症见关节红肿热痛、发热、口渴等。多见于风湿性关节炎、类风湿性关节炎、痛风等。

Heat-Type Bi a variety of arthritis including rheumatic arthritis, rheumatoid arthritis and gout due to invasion of joints by toxious heat or by accumulated heat and further complicated by pathogenic wind, cold and dampness, characterized by pain, redness, heat and swelling of the joints, thirst and fever.

热产 【rè chǎn】(暑产)指盛暑之月分娩,此时产妇应温凉适宜,否则易患他疾,如热甚则出现头痛、面赤昏晕等。

Delivering in Hot Weather referring to delivery in hot summer during which the parturient must be kept comfortably warm and cool, otherwise she could be easily affected, for

热喘 【rè chuǎn】指肺受热灼，痰火壅阻，肺气壅逆所致的喘证。症见喘急、喉有痰鸣、咳痰黄稠、烦热胸满、口渴喜饮等。

热疮 【rè chuāng】好发于口唇、口角和鼻孔周围的小疮疹，水泡成群，可伴有瘙痒和灼痛，一周左右消退，易复发。多由风热外感或肺胃积热上蒸所致。

热毒 【rè dú】1、多指外科痈疡（化脓性感染）等病的主要致病因素。2、见温毒。

热呃 【rè è】因胃火上逆，或痰火郁遏所致的呃逆。症见呃声有力、面赤烦渴、口干舌燥、舌苔黄、脉洪大而数等。

热敷止痛法 【rè fū zhǐ tòng fǎ】即在未破皮的软组织损伤处用药物进行热敷，藉以散瘀消肿，活络止痛的一种外治法。

instance, if too hot, headache, flushed face and faint might occur.

Dyspnea Caused by Heat dyspnea due to attack of the lung by pathogenic heat and obstruction of the lung-qi by phlegm-fire with the manifestations of rapid respiration, wheezing, yellowish thick sputum, dysphoria, fever, distention in the chest, thirst and desire for drinking.

Herpes Simplex small herpes mostly seen on the lips, mouth corners and round the nostrils in the form of blisters in groups accompanied by itching and burning pain, usually caused by exposure to wink-heat, upwards attack of accumulation of heat in the spleen and stomach, and often disappearing in a week with the tendency of high recurrence.

Heat-Toxin 1. mostly referring to the pathogenic factors for surgical large carbuncle (supurative infection). 2. violent heat.

Hiccup due to Heat hiccup due to upward adverse movement of the stomach fire or due to hinderance by accumulated phlegm-fire, characterized by hiccup with loud sounds, flushed face, thirst, dryness of lips and tongue, yellowish coating of the tongue and full, fast pules.

Relieving Pain by Hot Compress external therapy by hot compress to dissipate blood stasis, promote the subsidence of swelling and activate

热伏冲任 【rè fú chōng rèn】热邪伏于冲脉和任脉的病理。症见低热、腰酸痛、下腹疼痛、崩漏等。

热服 【rè fú】汤剂煎好后，趁热将药服下，一般适用于大寒证。

热膈 【rè gé】噎膈之属热性者。症见吞咽困难、胸痛短气、腰背痛、水谷不消、消瘦、口烂生疮、五心烦热或发热、四肢沉重等。

热烘 【rè hōng】是在病变部位涂上药物后，再加火烘的方法，适用于四肢寒冷、怕冷、腹部冷痛等。

热化 【rè huà】1、指在疾病发展过程中，寒邪化热入里的病理现象。2、指伤寒少阴病人一身手足厥冷转为一身手足尽热的热化证。3、五运六气术语。

collaterals to stop pain by applying pyrogenic drug to the injured soft tissues with the skin still intact.

Heat Gathering in Thoroughfare and Conception Vessels a morbid condition in which pathogenic heat stays in the TV and CV, marked by low fever, lumbago, pain in the lower abdomen and uterine bleeding.

Decoction to Be Taken Hot taking the decoction while it is hot, usually applied for the cases with serious cold syndrome.

Dysphagia with Internal Heat a morbid condition which is charaterized by difficulty in swallowing, chest pain, shortess of breath, lumbago, aphthous stomatitis, dysphoria with feverish sensation in chest, palms and soles, or fever and sense of heaviness of limbs.

Baking the Affected Part after Applying Some Drugs a therapeutic method to bake the affected part after applying some drugs, indicated by clammy limbs, fear or cold and coldpain in the abdomen.

Heat Transformation 1. a pathological process by which pathogenic cold is transformed into heat after invading interiorly of the body. 2. the process during which the limbs turn from cold to hot in a febrile disease of shaoyin meridian. 3. one of the terms in describing the five elements' motion and six kinds of natural factors.

热霍乱 【rè huà luàn】（热气霍乱）指因内伤饮食厚味；或外感暑热、湿热，秽臭郁遏中焦所致的一种疾病。症见腹中绞痛、呕吐泄泻、泻下热臭、胸闷、发热、口渴、小便黄赤、舌苔黄腻、脉洪数等。可见于细菌性食物中毒等疾病。

Summer Cholera a morbid condition caused by improper diet or by exposure to summer-heat, damp-heat or retained fetidness in the middle energizer, characterized by abdominal colic, vomiting, diarrhea, fetid hot stool, fullness in the chest, fever, thirst, dark urine, yellow and sticky tongue coating, full and fast pulse, which can be seen in diseases due to bacterial food poisoning.

热极生寒 【rè jí shèng hán】当热证病情发展到热极阶段，因热邪内盛，阳气闭郁于内，不能外达四肢而出现四肢逆冷、脉沉等假寒的现象。

Occurrence of Cold Syndrome in Case of Extreme Heat a pseudo-cold syndrome charaterized by cold limbs and sunken pulse due to extreme heat inside the body and the inability of yang-qi to reach the limbs because of the obstruction to its flow.

热剂 【rè jì】具有温热作用的方剂。

Prescription Containing Drugs of Hot Nature prescriptions indicated for the treatment of cold syndrome.

热结 【rè jié】热邪结聚于里的病理。常因结聚的部位不同而出现相应的症状，如热邪结于胃肠则可出现腹痛、大便秘结，甚则潮热、谵语等症。

Heat Accumulation a morbid condition due to the accumulation of pathogenic heat interiorly marked by the relative symptoms for the different positions of its accumulation; if it accumulates in the stomach and intestines, symptoms such as abdominal pain, constipation, or even tidal fever and delirium may appear.

热结膀胱 【rè jié páng guāng】热邪结于膀胱的病理。症见下腹部硬满、拘急不舒、小便自利、发热而不恶寒、神志如狂等。

Accumulation of Heat in the Bladder a morbid condition in which pathogenic heat accumulates in the bladder manifested by distention and fullness of the lower abdomen with subjective sensation of contraction,

热结下焦 【rè jié xià jiāo】热邪结于下焦的病理。症见下腹胀痛,大便秘结、尿少、尿痛甚至尿血等。

热结胸 【rè jué xiōng】即热实结胸。指热邪结于胸中,症见脘腹胀满硬痛、发热烦渴、懊憹、口燥便闭、脉沉滑等。

热厥 【rè jué】由于热邪过盛,津液受伤,阳气运行受阻,不能透达四肢而致手足厥冷的证候。常兼见胸腹灼热、口渴、烦躁、甚则神志昏愦、尿赤、便秘、舌红苔黄等。

热泪 【rè lèi】眼肿涩痛而泪常流出,泪下有热感,甚至泪热如汤,常伴有赤肿羞明。多由风热外袭,肝肺火炽或阴虚火炎所致,异物入目亦可引起。

frequency and urgency of urination, fever but without chills and restlessness.

Heat Accumulating in the Lower Energizer a morbid condition due to heat accumulation in the lower energizer manifested by distention and pain in the abdomen, constipation, oligura, urodyria, and even hematuria.

Accumulation of Heat in the Chest a morbid condition caused by the heat accumulating in the chest, characterized by distress in the chset, fullness and tenderness of the epigastrium, fever, dire thirst, fidget, dryness in the mouth, constipation, sunken and slippery pulse.

Cold Extremities Caused by Dominant Heat a morbid condition in which excessive pathogenic heat leads to consumption of body fluid which impairs the normal circulation of yang-qi and results in cold limbs with the accompanying symptoms of burning pain in the chest and abdomen, thirst, fidgets or even mental confusion, dark urine, constipation, red tongue with yellowish coating.

Warm Tear a condition marked by swelling and pain of the eyes with frequent tears and warm or even hot sensation, accompanied by photophobia, mostly due to the exterior attack by wind and heat, lung-fire mingled with liver-fire, or hyperactivity of fire

热痢 【rè lì】指痢疾之属热者。多因邪热侵入肠腑,积滞不清所致。症见身热腹痛、里急后重、痢下赤白、烦渴引饮、小便热赤、舌苔黄腻、脉滑数有力等。

热淋 【rè lín】因湿热蕴结下焦所致的淋证。症见小便短数、热赤涩痛,伴有寒热、腰痛、小腹拘急胀痛等。类似急性泌尿系感染。辨证分类1、湿热蕴结证;2、阴虚湿热证;3、脾肾两虚证。

热能去寒 【rè néng qù hán】用温热的药物,能够去除寒邪,治疗寒证。如治疗脾胃虚寒,症见食不消化、呕吐清水、大便清稀等,可用附子理中丸。

热呕 【rè ǒu】因脾胃积热,或热邪犯胃所致的呕吐。症见食入即吐、吐多涌猛、面赤、心烦喜冷、口渴便秘、小

due to yin deficiency, or even caused by foreign bodies.

Heat-Type Dysentery dysentery with heat syndrome due to the invasion of, or accumulation in the intestines by pathogenic heat, charaterized by fever, abdominal colic, tenesmus, diarrhea with mucous-bloody feces, fidgets, thirst and desire for drinking, hot sensation on the discharge of concentrated urine, yellow and greasy tongue coating, foreful, slippery and fast pulse.

Strangury due to Heat urination disturbance due to accumulation of damp-heat in the lower energizer manifested as frequency in urination, oliguria, hot and painful discharge of reddish urine, chills and fever, lumbago, distention, stiffness and pain in the lower abdomen, resembling acute infection of urinary tract. Types of differentiation: 1. syndrome due to damp-heat accumulation 2. damp-heat syndrome due to yin deficiency 3. syndrome due to insufficiency of both the spleen and kidney.

Dispelling Cold with Drugs of Warm and Heat in Nature a method to treat cold syndrome such as the treatment of insufficiency of the spleen-yang marked by indigestion, watery vomits as well as watery stool.

Vomiting due to Heat a type of vomiting commonly seen in acute gastritis, cholecystitis and pancreatitis,

便黄赤、脉多洪数等。多见于急性胃炎、胆囊炎、胰腺炎等。

due to accumulation of heat in the spleen and stomach, or the attack of pathogenic heat to the stomach characterized by vomiting in large quantity immediately after eating, flushed face, dysphoria, preference for cold, thirst, constipation, dark urine, full and fast pulse.

热迫大肠 【rè pò dà cháng】湿热邪气伤及肠胃,致大肠功能紊乱的病理。症见腹痛、泄泻如注、粪便黄臭、肛门灼热、小便短黄、舌苔黄腻、脉滑数等。

Invasion of the Large Intestine by Heat a morbid condition in which pathogenic damp-heat impairs the intestine and stomach, resulting in their functional disturbances, characterized by abdominal pain, severe diarrhea, yellow and fetid feces, burning sensation of the anus, scanty dark urine, yellow geasy coating of the tongue, slippery and fast pulse.

热入心包 【rè rù xīn bāo】在热性病过程中,出现高热、神昏、谵语等症的病理。一般表示热性病的严重阶段。

Attack of Pericardium by Heat a morbid condition usually occuring in severe cases of epidemic febrile disease marked by hish fever, and delirium.

热入血分 【rè rù xuè fèn】热邪侵入血分,温热病发展到严重阶段的病理。症见发热夜重、神志昏沉、躁扰不安、斑疹、舌绛紫等。有出血倾向甚则出现抽搐等。

Pathogenic Heat Attacking the Blood a morbid condition occurring in severe case of epidemic febrile disease with invasion of blood system by pathogenic heat, charaterized by high fever during the night, impairment of consciousness, restlessness, eruptions, dark red tongue with the tendency to bleed or even the appearance of convulsion.

热伤肺络 【rè shāng fèi luò】肺脏血络为热邪所伤,引起咳血或咯血的病理。临床上常有实热和虚热之分。

Lung-Collaterals Damaged by Heat a pathological change due to invasion of lung collateral by pathogenic heat, marked by bloody expectoration or hemoptysis, usually classified as excess syndrome and deficiency syndrome clinically.

热入血室 【rè rù xuè shì】妇女在月经期或产后感受外邪的病理。症见下腹部或胸胁部胀满而硬、寒热往来、神志异常等。

Invasion of the Blood Chamber by Heat a morbid condition in which the uterus is affected by exopathic heat during menstruation or after delivery, marked by tenderness and fullness in the lower abdomen or hypochondriac regions, recurret chills and fever, and mental abnormalities.

热伤筋脉 【rè shāng jīn mài】因高热或久热不退，灼伤营阴，致筋脉失养的病理。症见四肢拘挛、痿软、瘫痪等。

Impairment of Muscles and Tendons by Heat a morbid condition in which high or long standing fever impairs the nourishment of the muscular system, leading to cramps, flacidity or paralysis of the limbs.

热伤气 【rè shāng qì】热邪多伤气分，因热邪入侵、腠理开而多汗，汗多则耗津伤气。

Injury of Qi by Heat a pathological change caused by the impairment of qi due to the excessive pathogenic heat characterized by profuse sweating due to the invasion of the striae of skin by heat which, as a result, leads to the impairment of body fluids.

热伤神明 【rè shāng shén míng】因高热而出现谵语、意识障碍甚或神志昏迷等症的病理。

Mental Disorder Caused by Heat a pathological condition caused by high fever, characterized by delirium, mental disturbance or even coma.

热深厥深 【rè shēn jué shēn】热邪越深伏，手足厥冷的程度越重的病理。通常指某些温热病的严重阶段，由于热邪过盛且深伏，阳气被郁，不能外达四肢所致。

The Deeper the Pathogenic Heat, the Colder the Limbs the pathogenic manifestations in febrile disease at its severe stage due to the excessive pathogenic heat which interferes with the distribution of yang-qi to the limbs, hence causing colder limbs as it

热甚发痉 【rè shèn fá jìng】由于邪热壅滞；或热甚伤阴，筋脉失养所致的痉病。症见壮热、项背强、口噤龂齿、手足挛急、腹满便秘、甚或角弓反张、神昏不清、舌红降、苔黄、脉洪数或沉滑有力等。

Convulsive Seizures due to High Fever convulsive seizure caused by impaired nourishment of muscles owing to accumulation of pathogenic heat or impairment of the yin fluid by intense heat, usually associated with high fever, stiff neck, trismus, grinding of teeth, rigidity and spasm of the extremities, abdominal distention, constipation, and even opisthotonos, loss of consciousness, deep red tongue with yellowish coating, full, fast or sunken, slippery and forceful pulse.

热胜则肿 【rè shèng zé zhǒng】阳热偏盛而出现局部肿痛的病理。热邪太过郁于肌肤腠理，气血壅塞，从而发生红肿热痛的症状，如痈疮、皮肤炎症等。

Excessive Heat Bringing about Swelling a pathological change characterized by local redness, swelling, heat and pain, such as carbuncle and skin inflammation due to obstruction to the flow of qi and blood caused by the excessive heat in the striae of skin.

热盛风动 【rè shèng fēng dòng】急性热病过程中，因高热而出现风证，如神志昏迷、狂躁、惊厥、抽搐等。

Wind-syndrome Resulting from the Domination of Heat wind-Syndrome occurring in the course of epidemic febrile disease caused by high fever, marked by coma, restlessness, convulsion or opisthotonos.

热盛气分 【rè shèng qì fèn】气分热邪炽盛的病理。症见高热、不恶寒、面红、心烦、大汗、口渴甚、舌苔黄干、脉洪大等。

Overabundance of Heat Located at Qifen a morbid condition occurring in the second stags (the qifen) of an epidemic febrile disease, characterized by high fever without chill, flushed face, dysphoria, profuse sweating, dire thirst, yellowish dry coating of the tongue and full pulse.

热嗽 【rè sòu】积热伤肺所致的咳嗽。

Heat-Type Cough cough caused by

症见咽喉干痛、鼻出热气、痰少难咳、色黄粘稠或痰带血丝，或有发热等。

accumulation of pathogenic heat in the lung, usually accompanied with dry and sore throat, hot air breathing out from the nose, less and difficult to expectorate sputum which is yellowish, sticky or streaked with blood and sometimes fever, dysphoria, profuse sweating, dire thirst, yellowish dry coating of the tongue and full pulse.

热痰 【rè tán】（火痰）1、素有痰疾，因饮食失宜或时邪所诱发，以喘咳咯痰为主症的一种疾病。2、指痰迷于心。多因痰热相搏，聚而不散所致。症见痰黄粘稠或带赤、咯之难出、面赤、烦热心痛、喜笑癫狂、怔忡、口干唇燥、脉洪等。

Heat-Phlegm also called fire-phlegm; 1. chronic phlegm syndrome when induced by improper diet or by seasonal pathogens with dyspnea and cough as its chief symptoms. 2. mental confusion due to heat phlegm, impairment of consciousness caused by heat-phlegm, mostly due to accumulation of phlegm and heat, marked by yellowish, thick, difficult to expectorated sputum or sometimes with blood, flushed face, fidget, epigastric pain, mania, palpitation, dry mouth and lips, and full pulse.

热无沉 【rè wú chén】热性药的作用，一般是向上向外，没有沉的趋向。

Hot Natured Drugs without the Property of Sinking the action of hot-natured drugs, usually going upward and outward but not sinking.

热无犯热 【rè wú fàn rè】如果不属寒证，在炎热的夏天，不要随便使用热性药物，以免伤津化燥，发生变证。

Avoiding Medicines of Hot Nature for Heat-Syndrome hot-natured drug should not be administered in hot weather unless there is cold syndrome so as to avoid the impairment of body fluids which causes syndrome of dryness, thus deteriorating the heat-syndrome.

热痫 【rè xián】内有积热所致的痫证。

Heat-Type Epilepsy epilepsy, com-

症见手足抽搐、口中吐沫、壮热啼哭、面赤气粗、尿赤便秘等。多见于小儿。由于胃肠积热、风痰壅盛所致。

热邪 【rè xié】病邪之一。其致病特点是导致热性、阳性的症状,如发热、息粗、红肿、热痛、便秘等。

热邪阻肺 【rè xié zǔ fèi】热邪壅阻于肺,发生喘咳的病理。主要症状有发热、咳嗽、痰黄稠或痰中带血、甚则呼吸急促、胸痛、舌红、苔黄干、脉洪数等。

热泻 【rè xiè】(热泄)因热迫肠胃所致的泄泻。症见肠鸣腹痛,痛泻阵作,泻下稠粘,或注泻如水,或水谷不化、肛门灼痛、后重不爽、口渴喜冷、小便赤涩、脉数等。

热心痛 【rè xīn tòng】(热厥心痛、火心痛)因感受暑邪;或常服热药、热食,热郁于内所致的胃脘痛。症见胃脘灼热剧痛、时作时止、畏热喜冷,或兼面目赤黄、身热烦躁、手心热、大便坚等。

monly seen in children due to internal accumulation of heat in the stomach and intestines, and excessive pathogenic wind-phlegm, manifested by spasm of limbs, foam at the mouth, high fever, crying, flushed face, snorty breath, dark urine and constipation.

Pathogenic Heat one of the pathogens which is characteristic of bringing about febrile diseases with positive symptoms such as fever, raucous breathing, redness, swelling, hotness and pain, as well as constipation.

Stagnation of Heat in the Lung a morbid condition marked by fever, cough thick, yellowish or blood-stained sputum and even dyspnea, chest pain, redness of the tongue with dry yellow coating, full and fast pulse.

Heat-Type Diarrhea a morbid condition due to invasion of the large intestine by heat, manifested as increased borborygmi, paroxysmal diarrhea with abdominal pain, mucous or watery stools, or with undigested food, burning pain and heavy sensation in the anus, thirst with preference for cold drink and fast pulse.

Epigastric Pain due to Heat epigastralgia caused by invasion of pathogenic summer-heat, or frequent uses of drugs in hot nature, eating hot food and interior heat stagnation, characterized by severe burning pain

热罨法 【rè yǎn fǎ】 罨法的一种。用棉织物浸在热水或热的药液中,稍拧干后,掩盖在局部。用于治疗某种肿胀或疼痛。

热夜啼 【rè yè tí】(热啼)小儿夜眠不宁,容易烦躁而啼哭不休,伴面红身热溺赤等的一种病证。多因受惊、风热或痰热内扰心神所致。

热因寒用 【rè yīn hán yòng】反治法之一。治寒证用温热药的同时,加用少量寒性的药物,或热药凉服,以更好地发挥药效作用。

热因热用 【rè yīn rè yòng】反治法之一。以热性的药物治疗属真寒假热的疾病。

热郁 【rè yù】由于情志不舒,肝气郁结,郁久化热的病理。症见头痛、头昏目眩、口干口苦、情绪急躁、胸闷

in the stomach with intervals between attacks, intolerance of hot and preference for cold, or complicated by flushed and yellowish face. fever, restlessness, hot palm and hard stool.

Hot Compress Method one of the compress methods used by applying a piece of cotton fabrics that has been soaked in hot water or hot drug fluid and wringed out slightly, to a local area, for the treatment of swelling and distention or pain.

Morbid Night Crying of Babies due to Heart-Heat a manifestation due to frightenedness, wind-heat, or exhaustion of heart blood caused by interior heat, marked by restless sleep, restlessness, continuous crying accompanied by flushed face, fever and dark urine.

Using Drugs of Cold Nature Treating Cold-Syndrome a contrary therapeutic method to treat cold syndrome with drugs in cold nature besides the use of warm-natured drugs, or with warm natured drugs taken cold for better effects.

Using Drugs of Warm Nature to Treat Pseudo-Heat a contrary therapeutic method treating cold syndrome accompanied by pseudo-heat manifestations with drugs of warm or hot nature.

Heat Stagnation a morbid condition in which liver-qi accumulated and retained due to emotional distress trans-

胁胀、大便秘结、小便黄赤、舌红苔黄、脉弦数等。

forms into heat, marked by headache, dizziness, dryness and bitter taste in the mouth, irritability and anxiety, distress and distention in the chest, constipation, dark urine, reddened tongue with yellow coating, fast and wiry pulse.

热胀 【rè zhàng】因伤于酒食厚味，湿热蕴结于中，或气郁化火，邪盛阴虚所致的腹胀。症见腹部胀满、大便干结、小便黄赤或见发热、脉洪数等。

Flatulence due to Heat abdominal distention caused by immoderate drinking, damp-heat in the middle energizer, or transformation of qi stagnation into fire, exuberant pathogen and yin deficiency, marked by distention and fullness in the abdomen, constipation, dark urine or fever, full and fast pulse.

热者寒之 【rè zhě hán zhī】属热性的疾病，一般宜用寒凉的方药治疗。临床上须按其表、里、虚、实之不同而采用相应的治疗措施，如表热者辛凉解表，疏散风热；虚热者宜用甘凉养阴透热或滋阴清热等。

Heat Syndrome Being Treated with Drugs in Cold Nature a syndrome of heat usually treated with cold-natured prescription, for which, different therapeutic methods are used according to the difference in interior or exterior, deficiency or sufficiency, with measures such as relieving the exterior syndrome with drugs pungent in flavor and cool in property to dispel wind-heat if for exterior heat, or nourishing yin with drugs sweet in taste, cool in nature to dispel heat or nourishing yang to dispel heat if for the case with asthenic heat.

热证 【rè zhèng】在致病因子的作用下，引起阳气亢盛的一种证候。症见身热烦躁、面目红赤、不恶寒反恶热、口干咽燥、大便秘结、小便短赤、舌质红、苔黄干或黑、脉数等。

Heat Syndrome syndrome due to attack of pathogenic heat or hyperactivity of yang-qi characterized by fever, fidget, flushed face, intolerance of heat but not cold, dry mouth and

热中 【rè zhōng】1、指以善饥能食，小便多为主症的疾病。2、指风邪侵入胃经化热所致的以目黄为主症的疾病。3、指由于饮食劳倦等损伤脾胃所致气虚火旺的证候。症见身热而烦、气喘、头痛、恶寒或口渴、脉洪大无力等。

热灼肾阴 【rè zhuó shèn yīn】热性病后期，肾阴被热邪所消耗的病理。症见低热、手足心热、口齿干燥、耳聋、舌质深红、无苔、脉细数或虚数等。

人痘接种（法） 【rén dòu jiē zhòng (fǎ)】是取天花患者的痘痂制成浆，接种于健康儿童，使产生免疫力以预防天花的方法。

人事不省 【rén shì bù xǐng】意识丧失的状态。

人迎 【rén yíng】1、诊脉部位之一。即结喉旁两侧颈动脉搏动处。又称人迎脉，该处的脉搏变化与胃有关。2、左手寸口脉的别称。3、穴位名称。

throat, constipation, scanty dark urine, reddened tongue with dry brownish or black coating, and fast pulse.

Heat in the Middle Energizer 1. a morbid condition chiefly charaterized by polyphagia and polyuria. 2. a morbid condition with jaundice due to accumulation and retention of pathogenic heat in the stomach. 3. a morbid condition marked by deficiency of qi and excess of fire due to impairment ot the spleen and stomach by improper diet and overstrain, with the symptoms such as fevre, fidget, dyspnea, headache, intolerance of cold or thirst, full but weak pulse.

Kidney-Yin Consumed by Heat a morbid condition in which yin fluid of the kidney is consumed by pathogenic heat, usually seen at the later stage of epidemic febrile disease, manifested as low fever, hot sensation in palms and soles, dry mouth, impairment of hearing, dry and deep red tongue without coating, thready and fast pulse or feeble and fast pulse.

Human-Pox Vaccination a method of vaccination for healthy children with the serous fluid made from dried or soaked crusts of smallpox lesions.

Unconsciousness a state of coma.

Renying 1. the pulsation of common carotid artery lateral to the laryngeal prominence where the pulse is felt for diagnosis and changes of the pulse are

人中疔 【rèn zhōng dīng】生于人中穴附近的颜面部疔疮。

妊娠喘 【rèn shēn chuǎn】妊娠期症见痰多喘急、夜卧不安等病状。多因感受外邪，肺气失宣；或痰热交结，气逆作喘；亦有肺气素虚，水湿不化，上乘于肺所致。

妊娠疮疡 【rèn shēn chuāng yáng】指孕妇患痈疽疔毒。

妊娠恶阻 【rèn shēn è zǔ】妊娠早期恶心、呕吐、食入即吐或不食亦吐，甚至吐出血液或胆叶。辨证分类1、肝胃不和证；2、脾胃虚弱证；、3、痰湿阻滞证；4、气阴两亏证。

妊娠小便不利 【rèn shēn xiǎo biàn bù lì】妊娠期小便量小而不畅。多因湿热下注膀胱，气化受阻；或脾肺气虚，

related with the stomach. 2. another name for cun kou pulse on the wrist of the left hand. 3. name of an acupoint (sq).

Boil on philtrum boils appeared near the renzhong point on the face.

Dyspnea during pregnancy a morbid condition during pregnancy marked by dyspnea with profuse sputum and restless sleep due to dysfunction of lung-qi resulting from the invasion by exopathic factors, or due to dyspnea because of the accumulation of phlegm-heat, or caused by insufficiency of qi and the retained water going up to the lung.

Inflammatory Skin Disease during Pregnancy referring to carbuncle and furunculosis that pregnant women suffer.

Morning Sickness a morbid condition occurring during the early stage of pregnancy marked by vomiting immediately after eating, or vomiting without eating, even vomiting of blood or bilious fluid. Types of differentiation 1. syndrome of incoordination between the liver and the stomach. 2. syndrome of weakness of the spleen and the stomach. 3. syndrome of stagnation of phlegm-dampness. 4. syndrome of deficiency of both qi and yin.

Dysuria during Pregnancy a condition marked by oliguria and difficulty in urination, mostly due to the distur-

运化转输失职，不能下输膀胱所致。bance in qi transformation because of the downward flow of damp-heat into the urinary bladder, or caused by dysfunction of the spleen in transport down to the bladder due to qi deficiency of the spleen and the lung.

妊娠心烦 【rèn shēn xīn fán】怀孕后出现烦躁不安、心悸胆怯。多由阴血不足或素有痰饮，复因郁怒忧思，致火热扰心，神志不宁引起。 **Restlessness during Pregnancy** disease marked by restlessness, palpitation and timidity after pregnancy, induced mostly by insufficiency of yin and blood or long-standing phlegm retention, complicated by fire due to mental depression, leading to the disturbance of the heart, and dysfunction of mental activity.

妊娠心腹胀满 【rèn shēn xīn fù zhàng mǎn】怀孕期间脘腹胀满。多因素有虚寒，孕后复感寒邪或内伤饮食，致浊邪内阻，胃气壅滞，升降失调引起。 **Flatulence during Pregnancy** a morbid condition marked by fullness and distention of the stomach, during pregnancy, mostly caused by long-standing cold of insufficiency type, complicated by the invasion of pathogenic factor of improper diet, complicated by the stagnation of turbid pathogens, excessiveness of stomach-qi, failure of the spleen-qi to ascend and the stomach-qi to descend.

妊娠眩晕 【rèn shēn xuàn yūn】怀孕期间出现头晕、眼花、耳鸣等症。多因肝肾阴虚，肝阳偏亢，上扰清窍所致。 **Dizziness during Pregnancy** a morbid condition occurring during pregnancy manifested by dizziness, dim eyesight, and tinnitus, mostly caused by yin deficiency of the liver and the spleen, hyperactivity of liver-yang which interferes the upper orifices.

妊娠腰痛 【rèn shēn yāo tòng】怀孕期间出现腰部酸痛无力，劳累后加甚等症。多因素体肾虚，孕后肾虚加重，腰 **Lumbago during Pregnancy** a morbid condition during pregnancy marked by aching pain and weakness

失所养所致；亦有因风冷乘袭，或跌仆闪挫，瘀血阻滞经络所致。

of the loin, more severe when one becomes tired, mostly caused by consistent kidney deficiency which is worsened after pregnancy and the failure in the nourishment of the loin, or caused by the attack of wind-cold as well as blockage of collaterals by blood stasis due to trauma.

妊娠药忌 【rèn shēn yào jì】指妊娠期间，对于某些可能引起流产，或损伤母子的药物，一般不得使用或慎用。

Drugs Contraindicated in Pregnancy referring to drugs that should be-contraindicated or used with caution in pregnancy for their possibility of inducing abortion or the harmfull effect to both the mother and fetus.

妊娠肿胀 【rèn shèn zhǒng zhàng】（妊娠水肿）妊娠六个月以后肌肤肢体肿胀。多因脾肾阳虚，水滞停聚，泛滥肌肤所致。

Edema during Pregancy a morbid condition marked by extremital hydrops appeared 6 months after pregnancy, mostly caused by consistent yang deficiency of the spleen and kidney, retention of water within the body, leading to the overwhelming of pathogenic water over the musclse and skin.

妊娠中风 【rèn shèn zhòng fēng】多因孕后血虚，经络脏腑失荣，中于风邪所致的疾病。临床上有中经络和中脏腑之分。

Apoplexy in Pregnancy a morbid condition caused by deficiency of blood after pregnancy, dysfunction of meridians, collaterals and zang-fu organs, clinically classified as apoplexy involving the meridians and collaterals, and apoplexy involving the zang-fu organs.

日晡发热 【rì bū fā rè】出现于下午三时至五时左右的发热。

Afternoon Fever fever occurring from about 3-5 in the afternoon.

日晒疮 【rì shài chuāng】由于烈日曝晒引起的皮肤损害。症见皮肤裸露部分出现红斑、肿胀、甚者发生水泡，有

Solar Dermatitis skin damage caused by burning sun marked by red spots on the exposed skin and

灼热、瘙痒、刺痛的感觉。相当于日光性皮炎。

柔痓 【róu jìng】（柔痓）痓病的一种。以发热汗出而不恶寒为特征。多因感受风湿之邪所致。

肉刺 【ròu cì】（鸡眼）因局部长期受压磨擦，致皮肤角质增厚而成。多生于足底端或足趾间，状如鸡眼、根部深陷，顶端硬凸，表面淡黄，受压则痛，影响行走。

肉分 【ròu fēn】指肌肉的纹理。

肉瘤 【ròu liú】多由思虑伤脾，脾气郁结所致的肿瘤。瘤体坚实柔韧、皮色不变、无热无寒，相当于肌纤维瘤。

肉轮 【ròu lún】即眼睑，配属于脾。它的病变与脾胃有关。

肉脱 【ròu tuō】严重肌肉瘦削的征象。多因精血内竭，中气虚衰所致。

肉痿 【ròu wěi】痿症的一种。症见肢体痿软无力，或兼微肿麻木、饮食少、

swelling, or even blisters with burning hot and itching sensations as well as stabbing pain.

Rigidity with Sweating one kind of the diseases with spasms, charaterized by fever and sweating, mostly due to pathogenic wind-dampness.

Clavus corns caused by thickened keratoderma due to consistent rubbing of certain local areas, usually seen on the front part of soles or between toes, shaped like chicken eyes which are deep-rooted with hard protruding points, light yellow in color, pain when presssed, causing difficulty in walking.

Muscular Striae texture and interspace of muscles.

Muscular Tumor a kind of tumor, solid and tough with normal skin color and with absence of fever or chillness, referring to myofibroma, mostly caused by impairment of spleen due to anxiety and stagnation of spleen-qi.

Muscle Wheel referring to the eyelid belonging to spleen, whose pathological changes are related to the spleen and stomach.

Emaciation a morbid condition marked by thinness, it is mostly caused by exhaustion of esscence and blood, and deficiency of qi in middle energizer.

Muscular Atrophy an atrophic debility manifested by weakness of the

大便溏等。多因脾胃虚弱,或湿热浸淫影响气血运行,肌肉筋脉失养所致。

肉瘿 【ròu yǐng】颈前结块,呈园形、椭园形、表面光滑,能随吞咽动作上下移动。无疼痛和压痛。如囊内出血时,肿块可迅速增大,伴有胀痛。肿块增大时,可有呼吸困难、吞咽困难、声音嘶哑等压迫症状。本病多见于青中年妇女。辨证分类1、气郁痰凝证 2、气阴两伤证。

如丧神守 【rú sàng shén shǒu】神志昏乱、心神不宁、惊惶不安的病状,多因热盛于内所致。

濡脉 【rú mài】浅表、细而柔软的脉象。轻按可触知,重按反不明显。多见于失血伤阴或湿邪滞留的患者。

乳蛾 【rǔ é】(喉蛾、乳鹅)以扁桃体为主的咽部疾病。急性乳蛾见有发热、咽痛、喉核燉红,或有黄白色渗出物。慢性乳蛾常无明显全身症状,

limbs or complicated by swelling and numbness, anorexia and loose stool, mostly caused by the interference of the circulation of qi and blood due to the invasion of damp-heat factors and failure in the nourishment of muscles.

Fleshy Goiter   mass in the front neck, commonly seen in middle-aged women, which is round-shaped and elliptic with a smooth surface and able to move up and down along with swallowing, painless and tender, increasing rapidly in size, accompanied by distention and pain when there is bleeding inside of the mass with the appearance of symptoms due to being pressed such as dyspnea, difficulty in swallowing and hoarseness; Types of differentiation 1. syndrome of stagnation of qi and phlegm 2. syndrome of damage of both qi and yin.

Mental Derangement   a condition due to excess of internal heat marked by unconsciousness, restlessness and nervousness.

Soft and Floating Pulse   a pulse felt shallow, floating, thready and soft by light touch, but faint on heavy press, usually seen in cases with the impairment of yin due to loss of blood and stagnation of pathogenic dampness.

Tonsillitis   a pharyngeal disease mainly involving tonsils, usually with repeated attacks due to colds, characterized, in its acute form, by fever,

有时可有低热,咽痛。常因感冒引起反复发作。辨证分类1、风热证 2、毒热证 3、阴虚证。

pain of the larynx, inflammatory throat or with white yellow-exudate; no marked general symptoms in its chronic form, sometimes with low fever and pain of the larynx. Types of differentiation 1. wind-heat syndrome 2. toxic heat syndrome 3. yin deficiency syndrome.

乳发 【rǔ fā】(发乳、脱壳乳痈)症见乳房硬结肿痛,溃则皮肉腐烂,迅速扩大,易形成漏管,且伴有发热、恶寒等全身症状。相当于乳房急性蜂窝织炎。

Suppurative Mastitis disease marked by hard and swelling breast with its skin and muscles decomposed rapidly if with ulcers, resulting in fistulas, accompanied by generalized symptoms such as fever and aversion to cold, referring to mammary cellulitis.

乳房胀痛 【rǔ fáng zhàng tòng】乳房及乳头胀痛不适,多连及胸胁。常发生在月经前。多由肝郁气滞,经脉壅阻所致。

Distending Pain of the Breast a condition manifested by pain of the breast and nipple, mostly involving the chest and hypochondrium, usually ocurring before the menstruation, and mostly caused by stagnation of qi in the liver, resulting in blockage of meridians and collaterals.

乳疳 【rǔ gān】乳房所生疮肿或结块,经年不愈;或腐去半截,状如莲蓬,痛楚难忍。包括乳岩、乳腺结核等慢性乳病。

Necrotic Mass of the Mamma a long-standing ulcer or necrotic mass, or with half of which decomposed shaped like a lotus receptacle, including cancer and tuberculosis of the mammary gland.

乳疖 【rǔ jié】乳部所生的疖肿。

Furuncle of the Breast referring to the furuncles appearing on the breast.

乳痨 【rǔ láo】多由肝气郁结,胃经痰浊凝结所致。初起乳房中肿块形如梅李,硬而不痛,皮色如常;数月后肿

Mammary Tuberculosis a morbid condition which might involve the chest and the subaxilliary part, most-

块逐渐增大,与皮肤粘连、隐痛,皮色转微红,肿块逐渐变软成脓,溃后脓汁稀薄,腐肉不脱,周围肤色暗红,病变可延及胸胁腋下。相当于乳房结核。

ly caused by stagnation of liver-qi, phlegm stagnation in the stomach meridian, first manifested by mammary mass shaped like aplum which is hard but painless with normal skin colour, and which becomes larger and larger several months later, adhensive to the skin with dull pain, reddened skin color, and with the mass softened due to the pus forming inside which becomes watery fluid when ulcerated, still with the decomposed muscles attached and dark red skin around.

乳瘘 【rǔ lòu】(乳漏)生于乳房或乳晕部的漏管。多由乳痈、乳发等疾患调治失当,以致疮口经久不愈引起。症见疮口时有清稀分泌物或腐败组织流出,不易收口,易反复发作等。

Mammary Fistula fistulas appearing in breast or areola of nipple, mostly caused by long-standing wound due to improper treatment of acute mastitis and suppurative mastitis, marked by the discharge of watery exudate or decomposed tissue with the fistula difficult to heal with repeated reccurrence.

乳衄 【rǔ nǜ】多由忧思过度,肝脾受伤,血失统藏所致的病证。相当于乳房腺管内乳头状瘤。

Bleeding from the Nipple a condition mostly caused by excessive melancholy, impairment of the liver and spleen, failure of the blood in its control and store, referring to mammary papilloma of the glandular dust.

乳食积滞 【rǔ shí jī zhì】婴儿由于喂养不当,致乳食积滞胃肠。症见脘腹胀满、纳呆厌食、呕吐酸腐、大便酸臭、伴烦躁易啼、睡眠不安,或低热不退、形体消瘦等。

Infantile Dyspepsia indigestion due to improper feeding characterized by distention and fullness of the abdomen, anorexia, sour vomitus, sour fetid stool, accompanied by fidgets, frequent crying, restless sleep, or persistent low fever and emaciation.

乳头皲裂 【rǔ tóu jūn liè】（乳头破碎）又称乳头风。乳头、乳颈及乳晕部破裂疼痛，揩之出血；或流粘性分泌物；或结黄痂。多由肝火不能疏泄，肝胃湿热蕴结而致。

乳细 【rǔ xì】把药末放在乳钵内研至极细。如点眼药、吹喉药都需乳细使用。

乳腺增生病 【rǔ xiàn zēng shèng bìng】本病多见于20—40岁之间妇女。一侧或两侧乳房发生多个大小不同的园形、韧硬的结节。结节常分散于整个乳房，也可局限在乳房的一部。肿块边界不清，与皮肤不相连，推之可动。肿块每随喜怒而消长，始终不会溃破。乳房部有明显胀痛，常在月经前加重，月经后减轻。辨证分类 1、肝郁气结证 2、冲任不调证。

乳岩 【rǔ yán】多见于中年以上妇女。由悲怒忧思，肝脾气逆所致。初起乳中结块大如枣栗，表面不平，坚硬不痛，后渐增大，始觉疼痛不止，未溃时，肿若堆栗，肿块处皮核相连，推之不移，乳头内陷。若顶透紫色，则

Cracked Nipple a morbid condition mostly due to failure in dispelling liver-fire, and accumulation of damp-heat in the liver and stomach, marked by cracks and pain of nipple, the neck or areola of nipple with bleeding; or discharging viscous secreta; or forming crusts.

Reduction to Fine Powder fine powder of medicinal herbs ground in an earthen bowl, such as drugs for the eyes and throat that must be ground before use.

Hyperplasia of Mammary Glands a disease commonly seen in women between the ages of 20-40 with nodules appearing in one or both breasts, hard in texture and different in size, usually scattering in the whole breast, or sometimes localized to a certain part with unclear margins and adhensive to the skin, movable on pushing and disappearing along with changes of moods but never broken, with the manifestation of distending pain which is more severe before menstruation and relieved after menstruation. Types of differentiation 1. syndrome of stagnation of liver-qi 2. syndrome of incoordination of TV and CV.

Breast Carcinoma a disease mostly seen in women over middle age, caused by anger, anxiety, reversed flow of liver- and spleen-qi, first marked by a mass in the breast, with an uneven surface which is hard,

渐溃烂,溃后状如岩穴,形似菜花,时流污水或血。即乳腺癌。辨证分类 1.肝郁气滞证 2.冲任失调证 3.正虚毒结证。

painless, but consistently painful as it grows larger with rough surface before it ulcerates, which is adhensive to the skin, unmovable when pushed with the nipple sunk and which will gradually ulcerates when the nipple becomes purple with the ulcerated wound appearing as a grotto, shaped like cauliflower, often discharging foul water or blood. Types of differentiation 1. syndrome of the liver-qi stagnation 2. syndrome of the disturbance of TV and CV 3. syndrome of weakened body resistence and accumulation of pathogenic factors.

乳痈 【rǔ yòng】(乳吹) 患者多是哺乳期妇女,尤以未满月的初产妇为多见。多由肝气郁结,胃热壅滞而成。初起乳房出现硬块、胀痛,乳汁不畅,全身可有恶寒发热,继则肿块增大,焮红剧痛,寒热不退,蕴酿成脓。辨证分类 1. 气滞热壅证; 2. 热毒酿脓证; 3. 正虚毒恋证。

Acute Mastitis a morbid condition commonly seen in breast feeding women, especially the primiparae in the first month after delivery, first manifested by breast mass with distending pain, galactostasis, systemic cold, fever, and later, by the mass increasing in size which is swelling, red and very painful, as well as consistent cold-heat, leading to the formation of pus, Types of differentiation 1. syndrome of stagnation of qi and accumulation of pathogenic heat 2. syndrome of pus formation due to toxic heat 3. syndrome of weakened body resistance and accumulation of pathogens.

乳汁不足 【rǔ zhī bù zú】乳汁分泌过少。多因产后气血亏虚,乳汁化源不足或肝郁气滞,乳汁壅滞不行所致。

Lack of Factation insufficiency of milk after labor, mostly caused by insufficiency of the source, stagnation of liver-qi and the resultant blackage

乳子 【rǔ zǐ】指肾气未盛,天癸未至的少年儿童。

蓐风 【rù fēng】产后风邪所中。症见角弓反张、口噤不开等。

蓐劳 【rù láo】因产后气血耗伤,调理失宜,感受风寒或忧劳思虑等所致。症见虚羸喘乏、寒热如疟、头痛自汗、肢体倦怠、咳嗽气逆、胸中痞、腹绞痛或刺痛。

入静 【rù jìng】练功者在气功锻练过程中,在意念集中的情况下,所出现的高度安静,轻松舒适的一种特殊练功功能态。

软坚除满 【ruǎn jiān chú mǎn】使用咸寒而有润下作用的药物,润下大便以消除因大便燥结所致的腹部胀满的一种治法。

软坚散结 【ruǎn jiān sàn jié】治疗因痰浊瘀血等结聚而形成的瘰疬症积等病的方法。如属痰浊所致者用消痰软坚散结法;属气滞血瘀者则宜用破瘀消症的方法。

of collaterals, marking the milk difficult to flow out.

Children at Their Early Youth referring to people under age whose kidney-qi has not yet formed.

Puerperal Tetanus a morbid condition caused by pathogenic wind, marked by opisthotonus and lockjaw.

General Debility during Puerperium a morbid condition occurring after delivery, caused by consumption of qi and blood, exposure to wind and cold, worry, anxiety or overstrain, characterized by weakness and emaciation, shortness of breath, malaria-like cold and heat, headache, night sweat, lassitude, cough with dyspnea, distention in the chest, colic or stabbing pain of the abdomen.

Entering Static State a kind of special state in practice of qigong characterized by peace of mind and relaxation, reaching a high level under the condition of concentrating will.

Softening the Dry Feces and Relieving Flatulence a therapy by applying the salty, cold drug to relieve abdominal fullness caused by dry stool.

Softening the Hard lumps and Dispelling the Nodes therapy for masses formed by accumulation of phlegm and blood stasis, by adopting phlegm eliminating, blood-stasis-resolving and mass-dissolving method for those caused by accumulation of phlegm, blood-stasis by lump-remov-

软瘫 【ruǎn tān】小儿由于发育不良而出现的驰缓性瘫痪。

软下疳 【ruǎn xià gān】下疳的一种。见下疳。

润下 【rùn xià】（缓下）使用性甘平、具有滋润津液或润滑作用的药物，治疗肠燥津枯便秘的一种方法。适用于老人肠燥津枯便秘或习惯性便秘、孕妇产后便秘等。

润燥 【rùn zào】（清燥、凉燥）用生津滋润的方药治疗燥证的方法。通常分轻宣润燥、甘寒滋润、清肠润燥、养阴润燥等。

润燥化痰 【rùn zào huà tán】（润肺化痰）治疗燥痰的方法。适用于感受温燥之邪或肺阴不足。症见咽喉干燥或疼痛、咳嗽痰稠难出、舌红、苔黄而干等。

弱脉 【ruò mài】深沉而细软无力的脉象。多因气血不足所致。

爇 【ruò】古代用火针、温针或石针加热，以刺激体表局部的一种治疗方

ing method for those caused by stagnancy of qi and blood stasis.

Flaccid Paralysis a disease occurring among children with dysplasia.

Soft Chancre a type of chancre.

Causing Laxation a therapeutic method to treat dry stool and consumption of body fluid by using drugs sweet in taste with moistening effect to loose bowel, applied for the old with constipation due to dryness of intestine and deficient body fluid or habitual constipation, as well as women with constipation after delivery.

Moistening a therapy by using medicine with moistening effect to treat illness caused by pathogenic dryness, usually classified as moistening, moistening with drugs sweet in taste, cold in nature, moistening by clearing the bowels, and moistening by nourishing yin.

Moistening the Lung and Resolving the Phlegm a therapy to treat dryness-phlegm due to pathogenic warm-dryness or deficiency of lung-yin, marked by dry or sore throat, cough with thick sputum which is difficult to expectorate, reddened tongue with yellowish, dry coating.

Week Pulse a pulse felt extremely soft, sunken and thready, caused by deficiency of qi and blood.

Stimulation Therapy with Warm Needle an ancient therapeutic

法。

塞法 【sāi fǎ】外治法之一。把药粉用纱布包裹扎紧，或将药制成锭剂，塞于鼻、阴道、肛门内等处，以达到治疗目的。

塞因塞用 【sāi yīn sāi yòng】反治法之一。对某些本质属虚的疾病，虽然有闭塞不通的症状，仍应使用补的方法治疗。如中气虚，脾阳不运所引起的腹胀，治宜补中健脾。

三宝 【sān bǎo】即精、气、神，是生命现象的根本。

三痹 【sān bì】行痹、痛痹及着痹三种痹证的合称。

三部 【sān bù】诊脉的三个部位。古代的三部是指头部及上、下肢。近代一般是指桡动脉的三个部位，即寸、关、尺三个部位。

三部九候 【sān bù jiǔ hòu】古代脉诊方法之一。1、指寸口部寸、关、尺

method to stimulate a local body area by heating with heat needle, warm needle or stone needle.

Plug-in Method one of the methods for external treatment by inserting medicinal powder packed in cotton or gauze or lozenges into the nostril, vagina or rectum.

Treating the Pseudo-Obstructive Disease by Tonification one of the methods to treat a disease contrary to the routine by applying tonifying method to treat diseases of deficiency with the symptoms of pseudo-obstruction. For instance, abdominal distention due to deficiency of qi in middle energizer, failure of the spleen-yang in performing its transporting and transforming function, the principle of treatment should be replenishing the spleen and stomach.

Three Treasures the three essentials-essence, qi and spirit-the basics of life.

Three Kinds of Bi a collective term for arthralgia, or arthritides with wandering pain, that with severe pain and that with fixed pain.

Three Regions for Pulse Feeling in ancient time, referring to the head, the upper limbs and the lower limbs, now referring to the three pulse locations on the wrist over the radial artery classified as cun, guan and chi.

Three Regions and The Nine Subdivisions for Pulse Feeling 1. refer-

三部,每部以轻、中、重的指力相应分为浮、中、沉三种,故称三部九候。2、全身遍诊法。即诊查人体头部、上肢、下肢三部及每部上、中、下共九处脉搏的变化,以了解头部、耳眼、口齿、胸中及五脏的病变。

ring to the three regions, cun guan and chi on the wrist over the redial artery where the pules is felt with each region further classified as floating, moderate and sunken pulse felt by light, moderate and heavy touches accordingly. 2. systemic diagnostic method, i. e. the examination of the pulse changes over the nine locations of the upper, middle and lower parts of each of the three regions: the head, the upper limbs and the lower limbs so as to diagnose the pathological changes of the head, ears, eyes, teeth, chest as well as the five zang organs.

三法 【sān fǎ】指发汗、涌吐及泻下三种治法。

Three Therapeutic Methods diaphoresis, emesis and purgation.

三伏 【sān fú】1、指初伏、中伏和末伏,是一年中最炎热的时候。2 指末伏。

Three Periods of Dog Days 1. referring to the first, second and third ten day periods of the hottest season. 2. the third period of dog days.

三焦 【sān jiāo】(外腑) 六腑之一。分上、中、下三个部位。具有调节各脏腑机能活动和参与调节体液代谢的功能。

Triple Energizer one of the six fu-organs, including the upper, middle and lower-energizer responsible for regulating the functional activities of zang and fu-organs, and the metabolism of body fluids.

三焦辨证 【sān jiāo biàn zhèng】按温热病的病理过程及其传变情况,以上焦、中焦、下焦三个阶段作为辨证施治的纲领,判断病变的部位、病情轻重及预后的一种辨证方法。

Differentiation of Syndrome According to the Pathological Changes of Triple-Energizer a method to assess the pathological changes, the seriousness, and prognosis of diseases with the three phases, the upper、middle and lower-energizer as a

三焦咳 【sān jiāo ké】伴有腹胀、不欲饮食的咳嗽。
Triple-Energizer Cough cough with abdominal fullness and anorexia.

三焦实热 【sān jiāo shí rè】实热之邪同犯三焦而出现心肺实热、脾胃实热及肝肾实热的病理。
Sthenia-Heat of Triple-Energizer heat syndrome of excess type occurring simultaneously in the three portions of tri-energizer, leading to excessive heat in the heart and lung, spleen and stomach as well as the liver and kidney.

三焦主决渎 【sān jiāo zhǔ jué dú】三焦功能之一。即三焦具有通调水道、运行水液、参与调节体液代谢的功能。当其功能失调时，可出现小便不利、水肿等症。
The Tri-Energizer Managing the Dredging of Water Pathway one of the three functions of the tri-energizer, i. e. dredging the water pathway, transporting qi and fluid, and participating in regulating the metabolism of body fluid; with the symptoms such as difficulty in urination and edema appearing if any functonal disturbances occur.

三品 【sān pǐn】是古代的一种药物分类法。按药物是否有毒性、能否久服，将其分为上品、中品及下品三类。
Three Grades of Medicines an ancient classification of drugs according to their toxicity and if they can be taken over a long period of time: top grade, middle grade and low grade.

三日疟 【sān rì nüè】表现为每隔两天发作一次的疟疾。
Quartan Malaria malaria with repeated attacks in every two days.

三调 【sān tiáo】即调身、调息、调心。
Tri-Regulation referring to regulation of body, regulation of breathing, regulation of mental activity. It is a term of qigong.

三消 【sān xiāo】（消渴病）按照病机、症状和病情发展阶段的不同，把消渴
Three Types of Diabetes a collective term for diabetes which are divided

病分为上消、中消及下消，三消是这三种类型的合称。

into three types--diabetes involving the upper-energizer, diabetes involving the middle-energizer and diabetes involving the lower-energizer according to their pathogenesis, symptoms and the different stages in the course of the disease.

三阳病 【sān yáng bìng】是三条阳经受病（太阳病、少阳病、阳明病）的总称。

Diseases of the Three Yang Meridians a collective term for the taiyang (major yang) disease, yangming (splendid yang) disease and shaoyang (minor yang) disease.

三阴痉 【sān yīn jìng】出现三阴经症状的痉病。除见手足厥冷、筋脉拘急、汗出不止、项强脉沉等表现外，还可见头不自主摇动、牙关紧闭（属厥阴）；四肢强直、发热腹痛（属太阴）；闭目嗜睡（属少阴）等三阴经症状。

Convulsion with Syptoms of Three Yin Meridians a morbid condition characterized by involuntary head-shaking and lockjaw (symptoms of the jueyin meridian), stretch of the limbs, fever and abdominal pain (symptoms of the taiyin meridian), closed eyes and sleepiness (symptoms of the shaoyin meridian), besides the manifestations such as cold limbs, spasm of muscles, incessant perspiration, neck rigidity and sunken pulse.

三阳合病 【sān yáng hé bìng】太阳与少阳之热邪同时侵入阳明经的一种病证。症见身热、口渴、汗出、腹胀、身体倦怠、语言不利、食欲不振，甚则神昏谵语、二便失禁等。

Disease Involving All Three Yang Meridians a morbid condition characterized by transmission of pathogenic heat into the yangming meridian both from the taiyang and shaoyang meridians with the manifestations such as fever, thirst, perspiration, abdominal distention, lassitude, retardation in speech, loss of appetite or even delirium and incontinence of urine and stool.

三因 【sān yīn】古代三因分类法的三

Three Categories of Etiological Factors

三阴病 【sān yīn bìng】是三条阴经受病（太阴病、少阴病、厥阴病）的总称。

三阴疟 【sān yīn nüè】1、即三日疟。2、发于夜间的疟疾。

散 【sǎn】（散剂）把药物研成粉末，分为内服和外用两种。

散脉 【sǎn mài】散而不聚，轻按有散乱之感，中按渐空，重按则无的一种脉象。主元气离散。见于病情垂危阶段。

散者收之 【sàn zhě shōu zhī】属气散不固的疾病，一般宜采用收敛固涩的方法进行治疗。如久咳多汗、肺气不固之证，常用收敛肺气止咳的方法治疗。

色部 【sè bù】指脏腑及肢体分布于面部的色诊部位。面部不同部位的颜色变化与脏腑及肢体生理病理状况有

a collective term for the thrree etiological factors which are included in the ancient three categories i. e. endopathic, exopathic and non-endo-exopathic.

Disease of the Three Yin Meridians a collective term for the taiyin (major yin) disease, shaoyin (minor yin) disease and jueyin (terminant yin) disease.

Three-yin Malaria 1. quartan malaria 2. malaria occurring during the night.

Powder a preparation of drug ground into powder for oral administration or external application.

Scattered Pulse a pulse that feels diffusing and feeble on light touch, gradual empty on moderate pressure, and faint on heavy pressure, seen in critical cases, indicating exhaustion of qi.

The Treatment of Syndrome in which Escence of life Fails to Retain in the Body with Astringent a treatment of diseases due to diffusion of qi by astringing to arrest discharge, for instance, those marked by long-standing cough, profuse sweating, and deficiency of lung-qi, usually treated by using astringent to arrest discharge, for the purpose of retaining the lung-qi.

Regions for Inspection of Skin Color different regions, for color inspection, on the face representing differ-

关。所以诊病时把面部划分为若干部分，以代表相应的脏腑和肢体，通过观察面部颜色的变化来帮助了解脏腑和肢体的病理和生理状况。ent zang-fu organs and limbs whose pathological changes are related with the color changes of the different parts of the face, the observation of which would aid in marking the pathological and physiological changes in the zang-fu organs as well as the limbs clear when making a diagnosis.

色悴 【sè cuì】面色憔悴无华，通常见于慢性病患者的病容。 **Sallow Complexion** a state usually seen in a chronic case.

色脉合参 【sè mài hé cān】在辨证过程中，必须把脉象和色泽病理性变化互相参照，进行分析综合，以判断病情。 **Consideration of Both Pulse Condition and Complexion** a diagnostic method of reviewing the patient pulse condition together with complexion and making overall analysis to assess the status of illness in the course of differentiation.

色随气华 【sè suí qì huá】体表，特别是面部的颜色，是五脏精气的外在表现，所以色泽的变化是随五脏精气的变化而变化的。 **Variation of Complexion Reflecting the Condition of Qi** color of the skin, especially of the face, as the symbol of the visceral qi, varying along with the condition of the latter.

色诊 【sè zhěn】望诊内容之一。通过观察面部及皮肤颜色的变化，帮助了解病情的方法。 **Inspection of the Color of the Skin** a method to assess the status of illness by observing the color of the face as well as the other parts of the skin.

涩肠止泻 【sè cháng zhǐ xiè】（涩肠固脱）收涩法之一。使用具有固涩、收敛作用的药物，治疗大便滑泄不禁的方法。常用于泄泻或久痢，致大便不能控制的患者。但本法不能过早使用，否则容易留邪。 **Relieving Diarrrhea with Astringents** a treatment with astringents for cases with lingering diarrhea due to fecal incontinence caused by diarrhea or consistent dysentery, but with the astringents given at a proper time, the application in early stage may possibly lead to the retention of pathogenic factors.

涩剂 【sè jì】用具有收敛性质的药物如龙骨、牡蛎、莲须、罂粟壳等组成的方剂。

Astringent prescription a prescription that consists of medicines of astringente nature, for instance, the one consisting of Os oraconis, Conch Ostreae, Stamen Nelumbinis and Preicarpium Papaveris.

涩可去脱 【sè kě qù tuō】用收涩的方剂可以治疗一些滑脱不固的疾病,如大便滑脱不禁、滑精、自汗等。

Arresting Discharges by Astringents a method to treat disease marked by discharges or deficiency, such as lingering sweat with prescriptions of astringents.

涩脉 【sè mài】脉搏不流畅,细而往来艰涩的一种脉象。多因津血亏损,气滞血瘀所致。

Uneven Pulse a weak pulse coming and going unsmoothly, indicating deficiency of blood essence and fluid, or stagnancy of qi and blood stasis.

杀血心痛 【shā xuè xīn tòng】又称失血心痛。指妇女因血崩而出现心痛的病证。多因失血过多、心脾失养,或瘀血凝滞所致。症见崩漏、心痛较剧、血色淡如水、小腹喜按等。若症见血色紫、有块、心痛巨按者,一般属瘀血凝滞。

Precardial Pain due to Metrorrhagia a morbid condition mostly caused by excessive loss of blood, poor nourishment of the heart and spleen and accumulation of blood stasis, characterized by metorrhagia, metrostasis severe epigastric pain, thin and light colored blood, and pain relieved by pressing the lower abdomen, those marked by purple colored blood with clots and abdominal tenderness usually caused by accumulation of blood stasis.

沙虱病 【shā shī bìng】因沙虱咬伤所致的发热性疾病。初被刺时皮肤不痛,摩之如芒刺状,原发灶上发疮(焦痂),约第五天出痧疹。

Tsutsugamushi Disease a febrile disease caused by the bites of shashiitsu, painless at the beginning after being bitten, when scrubbed to shapes like prickles, carbuncles (eschars) appeared on the fifth day after the bites.

砂石淋 【shā shí lìn】(砂淋)为砂淋与石淋的统称。见石淋。

Stranguria Resulting from Urinary Stone

痧 【shā】 1、(痧气、痧胀）见痧胀。2、指皮肤出现红点如粟，以指循皮肤稍有阻碍的疹点。

痧块 【shā kuài】 痧症放痧后，痧毒未尽，聚结成块作痛，或现于肋下，或结于胸腹的一种病变。

痧胀 【shā zhàng】 (痧）因夏秋之间感受风寒暑湿之气，壅阻经络所致的病证。症见恶寒发热、全身胀痛，或上吐下泻，或手足硬直麻木等。

闪挫 【shǎn cuò】 闪伤和挫伤的合称。

闪跌血崩 【shǎn diē xuè bēng】 因跌仆或闪挫受伤，致冲任失调所引起的血崩症。

闪罐法 【shǎn guàn fǎ】 拔罐法的一种。当火罐吸着皮肤后，随即取下，又立刻再吸上，反复多次，直至局部皮肤充血为止。

闪伤 【shǎn shāng】 因急剧运动，腰部的筋肌受到突然牵拉而引起的损伤。

疝 【shàn】 1、泛指体腔内容物向外突出的病。2、指生殖器、睾丸、阴囊部

Sha   1. eruptive disease 2. skin eruptions red in color, which can be felt by the fingers moving along the skin.

Skin Eruptions Concentrated in One Place   a morbid condition in which the remaining measeals toxicity after the eruptions accumulates, resulting in pain, or retains in the subhydrochondrium or in the chest and abdomen.

Acute Filthy Disease   a disease occurring at the end of summer and the beginning of autumn caused by the blockage of meridians and collaterals due to the infection of pathogenic wind, coldness, heat and dampness, marked by severe cold, fever, generalized distending pain or vomiting and diarrhea, stiffness and numbness of the limbs.

Sudden Sprain and Contusion   a collective term for sprain and contusion.

Vaginal Hemorrhage due to Trauma   a condition caused by the disturbance of TV and CV due to traumatic injuries.

Quick Cupping   a cupping method to apply repeatedly and romove swiftly the cup over the same area until the skin of that area becomes hyperemic.

Sudden Sprain   injury to the lumbus caused by sudden violent traction of foscia, ligament or tendon.

Hernia   1. any condition with the internal tissues or organs bulging out-

位的病变。3、指腹部的剧烈疼痛，兼有二便不通的病。side 2. a term for diseases of the external genitalia, testicle and scrotum 3. severe abdominal pain accompanied by difficulty of urination and constipation.

善饥 【shàn jī】指容易饥饿的症状。多因胃热所致。是消渴病主证之一。
Bulimia a symptom of easily becoming hungry which is the major manifestation of diabetes, usually caused by stomach heat.

善恐 【shàn kǒng】指患者易产生胆怯恐怖的症状。多因心、肾、肝的内伤致心气不足或肝肾亏损引起。
Susceptible to Fear a disease characterized by fear, mostly caused by deficiency of heart-qi due to the internal impairment of the heart, kidney and liver or deficiency of liver-yin and kidney-yin.

善惊 【shàn jīng】指遇事容易惊吓，或经常自觉惊慌的病证。由心气虚，心火旺、肝阳上亢、胆虚或气血亏损所致。
Susceptible to Fright a state in which one is susceptible to fright or consciously aware of fright, caused by deficiency of qi, excessive heart fire, excess of liver-yang, insufficiency of the gallbladder or deficiency of qi and blood.

善怒 【shàn nù】指容易发怒。多因肝气郁结，肝血不足；或肝肾阴虚，肝火偏旺所致。
Susceptible to Anger a state in which one gets angry easily, mostly caused by stagnation of liver-qi, insufficiency of liver blood or deficiency of liver-yin and kidney-yin, or excessive liver-fire.

善色 【shàn sè】疾病反映在面部的色泽表现为明润而柔和者，表示脏气未衰，病情较好，预后较好。
Well-Meaning Complexion bright and mild color on the face, as the reflection of diseases, indicating the inexhaustion of the visceral qi and therefore the status of illness is mild with a good prognosis.

鳝漏 【shàn lòu】由于湿热内搏，外感风邪，滞于肌肤，留于血脉而成的病
Fistula of the Calf a morbid condition caused by cojoint invasion of

证。常发于小腿肚。dampness and heat, exposure to pathogenic wind, and their lingering in the muscles and skin as well as in the blood vessels, usually occurring in the calf.

伤风 【shāng fēng】1、指普通感冒。2、见太阳中风。
Invasion by Wind 1. common cold 2. syndrome of taiyang meridian affected by the wind.

伤风发痉 【shāng fēng fā jìng】受风邪所致的痉病。多见于小儿。症见发热、四肢痉挛、目上视、头痛、汗出、鼻鸣及干呕等。
Common Cold Complicated by Spasm a morbid conditon due to pathogenic wind, mostly seen in children, marked by fever, spasm of the limbs, upward staring of the eyes, headache, sweating, nostril wheezing and retching.

伤风咳嗽 【shāng fēng ké sòu】因风邪伤肺所致的咳嗽。症见恶风自汗或恶寒发热、鼻塞流涕、声重、喉痒咳嗽及脉浮等。
Cough due to Common Cold cough during common cold, usually accompanied by aversion to wind, spontaneous sweating or chills and fever, stuffy and running nose, hoarseness, itchy throat and floating pulse.

伤寒 【shāng hán】1、指广义伤寒。为多种外感热病的总称。2、指狭义伤寒。为感受寒邪而即发的病证。症见恶寒、体痛、呕逆、脉紧、可有发热或不发热。3、指病因。即冬天感受的寒邪。
Febrile Disease 1. exogenous febrile disease 2. effection by cold, marked by severe cold, generalized pain, vomiting, rigid pulse and with or without fever 3. referring to the cause of the disease, i. e. affected by cold in winter.

伤寒表证 【shāng hán biǎo zhèng】伤寒病邪在表的病证。《伤寒论》称为太阳表证。
Superficies-Syndrome of Exogenous Febrile Disease syndrome indicating the presence of pathogenic factor in the superficial part of the body, which is called "taiyang meridian syndrome" in Treatise on Febrile Disease.

伤寒里证 【shāng hán lǐ zhèng】伤寒
Interior Syndromes of Febrile Disease

病外邪由表入里所引起的病证。一般指阳明里证和三阴里证，前者属实热，后者属虚热。

a condition caused by the invasion of pathogenic factor from superficies to interior, usually referring to the interior syndrome of yangming and interior syndrome of three-yin with the former being excess syndrome and the latter, deficiency syndrome.

伤寒蓄水证 【shāng hán xù shuǐ zhèng】太阳病腑证之一。太阳病不解，邪热随经入膀胱与水相结，气化不行所致。症见发热、渴而小便不利、少腹满、水入即吐、脉浮等。

Febrile Disease with Fluid Retention one of the syndromes of taiyang fu-organ caused by the combination of pathogenic heat and water with the former invading the gallbladder by taiyang meridian due to its unrelieved syndrome, characterized by fever, thirst, oliguria, distension of the lower abdomen, vomiting immediately after drinking water, and floating pulse.

伤寒蓄血证 【shāng hán xù xuè zhèng】太阳腑证之一。太阳邪热随经入腑，瘀热结于下焦所致。症见少腹急结或少腹硬满、如狂或发狂、善忘、大便溏而黑如漆、小便自利等。

Febrile Disease with Accumulation of Blood one of the syndromes of taiyang fu-organ caused by the accumulation of heat in the lower energizer due to pathogenic heat which enters the fu-organ by the taiyang meridian, characterized by spasmatic distention and fullness or rigidity and distention of the lower abdomen, manic state or mania, forgetfulness, loose bowels with sticky dark stool and normal amount of urine.

伤津 【shāng jīn】一般指热性病过程中，由于高热，出汗过多或感受燥邪，肺胃津液耗伤而出现的证候。

Consumption of Body Fluid impairment of fluids in the lung and stomach due to high fever, profuse perspiration or affection of pathogenic dryness.

伤筋 【shāng jīn】指软组织损伤。多

Injury of the Soft Tissues including

因跌打、扭挫所致。traumatic injury, sprain and contusion.

伤酒头痛 【shāng jiǔ tóu tòng】由嗜酒过量所致的头痛。症见头痛昏眩、恶心呕吐、口渴,甚则神昏、脉数等。
Headache due to Excessive Drinking a condition characterized by headache, dizziness, nausea, vomiting, thirst, or even coma and fast pulse.

伤科 【shāng kē】诊治跌打损伤的一门专科。伤科诊治疾病的范围有金创、跌仆、骨折、脱臼、汤火伤及虫兽伤等。
Department of Traumatology a department responsible for the treatment of traumatic injury including incised wound, injuries caused by fall and stumble, fracture, joint dislocation, scald, burn and animal bite.

伤力症 【shāng lì zhèng】因负重物所压或持重远行,致使有关内脏气血伤损而成的病证。
Injury due to Overload injury caused by the impairment of qi and blood in the internal organs due to physical overload.

伤乳食 【shāng rǔ shí】婴幼儿哺育不当或饮食不节,损伤脾胃,引起呕吐、腹痛、腹胀、发热或泄泻等症。
Dyspepsia due to Improper Feeding a morbid condition in infancy caused by the impairment of the spleen and stomach due to improper feeding, resulting in vomiting, abdominal pain and distention, fever or diarrhea.

伤乳食吐 【shāng rǔ shí tù】(伤乳吐、嗌乳)指哺乳儿因乳食过饱或饮食不节引起的呕吐。吐出物多夹奶片。伴发热、腹胀等。
Milk Vomiting a condition caused by excessive or improper feeding in infants with mild pieces seen in the vomitus, accompanied by fever and abdominal distention.

伤湿 【shāng shī】指受湿邪所伤而发病,分为外感湿邪和湿浊内阻。
Affection by Dampness morbid conditions caused by dampness, usually classifed as affection by exogenous dampness and condition caused by interior accumulation of pathogenic dampness.

伤湿咳嗽 【shāng shī ké sòu】指因感受湿邪,痰湿壅肺所引起的咳嗽。症
Damp Cough cough caused by the accumulation of phlegm-dampness in

见咳嗽痰多、关节疼痛、面部及四肢浮肿、小便不利等。the lung due to the affection by damp with the manifestations such as cough with profuse sputum, joint pain, edema of the face and limbs, and dysuria.

伤湿腰痛【shāng shī yāo tòng】(湿腰痛)因久坐寒湿之处或为雨露所着而致的腰痛。症见腰部冷痛沉重,如坐水中,逢阴雨或久坐则增剧;或见身肿、脉缓等。

Lumbago due to Dampness lumbago, usually as a result of staying in a damp and cold place for a long period or caught in the rain, marked by pain and sensation of coldness and heaviness in the lumbar region, like sitting in water, often aggravated during rainy days or by sitting for a long time; or with the symptoms of systemic edema and soft pulse.

伤湿自汗【shāng shī zì hàn】由湿邪阻遏所致的自汗。症见自汗恶风、声音重浊、身重体倦、关节疼痛、天阴转甚等。

Spontaneous perspiration due to Dampness a condition caused by retention of pathogenic dampness, marked by spantaneous sweatig, aversion to wind, low and hoarsened voice, heaviness sensation in the body, fatigue, joint pain, aggravated during cloudy days.

伤食【shāng shí】(食滞)因饮食损伤脾胃所致的病证。症见上脘腹痞满、嗳气腐臭、厌食、恶心、呕吐、泄泻及苔腻等。

Impairment by Overeating disease due to immoderate eating and drinking which causes the impairment of the spleen and stomach, with symptoms such as fullness in the abdomen, anorexia, nausea, vomiting, diarrea and greasy coating of the tongue.

伤食头痛【shāng shí tóu tòng】由饮食不节,宿食不化所致的头痛。症见头痛、胸脘满闷、嗳腐吞酸、厌食、脉滑实等。

Headache due to Improper Diet headache caused by immoderate eating and drinking, and the stagnancy of food in the stomach marked by heachache, stuffiness and fullness sensation in the chest and abdomen,

伤食吐 【shāng shí tù】指饮食不节引起的呕吐。吐出的多为不消化的食物，气味酸臭、伴有发热、厌食、口臭等。

伤暑 【shāng shǔ】1. 夏月中暑病证的总称。2. 指暑证之轻者。

伤损腰痛 【shāng sǔn yāo tòng】因跌打损伤致腰部经络循行受阻而引起的腰痛。

伤阳 【shāng yáng】即阳气受伤。多因过用苦寒或发汗、泻下不当，或阴寒之邪内盛以及情志刺激过度等损伤阳气。

伤阴 【shāng yīn】即耗损真阴。由于阳气偏亢，灼伤阴液或温热病后期热邪耗伤真阴所致。常见有低热、手足心热、神倦、消瘦、口干燥或咽痛、耳聋、颧红、舌深红而干、脉细数无力等症状。

伤燥咳嗽 【shāng zào ké sòu】因外感燥邪耗伤肺津所致的咳嗽。多发于秋

acid regurgitation, belching with fetid odor, anorexia, slippery and smooth pulse.

Vomiting due to Improper Diet vomiting caused by immoderate eating and drinking with the vomitus being mostly undigested food with sour and fetid odor, accompanied by fever, anorexia and halitosis.

Sunstroke 1. a collective term for conditions affected by summer-heat 2. mild form of summer-heat syndrome.

Lumbago due to Injury a condition by the blockage of meridians and collaterals due to traumatic injury.

Impairment of Yang a morbid condition mostly caused by overdose of drugs of bitter-cold nature, overuse of diaphoretics and cathartics or excessiveness of internal cold as well as emotional stress.

Impairment of Yin a morbid condition due to the impairment of yin fluid due to excessive yang-qi or impairment of genuine yin by the pathogenic heat in the advanced stage of a febrile disease, usually manifested as low fever, heat sensation in palms and soles, mental fatigue, emaciation, dryness in the mouth or sore throat, deafness, flushed cheeks, dry and deep red tongue, thready, feeble and fast pulse.

Cough due to dryness dry cough due to consumption of lung fluid by

季。症见干咳少痰、口干咽燥、大便干结、舌红而干等。 the attack of exopathogenic dryness, usually occurring in summer, with the manifestations of dry cough with little sputum, dryness of the mouth and throat, constipation, red and dry tongue.

上胞下垂【shàng bāo xià chuí】（睢目、侵风）上眼睑无力提起，以致经常处于下垂位置的一种病证。严重者可遮盖瞳孔，妨碍视线。常因先天发育不全或脾虚气弱、风邪客于眼睑所致。 **Blepharoptosis** a condition in which the upper eyeild fails to go upward, resulting in long-standing ptosis with the pupils covered by the eyelid in severe cases, usually caused by congenital aplasia or invasion of the eyelid by pathogenic wind due to deficiency and weakness of the spleen-qi.

上病下取【shàng bìng xià qǔ】疾病的表现偏于上部，用针灸或药物从下部进行治疗的方法。如眩晕属阴虚火旺者，往往采用滋肾阴降虚火的治法。 **Treating Diseases in the Upper Part by Managing the Lower** a therapeutic method of treating diseases in upper part of the body by administering drug or acupuncture to the lower part, treating vertigo due to deficiency of yin and excess of pathogenic fire, usually by nourishing kidney-yin and descending asthenic-fire.

上丹田【shàng dān tián】两眉之间的部位。 **Upper Dantian** the site between eyebrows.

上腭痈【shàng è yōng】位于上腭的脓肿。 **Abscess on Palate** referring to abscess of the upper palate.

上发背【shàng fā bèi】位于上背部的有头疽。 **Carbuncle of the Nape**

上寒下热【shàng hán xià rè】在疾病的某一阶段出现寒热错杂的病理表现。如上见恶寒、呕吐、苔白等寒的症状；下见腹胀便秘、小便赤涩等热的症状。 **Cold Syndrome in the Upper but Heat in the Lower** a complicated condition, during certain stage of disease, with the simultaneous occurrence of cold and heat syndromes, e. g. invasion of the upper part of the body by pathogenic cold causing chills, nause-

上焦 【shàng jiāo】三焦的上部，从咽喉至胸膈，心肺位于其中。具有将脾胃转输而来的营养物质均匀地分布到全身的作用。

Upper-Energizer the upper portion of tri-energizer, the part from the throat to the diaphragm with the heart and lung being included, the function of which is to distribute the nutrients from the spleen and stomach, evenly to the whole body.

上焦如雾 【shàng jiāo rú wù】喻上焦的功能特点。因上焦具有象雾露的分布作用，能把脾胃转输而来的营养物质均匀地分布到全身。

The Upper-Energizer Resembling a Sprayer analogizing the function of the upper-energizer which can spread water and food essence from the spleen and stomach throughout the whole body.

上焦主纳 【shàng jiāo zhǔ nà】上焦功能之一。即空气与饮食均需通过上焦而进入人体内。

The Upper-Energizer is in Charge of Receiving air is inhaled and food is ingested through the uppper-energizer.

上厥下竭 【shàng jué xià jié】指由于下部真阴真阳衰竭而出现的阴阳平衡失调的病理。症见突然昏倒不省人事。

Syncope due to Exhaustion below a morbid condition caused by the imbalanec of yin and yang due to the exhaustion of genuine yin and yang in the lower part of the body, marked by sudden fall-down because of syncope and loss of conciousness.

上品 【shàng pǐn】古代认为没有毒性可以多服、久服也不会损害人体的药物，称为上品。

The-Grade Medicines medicines with no toxicity and no harm to the body if taken excessively or over a long periold of time, regarded as very good medicines.

上气 【shàng qì】1、由于肺气上逆，所

Abnomal Rising of Qi 1. dyspnea

致的呼多吸少、气息急促的证候。2、指上焦心肺之气。

上窍 【shàng qiào】指头面部的孔窍，如鼻、眼、口、耳等。

上热下寒 【shàng rè xià hán】患者同时表现为热邪感于上，寒邪发于下的症候。如上有咽喉疼痛，甚则咳咯黄痰或血痰的热证；下有泄泻、肢冷、脉沉迟的寒证。

上盛 【shàng shèng】1、指人体上部邪气盛。2、指人迎脉浮盛的脉象。

上实下虚 【shàng shí xià xū】1、指邪气实于上，正气虚于下的一种病理现象。2、指肝肾阴虚，肝阳上亢的病理。

上损及下 【shàng sǔn jí xià】指五脏久虚而产生的衰弱性疾病，由上部发展到下部的病理过程。即自肺损开始而累及心、脾、肝、肾。

due to upward adverse flow of the lung-qi with less air breathed in and more breathed out. 2. The Heart-qi and Lung-qi in the Upper Energizer.

Upper Orifices orifices on the head, i. e. nose, eyes, mouth and ears.

Heat Syndrome in the Upper but Cold in the Lower heat symptoms occurring in the upper part of the body with cold symptoms simultaneouly appearing in the lower, one of the jueyin syndromes, symptoms such as sore throat, or even yellowish sputum or bloody sputum, seen in heat syndrome while manifestations such as diarrhea, cold limbs, sunken and soft pulse, seen in cold syndrome.

Excess in the Upper 1. excess of pathogenic qi in the upper part of the body 2. referring renying pulse which is floating and strong.

Sthenia-Syndrome in the Upper Part of the Body and Asthenia in the Lower 1. a morbid condition with deficiency of genuine qi in lower part of the body and a preponderance of pathogenic factors in the upper. 2. referring to deficiency of yin of the kidney and liver with exuberance of liver yang in the upper body.

Asthenia Diseases in the Upper Involving the Lower spread of pathological changes of deficiency from the upper part of the body to the lower in asthenia diseases caused by persistent deficiency of the five visceras, i. e.

上吐下泻 【shàng tù xià xiè】即呕吐和腹泻交作的症状。多由饮食不节或不洁，或兼感外邪致肠胃受伤所致。若吐泻突然发作，腹绞痛，甚则出现失水虚脱等，则类似霍乱，多因感受时邪所致。

上脘 【shàng wǎn】1、胃脘上口贲门的部位。2、穴位名称。

上消 【shǎng xiāo】（膈消、隔消）是以口渴多饮为特征的消渴病。

上虚下实 【shàng xū xià shí】正气虚于上，邪气实于下的一种病理现象。如原有心血虚损（上虚），又湿热积于大肠（下实），患者既有心悸怔忡，又有腹痛、便脓血、苔黄腻等症。

烧存性 【shāo cún xìng】指把植物制成炭时，要掌握好火候，使药物外部炭化，而保存药物原性的一种炮制方法。

烧山火 【shāo shàn huǒ】古代针刺手

from the lung to the heart, spleen, liver and kidney.

Vomiting and Diarrhea alternate attacks of vomiting and diarrhea, mostly caused by improper diet or by taking polluted food, or impairment of stomach and intestines due to the coplicated affection by exopathic factors; resembling chlora if marked by sudden attacks of vomiting and diarrhea, abdominal colic or even collapse due to dehydration.

1. **Cardia** 2. **Shangwan acupoint** (ren 13).

Diabetes Involving the Upper-Energizer diabetes markd by thirst and polydipsia

Deficiency in the Upper and Excess in the Lower a morbid condition with deficiency of genune qi in the upper part of the body and preponderance of pathogenic factors in the lower, e. g. a case with deficiency of the heart blood (upper deficiency) complicated by accumulation of pathogenic damp-heat in the large intestine (lower excess), with the symptoms such as both cardiac palpitation and abdominal pain, supurative blood in the stool, yellowish and greasy coating of the tongue.

Drug-Scorching broiling medicinal herbs or drugs in charcoal fire until its crust chars while its original properties are retained.

Heat-Producing Needling one of

法之一，属补法，用于治疗寒证。操作方法为：病人呼吸时，迅速将针刺入皮下浅表，并重按穴位周围皮肤，强度捻转多次，稍行进针，作同样捻转一直刺入一定深度，再作同样捻转，待病人感觉局部或全身有温热感后，将针缓缓捻转退出。

the ancient acupuncture methods for reinforcement, usually applied for cold-syndromes. Method: rapidly insert the needle into the subcutaneous superficial layer while the patient is breathing, press hard the skin around the acupoint, and then twirl the needle forcefully for many times; advance it slowly along with the same twirling till it reaches a certain depth; twirl the needle in the same way and withdraw it slowly by twirling when hot sensation is produced locally or systemically for the patient.

烧伤 【shào sháng】（火疮、烫火伤）由于接触物理或化学因素之高热引起的外伤。皮肤局部呈现红晕、起疱或腐烂。

Burn wound produced by exposing to physical or chemical heat, causing redness of the local skin, blisters and even decomposition.

少腹拘急 【shào fù jū jí】指病人自觉脐下有拘挛急迫的感觉。多因肾气虚寒，膀胱气化不利所致。

Cramping Sensation of the Lower Abdomen cramping sensation which the patient experiences conciously in the lower abdomen, mostly caused by asthenic-cold of the kidney-qi and hypofunction in qi transformation in the gallbladder.

少腹如扇 【shào fù rú shàn】下腹部自觉寒冷感。多因妊娠六、七个月时，下焦虚寒、阳气不能温养胞胎所致。

Cold Feeling of the Lower Abdomen chilly sensation of the hypogastrium, mostly caused by cold of insufficiency type in the lower-energizer and failure of yang to warm and nourish the fetus during the 6th or 7th month of pregnancy.

少腹硬满 【shào fù yìng mǎn】下腹部坚硬胀满的症状。由于瘀血与邪热互结，阻滞于下腹；或膀胱气化失常，水停下焦所致。

Muscular Rigidity and Fullness of the Lower Abdomen a symptom produced by blood stasis complicated by invasion of pathogenic heat and re-

少火 【shào huǒ】指正常的、具有生气的火,是维持人体生命活动的阳气。

Physiological Fire referring to the normal vigorous fire-yang qi which maintains normal life.

少阳 【shào yáng】经脉名称之一。位于太阳和阳明之间。少阳有阳气减弱的意思。

Shaoyang one of the meridians located between taiyang and yangming meridians. Shaoyang also implies the weakening of yang-qi.

少阳病 【shào yáng bìng】病邪在半表半里的一种病证。症见往来寒热、胸胁苦满、食欲不振、口苦咽干、目眩、心烦喜呕、脉弦细等。通常分少阳经证和少阳腑证。

Shaoyang Disease a syndrome with the pathogenic factors located half exterior and half interior, markde by alternate fever and chills, fullness of the chest and hypochondrium, loss of appetite, bitter taste in the mouth, dryness of the throat, dizziness, dysphoria, nausea and vomiting, wiry pulse, usually classified as syndrome of shaoyang meridian and syndrome of shaoyang-fu.

少阳腑病 【shào yáng fǔ bìng】少阳病热郁胆腑的病证。以口苦咽干、目眩、胸闷呕吐为主症。

Syndrome of Shaoyang-Fu shaoyang syndrome with heat accumulated in the gallbladder, marked by bitterness in the mouth, dryness of the throat, dizziness, distress in the chest and vomiting.

少阳经病 【shào yáng jīng bìng】热邪郁少阳经,而产生胸胁苦满、往来寒热、心烦胁痛为特征的一种病证。

Syndrome of Shaoyang Meridian shaoyang syndrome with accumulation of pathogenic heat which produces distress in the chest, alternate chills and fever, dysphoria and hypochondriac pain.

少阳头痛 【shào yáng tóu tòng】1、伤寒少阳病的头痛。以头痛兼有寒热往来,脉弦细为特征。2、位于少阳经循

Shaoyang Headache 1. headache due to shaoyang disease caused by attack of cold with the characteristic

行部位（即两侧颞部）的头痛。

少阴　【shào yīn】经脉名称之一。位于太阴和厥阴之间。有阴气减弱的意思。

少阴病　【shào yīn bìng】六经病变发展过程中最后和最危重阶段，是以心肾两伤，阴阳气血均虚为主要病理变化的一种病证。可从三阳病转变而来，也可因外邪直接侵袭少阴引起。症见脉微细、精神萎靡不振、恶寒蹉卧、四肢厥冷、大便泄泻，甚则汗出亡阳等。

少阴寒化　【shào yīn hán huà】病邪传入心肾，心肾功能低下，导致阴寒内盛，阳气衰弱的病理。症见精神萎靡、恶寒、四肢厥冷、大便泄泻、完谷不化、脉微细等。

少阴热化　【shào yīn rè huà】病邪侵入心肾、灼伤阴液的病理。症见心烦、不眠、咽痛、舌红、脉细数等。

symptom of headache coplicated by alternate chills and fever, wiry and thready pulse. 2. headache characterized by pain in the temples.

Shaoyin　one of the meridians located between taiyin and jueyin meridians. Shaoyin also implies the weakening of yin-qi.

Shaoyin Disease　the last and most serious stage of the six-meridian diseases in the course of their pathological changes which is characteristic of damagement of both the heart and kidney, and deficiency of yin, yang, qi and blood, possibly developing from three yang diseases, or directly caused by invasion of shaoyin by exopathic factors, marked by faint and thready pulse, mental distress, aversion to cold, sleep with the knees drawn up, cold limbs, diarrhea, or even sweating and yang depletion.

Cold Syndrome Resulting from Damage of Shaoyin　pathological changes due to dysfunction of the heart and kindney caused by the invasion of pathogenic factors, leading to internal excess of cold and deficiency of yang, manifested by mental distress, aversion to cold, cold limbs, diarrhea, undigested food, faint and thready pulse.

Heat Syndrome Resulting from Damage of Shaoyin　pathological changes due to invasion of the heart and kidney by pathogenic heat result-

少阴头痛 【shào yīn tóu tòng】寒邪侵犯少阴经引起的头痛。兼见气逆、肢冷、心痛烦闷、脉沉细等症状。

舌 【shé】在口腔内活动的肌性器官，对气味有特别的感觉，有助于咀嚼、吞咽、发音。与心的功能有密切关系。观察舌的色、质、形态及舌苔变化是中医望诊的重要内容这一。

舌本 【shé běn】1、见舌根。2、风府穴和廉泉穴的别称。

舌痹 【shé bì】（舌自痹）舌体麻木不仁的疾病。实证多因七情郁结，心火灼痰、滞涩经络所致。兼见舌肿大而舌质紫赤或有疼痛；虚证多无故自痹，兼见脉虚无力。

舌边 【shé biān】舌的边缘。该部位与肝胆有关，观察该部形态颜色的变化可以帮助了解肝胆的生理病理状况。

ing in impairment of yin-fluid, characterized by dysphoria, insomnia, dry and sore throat, deep red tongue, thready and fast pulse.

Shaoyin Headache headache caused by invasion of shaoyin meridian by pathogenic cold with accompanying symptoms such as adverse flow of qi, cold limbs, precordial pain vexation, sunken and thready pulse.

Tongue a muscular organ moving about in the mouth, which is specially sensive to taste and aids greatly in chewing, swallowing and enunciating, and which is closely related to the heart. Observation of the tongue is one of the important respects in TCM inspection.

Root of the tongue another name for acupoints of Fengfu (Du 16) and Lianquan (Ren 23).

Numbness of the Tongue a disease of the tongue, if of excess type, mostly due to seven emotion upsets, phlegm-stagnancy in meridians and collaterals due to heart-fire, with accompanying symptoms such as enlargement of the tongue, purplish red tongue or pain; if of deficiency type mostly marked by numbness of no reasons, accompanied by weak pulse.

Margin of the Tongue a part which is related to the liver and gallbladder, observation of which on its shape and color would aid in understanding the physiological and pathological condi-

舌颤 【shé chàn】(战舌)指舌头颤动。多因内风或酒毒所致。

舌出 【shé chū】舌伸出口外不收,肿胀多涎的证候。多因心火炽盛所致。也可因热病后阴液受伤,或胃气虚寒所致。

舌疮 【shé chuāng】多因心胃积热熏蒸或胎毒上冲所致的病证。症见舌上生疮、舌裂舌肿、时流鲜血、口臭、便秘、脉实有力等。有虚实之分。

舌抵上腭 【shé dǐ shàng é】(舌顶上腭、舌柱上腭)是指以舌尖抵着上腭。

舌疔 【shé dīng】(卷帘疔)多由心经火毒所发或瘟疫病所致的疾病。症见舌生紫泡、坚硬疼痛、继而化脓,可发展为舌痈。

舌短 【shé duǎn】(舌缩)即舌体紧缩难以伸出的症状。寒邪凝滞、热邪伤津、心脾积热、痰湿阻闭等均可引起。

舌根 【shé gēn】舌体靠近咽喉的部位,数条经脉行经该部,与各经脉及内脏tions of the liver and gallbladder.

Tremor of the Tongue a morbid state mainly caused by endogenous wind or alcoholism.

Protrusion of the Tongue enlarged tongue with a salivation chiefly resulted from the hyperactivity of heart fire, consumption of yin fluid after febrile disease or asthenia-cold of the stomach-qi.

Tongue Sore a condition mostly caused by accumulation of heat in the heart and stomach or upsurging of fetal toxin, manifested as lesions, fissures and swelling of the tongue with occassional bleeding, foul breath, constipation, full and strong pules.

Putting the Tongue on the Palete referring to sticking the tip of the tongue on the palate.

Pustule of Tongue a disorder caused by the accumulation of fire in the heart meridian or as a sequelae of an infectious disease manifested as a purplish indurated and painful blisters on the tongue with pus collection or even abscess formation.

Shortened Tongue a sign characterized by contracture of the tongue with inability to stretch caused by the stagnation of cold, the consumption of body fluid by heat accumulated heat in the heart and spleen or the retention of phlegm-damp.

Root of Tongue the part of the tongue attached to the hyoid bone

有密切的关系。

舌根痈 【shé gēn yōng】生于舌根的痈。

舌红 【shé hóng】舌质比正常的淡红色较深，多主热证。

舌尖 【shé jiān】舌之尖部。该部形态色泽的变化与生理和病理状况有关。

舌謇 【shé jiǎn】因脾胃积热，津液灼伤所致的病证。症见舌体卷缩、转动不灵、言语不清。

舌绛 【shé jiàng】舌质呈深红色，是温病热邪侵入营分的舌象。深红而中心干，是胃火伤津；深红光亮而无苔，属胃阴已亡，深红而干枯不鲜者，是肾阴涸竭的征象。

舌卷 【shé juǎn】指舌体卷曲不能说话。由心火上炎，或肝经积热，或温邪内陷心包所致。

and the mandible through which several meridians pass. It is closely related to the condition of various meridians and organs.

Abscess on the Root of Tongue

Red Tongue a tongue colour deeper than normal, usually indicating a heat-syndrome.

Tip of the Tongue the changes of appearance and colour of this portion is corresponding to pathological and physiological state of the heart.

Stiffness of the Tongue a disorder due to accumulation of heat in the spleen and stomach causing consumption of body fluid, manifested as contracture and stiffness of the tongue, and dysphasia.

Crimson Tongue deep red color of the tongue, indicating the attack of heat to the yingfen during a febrile disease that with dryness at the center signifies the consumption of the body fluid by stomach fire, that with bright and uncoated appearance signifies the exhaustion of stomach-yin; that with dryness all over the tongue sygnifies the exhaustion of kidney-yin.

Curled Tongue a condition with inability to extend the tongue and hindrance from speaking; due to flamming up of heart-fire, accumulation of heat in the liver meridian, attack of febrile pathogen to the pericardium.

舌卷囊缩 【shé juǎn náng suō】舌体卷曲，不能伸直，并见阴囊上缩的症状。常见于热性病的危重阶段。亦可因少阴虚寒所致。

舌菌 【shé jūn】（舌岩）由于七情郁结心脾二经，化火化毒所致的病证。初起舌面肿起如菌如豆、头大蒂小、继而发红糜烂，疼痛不已。类似于舌癌肿。

舌烂 【shé làn】（烂舌边）舌的任何部位发生溃烂、肿痛的病证。多由于肝胃湿热或心脾热毒熏蒸所致。

舌裂 【shé liè】舌体表面有裂纹，多为伤阴所致。若见舌深红光燥无苔且裂纹显著，为热盛伤阴所致；若舌淡质软而有裂纹，多为久病阴阳俱虚，气阴两伤所致。

舌面如镜 【shé miàn rú jìng】舌质表面无苔，光滑如镜。常是肝肾真阴亏损或胃阴不足的征象。

舌衄 【shé nǜ】（舌体出血、舌本出血）因心经蕴热引起者，症见舌肿大

Curled Tongue and Shrunken Scrotum   a sign usually seen in critical stage of febrile diseases or in the patient suffering from asthenia cold syndrome of shaoyin.

Carcinoma of the Tongue   a disorder due to formation and stagnation of toxic material resulted from the emotional upset involving the heart and spleen meridians; manifested as mushroom, or bean-shaped swelling of the tongue with broad head and narrow base followed by red colouration ulceration and severe pain.

Erosion of Tongue   a disorder usually accompanied with white spot swelling and pain over the tongue due to accumulation of damp-heat in the stomach and liver or virulent heat attacking the heart and spleen.

Fissured Tongue   a sign indicating the damage of yin that with deep fissures and dark red smooth and dry apppearance suggests damage of yin by the overabundance of heat; that with pale and soft appearance suggests deficiency of both yin and yang or damage of both qi and yin after prolonged illness.

The Tongue Surface Becoming Smooth as a Mirror   a sign usually indicating the consumption of the original yin of the liver and kidney or the deficiency of stomach-yin.

Bleeding of Tongue   a disorder caused by the accumulation of fire in

木硬，出血如泉涌；因脾肾二经虚火上炎所致者，症见舌上渗血，或有潮热、盗汗。

舌胖 【shé pàng】舌体胖大。若伴舌质色淡，边有齿痕，多属脾虚；若伴舌质深红，是心脾有热。

舌胖齿形 【shé pàng chǐ xíng】舌体肿大，边有齿痕。多因脾虚或寒湿壅盛所致。

舌起芒刺 【shé qǐ máng cì】舌苔突起如刺状，是热极的征象。往往视其颜色及所在的部位不同而反映不同的病变。如舌尖部位芒刺为心热等。

舌强 【shé qiáng】舌体强硬，运动不灵。多兼见语言謇涩不清。若伴体胖瘫痪、口眼㖞斜等症，多属中风；若舌强硬、舌质红绛、神昏谵语者，多属于温病热入心包或高热伤津所致。

舌色 【shé sè】舌质的颜色。是舌诊重

the heart meridian; manifested as profuse bleeding from the tongue which is swollen and stiff; or by flaming up of asthenic-fire in the spleen and kidney meridians, manifested as blood oozing from the tongue, probably accompanied with hectic fever and night sweat.

Corpulent Tongue   a condition with pale colour and teeth marks along the lateral margin is indicative of spleen-deficicncy, while that with dark red colour is indicative of accumulation of heat in the heart and spleen.

Corpulent Tongue with Teeth Marks on Its Margin   a sign indicative of spleen asthenia or that associated with overabundance of cold-damp.

Rough and Prickly Fur   a sign indicative of the overabundance of heat, the diagnosis is made according to the colour and the location of the fur, e. g. heart-heat should be considered when it appears over the tip of the tongue.

Stiff Tongue   immovability of the tongue usually associated with disturbance of speech that accompanied with paralysis of the extremities and distortion of the face may be seen in apoplexy while that accompanied with delirium and crimson tongue may be seen in seasonal febrile diseases when the pericardium is attacked by the heat

Colour of the Tongue   an important

要内容之一。观察舌色的变化可以作为判断病变的性质、病邪深浅及病情虚实等的依据。

舌神 【shé shén】舌的荣枯及舌的活动情况。如舌红润鲜明，活动灵活，即所谓有神。

舌生泡 【shé shēng pào】由脾肾虚火上炎或心脾积热所致的病证。症见舌生白泡，大小不一，连绵而发，可出现红、黄等色，疼痒溃烂。

舌笋 【shé sǔn】小儿舌上起白泡，妨碍吮乳，以致啼哭不止的病证。

舌苔 【shé tāi】舌质表面的一层苔状物。观察舌苔的变化可以判断病情的轻重，病邪的深浅以及津液的存亡等，是望诊的重要内容之一。

舌苔厚 【shé tāi hòu】超过正常舌苔厚度的病理性舌苔。

舌体 【shé tǐ】（舌质）即由舌质的肌肉、血管等组织组成的舌实体。观察舌形态、色泽、湿润度及活动情况可以了解脏腑的虚实和正气的盛衰。

aspect of tongue inspection, Inspection of changes of the colour is helpful for distinguish the nature of the disease the depth of the invasion and asthenia of the patient.

Expression of the Tongue the condition concerning with the lustrousness and mobility of the tongue when it looks red, moist and bright and moves freely, it is considered as full of expression.

Lingual Blisters a disorder due to flaming up of asthenic fire from the spleen and kidney or accumulation of heat in the heart and spleen manifested as blisters on the tongue, white or occasionally reddish and yellowish in colour which are painful and itching and repture easily, various in size, occuring in cluster.

Blisters of the Tongue a disorder in infants which hampers sucking of milk and renders them irritated.

Fur a coating over the surface of the tongue serving as an important criteria for the diagnosis, prognosis of a disease and the estimation of fluid amount of the body.

Thick Fur an abnormal fur on the tongue which is thicker than normal.

Body of the Tongue the consisting of muscles, vessels, etc. observation of its feature, color, moisture and mobility is necessary for the investigation of the conditions of viscera and original qi.

舌歪 【shé wāi】舌伸出时偏于一侧，歪斜不正。常与四肢偏瘫或口眼㖞斜同时出现，多因肝风内动或风邪中络所致。

Crooked Tongue a sign characterized by the deviation of the tongue to one side, usually accompanied with paralysis and distortion of the face, caused by the liver-wind stirring in the interior or the wind invading the collaterals.

舌痿 【shé wěi】指舌的肌肉萎缩。因脾虚或阴液耗损，筋脉失养所致。

Atrophy of the Tongue a disorder due to failure to nourish the muscles and vessels resulting from asthenia of the spleen or consumption of yin fluid.

舌形 【shé xíng】指舌的形态，包括舌质的老嫩、裂纹、起芒刺、胀瘪等变化。观察舌形的变化，能了解病情，帮助诊断。

Status of the Tongue the signs including certain features, such as tenderness or toughness, swelling or shrinkage, fissure, prickly-looking papillac etc, which are helpful to make a diagnosis.

舌瘖 【shé yīn】舌体转动不灵而致语言障碍的病证。急病多由风痰壅盛所致，兼见痰声辘辘、脉大有力，久病多因血虚风动所致，兼见舌痿、形体消瘦。

Dysphonia due to Tongue Disorder a condition with immobillity of the tongue and difficulty in speaking, the acute case is caused by the attack of wind phlegm accompanied with noisy breathing and large vigorous pules, the chronic case is caused by blood deficiency and the stirring of wind, accompanied with flaccidity of the tongue, and emaciation.

舌痈 【shé yōng】（卷舌痈）舌上的化脓性感染。由于心火积盛，胃中伏热，化毒凝滞而成。初起舌红而肿痛，妨碍饮食和言语，继而逐渐成脓，甚至溃烂流脓、口中臭腐。

Pyogenic Infection of Tongue a disorder due to formation and stagnation of toxic material resulting from the hyperactivity of heart-fire and accumulation of heat in the stomach, manifested as redness and swelling of the tongue with hindrance of eating and speaking followed by formation

...and discharge of pus with foul smell in the mouth.

舌胀大 【shé zhàng dà】舌体肿胀增大。色红、肿大满口，是心脾有热所致；舌肿青紫晦暗常见于食物中毒；舌肿而质淡，边有齿痕者，多属脾虚而寒湿壅盛所致。

Swollen Tongue enlargement of the tongue with red color is considered as the presence of heat in the heart and spleen, that with purplish blue color and luster less appearance suggests food poisoning; that with pale color and teeth marks on its margin is indicative of spleen asthenia with accumulation of cold-damp.

舌诊 【shé zhěn】望诊的重要内容，即通过观察舌质、舌苔、形态等的变化，来判断病情，帮助诊断。

Inspection of the Tongue a major item of inspection by observing the nature, fur, appearance of the tongue for making a diagnosis.

舌中 【shé zhōng】舌体的中央部分，该处与脾胃有密切关系。

Middle Surface of Tongue a major item of inspection by observing the nature, fur, appearance of the tongue for making a diagnosis.

舌肿 【shé zhǒng】以舌渐肿大满口，坚硬疼痛为主症的病证，常由七情郁结，心火暴盛，痰浊瘀血滞于舌间所致。

Glossoncus Swelling of the tongue due to the stagnation of phlegm and blood stasis in the tongue resulting from accumulation of emotional upsets and hyperactivity of heart fire.

蛇腹疔 【shé fù dīng】（鳅肚疔、鱼肚疔、中节疔）即生于中指中节掌面的疔疮，形如鱼肚，色赤疼痛。

Snake-abdomen-like Furuncle furuncle occuring at the ventral surface of the middle segment, shaped like fish abdomen, red in color and pain.

蛇节疔 【shé jié dīng】 生于手指中节，绕指俱肿的疔疮。

Furuncle on the Middle Segment of the Finger

蛇窠疮 【shé kē chuāng】多发于胸胁、脐腹，其形如蛇绕身，皮肤疼痛，轻则腐浅，重则深烂的病证。多见于带状疱疹兼有溃破感染的情况。

Herps Zoster Complicated by Infection a morbid condition often seen in hypochondrium or around the umbilicus shaped like a snake reeling around the trunk which is painful in skin in slight case with a shallow ulceration

蛇头疔 【shé tóu dīng】（手指毒疮、发指）生于手指尖的疔疮，肿似蛇头。相当于化脓性指头炎。

伸舌 【shēn shé】舌伸出口外，不能回缩口内的一种证候。伸舌而舌觉灼热，神志不清者，多因痰热扰乱心神所致；伸舌而痿软无力、麻木不仁者，多属气虚。

身热 【shēn rè】指全身发热。

身瘦不孕 【shēn shòu bù yùn】某些瘦弱的人，因阴虚火旺，精血不足，冲任亏损，胞脉失养，不能摄精成孕所致的不孕症。

身痒 【shēn yǎng】皮肤发痒，游走不定，或起风热疹子，甚则遍身奇痒难忍。多由体虚，腠理不密，风邪侵入肌肤而成。

身重 【shēn zhòng】指肢体重着，活动不便的症状。多因脾肾阳虚，水湿留滞所致。

神 【shén】（神明）1、是人体生命活动的总称，包括生理性或病理性的显露于外的征象，是望诊的重要内容之一。2、指思维意识活动。

and deeper in severe case.

Snake-head-like Felon a purulent infection or abscess involving the pulp of the distal phalanx of the finger.

Persistent Protrusion of the Tongue a condition that accopanied with hot sensation and the unconsciousness is usually due to attack of the heart by phlegm-heat, while that accompanied with flaccidity and numbness of the tongue is due to deficiency of qi.

Fever

Sterility in Asthenic Women the inability to conceive seen in some asthenic woman, due to impairment of thoroughfare and conception vessels failing to nourish the vessels on uterus, resulting from yin-deficiency with fire-hyperactivity and insufficiency of essence blood.

Pruritis a condition manifested as itching here and there or all over the whole body or accompanied with skin eruption, which is due to general debility and the wind attacking the skin.

Heavy Sensation of the Body a symptom of lassitude and immobility of the extremities, resulting from the deficiency of spleen-yang and kidney-yang leading to retention of water and damp in the body.

Spirit 1. a general term for the life activities, including the external appearance of the physiological condition of the body, which are major cri-

神不守舍 【shén bù shǒu shè】因病邪犯心或精神过度刺激而出现的神志异常的状态。

Mental Derangement a state of mental confusion caused by the pathogenic factors attacking the heart, or by mental upsets.

神昏 【shén hūn】指神志昏迷，意识不清的症状。往往由邪热内陷心包，或湿热、痰浊蒙蔽清窍所引起。

Coma a state of unconsciousness usually caused by heat attacking the pericardium or by damp-heat, phlegm blocking the upper orifices.

神门脉 【shén mén mài】古代诊脉部位之一。即掌后锐骨端陷中的动脉搏动处。

Shen Men Pulse a position for pulse feeling located at the depression proximal to the first metacarpal bone.

神阙 【shén què】1、脐的别名。2、穴位名称。

1. **Umbilicus** 2. **A Name of Acupoint**, RM CV8.

神脏 【shén zàng】指与人体的精神思维活动有密切关系的五脏。

Organ of Mind referring to the five zang organs which are responsible for the mental activities.

神志不清 【shén zhì bù qīng】指病人由于某些原因使意识丧失的症状。

Unconsciousness a state of loss of consciousness.

审苗窍 【shěn miáo qiào】观察舌、鼻、眼、口唇、耳等器官的变化，作为识别内脏病变的参考。

Inspection of Signal Orifices a method of physical examination serving as a reference for the diagnosis of visceral diseases by the observation of the changes, of the tongue, nose, eyes, lips and ears.

肾 【shèn】五脏之一。它的主要功能是：(1) 主藏精，滋养脏器、骨和脑。肾精的盛衰对个体的生长发育（包括胚胎时期）有着极重要的意义；(2) 与肺、脾两脏共同参与人体水液的代谢，是调节人体水液代谢的重要器官。肾包括了现代医学中泌尿生殖系统、及内分泌系统、造血系统、中枢神经系统的部分功能。

Kidney one of the five zang organs in TCM, the main functions are following 1. storing the essence of life so as to nourish the viscera, bones and brain, the kidney-essence is important for the growth and development of an individual, including the enbryonic stage. 2. being an important organ in participating in the metabolism of body fluids together with the lung and spleen. In general, the kidney in TCM mainly performs the functions of urogenital system, hematopoietic system and central nervous system of western medicine.

肾痹【shèn bì】由骨痹日久不愈，复感外邪，或过劳伤肾所致的痹证。症见腰背佝曲不能伸、下肢挛曲、运动障碍、腰痛、遗精等。

Kidney-Bi Syndrome a type of bi syndrome due to intractable bone bi syndrome complicated by the attack of exogenous factors leading to the impairment of the kidney-qi, manifested as bending of the back with inability to stretch, contracture and dyskinesia of the lower limbs, akinesia, lumbago, nocturnal emission, etc.

肾病【shèn bìng】五脏病候之一。泛指肾脏发生的多种病证。肾病以虚证为多，常由精气耗伤所致。症见头晕、耳鸣、精神不振、腰膝痿弱、腰酸遗精等。

Kidney Diseases a general term referring to the diseases involving the kidney, usually attributive to the asthenia-syndrome of the kidney caused by the consumption of the kidney-essence and original-qi clinically manifested as dizziness, tinnitus, listlessness, weakness of the lower extremities, soreness of the loins, nocturnal emission, etc.

肾藏精【shèn cáng jīng】肾的主要功能之一。包括：(1)藏生殖之精，主管人的生育繁殖；(2)藏五脏六腑之精，具有营养其他脏腑及促进机体生长发育的作用。

Kidney Stores Essence one of the chief functions of the kidney, including 1. storage of the essence for reproduction. 2. storage of the essence derived from the zang and fu organs, which nourish the other viscera and promote the growth and development of the body.

肾喘【shèn chuǎn】由肾经聚水，水气逆行，上乘于肺所致的气喘。症见气逆喘急、不得平卧、咳而呕吐等。

Dyspnea due to Disorder of the Kidney a type of dyspnea due to involvement of the lung by the retention of

肾疳 【shèn gān】 （骨疳、急疳）多因伏热内阻，或由肾气不足所致的疳症。症状见形体羸瘦、齿龈出血或溃烂、寒热时作、多汗、乳食减少，四肢无力等。

肾合膀胱 【shèn hé páng guāng】指肾与膀胱之间的互相关联和影响。它们通过经络的联系，互为表里，在生理上互相协调，在病理上互相影响。如肾与膀胱互相配合共同完成尿的生成、贮藏和排出。若肾的功能失常、往往影响到膀胱的功能而出现尿液排泄障碍。

肾火偏亢 【shèn huǒ piān kàng】（命门火旺）指肾阴不足，虚火偏亢的病理。常见有性欲亢进、遗精早泄等症状。

肾间动气 【shèn jiān dòng qì】指命门的功能。有人认为命门位于两肾之间，因此，把命门的功能称为肾间动气。

fluid in kidney meridian, abnormal circulation of body fluid, characterized by difficulty in breathing with inability to lie flat, cough, vomiting, etc.

Infantile Malnutrition due to Disorder of the Kindey a type of malnutrition due to accumulation of heat in the body or insufficiency of kidney-qi, manifested as marked emaciation, bleeding or ulceration of the gum, intermitent fever and chilliness, profuse sweating, poor appetite, weakness of the limbs, etc.

Kidney is Connected with the Bladder the paired-relationship between the kidney and the bladder which are connected with each other by the network of meridian. They cooperate in functioning and involve each other, when diseased. For instance, the formation, storage, and discharge of urine are completed by the kidney and bladder coordinately and dysfunction of the kidney may cause disorders of the bladder leading to the impediment of urination.

Hyperactivity of Kidney-Fire a morbid condition of deficiency of kidner-yin and hyperactivity of asthenic fire; manifested as excessive sexuality, nocturnal emission, spermpa, etc.

Energy Stored in the Place between the Two Kineys referring to the function of the gate of life which lies between the two kidneys. Function of the Life Gate a term referring to the

肾精 【shèn jīng】肾脏所藏的具有生殖功能和滋养其他脏腑作用的物质，属肾阴。

Kidney Essence a substance stored in the kidney, possessing the function of nourishing other organs and reproduction, attributive to kidney-yin.

肾厥头痛 【shèn jué tóu tòng】由于下虚上实，肾气厥逆所致的头痛。症见头顶痛不可忍、四肢逆冷、胸脘痞闷、多痰、脉弦等。

Headache due to Disorder of the kidney a morbid condition caused by asthenia in the lower part and sthenia in the upper part and adverse rising of kidney-qi; manifested as intense headache at the vertex, cold limbs, fullness sensation in the chest, profuse expectoration, wiry pules, etc.

肾开窍于耳 【shèn kāi qiào yú ěr】（肾气通于耳、肾主耳）指肾与听觉有密切关系。中医学认为听觉正常与否和肾的精气的盛衰有关。通过听觉的变化有助于了解肾的功能变化。

Ears are Orifies to the kidney the close relationship between the kidney and ears through which the action of kidney essence is responsible for the normalcy of the auditognosis. Hence the changes of auditognosis may be helpful to understand the function of the kidney.

肾开窍于二阴 【shèn kāi qiào yú èr yīn】指肾与尿道和肛门有密切关系。肾开窍于二阴主要是指肾与二便的关系。通过对二便的调节是肾对机体进行水液代谢调节的途径之一。肾阴或肾阳的不足都可导致大小便的异常。

Anus and Urethra are Orifices to the kidney the close relationship between the kidney and the anus and urethra through which the regulation of urination and defecation serves as a way for the kidney to regulate body fluids. Deficiency kidney yin or kidney-yang may lead to various disturbances of urination and defecation.

肾咳 【shèn ké】（肾经咳嗽）由肾的病变影响到肺而引起的咳嗽。往往伴有气喘，腰膝酸软等症。

Cough due to Disorder of Kidney Meridian a symptom due to disorder of the kidney involving the lung usually accompanied with dyspnea,

肾劳 【shèn láo】五劳之一。指由于性欲过度损伤肾气所致的一种疾病。症见遗精、盗汗、骨蒸潮热, 甚则腰痛如折、下肢痿弱等。

Kidney Exhaustion-Syndrome one of the five visceral exhaustion-syndromes due to impairment of the kidney-qi by excessive sexuality, which is manifested as nocturnal emission, night sweat, hectic fever or even severe lumbago, flaccidity of lower limbs etc.

肾囊风 【shèn náng fēng】(绣球风) 由肝经湿热下注, 风邪外袭而成的病证。初起肾囊干燥作痒, 甚则起疙瘩, 形如粟米、色红, 搔破浸淫脂水, 热痛如火燎, 经久不愈。见于阴囊湿疹、神经性皮炎、核黄素缺乏等病。

Dermatitis of Scrotum a condition caused by the attack of damp heat in the liver meridian and exposure to exogenous wind, characterized by dryness and itching of the skin of the scrotum, miliary red rashes, profuse discharge after scratching, burning pain and its chronicity; seen in eczema neurodermatitis, ariboflavinosis.

肾, 其华在发 【shèn, qí huá zài fà】指肾的功能盛衰可以从毛发显露出来。肾的功能旺盛, 头发茂密而有光泽; 肾的功能衰退, 头发稀疏易脱落且没有光泽。

Hair Reflects the Condition of the Kidney observation of the hair may be helpful for the estimation of the condition of the kidney when kidney qi is vigorous, the hair will always be thick and sheeny while kidney qi is deficient, the hair will be thin withered and dropped easily.

肾气 【shèn qì】指肾的功能活动。如生长、发育及性机能的活动。

Kidney-Qi referring to the functional activities of the kidney, e. g., growth and development of the body and sexual activity.

肾生骨髓 【shèn shēng gǔ suǐ】中医认为骨髓是由肾的精气所化生。

Kidney Produces Bone Marrow a term signifying that the bone marrow is derived from the essence and qi of the kidney and nourishes the bones and brain, hence the growth, develop-

肾俞漏【shèn shù lòu】为漏管生于肾俞穴部位。相当于腰椎寒性脓疡破溃的病证。

肾俞虚痰【shèn shù xū tán】流痰病的一种。常继发于胸腰椎结核。起于腰部肾俞穴，色白漫肿而硬，酸胀不舒，疼痛，日久溃脓，脓液清稀或如见败絮，不易收口。

肾哮【shèn xiāo】因肾阳虚衰或肾阴不足所致的哮证。

肾消【shèn xiāo】(1) 见下消。(2) 指渴而饮不多，腿肿而脚先瘦小、阴痿弱、小便数者。(3) 指内消。即多食、多尿而不渴的消渴病。

肾泄【shèn xiè】泄泻日久不愈，常在黎明前发作，粪便清稀，常伴腹部畏寒，腰膝时冷、面色黧黑、舌淡苔白、脉沉细等。多因久病或久泄，损伤肾阳，肾阳不足，脾失温煦所致。

ment and functions of the bones and brain are closely related to the condition of kidney essence and kidney-qi.

Fistula at Shen Shu   fistula formed by the rupture of cold abscess of lumbar vertebrae.

Asthenic phlegm at Shen Shu   a cold abscess secondary to tuberculosis of the spine characterized by slow development of whitish indurated and painful swelling over the shenshu point, followed by rupture with thin discharge, containing necrotic tissue.

Asthma due to Kidney Disorder   asthma caused by the deficiency of kidney-yang or insufficiency of kidney-yin.

Diabetes Involving the Kidney   1. diabetes involving the lower energizer 2. a syndrome characterized by thirst but drinking a little, edema of the legs but gaunt feet, atrophy of the external genitals. 3. referring to the diabetes characterized by polyphagia polyuria but on polydipsia.

Diarrhea due to kidney Disoredr   a disease characterized by lingering morning diarrhea with greenish watery stools, accopanied with intolerance of cold in the abdomen, coldness of the loins and the knees, blackish complexion, pale tongue with whitish fur, sunken and thready pulse, etc; due to impairment of the kidney-yang during a chronic illness or prolonged diarrhea leading to the insufficiendy

肾虚 【shèn xū】（肾亏）通常指肾脏精气不足。症见精神疲乏、头晕耳鸣、健忘、腰酸、遗精等。

Asthenia of kidney a morbid state of insufficiency of essence and qi of the kidney manifested as fatigue dizziness, tinnitus, amnesia, lumbago, nocturnal emission, etc.

肾虚不孕 【shèn xū bù yùn】因肾虚精血亏少引起的不孕症。多由禀赋素弱或久病、房劳等而致肾气损伤，精亏血少，冲任胞脉失养，不能受孕。多伴神疲、头晕耳鸣、腰酸腿软、月经不调等症。

Sterility due to kidney-Asthenia inability to conceive due to congenital insufficiency, prolonged illness and frequent sexual intercourse leading to kidney-asthenia, deficiency of essence and blood, and impairment of thoroughfare, conception, bao vessels, usually accompanied with listlessness, dizziness, tinnitus, lumbago, weakness of the limbs, irregular menstruation, etc.

肾虚滑胎 【shèn xū huá tāi】因肾虚而致胎失所系引起的滑胎。症状头晕、耳鸣、腰膝酸痛、小腹有下坠感，或见阴道流血等。

Habitual Abortion due to kidney-Asthenia a disorder caused by the asthenia of kidney which fails to nourish the fetus, marked by dizziness, tinnitus, soreness and weakness of the loins and knees, bearing down sensation over the lower abdomen or vaginal bleeding, etc.

肾虚经闭 【shèn xū jīng bì】多因先天不足，早婚多育，或房室不节等，使肾气受损，冲任不足，胞宫血虚而致的闭经。症见头晕耳鸣、腰膝酸软、小便清长等。

Amenorrhea due to Kidney-Asthenia stoppage of menstruation resulting from the impairment of kidney-qi, hypofunction of thoroughfare and conception vessels and deficiency of uterus blood, which is manifested as dizziness, tinnitus, soreness and weakness of the loins and knees, polyuria with watery urine, etc.

肾虚经行后期 【shèn xū jīng xíng hòu

Delayed menstruation due to Kidney

qī】多因先天不足，或因病损伤肾气，精亏血少，冲任不足，胞宫不能按时满溢所致的月经延期。症见月经错后、量少质稀、色淡红，伴头晕耳鸣、腰部酸痛、小腹空坠、脉沉细等。

肾虚水泛　【shèn xū shuǐ fàn】(肾虚水肿）指肾阳亏损，不能温化水湿，致水湿停聚引起的水肿的病理。症见全身浮肿，下肢尤甚，按之凹陷，腰痛酸重、畏寒肢冷、舌淡胖、苔白润、脉沉细等。

肾虚头痛　【shèn xū tóu tòng】由肾虚所致的头痛。属肾阴虚者，症见头脑空痛、头晕耳鸣、腰膝无力、舌红、脉细；属肾阳虚者，症见头痛畏寒、四肢不温、面色白、舌淡、脉沉细。

肾虚眩晕　【shèn xū xuàn yūn】因肾精不足，不能上充脑髓所致的眩晕。症见头晕耳鸣、神疲、健忘、腰膝酸软、

Asthenia　a disorder due to deficiency of essence and blood and hypofunction of thoroughfare and conception vessels failing to fill the uterus regularly, resulting from the congenital insufficiency or secondary damage of kidney-qi manifested as postponed menstrual cycle with scanty and pink menses accompanied with dizziness, tinnitus, lumbago, bearing down sensation over the lower abdomen, sunken and thready pulse, etc.

Edema due to kidney-Asthenia　accumulation of body fluid resulting from the deficiency of kidney-yang manifested as general anasarea with pitted edema over the lower limbs, lumbago, intolerance of cold, cold limbs, pale and corpulent tongue with whitish and moist fur, sunken and thready pulse.

Headache due to kidney-Asthenia　a type of headache caused by the hypofunction of kidney, that due to deficiency of kidney-yin is accopanied with headache with the brain-empty sensation, dizziness, tinnitus, weakness of the loins and knees, red tongue and thready pulse, that due to deficiency of kidney-yang is accompanied with headache, aversion to cold, cold extremities, pale complexion, pale tongue, sunken and thready pulse.

Dizziness due to kidney-Asthenia　a condition due to deficiency of kidney-essence which fails to nourish

脉细等。可见于神经衰弱、脑动脉粥样硬化症、贫血等病证。the brain; manifested as dizziness, tinnitus, languor, amnesia, soreness and debility of the loins and knees, thready pules, etc. seen in neurasthenia, cerebral atherosclerosis, anemia, etc.

肾虚阳痿 【shèn xū yáng wěi】指肾虚所致的阳痿。症见阴茎不举或举而不坚,常伴有腰酸肢冷、脉沉细等症。多因房劳过度或手淫,使肾阳受伤所致。

Impotence due to kidney-Asthenia a condition manifested as lack of copulative power in the male, with inability to achieve penile erection or to achieve ejaculation, usually accompanied with lumbago, cold limbs, sunken and thready pulse, etc; which is due to impairment of kidney-yang resulting from frequent sexual intercourse or mastrubation.

肾虚腰痛 【shèn xū yāo tòng】因肾脏虚衰所致的腰痛。症见腰痛酸软、腿膝无力、遇劳更甚、脉弱无力等。

Lumbago due to kidney-Asthenia a type of lumbago manifested as aching and debility of the loins and weakness of the legs, which are aggravated by ovrstrain, weak pulse, etc.

肾虚遗精 【shèn xū yí jīng】肾阴不足或肾气虚所致的遗精。

Nocturnal Emission due to Kidney-Asthenia a disorder caused by insufficiency of kidney-yin or deficiency of kidney-qi.

肾虚月经过少 【shèn xū yuè jīng guò shǎo】因平素肾精不足;或因病损伤肾精,致冲任亏损,血海不盈引起的月经量过少。症见月经如期而至但量少、色淡红、质清稀、伴有头晕、耳鸣、腰膝酸软等。

Hypomenorrhea due to kidney-Asthenia a disorder due to impairment of thoroughfare and conception vessels and emptiness of blood-sea resulting from the primary insufficiency or secondary damage of kidney essence; manifested as regular menstruation with scanty and pink discharge accompanied with dizziness, tinnitus, soreness amd weakness of the loins

肾岩 【shèn yán】多因肝肾素亏；或忧思郁怒，肝经血燥，火邪郁结而成的病证。症见龟头或阴茎冠状沟附近发生结节，坚硬痒痛，或呈菜花样，晚期腹股沟部有坚硬如石的肿块，甚则危及生命。相当于阴茎癌。

Penial Carcinoma a critical condition due to asthenia of the liver and kidney, or accumulation of emotional upsets, blood dryness in the liver meridian leading to retention of fire; manifested as a itchy, painful and indurated node over the glans penis or the coronary sulcus of the penis, in the later stage marked by indurated enlatgement of the inguinal lymphnodes.

肾阳 【shèn yáng】（肾火、真火、真阳）是肾生理功能的动力，也是人体生命活动力的源泉。

Kidney-Yang the motive force for the physiological functions of the kidney and also the source of life activities of the human body.

肾阳衰微 【shèn yáng shuāi wēi】（命门火衰）是肾阳虚的进一步发展，除肾阳虚的症状加重外，尚可见精神痿靡、五更泄泻、水肿、脉沉迟微弱等症状。

Declination of Kidney-Yang a morbid state of further development of kidney-yang deficiency, manifested as listlessness, morning diarrhea, edema and sunken slow weak pulse in addition to the symptoms of kidney yang deficiency.

肾阳虚 【shèn yáng xū】肾脏生理功能低下，也是人体生命活动功能低下的病理。症见身寒、怕冷、腰痛、阳痿、夜尿多，甚则浮肿、气喘等。

Deficiency of kidney-Yang a morbid state of renal hypofunction and hypofunction of vital activities; which is manifested as low body temperature, intolerance of cold, lumbago, impotence, frequency of urination at night or even edema, dyspnea, etc.

肾阴 【shèn yīn】（元阴）肾的阴液及其所藏之精，是肾功能活动的物质基础。它与肾阳互相依附、互相制约，共同完成肾的生理功能。肾阴不足可引起肾阳偏亢。

Kidney-Yin the yin fluid and essence stored in the kidney which serve as the materials for the functional activities of the kidney-yang, it coordinates and inhibits each other with kidney-yang to carry out the

肾阴虚 【shèn yīn xū】（肾水不足、肾阴不足）即肾脏阴精的不足，引起肾脏功能病理性亢进的病理。症见腰酸疲乏、头晕耳鸣、遗精早泄、口干咽痛、五心烦热或午后潮热、舌红少苔、脉细数等。

肾与膀胱相表里 【shèn yǔ páng guāng xiāng biǎo lǐ】见肾合膀胱。

肾之府 【shèn zhī fǔ】指腰部。

肾主骨 【shèn zhǔ gǔ】中医学认为骨依赖于骨髓的营养而生长、发育，而骨髓由肾精气化生，所以，骨骼的发育、生长、荣枯，与肾的精气盛衰有着密切的关系。

肾主伎巧 【shèn zhǔ jì qiǎo】肾藏精，主骨、生髓。因此，肾气旺盛能使人精神饱满，动作敏捷。

肾主纳气 【shèn zhǔ nà qì】指肾与吸气功能有关，它和肺互相配合，保证呼吸的正常。一般认为某些表现为呼吸不全的疾病与肾主纳气的功能失常有关。

functions of the kidney. Deficiency of kidney yin may cause hyperfunction of kidner-yang.

Deficiency of kidney-Yin a morbid state of insufficiency of kidney yin fluid usually leading to pathological hyperfunction of kidney-yang; manifested as lumbago, tinnitus, nocturnal emission, precocious ejaculation, dry mouth, sore throat, feverish sensation of the palms, soles and chest, or afternoon fever, red tongue, uncoated fur, thready and fast pulse, etc.

Kidney and the Bladder Share a Paired Relationship

House of Kidney referring to the loins.

Kidney Dominating the Bones one of the functions of the kidney by which the growth and the normal function of the bone are maintained, since the kidney essence produces the marrow substance which nourishes the bone.

Kidney is in charge of Agility one of the functions of the kidney by which the individual is kept energetic and nimble in action since the kidney stores the essence of life and dominates the bones and produces marrow.

Kidney Recepts Qi one of the functions of the kidney, but which respiration is maintained with the cooperation of the lung. In general, some cases of respiratory insufficiency are

肾主水 【shèn zhǔ shuǐ】肾的主要功能之一。指肾主持体内水液的分布与排泄,并在调节体液平衡中起着重要的作用。

Kidney Dominates Water Metabolism one of the main functions of the kidney by which the distribution and excretion of body fluid are controlled, and an important role in the regulation of body fluid equilibrium is played.

肾主先天 【shèn zhǔ xiān tiān】肾藏精。对人体(包括胚胎时期)的生长和发育起着极重要的作用。

Kidney Dominates Congenital Essence a term signifying the important role of the kidney in dominating the growth and development of an individual, including the embryonic stage, through the action of kidney essence.

肾着 【shèn zháo】由肾虚寒湿内著所致的病证。症见腰部冷痛重着、转侧不利,虽静卧亦不减,遇阴雨则加重。

Retention of Damp-Cold in the Kidney disorder resulting from kidney asthenia; manifested as pain, cold and heavy feeling in the loins which are not relieved by rest and aggravated in rainy season.

甚者从之 【shèn zhě cóng zhī】对病情重而复杂的疾病,应采用从症状而治的治法。

Treating the Serious Case Based on the False Symptoms a therapeutiic principle, contrary to the routine treatment, for treating the serious and complicated diseases aiming at the relief of symptoms.

甚者独行 【shèn zhě dú xíng】对于病情严重的病证,应采用药力较强,功用专一的方剂来治疗。

Treating a Serious Case with the Formular of Strong and Specific Action

胂 【shèn】夹脊肉。

Group of Muscles along the Spine.

升剂 【shēng jì】用有升提作用的药物(如升麻、柴胡之类)组成的方剂。

Prescription with Ascending Effect the prescription composed of

升降浮沉【shēng jiàng fú chén】指药物作用的趋向性。升是上升,降是下降,浮是发散上行,沉是泻利下行。升浮药上行而向外,有升阳、发表、散寒等作用;沉降药下行而向内,有潜阳、降逆、收敛、清热、渗湿、泻下等作用。

Ascending Descending Floating Sinking referring to the actions of Chinese materia medica, the ones in ascending natures act upwards and outwards, and possess the actions of ascending yang, producing sweating and expelling exogenious factors; the ones in descending and sinking natures act downwards and inwards and possess the actions of calming yang, descending the adverse rising of qi astringing, clearing away heat, eliminating damp and purging.

medicines with ascending effect, such as Rhizoma Cimicifugae, Radix Bupleuri, etc.

升降失常【shēng jiàng shī cháng】指脾胃功能失调,致脾气不升,胃气不降的病理。症见腹胀、嗳气、呕吐、泄泻等。

Abnormal Ascending and Descending of the Visceral Qi a functional disorder of the stomach and spleen, in which the spleen-qi fails to ascend and the stomach qi fails to descend normally, which is manifested as flatulence, belching, vomiting, diarrhea, etc.

升可去降【shēng kě qù jiàng】具有升提作用的药物,可以治疗因气虚下陷而引起的病证,如脱肛,子宫下垂等。

Prescription with Ascending Effect Treating Collapes-Syndrome the prescription with effect of ascending qi is applied for the treatment of the disease due to deficiency of qi and collapse of qi, such as prolapse of rectum, hysteroptosis.

升提中气【shēng tí zhōng qì】治疗中气下陷的方法。适用于脾虚中气下陷引起久泻、脱肛、子宫脱垂等病证。

Ascending up the Middle-Energizer Qi a treatment for the collapse of middle-energizer qi. applicable to the case caused by spleen deficiency and collapse of middle-energizer qi, such

生津　【shēng jīn】（养津液）即用滋养津液的药物，治疗热性病津液受伤或久病阴伤者，症见发热、口干渴、舌红、唇燥等。

生殖之精　【shēng zhí zhī jīng】（先天之精）是人体生殖功能的基本物质。

声如拽锯　【shēng rú zhuài jù】指呼吸时喉中痰鸣如拉锯样的声音。常见于昏迷病人，亦见于一些喉头梗阻的疾病。

胜气　【shèng qì】运气学说术语。指偏胜之气。如上半年发生某种超常的气候，或五运中某运偏胜，均称胜气。

尸厥　【shī jué】突然昏倒失去知觉，状如死尸的一种严重证候。

失精家　【shī jīng jiā】平素患有遗精的人。

失眠　【shī mián】（不寐）指经常入睡困难甚至彻夜难眠，或睡后易醒的病证。本症多由阴血亏损、中气不足、心脾两虚或痰饮内停等多种原因使心神不安所致。

as chronic diarrhea, prolapse of rectum, uterine prolapse, etc.

Promoting the Production of Body Fluid　a treatment for the consumption of body fluid, in the case of febrile diseases manifested as fever, dry mouth and lips, reddish tongue, etc. by the application of drugs of increasing the production of body fluid.

Essential Substance for Reproduction　also named as congenital essential substance. It is the basic substance for reproductive function of the human body.

Sounding as Sawing　a characteristic respiratory sound in the dyspneic state, usually seen in coma and laryngeal obstruction.

The Climate Changing beyond Regularity　a term of science of five elements motion; the changes of the climate in a year proceed with regularity, it means the changes are beyond its regularity in the first half of the year.

Syncope　a serious condition characterized by sudden loss of consciousness.

Patients Suffering from Frequent Emission

Insomnia　a condition of inability to sleep or abnormal wakefullness due to irritability resulting from deficiency of yin blood, insufficiency of middle energizer-qi, asthenia of the heart and spleen or retention of phlegm.

失气 【shī qì】1. 指机体生命动力的衰竭。2. 又称矢气，俗称放屁。

失荣 【shī róng】因情志所伤，肝郁络阻，痰火凝结所致的颈部肿瘤。肿块逐渐增大，坚硬如石，固定难移，溃烂后流出血水。患者形容瘦削，宛如树木失去荣华。

失神 【shī shén】（脱神）即神气衰败，指机能严重障碍，五脏精气衰败的病态，如目光昏暗、形体消瘦、剧烈泄泻不止、神志异常或突然昏倒等。

失血 【shī xuè】 泛指因火热、虚寒、外伤、瘀阻等使血不循经所引起的出血。如衄血、呕血、咯血、便血、尿血等。

失血心痛 【shī xuè xīn tòng】妇女因血崩而出现以心痛为主症的病证。多因出血过多，心脾失养，或血瘀凝滞所致。

失血眩晕 【shī xuè xuàn yūn】因失血过多而引起眩晕的一种病证。

失音 【shī yīn】（暗或瘖）即发音困难。若突然失音，多因外感风寒、风热所致，属实证；若慢性失音反复发作，多因肺肾受伤，阴精亏损所致，属虚证。

Loss of Qi　　1. a condition of exhaustion of the motive force in the human body.　2. break wind.

Malignant Tumor of the Nck　　cervical mass caused by emotional upsets leading to stagnation of liver-qi with obstruction of collaterals and accumulation of phlegm-fire, the tumor gradually enlarges and becomes hard like a stone immovable with bloody discharge, the patient appears haggared like a tree lossing its flourish.

Depletion of Spirit　　a morbid state due to serious impairment of the vital activities of human body and the exhaustion of essence qi of the five zang organs; manifested as lusterless of the eyes, emaciation, intractable diarrhea, mental disorder, sudden syncope, etc.

Loss of Blood　　generally referring to extravasation of blood, which results from fire-heat, asthenia-cold, injury, or blood stasis, such as epistaxis, hematemesis, hemoptysis, hematochezia, hematuria, etc.

Precordial Pain due to Loss of Blood　　a woman disease with precordial pain as the major symptom due to metrorrhagia, bleeding, innourished spleen and heart or blood stasis.

Dizziness due to Loss of Blood.

Dysphonia　　a condition marked by difficulty in speaking with sudden onset, in consequence of exposure to wind-cold or wind-heat generally be-

失枕 【shī zhěn】（落枕、失颈）因睡卧姿势不当或颈部感受风寒或外伤引起颈部疼痛、转动不灵的病证。

湿痹 【shī bì】（着痹）1、痹证的一种。指风寒湿邪侵袭肢节，经络，湿邪偏盛的痹证，症见肢体重着、肌肤顽麻或肢节疼痛、痛处固定。2、脚气病的一种。指脚气病见下肢疼痛不仁者。

湿病 【shī bìng】泛指因湿而引起的疾病。主要表现为身体重着、肢体酸痛、胃纳不佳、泄泻、腹胀，甚至面目四肢浮肿。

湿毒 【shī dú】湿气郁积成毒。其致病特点为慢性过程，病灶渗出物多，经久不愈。如湿毒积于肠而下注，可致湿毒便血；湿毒流于肌肤，则可致局部溃烂流水。

湿毒带下 【shī dú dài xià】带下证型之一。多因经期或产后阶段，胞脉正虚，湿毒秽浊之邪乘虚内侵、伤及胞

longs to sthenia syndrome, while that with recurrent relapses in consequence of the impairment of the lung and kidney or the consumption of yin-essence generally belongs to asthenia-syndrome.

Torticollis a disorder due to improper posture or attack of wind-cold involving the neck, or trauma, which is manifested as pain and immobility of the neck.

Damp-Type Arthralgia 1. a syndrome due to wind-cold-damp with damp as predominant factor attacking the joints, and meridians, manifested as heaviness and numbness of the limbs and localized arthralgia, 2. a type of beriberi with pain and numbness of the lower extremities.

Diseases due to Damp a disease caused by the attack of damp, which is manifested as heavy feeling of the body, soreness of limbs, poor appetite, diarrhea, abdominal distension, even edema of face and limbs.

Toxic Material Produced by Damp a pathogenic factor which causes disease characterized by its chronicity, intractability and copiors exudation, that stagnate in the intestines may cause hematechezia, while that distribute to the skin may cause local erosion and exudation.

Leukorrhagia due to Damp-Toxin profuse luekorrhagia caused by the impairment of thoroughfare, concep-

脉及冲任所致。症见带下色如米泔或黄绿如脓汁或五色杂下、气味臭秽、阴部痒痛，或有发热腹痛、小便短赤等。

tion and bao vessels resulting from the attack of damp during the menstral period or puerperium characterized by whitish or greenish yellow or multi-coloured vaginal discharge with foul odour; accompanied with itching and pain of the vulva of fever and abdominal pain or oliguria with reddish urine, etc.

湿毒下血 【shī dú xià xuè】便血的一种。多由湿毒蕴结大肠所致。症见便血颜色不鲜或紫黑如赤豆汁、腹不痛、胸膈胀闷、饮食减少、小便不利等。

Hematochezia due to Virulent Damp a disorder caused by the retention of virulent damp in the large intestine, manifested as discharge of purplish dark stool, absence of abdominal pain, feeling of distention and oppression over the chest, poor appetite, dysuria, etc.

湿剂 【shī jì】具有滋润作用的方剂，含有润肠药，如麦门冬、地黄之类。

Prescription with Moisturizing Effect prescription of increasing the production of body fluid, containing medicines of moisturizing effect, such as Radix Ophiopoganis, Radix Rehmanniae, etc.

湿家 【shī jiā】平素患湿的病人。

Patients Suffering from Damp-Syndrome

湿脚气 【shī jiǎo qì】指以膝浮肿为主症的脚气病。多因水湿外袭，经络不得宣通所致。症见足胫肿大、麻木重着、软弱无力、小便不利、舌苔白腻、脉濡缓等。

Damp Beriberi a form of beriberi characterized by edema of the lower limbs due to attack of damp causing obstruction of the meridians; manifested as swelling, numbness and weakness of the lower limbs, dysuria, whitish and greasy fur on the tongue, slow and soft, floating pulse, etc.

湿疥 【shī jiè】疥疮的一种类型。疥疮抓破后有滋水。

Damp Scabies scabies characterized by oozing from the skin lesions.

湿痉 【shī jìng】感受湿邪而致的痉证，多见于小儿。症见神昏、痉厥、身热不扬、舌苔白厚等。

Convulsive Disease due to Damp a disease usually seen in children, which is manifested as coma, convulsion, fever without hot sensation over the body, thick, whitish fur on the tongue, etc.

湿咳 【shī ké】（湿嗽）咳嗽的一种。因感受湿邪，湿痰壅肺所致。症见咳嗽多痰、骨节疼痛、四肢沉重、面浮肢肿、小便不利等。

Cough due to Damp a disease due to retention of damp in the lung; manifested as productive cough, arthralgia, lassitude, swelling of the face and limbs, dysuria, etc.

湿可去枯 【shī kě qù kū】用滋润的药物，可以治津血枯燥、阴液不足所引起的一些疾病。

Medicine with Moisturizing Effect Promoting the Production of Body Fluid the prescription that increase yin fluid production is used for the diseases due to dryness of body fluid or blood or insufficiency of yin fluid.

湿困脾阳 【shī kùn pí yáng】指因水湿之邪影响脾的运化功能的病理。症见食欲减退、上腹部胀闷、口渴喜热饮、小便短赤、舌苔厚腻、脉缓等。

Spleen-Yang Impaired by Damp a morbid condition due to invasion of damp into the body affecting the function of the spleen; manifested as poor appetite, epigastric distention, thirst and appeal to warm drink, dark short urine, thick greasy fur and slow pulse.

湿疟 【shī nüè】1. 见暑疟。2. 指湿邪内伏，复感风寒引起的疟疾。症见恶寒发热不甚、一身尽痛、四肢沉重、脘满呕恶、或面浮尿少、舌苔白腻、脉濡缓。

Damp-Type Malaria 1. summer-malaria 2. malaria caused by the attack of wind-cold to a patient with retention of damp in the body; manifested as mild chilliness and fever, general pain, heaviness of limbs, nausea, edema of face, oliguria, whitish and greasy fur on the tongue, and slow, soft and floating pulse.

湿热 【shī rè】1. 湿与热相结合形成的一种致病因子，如湿热之邪所致的

Damp-Heat 1. pathogenic factor formed by blending of heat and damp

黄疸。2. 湿病中的一种。症见发热、头痛、身重而痛、怠倦、腹满、食欲减退、小便短少而黄、舌苔黄腻、脉濡数等。

such as jaundice due to damp-heat. 2. one of the seasonal febrile diseases manifested as fever, headache, pantalgia fatigue, distention of abdomen, anorexia, oliguria, yellowish urine, yellow and greasy fur, floating and fast pulse, etc.

湿热腹痛 【shī rè fù tòng】由于湿热蕴结脾胃所致的腹痛。症见腹痛时作时止、痛而拒按、胸闷纳呆、呕吐、口苦而腻、恶寒发热、身目发黄、大便秘结或下痢、小便黄短、舌苔黄腻、脉濡数或洪数等。

Abdominal Pain due to Damp-Heat a disorder caused by accumulation of damp-heat in the spleen and stomach; manifested as intermittent abdominal pain and tenderness, feeling of oppression over the chest, anorexia, vomiting, chilliness, fever, jaundice, constipation or diarrhea, oliguria with yellowish urine, yellowish and greasy fur on the tongue, fast and soft, floating or bounding pulse, etc.

湿热黄疸 【shī rè huáng dǎn】阳黄的一种。指因湿热蕴结脾胃熏蒸肝胆所致的黄疸。症见身热、烦渴、脘腹胀满或躁扰不宁、小便热痛赤涩或大便秘结、脉洪滑有力等。

Jaundice due to Damp-Heat a type of yang jaundice caused by damp heat accumulating in the spleen and stomach and attacking the liver and gall bladder; manifested as fever, thirst, abdominal distension, irritability, painful and difficult urination with hot and reddish urine, constipation, full and smooth pulse, etc.

湿热内蕴 【shī rè nèi yùn】指湿热之邪蕴酿于脾胃肝胆而引起的病理。症见发热经久不退、午后热高、身重、神疲、胸脘痞闷、恶心、纳呆、腹胀、便溏或见黄疸、小便不利、舌苔多黄腻等。

Retention of Damp-Heat a morbid condition caused by the accumulation of damp-heat in the spleen stomach, liver and gall bladder; manifested as persistent fever higher in the afternoon, lassitude, feeling of oppression over the chest and epigastrium, nausea, poor appetite, flatulence, loose bowels, jaundice, dysuria, greasy and

湿热头痛 【shī rè tóu tòng】指由湿热熏蒸，上蒙清窍所致的头痛。症见头痛而重、心烦身重、肢节疼痛或面目及四肢浮肿、舌苔黄腻、脉濡数等。

湿热痿 【shī rè wěi】痿证的一种。因湿热浸淫，伤及筋脉所致的痿证，症见两足痿软、微肿或足指麻木，伴有身重胸闷、小便赤涩、舌苔黄腻、脉濡数等。

湿热下注 【shī rè xià zhù】指湿热流注于下焦。症见小便短赤、身重疲乏、胃纳不佳、舌苔黄腻。

湿热胁痛 【shī rè xié tòng】指因湿热熏蒸，肝胆络脉气滞所致的胁痛。症见胁肋持续胀痛或阵发性剧痛、痛引心下或胸背、恶心呕吐、胸闷纳呆、或有寒热、身目发黄、小便短赤等。

yellowish fur on the tongue, etc.

Headache due to Damp-Heat a disorder caused by damp-heat attacking the upper orifices; manifested as headache with heavy sensation, restlessness, lassitude, pain in the joints, greasy fur on the tongue, soft and floating, fast pulse, etc.

Flaccidity-Syndrome due to Damp-Heat a type of flaccidity syndrome due to impairment of muscles and vessel by damp-heat, manifested as flaccidity and swelling of the lower extremities, numbness of toes accompanied with lassitude, feeling of oppression over the chest, dysuria with reddish urine, yellowish and greasy fur on the tongue, soft, floating and fast pulse, etc.

Damp-Heat Attacking the Lower Energizer a morbid condition manifested as oliguria with reddish urine, fatigue, poor appetite, yellowish and greasy fur on the tongue, etc.

Hypochondriac pain due to Damp-Heat a disorder due to stagnation of qi in the collaterals of the liver and gall bladder resulting from the accumulation of damp-heat; manifested as continuous distending pain or paroxymal sharp pain over the hypochondrium, radiating to the epigastrium chest and back, nausea, vomiting, feeling of oppression over the chest, loss of appetite or accompanied with chills and fever.

湿热眩晕 【shī rè xuàn yūn】指暑令感受湿热之邪所致的眩晕。症见头昏目眩、身热、自汗、烦渴引饮、脉虚数。

Dizziness due to Damp-Heat a disorder resulting from damp-heat in summer manifested as dizziness, fever, spontaneous perspiration, extreme thirst with desire for drinking, feeble and fast pulse, etc.

湿热腰痛 【shī rè yāo tòng】腰痛的一种。指因湿热之邪阻遏经络所致的腰痛。症见腰部疼痛、痛处伴有热感、小便短赤、脉弦数等。

Lumbago due to Damp-Heat a symptom caused by the stagnation of damp-heat in the meridians; manifested as pain with feverish sensation over the lumbar region, oliguria with discharge of reddish urine, fast, wiry pulse.

湿胜阳微 【shī shèng yáng wēi】湿邪偏胜,伤害阳气,致阳气衰微的病理。症见面色苍白、胸闷、腹胀、泄泻或水肿等。

Hyperactivity of Damp Causing Declination of Yang a morbid condition of deficiency of yang-qi, due to impairment of yang-qi by the hyperactive damp; manifested as pallor, feeling of oppression over the chest, fullness of the abdomen, diarrhea, etc.

湿胜则濡泻 【shī shèng zé rú xiè】湿邪偏胜,脾阳受困,运化功能障碍而出现大便泄泻。

Hyperactivity of Damp Cauing Watery Diarrhea a morbid condition with hypofunction of the spleen due to suppression of spleen-yang by the hyperactive damp; manifested as watery diarrhea.

湿痰 【shī tán】由脾失健运,湿浊内蕴,日久成痰所致的痰证。症见痰多稀白或痰浊滑而易出、身重、倦怠、腹胀、食不消化或兼腹痛、腹胀、泄泻、脉缓滑等。

Damp-Phlegm Syndrome a syndrome resulting from dysfunction of the spleen leading to the accumulation of damp with formation of phlegm; manifested as copious expectoration of thin, whitish or yellowish sputum, fatigue, abdominal pain and flatulence, indigestion, edema, diarrhea, slow and smooth pulse, etc.

湿痰脚气 【shī tán jiǎo qì】指由湿盛生痰、湿痰下注所致的脚气病。常见大小便滑泄。

湿痰流注 【shī tán liú zhù】指脾虚气弱，湿痰内阻，复感邪毒，流溢于肌肤所致的流注。

湿痰痿 【shī tán wěi】痿证的一种。指湿痰客于经脉所致的痿证。症见四肢痿弱、腰膝麻木、脉象沉滑等。

湿温病 【shī wēn bìng】指因感受时令湿热所致的病证。多发于夏秋季节。症见身热不扬，有汗不畅，午后热甚，面色垢滞、表情淡漠，伴有胸脘痞闷、纳呆恶心、腹胀便溏、苔腻、脉缓。辨证分类：1、湿郁卫气证 2、气分湿热证。3、邪入营血证。

湿泻 【shī xiè】（濡泻）指因湿气伤脾所致的泄泻。症见泻下如水或大便溏薄、苔腻、脉濡等。

Damp-Phlegm Beriberi   a form of beriberi due to attack of damp-phlegm to the lower part of the body usually accompanied with diarrhea.

Multiple Abscess due to Damp-Phlegm   formation of superficial abscess occuring in debilitated patient due to deficiency of spleen-qi, accumulation of damp-phlegm and affected by toxic factor.

Flaccidity Syndrome due to Damp-Phlegm   a syndrome caused by the retention of damp-phlegm in meridians and collaterals; manifested as flaccidity of extremities, numbness of loins and kness, sunken and smooth pulse, etc.

Damp-Warm Syndrome   a morbid condition due to attack of epidemic damp-heat, mostly seen in summer, marked by moderate fever, sweating but partially obstructed, dirty complexion, listlessness, accompanied by stuffiness in the chest and epigastrium, loss of appetite, nausea, abdominal distension, loose stools, greasy coating of the tongue, soft and relaxed pulse. Types of differentiation 1. accumulation of pathogenic dampness in wei qi system 2. pathogenic damp-heat in qi fen system 3. invasion of pathogens in the ying and blood.

Diarrhea due to Damp   a disease due to damage of the spleen by damp; manifested as diarrhea with watery or

湿癣 【shī xuǎn】风湿邪热侵于肌肤而发的病证。患处皮损潮红糜烂。瘙痒不止。搔破滋水淋漓、浸淫不断扩大。 **Damp-Type Dermatitis** a skin disease caused by the attack of wind-damp-heat to the skin; characterized by redness, erosion, intense itching, oozing of the lesion and later becoming sidespread.

湿郁 【shī yù】多因湿邪郁困而使气机不畅所致的郁证。症见全身疼痛、身重、头昏重、倦怠、苔薄腻,遇阴天或寒冷即发。 **Retention of Damp** a disorder caused by the retention of damp leading to the sluggishness of qi, commonly seen in the wet or cold weather; manifested as general aching, dizziness, fatigue, thin and greasy fur on the tongue, etc.

湿郁热伏 【shī yù rè fú】湿邪阻遏所引起热邪不易散发的病理。症见发热不高但缠绵不愈、午后热甚、汗出热不退、疲乏、胸闷腹胀、食欲不振、小便黄赤等。 **Stagnation of Damp Causing Retention of Heat** a morbid condition of stagnation of damp interfering in the dispersion of heat; manifested as prolonged moderate fever with daily rise in the afternoon, and not subsided after sweating, fatigue, thin and greasy fur on the tongue, etc.

湿浊 【shī zhuó】(湿气) 其性重浊粘腻,每于病位停留滞着,阻碍阳气的活动。 **Damp** it with thick and sticky nature is liable to be retained in the diseased part and to impede the activity of yang qi.

湿阻气分 【shī zǔ qì fèn】湿邪滞留气分的病理。症见发热、头重、全身酸重、关节疼痛、胸闷、食欲不振、腹胀或腹痛、呕吐或泄泻、舌苔滑腻、脉象濡缓等。 **Damp Stagnated in Qifen** a morbid condition manifested as fever, heaviness of the head, fatigue, general aching, arthralgia, feeling of oppression over the chest, poor appetite, fullness of the abdomen, abdominal pain, vomiting or diarrhea, moist and greasy fur on the tongue, soft and floating slow pulse, etc.

湿阻中焦　【shī zǔ zhōng jiāo】湿邪滞留脾胃影响运化功能的病理，症见头重、倦怠、脘闷、腹胀、食欲不振、口粘渴喜热饮、小便短赤、舌苔厚白，脉缓等。

Damp Stagnated in the Middle Energizer　a morbid condition due to retention of damp in the spleen and stomach; manifested as heaviness of the head, fullness of abdomen, poor appetite, thirst and desire for hot drinking, oliguria with deep coloured urine, thick and whitish fur on the tongue, slow oliguria with deep coloured urine, thick and whitish fur on the tongue, slow pulse, etc.

十八反　【shī bā fǎn】中药配伍禁忌的一类。相传下来有十八种药的药性相反，即甘草反大戟、芫花、甘遂、海藻；乌头反贝母、瓜蒌、半夏、白蔹、白芨；藜芦反人参、丹参、沙参、苦参、细辛、芍药。

Eighteen Incompatible Medicaments　a kind of incompatibility of drugs in prescription, the following durgs are believed to give rise to serious side effects, if given combination Radix Glycyrrhizae being incompatible with Radix Ginseng, Radix Euphorbiae Kansui, Radix Euphorbiae Pekinesis, Flos Genkwa and Sargassum; Radix Aconiti incompatible with Bulbus Fritillariae Fructus Trichosanthis, Rhizoma Pinelliae, Radix Ampelopsis, Rhizoma bletillae; Radix Veratro Nigri incompatible with Radix Glehniae, Radix Saoviae Miltiorrhizae, Radix Sophorae, Flavescenits, Herba Asari and Radix Paeoniae.

十二剂　【shī èr jì】按不同功用将方剂分为十二类，称为十二剂。

Twelve Kinds of Formulars　a classification of formulars based on their different effect.

十二时　【shī èr shí】中国古代计时单位，即子、丑、寅、卯、辰、巳、午、未、申、酉、戌、亥十二个时时辰，每个辰相当于二小时。

The Traditional Twelve Hour Periods　the twelve two-hour periods into which a day was traditionally devided, each being given the names, as zi, chow, yin, mao, chen, si, wu, wei, shen, you, xu and hai.

十二脏 【shí èr zàng】指心、肝、脾、肺、肾、心包络、胆、胃、大肠、小肠、三焦、膀胱。

Twelve Viscera referring to the heart, liver, spleen, lung, kidney, pericardium, gallbladder, stomach, large intestine, small intestine, triple energizer and bladder.

十九畏 【shí jiǔ wèi】中药配伍禁忌的一类。相传有十九种药相畏,即硫黄畏朴硝,水银畏砒霜,狼毒畏密佗僧,巴豆畏牵牛,丁香畏郁金,牙硝畏三棱,川乌草乌畏犀角,人参畏五灵脂,肉桂畏赤石脂。

Mutual Inhibition among the Nineteen Chinese Materia Medica the incompatibility between two drugs recorded in the ancient medical works, such as Sulfur and Sodium nitrite; Mercury and Arsenics; Radix Enphorbiae Ebracteolatae and Lithargyrum; Fructus Crotonis and Herba pharibitidis; Flos Syzgii Aromatici and Radix Curcumae; Mirablite and Rhizoma Sparganii; Radix Aconniti, Radix Aconiti Kusnezoffii and Cornu Rhinoceri. Radix Ginseng and Faeces Trogopterorum; Cortex; Cinnamoni and Halloysitum Rubrum.

十问 【shí wèn】问诊的十项重点内容,包括(1)发热恶寒;(2)出汗;(3)头部及躯干肢体;(4)大小便;(5)饮食;(6)胸腹;(7)听力及睡眠;(8)口渴;(9)妇女月经、带下、妊娠、产褥及小儿生长发育、喂养等;(10)既往病史及发病原因。

Inquiring Ten Aspects of the Patient the important contents during inquiry, including:(1) fever and chilliness (2) perspiration (3) the condition of the head, trunk and limbs (4) urination and defecation (5) appetite (6) the condition of the chest and abdomen (7) hearing and sleeping (8) thirst (9) manstruation, leukorrhea, pregnancy and puerperium of the women and the growth and feeding of her children; (10) the past history of illness and the cause of disease.

石蛾 【shí é】即慢性扁桃体炎。
Chronic Tonsillitis

石瘕 【shí jiǎ】因寒气入侵,致恶血停
Stony Mass of Uterus retention of

积子宫内的病证。以子宫日渐增大，状如怀子及闭经等为特征。

石疽 【shí jū】因寒凝气滞所致的皮下肿块，形如桃李，皮色不变，坚硬如石，逐渐增大，难消难溃，多发于颈项、腰胯和膝部。

石淋 【shí lín】因下焦积热，煎熬水液杂质所致的淋证。症见发作时腰腹绞痛，痛及前阴，甚则面色苍白、冷汗、恶心呕吐。可伴有发热；尿频尿急刺痛，或排尿中断，可见血尿或小便有砂石排出。辨证分类：1、湿热蕴结证 2、瘀血阻滞证 3、肾元亏虚证。

石女 【shí nǚ】1、患先天性阴道狭窄的妇女。2、患原发性闭经的妇女。

石水 【shí shuǐ】1、因肝肾阴寒，水气凝聚下焦，致以腹水为主症的水肿病。症见少腹肿大坚如石、胁下胀痛、腹满、脉沉等。2、即单腹胀。

extravasated blood in the uterus caused by the invasion of cold; manifested as gradual becoming large, just like pregnancy, amenorrhea, etc.

Indurated Subcutaneous Mass a plum like mass due to stagnation of cold and qi as hard as stone, covered with normal skin, growing gradually, and seldom to subside spontaneously and rupture, mostly appearing on the neck, waist, hip and knee.

Stranguria Caused by the Passage of Urinary Stone a morbid condition caused by accumulation of heat in the lower energizer, which caused consumption of fluid with impurities, marked by the stabbing lumbar pain that involves both the lower abdomen and external genitalia, or even pale complexion, cold sweating, nausea, vomiting, accompanied by fever, frequent and hasty urinary discharge with painful sensation, or on and off urinary discharge, occasionally with blood, or with sandy substance in the urine. Types of differentiation 1. accumulation of damp-heat 2. obstruction due to blood stasis 3. deficiency of the kidney.

1. **Female with Congenital Stricture of Vagina** 2. **Female with Primary Amenorrhea**

Indurated Edema a type of edema with ascites as the major sign, caused by asthenic cold in the kidney and liver and retention of fluid in the low-

石瘿 【shí yǐng】因气郁、痰湿或瘀血凝滞所致,以甲状腺增大为主证的病症。症见甲状腺肿大,较硬。表面凹凸不平,不能移动;并伴有易怒、多汗、胸闷、心悸等;肿块增大可发生气管、食道和声带压迫症状。

Indurated Goiter enlargement of the thyroid caused by stagnation of qi or damp phlegm, and its surface is uneven; associated with symptoms of irratability, profuse sweating, feeling of oppression over the chest, palpitation, etc, or accompanied with pressure symtoms of the trachea, esophgus and vocal cords when it is significantly enlarged.

时病 【shí bìng】指与四时气候变化有较密切关系的外感发热性疾病。

Seasonal Disease seasonal febrile disease caused by exogenous pathogenic factors, related to the change of climate in different seasons.

时毒 【shí dú】1、(时毒发颐)时邪疫毒客于三阳经络,发于项腮颌颐等部位,形成肿块的疾患。症见恶寒发热,肢体酸痛,或有咽痛,一、二日间,腮颐漫肿,焮红疼痛。2、指具有较强烈致病作用的、可引起季节性流行疾病的病邪。3、即温毒。

Seasonal Virulent Pathogenic Factor 1. epidemic parotitis, a disease caused by the attack of seasonal pathogenic factor in the three yang meridians; manifested as chillness, fever, aching of limbs or sore-throat, and marked swelling redness and pain of the cheeks. 2. virulent, exogenous factor that causes seasonal contagious disease. 3. epidemic heat-syndrome.

时毒发颐 【shí dú fa yí】见时毒。

Epidemic Parotitis see "seasonal virulent pathogenic factor".

时方 【shí fāng】汉代张仲景以后医学家所制定的方剂。它是在经方基础上发展起来的。

Non-Classical Prescription prescriptions designed by the doctors after Zhang zhong jing in Han Dynasty, based on the classical prescription.

时令 【shí lìng】1、每一季节的气候特点。2、按季节制定有关农事、医事的措施。

Seasonal Characteristics 1. the characteristics of the climate in different seasons. 2. Seasonl Work the measures suited for the agriculture and medical works accordig to the climate of different seasons.

时邪 【shí xié】泛指与四时气候相关的病邪,是季节流行病致病因素的统称。

Seasonal Factors pathogenic factors prevalent in particular season, seasonal epidemic diseases are all called seasonal factors.

时行感冒 【shí xíng gán mào】病情较重而广泛流行的感冒。多因感受时邪所致。症见恶寒高热、头痛、骨节酸痛、神疲乏力、口渴、咽痛、舌苔白、舌质红、脉数等。

Influenza an epidemic disease usually caused by seasonal factors, manifested as chillness, high fever, headache, arthralgia, lassitude, thirst, sore throat, red tongue with whitish fur, fast pulse, etc.

时行寒疫 【shí xíng hán yì】春夏季节因暴寒而引起的一种流行性疾病。症见头痛身疼,寒热无汗,或见呕逆、苔白不渴、脉浮紧等。

Seasonal Epidemic Disease due to Exogenous Coldness an epidemic disease occuring in spring and summer, manifested as headache, general aching, chills, fever without sweating, nausea or vomiting, whitish fur on the tongue, floating and tense pules, etc.

时行戾气 【shí xíng lì qì】即具有强烈流行性的致病因素。

Cotagious Factors pathogenic factors which are epidemic and virulent.

时行嗽 【shí xíng sòu】(时行暴嗽)因感时行之气而引起以咳嗽为主症的病证。常伴有发热恶寒、头痛鼻塞、咳嗽连声不已等,往往呈流行性。

Epidemic Disease Characterized by Cough an epidemic disease caused by epidemic factors, characterized by paroxymal cough, accompanied with chillness, headache, stuffy nose, etc.

时疫 【shí yì】指季节性的流行病。如在夏秋季多发生某些肠道传染病。

Epidemic Disease referring to the seasonal, widespread diseases, such as the intestinal infectious diseases occuring in summer and autumn.

时疫发斑 【shí yì fā bān】(温疫发

Epidemic Eruptive Disease appear-

实秘 【shí bì】指实证便秘。包括热秘、痰秘、气秘等。

Constipation of Sthenia-Type the constipation occuring in sthenia-syndrome including constipation due to accumulation of heat, constipation due to phlegm retention, constipation due to stagnation of qi, etc.

实喘 【shí chuǎn】因邪气盛引起的气喘。多因外感六淫邪气,痰火郁热,水饮凌肺致肺气壅阻,气道不利所致。一般起病急,病程较短。常因病因不同而有不同的临床表现。

Dyspnea of Sthenia-Type a type of dyspnea due to stagnation of lung-qi, resulting from the exposure to six factors, phlegm-fire, stagnation of heat, and retention of fluid invading the lung, characterized by sudden onset and short duration. Its manifestations vary with its etiology.

实火 【shí huǒ】热邪炽盛所致的属于实、热的病证,症见高热、目赤、口渴、烦燥、腹痛拒按、便秘、口苦、舌苔黄厚、干燥、脉滑数有力等。

Sthenic Fire-Syndrome a morbid state of sthenia and heat in nature, caused by the hyperactivity of heat; manifested as high fever, red eyes, thirst, irritability, abdoninal pain and tenderness, constipation, bitter mouth, thick yellowish and dry fur on the tongue, smooth and fast, vigorous pulse, etc.

实脉 【shí mài】浮、中、沉取寸、关、尺三个部位均指感有力的一种脉象。主实证,多因实热内结,痰食停积所致。

Solid Pulse a pulse condition with forceful beats while pressing slightly, moderately or heavily the three regions of cun, guan and chi, which indicates sthenia-syndrome caused by the accumulation of sthenic-heat and phlegm or indigestion.

实痞 【shí pǐ】由外邪内侵;或湿浊内

Lump-Syndrome of Sthenic Type a

阻、寒滞脾胃；或痰食内结；或肝气郁遏所致的痞证。症见胃脘痞满，可兼见疼痛呕逆、不思饮食、大便秘结等。

type of lump-syndrome caused by the invasion of exogenous factors, the retention of dampness in the spleen and stomach, the accumulation of phlegm and indigested food, or the stagnation of liver-qi; manifested as feeling of oppression and fullness over the epigastrium, probably accompanied with stomachache, vomiting, anorexia, constipation, etc.

实热 【shí rè】外邪化热入里，邪气盛，正气尚足，邪正斗争剧烈所表现的证候。如高热、烦渴引饮、便秘、或腹痛拒按，尿色深黄、舌质红、苔黄干、脉洪数有力等。

Sthenic Heat-Syndrome a syndrome appearing in the case of violent conflict between the pathogenic factor and the healthy qi when the exogenous factors changes into heat in the interior and the healthy qi is still sufficient; manifested as high fever, excessive thirst, desire for drink, constipation, abdominal pain and tenderness, deep yellow urine, red tongue with yellowish and dry fur, full and fast, vigorous pulse, etc.

实则太阳，虚则少阴 【shí zé tài yáng, xū zé sháo yīn】指感受外寒发病后两种不同的病理变化。机体抗病能力强，与外感寒邪相争于表，出现头项强痛、恶寒发热、脉浮等太阳证；若机体抗病力低下，感受寒邪之后可内陷少阴，而出现虚寒证。

Sthenia-Syndrome is Taiyang and Asthenia-Syndrome is Shaoyin referring to the two different pathological changes after the attack of exogenous cold. If the body resistance is strong enough to limit the cold on the superficies, the symptoms of taiyang appear, such as stiff neck, fever, chillness, floating pulse, etc. If the body resistance is weak and cold invades into the interior, the symptoms of shaoyin, i. e. asthenia-cold syndrome appear.

实胀 【shí zhàng】因气滞湿阻、湿热

Abdominal Distention of Sthenia-Type

蕴结，瘀血，食积于胃的病证。症见腹胀坚硬拒按、便秘、小便黄赤、脉滑数有力等。

a disorder caused by the stagnation of qi, retention of damp or damp-heat, blood stasis, or accumulation of indigested food in the stomach, manifested as abdominal flatulence, regidity and tenderness, constipation, radden and yellowish urine, smooth and fast, strong pulse, etc.

实者泻其子 【shí zhě xiè qí zǐ】运用五行相生和五脏母子关系的理论，指导治疗五脏实证的一种方法。如肝为母、心为子，所以治疗肝脏实证时，不仅要泻肝还要泻心火。

Treating the Sthenia-Syndrome of the Mother-organ by Purging the Child-organ a principle for treating sthenia-syndrome of the five zang organs, based on the theory of generation and mother-and-child relationship of the five elements. For instance, the sthenia-syndrome of the liver (mother-organ) should be treated by purging the fire of the liver and the fire of the heart (child-organ) as well.

实者泻之 【shí zhě xiè zhī】属邪实的疾病，宜用泻法去其邪气。临床上一般宜按病邪的性质以及所在的部位而采用不同的泻法。如属热结大肠，宜寒下；属寒积，宜温下等。

Sthenia-Syndrome Should Be Treated with Purgation a therapeutic principle for treating the case with sthenic factors. Different types of purgation are applied according to the character and the location of factors, e.g.; the accumulation of heat in the large intestine should be purged with cold-nature drugs, while the coldness accumulation should be purged with warm natured drugs.

实证 【shí zhèng】病邪亢盛而患者体质较好，正邪斗争剧烈，或脏腑功能障碍引起气血郁结，痰饮内停，食积等所致的一种证候。症见高热、口渴、烦燥、谵语、腹胀、腹痛而拒按、便

Sthenia-Syndrome a syndrome occuring in a relatively strong patient exposed to virulent factors or dysfunction of the viscera leading to the stagnation of qi and blood, phlegm-

秘、尿少而深黄、舌红、苔黄而干糙、脉实有力等。

实中夹虚 【shí zhōng jiá xū】属实邪结聚的疾病,同时伴有正虚的临床表现。多属邪盛正虚的一种病理现象。

食痹 【shí bì】指进食后引起的胃脘胀痛不适连及两胁,重者呕吐后疼痛才能缓解的一种疾病。多因肝气横逆犯胃或痰饮恶血停留胃脘所致。

食复 【shí fù】久病或大病初愈,不注意饮食的调节,影响脾胃的消化和吸收,致使旧病复发。

食积 【shí jī】因脾胃运化失常,食物积滞不化所致的一种疾病。症见胸脘满闷、胀痛拒按、或有痞块、大便秘结、纳食减少、嗳腐吞酸、舌苔厚腻等。

retention, indigestion, etc; manifested as high fever, thirst, irritability, delirium, abdominal distension, pain and tenderness, constipation, oliguria with deep-coloured urine, red tongue with rough, dry and yellowish fur, solid and strong pulse, etc.

Sthenia-Syndrome Accompanied with Asthenia-Syndrome a morbid condition with the clinical manifestations of the accumulation of sthenic factors and accompanied with deficiency of healthy qi.

Stomachache after Food Intake a disorder characterized by distending pain in the stomach radiating to the hypochondria, provoked by food intaking and relieved by vomiting due to the attack of the hyperactive liver qi to the stomach, or retention of phlegm or blood stasis in the stomach.

Recurrence of Illness due to Immoderate Diet a phenomenon occuring during the convalescence of advanced or serious illnesses, resulting from the impairment of digestive function by immoderate diet.

Dyspepsia a disease caused by indigestion resulting from the functional disorder of the spleen and stomach; manifested as fullness over the chest and upper abdomen, abdominal pain and tenderness, or palpable mass, constipation, poor appetite, eructation with fetid odor, acid regurgitation,

食积腹痛 【shí jī fù tòng】因饮食不节，脾虚不运，食物停滞肠胃所致的腹痛。症见腹部胀满疼痛、便后痛减、厌食、嗳气吞酸、便秘、苔腻、脉弦或沉滑等。

Abdominal Pain due to Indigestion a disorder due to rentention of indigested food in the gastrointestinal tract resulting from immoderate eating and drinking, and asthenia and hypofunction of the spleen; manifested as abdominal distending pain which may be relieved after defecation, anorexia, eructation acid regurgitation, constipation, greasy fur on the tongue, wiry or sunken and smooth pulse etc.

食疟 【shí nüè】疟疾的一种，往往由饮食停滞所诱发。常伴有嗳气、纳呆、食则吐逆、腹胀脘闷等症。

Malaria with Prominent Digestive Disoredr a type of malaria usually provoked by indigestion, accompanied with belching, loss of appetite, vomiting after intaking, abdominal fullness, etc.

食呕 【shí ǒu】由于脾胃损伤，食积不化所致的呕吐。症见脘腹满闷，甚则胀痛，嗳气腐臭、厌食、食入即吐，或朝食暮吐、舌苔腻、脉多弦滑等。

Vomiting due to Improper Diet a disorder caused by the impairment of the stomach and spleen and indigestion, which is manifested as fullness and pain over the epigestrium and abdomen, eructation with fetid odor, anorexia, vomiting upon ingestion or a long interval afetr meal, greasy fur on the tongue, wiry and smooth pulse.

食气 【shí qì】（服气）是指通过呼吸锻炼，以吸纳天地清气，以求延年益寿的气功方法。

Eating Qi referring to absorb pure qi in nature, through breathing training so as to reach the aim of longevity.

食肉则复 【shí ròu zé fù】（食肉则遗）指在某些热性病恢复期，病人消

Recurrence of Iiiness due to Excessive Intake of Meat a phenomenon of

化功能低下，若多食腥荤肥腻会使病情反复的现象。

食痫 【shí xián】1、指因伤食而诱发的痫疾。2、指小儿伤食发热所致之抽搐。症见腹泄、呕吐、下利酸臭、时时抽搐等。

Epileptic Seizures Induced by Improper Diet 1. epilepsy provoked by improper diet 2. infantile convulsion caused by improper feeding and fever, accompanied with diarrhea with foul stool, vomiting, etc.

食蟹中毒 【shí xié zhòng dú】因食螃蟹所致的中毒症状。症见胸闷烦乱、精神不安、或腹痛、呕吐、腹泻不止等。

Crab Poisoning intoxication caused by eating crab, manifested as feeling of oppression over the chest, restlessness, or even abdominal pain, frequent vomiting and diarrhea, etc.

食心痛 【shí xīn tòng】因伤于饮食所致的胃脘痛，常伴有嗳腐吞酸、厌食胀满、胸闷、脉滑实等。

Stomachache due to Improper Diet stomachache due to damage of the stomach by the indigested food usually accompanied with eructation with fetid ordor, acid regurgitation, anorexia, flatulence, feeling of oppression over the chest, smooth and solid pulse, etc.

食蕈菌中毒 【shí xùn jùn zhòng dú】因误食毒蕈菌所致的中毒，症见头痛、呕吐、腹泻、昏睡、幻视、精神错乱等，严重者可致死亡。

Fungus Poisoning intoxication caused by eating poisonous mushroom, manifested as heahache, vomiting, diarrhea, stupor, visual illusions, mental confusion, and even death in severe cases.

食医 【shí yī】指古代为帝王管理饮食卫生的医生。

Dietetic Officer a medical officer who was responsible for the dietetic hygiene of the imperial court in the ancient time.

食亦 【shí yì】指多食而形体消瘦的疾病。多因肠胃和胆有燥热所致。

Polyphagia-Emaciation Syndrome a condition of voracious eating but progressive leanness, caused by the accumulation of dryness-heat in the

食 shi

stomach, intestines and gallbladder.

食郁 【shí yù】由于食滞不消，气机不利所致的一种病证。症见脘腹饱胀，嗳气酸腐、食欲不振、大便不调、脉多滑而紧盛，甚至黄疸、痞块、膨胀等。

Stagnation-Syndrome due to Indigestion a syndrome due to indigestion and dysfunction of qi; manifested as fullness of the stomach and abdomen, erucation with fetid odor, anorexia, irregular bowel movement, smooth and tense pules, or oven jaundice, abdominal mass, tympanites, etc.

食郁肉中毒 【shí yù ròu zhòng dú】指肉类食物放置在密闭器内生热变质，进食后引起的中毒，如呕吐、腹泻，烦乱不安等。

Putrid Meat Poisoning poisoning caused by the ingestion of puterfactive meat, manifested as vomiting, diarrhea, irrability.

食远服 【shí yuán fú】即离正常进食时间较远时服药，通常用于治疗脾胃病。泻下药也可以采用这种服药方法。

Be Taken at a Longer Interval after Meal the suitable time for taking decoction, such as those for treating the spleen and stomach disorders and those for purgation.

食胀 【shí zhàng】因过食生冷；或饥饿不调，谷食不化所致的腹胀。症见脘腹胀满坚硬，甚则胀痛拒按、嗳气泛酸、畏食、自利或便秘等。

Flatulence due to Indigestion a disorder caused by over intake of cold and uncooked food, or immoderate eating leading to indigestion; manifested as abdominal flatulence and rigidity or even pain and tenderness, belching, acid regurgitation, anorexia, diarrhea or constipation etc.

食治 【shí zhì】(食疗)用适当的食物对某些疾病进行治疗或调理。

Dietotherapy the dietetic treatment for the patients in the course of diseases or during convalescence.

食滞胃脘 【shí zhì wèi wǎn】因饮食不节，脾胃运化失职所致的病证。症见胃脘胀痛、嗳腐、呕吐、舌苔厚腻、脉滑等。多见于消化不良、急性胃炎等。

Retention of Indigested Food in the Stomach a disorder due to functional disturbances of the spleen and stomach resulting from immoderate eating and drinking; manifested as epigastric distending pain, eructation

食诸鱼中毒 【shí zhū yú zhòng dú】因误食有毒或变质鱼类引起的中毒。症见头晕、面肿、肤红起瘰瘙痒、心腹闷满烦乱；严重者心悸、气急、甚至休克。

Fish Poisoning intoxication caused by eating poisonous or putrid fish, manifested as dizziness, swollen face, itching and red skin, fullness of the chest and abdomen, irritability, even palpitation, dyspnea and shock in severe cases.

视赤如白 【shì chì rú bái】（视物易色）不能正确识别某些颜色或全部颜色的病证。相当于色盲或色弱。

Colour Blindness inability to recognize one or more of the seven primary colours.

视一为二症 【shì yī wéi èr zhèng】指一物而目视为二的病证。即复视。多由脏腑精气不足,风火、痰邪攻上,或外伤等引起。

Diplopia the perception of two images of a single object, which is due to insufficiency of essence and energy of the viscera and attack of wind, fire phlegm to the eyes, or due to injury.

视衣 【shì yī】 相当于视网膜、脉络膜等组织。内属心、肝、肾等经。

Coats of the Eyeball the eye structure including retina and choroid, attributive to the heart, liver and kidney meridians.

视瞻昏渺 【shì zhān hūn miǎo】多由神劳精亏,血虚气弱引起的视物昏蒙不清。常见于各种内障眼病。

Poor Vision a condition due to overstrain, essence consumption, qi and blood deficiency, seen in various kinds of internal ocular diseases.

室女 【shì nǚ】即未婚的女子。

Home Girl unmarried woman.

室女经闭 【shì nǚ jīng bì】（室女月水不通）指未婚女子经闭。因体质羸弱,肝脾失调,冲任血虚,或因情志不遂,心怀抑郁,气血凝结所致。

Primary Amenorrhea a condition due to general debility, dysfunction of the liver and spleen, blood deficiency of thoroughfare and conception vessels, or emotional upsets leading to stagnation of qi and blood.

嗜偏食 【shì piān shí】偏嗜吃某些食物的一种病态,常与胃肠的病理变化

Special Food Hobby a morbid state usually related to the gastrointestinal

有关。如嗜食辛辣，多属胃寒。 disorders, e. g. a hobby of acid and purgent food is suggestive of stomach-cold syndrome.

嗜卧 【shì wò】指困倦欲睡的一种症候。多因湿胜、脾虚、胆热所致。素体虚弱及病后元气未复也可引起。
Somnolence a condition of sleepiness, usually due to accumulation of dampness, spleen-asthenia, gallbladder-heat or insufficiency of primordial qi during convalesence.

嗜卧欲寐 【shì wò yù mèi】(多寐)困倦欲睡的一种症状。湿邪偏胜、脾虚、胆热等均可引起；亦见于素来身体虚弱，不能适应气候变化的患者。
Drowsiness a symptom caused by the domination of dampness, asthenia of the spleen, or heat-syndrome of the gallbladder and also seen in the debilitated person with inability to accommodate to the climatic variations.

收涩 【shōu sè】(固摄，固涩) 治疗精气耗散，滑脱不收的方法。常与补益药同用。
Astringent Therapy a treatment for excessive loss of essence-qi and body fluid, usually applied together with tonics.

手部疔疮 【shǒu bù dīng chuāng】指生于手部的疔疮。根据其部位不同分为蛇眼疔、蛇头疔、蛇腹疔、托盘疔。多因饮食不节，外感风邪火毒，或创伤引起，辨证分类：1、火毒凝结证 2、腐筋损骨证。
Pustule of the Hand pustules that can be classified as snake-eye-like infection, pustule of the finger tip, thecal whitlow, and palmar pustule by their positions, mostly caused by improper diet, exogenous pathogenic wind-heat, or traumatic injuries. Types of differentiation 1. accumulation of noxious fire 2. puterfaction of the muscles and impairment of bones.

手发背 【shǒu fā bèi】(手背毒)指手掌背面的皮肤感染。
Infection of the Back of the Hand

手心毒 【shǒu xīn dú】指手掌面的皮肤感染。
Infection of the Palm

手指麻木 【shǒu zhǐ má mù】多因气虚而兼有湿痰、瘀血阻滞所致手指麻木不适的一种症状。
Numbness of Fingers a symptom usually caused by deficiency of qi with retention of dampness-phlegm

手指脱臼 【shǒu zhǐ tuō jiè】即手指关节脱臼。

Dislocation of Phalangeal Joints

手足汗 【shǒu zú hàn】因脾胃湿蒸,旁及四肢所致的手足潮湿,多汗症。如见手足心热者属阴亏血虚;手足发凉者属中阳不足。

Polyhidrosis of Hands and Feet a disorder caused by the attack of dampness to the spleen and stomach involving the extremities. That accompanied with warm hands and feet is attributable to the deficiency of yin and blood; and that with cold hands and feet to the insufficiency of middle-energizer.

手足厥冷 【shǒu zú jué lěng】(手足逆冷)四肢肘膝以下厥冷的症状。由阳气衰微,阴寒内盛所致者,常伴有怕冷、下利清谷、脉沉微等;由热邪阻遏,阳气不能通达四肢所致者,常伴有胸腹烦热、口渴等。

Cold Hands and Feet coldness of the extremities below the elbows and knees, that caused by the deficiency of yang-qi and overabundance of yin-cold is usually accompanied with intolerance of cold, lienteric diarrhea, sunken and weak pulse, that caused by the retention of heat and yang-qi failing to flow to the extremities is usually accompanied by feverishness in the chest and abdomen, thirst, etc.

手足心热 【shǒu zú xīn rè】因阴虚内热或火热内郁所致的手足心发热感。

Feverish Sensation over the Palms and Soles a symptom caused by internal heat derived from yin-deficiency or by the stagnation of fire-heat inside the body.

首风 【shǒu fēng】指以头面多汗、头痛、恶风、遇风易发为主要症状的一种疾病。多由洗头后感受风邪所致。

Head-Wind Syndrome a syndrome due to attack or wind after having a shampoo; manifested as sweating over the head and face, aversion to wind, headache, and liability to relapse after exposure to wind.

寿夭 【shòu yāo】从人体形体、气血、骨肉的情况来判断寿命的长短。如形

Life Expectancy the life expectancy of an individual may be

体壮实，肌肉发达者寿命较长；形体虽肥胖，但肌肉不发达者，寿命较短。judged according to the physique and the condition of qi, blood, bones and muscles. In general, a person with strong physique and muscles has a longer life while a fat person with weak muscles has a shorter life.

受盛之腑 【shòu chéng zhī fǔ】指小肠是承受胃腐熟的食糜进行泌别清浊的消化器官，故称。 **Fu Organ in Charge of Reception** referring to the small intestine. It is so called because the small intestine receives the digested food from the stomach.

受盛之官 【shòu chéng zhī guān】指小肠。见受盛之腑。 **Official in Charge of Reception** see "fu organ in charge of reception".

疏表 【shū biǎo】即疏解表邪。使用发散解表作用较弱的药物，治疗症状较轻的外感病的一种方法。 **Dispersing the Factors from the Superficies** a treatment for the exogenous febrile disease with mild symptoms by the application of mild disphoretics.

疏表化湿 【shū biǎo huà shī】治疗湿邪在上焦卫分的方法。症见头重而胀、肢体酸疼、口不渴、苔白腻、脉浮濡等。 **Dispersing the Superficies to Eliminates the Dampness** a treatment for the accumulation of dampness in weifen of the upper energizer, applicable to the case manifested as feeling of haviness and distension of the head, sorness of the extremities, no thirst, whitish and greasy fur on the tongue, floating and soft pules, etc.

疏风 【shu fēng】用祛风解表药疏散风邪的一种治法。临床上常视风寒表证、风热表证或风湿表证的不同，运用相应的药物，如风寒表证常用防风、桂枝、藁本等。 **Dispersing Wind** a treatment for dispersing wind in the superficies by the application of different drugs varying with the presence of cold or heat, e.g., Rhizoma Ledebouriellae, Ramalus Cinnamomi, Rhizoma Ligustici, etc. used for wind-cold syndrome in the superficies.

疏风泄热 【shū fēng xiè rè】即解表清 **Eliminating Wind and Heat** a

热。用具有疏散表邪的清热作用的药物，治疗外感风邪兼有里热的方法。适用于头痛鼻塞、咳嗽、咽痛口渴、舌质红、苔薄黄、脉浮数等症。

treatment for the exposure to wind accompanied with heat-syndrome in the interior by the application of drugs of eliminating the wind in the superficies and clearing away the heat, applicable to the case manifested as stuffy nose, cough, sore throat, thirst, reddish tongue with thin and yellowish fur, floating and fast pulse, etc.

疏肝 【shū gān】(舒肝、疏肝理气、泄肝) 疏散肝气郁结的治法。常用于肝气郁结。症见两胁胀痛、胸闷不舒或恶心、呕吐酸水、食欲不振、腹痛腹泻、舌苔薄、脉弦等。

Dispersing the Stagnated Liver-Qi a treatment for the stagnation of liver-qi, applicable to the case with manifestations as distending pain over the hypochondrium, oppressive feeling over the chest, nausea, acid regurgation, loss of appetite, abdominal pain, diarrhea, thin fur on the tongue, wiry pulse, etc.

疏通经络 【shū tōng jīng luò】用行气活血及具有温通作用的药物组成方剂，以治疗因气血凝滞致经络阻塞的一种方法。

Dregding the Meridian Passage a treatment for the obstruction of meridians resulting from the stagnation of qi and blood, by the application of prescriptions composed of drugs with the action of promoting qi and blood circulation and with warming and dispersing effects.

疏郁理气 【shū yù lǐ qì】是治疗因情志抑郁而引起气滞的方法。适用于胸膈痞满，两胁及下腹部胀痛等症。

Regulating Qi by the Alleviation of Mental Depression a treatment for the stagnation of qi due to mental depression, applicable to the disorder with feeling of oppression over the chest and distending pain of hypochondria and lower abdomen.

暑 【shǔ】六淫之一。暑为阳邪，多在夏季致病。感受暑邪后表现为高热、

Summer-Heat one of the six pathogentic factors, yang in nature,

口渴、多汗、心烦、体倦、脉洪等。usually in summer time, and causing the syndromes manifested as high fever, thirst, profuse sweating, restlessness, fatigue, bounding pulse, etc.

暑病 【shǔ bìng】泛指夏天感受暑热邪气所发生的多种热性病。一般多指暑温、中暑等病证。

Summer-Heat Disease febrile diseases due to attack of summer-heat in summer time, which usually refers to summer-heat warm syndrome and sunstroke.

暑风 【shǔ fēng】1、指伤暑后又感风邪,以致手足时有搐搦者;2、暑温病,因热盛而见昏迷抽搐等症。3、指暑天身痒如针刺或见皮肤红肿。

Summer-Heat Wind Syndrome 1. a syndrome due to attack of summer-heat followed by the exposure to wind, manifested as muscular cramps of the extremities; or due to hyperactivity of heat in a case of summer-heat warm syndrome, manifested as coma and convulsion. 2. general itching or redness and swelling of the skin in summer time.

暑厥 【shǔ jué】因暑热闭窍所致的厥证。症见卒然昏倒,昏不知人、身热、手足厥冷、牙关微紧或口开、脉洪大或滑数等。

Syncope due to Summer-Heat a disorder resulting from the obstruction of upper orifices by summer-heat; manifested as sudden syncope, fever, cold extremities, lock jaw or open mouth, bounding and large pulse or smooth and fast pulse, etc.

暑咳 【shǔ ké】指暑邪伤肺而致的咳嗽。症见身热、咳嗽无痰或少痰,气急面赤、口渴、胸闷胁痛。脉濡而数等。

Cough due to Summer-Heat a disease manifested as watery diarrhea, nausea, vomiting, abdominal pain, thirst, discharge of reddish urine, spontaneous perspiration, dirty complexion, greasy or yellowish fur on the tongue, etc.

暑痢 【shǔ lì】由于感受暑热所致的痢疾。症见腹痛下痢发热。或见汗出、面垢、渴欲引饮,小便不利,脉虚等。

Dysentery due to Summer-Heat a type of dysentery accompanied with abdominal pain, diarrhea, fever,

暑疟 【shǔ nüè】1、指受暑邪而得疟者。症见但热不寒或壮热，烦渴而呕、肌肉消瘦、背寒、面垢等。2、见湿疟。

暑热 【shǔ rè】1、即暑邪。2、外感暑邪的发热病证。

暑热胁痛 【shǔ rè xié tòng】指暑证兼见胁肋疼痛之症。

暑热证 【shǔ rè zhèng】外感暑邪的热证。

暑痧 【shǔ shā】因暑天感受秽浊痧邪所致的一种病证。症见呕吐、恶心、泻下臭秽、腹痛时紧时缓、头晕、汗出如雨、脉洪等。

暑湿 【shǔ shī】为夏季常见病，是暑热挟湿所致的病证。症见胸脘痞闷、心烦、身热、怠倦、舌苔黄腻等。

暑湿眩晕 【shǔ shī xuàn yūn】指暑令感受湿邪所致的眩晕。症见头昏目眩、身热自汗、面垢背寒、烦渴引饮、脉虚数、或恶寒、身重且痛、脉虚缓

sweating, dirty complexion, thirst with desire for drinking, dysuria, feeble pulse, etc.

Summer-Heat Malaria 1. malaria caused by attack of summer-heat; manifested as fever without chills or high fever, thirst and vomiting, emaciation, feeling of cold over the back, dirty complexion, etc. 2. referring to damp-type malaria.

Summer-Heat 1. summer-heat 2. a febrile disease caused by the attack of summer-heat.

Hypochondrium due to Summer-Heat

Febrile Disease due to Summer-Heat

Sha-Syndrome due to Summer-Heat

a disease caused by the attack of summer-dampness; manifested as vomiting, nausea, diarrhea with foul stools, intermittent abdominal pain, dizziness, profuse perspiration, bounding pulse, etc.

Summer-Heat-Dampness Syndrome

a common disease seen in summer which is caused by summer-heat and dampness, manifested as feeling of fullness and oppression over the chest and epigastrium, restlessness, fever, fatigue, yellow and greasy fur on the tongue, etc.

Dizziness due to Attack of Dampness in Summer Days a syndrome manifested as dizziness, fever, spontaneous perspiration, dirty complexion, cold-

等。

暑温 【shǔ wēn】指感受暑热之邪而发生的一种急性热病。症见高热、口渴、面赤、自汗、少气等。

暑痫 【shǔ xián】指感受暑邪，暑热动风所致的病证。症见发热、昏迷、抽搐等。

暑泻 【shǔ xiè】因感受暑邪所致的泄泻。症见泄泻如水、恶心、呕吐、腹痛、烦渴尿赤、自汗、面垢、苔腻或黄腻等，有偏湿和偏热之分。

暑瘵 【shǔ zhài】因感受暑热所致的突然咳嗽咯血的病证。由暑热之邪灼伤肺络引起，常伴烦热口渴、气喘、头目不清、脉洪无力等。

鼠疫 【shǔ yì】因疫毒侵入血分，瘀阻不行所致的烈性传染病。

漱涤 【shù dí】用各种药物加水煎成药液，使用时用温水配成一定浓度，

ness of the back, extreme thirst and feeble, fast pules; or as chillness, fatigue, general pain, feeble and slow pules, etc.

Summer-Heat-Warm Syndrome an acute febrile disease caused by summer-heat; manifested as high fever, thirst, flushed face, spontaneous persperation, shortness of breath, etc.

Convulsive Seizures Caused by Summer-Heat a disorder due to the wind activated by summer-heat; manifested as fever, coma, convulsion, etc.

Diarrhea due to Summer-Heat a disease manifested as watery diarrhea, nausea, vomiting, abdominal pain, thirst, discharge of reddish urine, spontaneous perspiration, dirty complexion, greasy or yellowish fur on the tongue, inclination to dampness or to heat.

Hemoptysis Caused by Summer-Heat hemoptysis due to damage of the lung collaterals by the summer-heat, usually accompanied with feverish sensation, thirst, shortness of breath, dizziness, bounding but weak pulse, etc

Plague an acute infectious disease with a high fatality rate, due to a virulent pestilent factor invading xuefen leading to the stagnation of blood circulation.

Gargle a treatment for the inflammation and ulcer of the buccal cavity

进行含漱，以清洁口腔咽喉部，并能治疗口腔咽喉的炎症、肿痛及溃疡等的一种治疗方法。

衰者补之 【shuāi zhě bǔ zhī】同虚者补之。

双乳蛾 【shuāng rǔ é】双侧急性扁桃体炎。

水不涵木 【shuǐ bù hán mù】肾阴不足而不能滋养肝脏，引起肝阴不足，虚风内动的病理。常见有眩晕、耳鸣、遗精、腰酸、口干、甚至出现抽搐等等。

水不化气 【shuǐ bù huà qì】水液代谢障碍的病理，与肺、脾、肾功能障碍有密切关系，症见小便不利、水肿等。

水喘 【shuǐ chuǎn】因水饮犯肺引起以气喘为主症的病证。伴见胸膈满闷、腹胀、怔忡、面目或四肢浮肿、小便不利等。

水痘 【shuǐ dòu】（水疮、水疱、水花、肤疹）是指以发热、皮肤及粘膜分批出现斑疹和丘疹为特征的一种急性儿童传染病。由外感时邪风毒、内蕴湿热，扰于卫分所致。辨证分类 1、风热证 2、热毒证。

and pharynx, by rinsing the mouth and throat with medicinal solution.

Asthenia-Syndrome Should Be Treated with Tonic Therapy

Bilateral Acute Tonsillitis

Water Fails to Nourish Wood a morbid condition of the deficiency of liver-yin with the hyperactivity of asthenic wind resulting from the inability of kidney-yin to nourish the liver, manifested as dizziness, tinnitus, nocturnal emission, thirst, even convulsion.

Disturbance of Body Fluid Metabolism a morbid condition attributed to the dysfunction of the lung, spleen and kidney, manifested as dysuria, etc.

Dyspnea due to Fluid Retention a disease with dyspnea as the feeling major symptom, which is caused by fluid retention in the lung, accompanied with oppressions over the chest, flatulence, palpitation, edema of face or extremities, dysuria, etc.

Chickenpox an infectious infantile disease markde by fever, respective appearance of papules and macules on skin and the mucous membrane, caused by exogenous epidemic noxious wind and interior accumulation of damp-heat disturbing weifen. Types of differentiation 1. syndrome of wind-heat 2. syndrome of notox-

水　shui

...ious heat.

水毒【shuǐ dú】指接触被某种致病微生物污染后的水而发生的一类疾病。常见有恶寒、头痛、心烦、发热、谵语、狂躁或下部生疮，不痛、不痒、脓溃等症。

Disease Caused by Contaminated Water the infectious diseases resulting from a contact with the water contaminated by pathogenic microorganisms, which is manifested as chilliness, headache, restlessness, fever, delirium, mania, ulcer without paining and itching in the lower part of the body, degeneration with pus, etc.

水毒病【shuǐ dú bìng】因接触疫水引起的一种流行性疾病。类似血吸虫病。

Poisonous Water Disease an epidemic disease due to contact with infectious water; similar to schistosomiasis.

水飞【shuǐ fēi】中药炮制的方法之一。先将药物碾成药末，放入乳钵内加水同研至极细，再加入多量水搅拌后，将含有药粉的水倾出、过滤、干燥、而得到极细的药粉，多用于矿物药。

Grinding in Water a method of processing crude traditional Chinese drugs, by cutting it into small pieces and then grinding into fine power by adding water at the same time, and finally by filtrating and drying.

水府【shuǐ fǔ】指膀胱。因它贮藏尿液，故称水府。

Water Storage referring to the bladder. It is so called because the bladder stores the urine.

水谷之海【shuǐ gǔ zhī hǎi】指胃。四海之一。指胃有接受容纳食物的功能。

The Sea of Water and Cereals one of the four seas, referring to the stomach, where the food is received and stored.

水谷之精【shuǐ gǔ zhī jīng】（后天之精）由饮食所化生的，构成人体，维持机体生命活动所需的营养物质。它可转化为生殖之精。

Essential Substance from Food also named as acquired essential substance. It is derived from foods and is necessary for the constitution of the human body and for the maintainance of health and physical activities. It can be converted to the essential substance for reproduction.

水臌【shuǐ gǔ】以腹水为主症的病证。

Ascites accumulation of fluid in the

常伴有小便不利、胁痛、面色萎黄、或黄疸。多由肝气郁结，脾失健运，或酒食不节，水湿结聚所致。

abdominal cavity due to stagnation of liver-qi, dysfunction of the spleen, or retention of water caused by immoderate drinking and eating; usually accompanied with dysuria, hypochondriac pain, sallow complexion, or jaundice.

水罐法 【shuǐ guàn fǎ】竹罐用水煮沸后进行拔罐的一种治疗方法。适用于风寒湿痹、痈肿等疾病。

Water Cupping Therapy a method of cupping with a hot bamboo cup from the boiling water, applicable to the diseases such as wind-cold-dampness type of arthralgia, carbuncle, etc.

水寒射肺 【shuǐ hán shè fèi】寒邪与水气侵犯肺脏引起的病理。症见咳嗽、气喘、痰多而稀白、舌苔白腻等。

Lung Attacked by Cold and Accumulated Fluid a morbid condition manifested as productive cough with thin, whitish sputum, dyspnea, whitish and greasy fur on the tongue, etc.

水火不济 【shuǐ huǒ bù jì】肾的水火或心火与肾水互相制约、互相协调功能丧失的病理。常出现心烦、失眠、遗精等。

Water and Fire Fail to Coordinate each other a morbid condition caused by the incoordination between kidney-yin and kidney-fire or kidney-yin and heart-fire, manifested as restlessness, insomnia, nocturnal emission, etc.

水火烫伤 【shuǐ huǒ tàng shāng】因开水或火接触皮肤所致。根据其程度分为Ⅰ度（红斑），Ⅱ度（水泡）包括浅Ⅱ度和深Ⅱ度，Ⅲ度（焦痂）。辨证分类 1. 火毒炽盛证 2. 火盛伤阴证 3. 火毒内攻脏腑，包括（1）热毒传心（2）热毒传肺（3）热毒传肝（4）热毒传脾（5）热毒传肾 4. 阴损及阳证 5. 气血两虚证 6. 阴伤胃败证。

Burn a condition due to exposure to hot water or fire, which can be classified according to the seriousness of the condition as three types; first-degree burn (redness of the skin), second-degree burn (blisters) including the superficial and deep types, third-degree burn (eschar). Types of differentiation 1. excess of noxious fire 2. impairment of yin due to excess of fire 3. invasion of zang-fu organs by noxious fire, including (1) invasion of the heart by noxious heat (2) invasion of the lung by noxious heat (3) invasion of the liver by noxious heat (4) invasion of the spleen by noxious heat (5) invasion of the kidney by noxious heat 4. impairment of yin and yang syndrome 5. deficiency of qi and blood 6. impairment of yin and dysfunction of the stomach.

水火相济 【shuǐ huǒ xiāng jì】肾的水火或心火与肾水互相制约、互相协调的生理功能，藉此以维持它们的正常活动。

Water and Fire Coordinate each other coordination between kidney-yin and kidney-fire, or kidney-yin and heart fire, a physiological function necessary for the maintainence of normal activities of the organs.

水火之脏 【shuǐ huǒ zhī zàng】即肾脏。因肾藏元阴、元阳，用水火来代表。

Viscera Attributed to Water and Fire referring to the kidney. It is so named because the kidney stores premier-yin and premier-yang, which are attributive to water and fire respectively.

水结胸 【shuǐ jié xiōng】因水饮结于胸胁所致的病证。表现为胸胁闷痛、心下怔忡、颈项强硬、头汗出等。

Sydrome Caused by Accumulation of Fluid in the Thorax a disorder manifested as dull pain in the chest, palpitation, stiffneck, sweating over the head, etc.

水精 【shuǐ jīng】即水谷所生的精微物质。

Refined Substances of Food the nutrients derived from the water and cereals.

水亏火旺 【shuǐ kuī huǒ wàng】1. 肾阴不足，致命门之火偏亢的病理。症见牙齿疼痛且有浮动感、性欲亢进、遗精等。2. 指肾阴不足、心火偏亢的病理。

An Excess of Fire due to Insufficiency of Fluid 1. a morbid condition of hyperactivity of fire from the gate of life caused by the deficiency of kidney-yin; manifested as toothache,

水轮 【shuǐ lún】即瞳神，配属于肾。它的病变与肾和膀胱有关。

水逆 【shuǐ nì】指胃有水饮停留，水气不化的病证。症见渴欲饮水，水入即吐。

水气 【shuǐ qì】1. 泛指出现水肿的疾病。2. 饮证，如水饮、痰饮等。

水气凌心 【shuǐ qì líng xīn】因脾肾功能低下，气化障碍，水液停留体内引起水肿、痰饮，进而导致心脏功能障碍的病理。症见心悸、气促等。

水疝 【shuǐ shàn】指单侧性阴囊肿大，逐渐增大，伴阴囊下坠感。多因水湿下注或感受风寒湿邪所致。辨证分类：1. 肾气不足证 2. 湿热下注证 3. 肾虚寒湿证 4. 瘀血阻络证。

swollen gum, excessive libido, nocturnal emission, etc. 2. a morbid condition of hyperactivity of heart-fire caused by deficiency of kidney-yin.

Water-Wheel referring to the pupil, which is linked closely with the kidney. Its disorders usually indicate the involvement of the kidney and bladder.

Adverse Rising of Fluid a disorder due to retention of fluid in the stomach, manifested as desire for drinking and vomiting immediately after drinking.

1. Edema 2. Fluid-Retention Syndrome referring to the disorders with retention of fluid, phlegm, etc.

Heart Involved by the Retention of Fluid a morbid condition with dysfunction of the heart due to retention of fluid or phlegm caused by the hypofunction of the spleen and kidney; manifested as palpitation, dyspnea, etc.

Hydrocele referring to the mass in the unilateral side of the scrotum, which gradually increases in size, accompanied by skining sensation in the scrotum, mostly caused by downward flowing of water or invasion of wind, coldness and dampness. Tyes of differentiation 1. deficiency of kidney-qi 2. downward flowing of damp-heat 3. deficiency of the kidney and invasion of cold-dampness 4. blood stasis blocking collaterals.

水土不服 【shuǐ tǔ bù fú】由于身体不能适应新到地区的气候、环境、饮食的改变而出现的各种病状。常见的有食欲不振、腹胀、腹痛、泄泻及月经不调等。

Unacclimatization a disorder caused by being unaccustomed to the changes of climate, environment and diet; manifested as loss of appetite, abdominal pain and flatulence, diarrhea, irregular menstruation, etc.

水泻 【shuǐ xiè】(注泻) 排出水样粪便的腹泻。

Watery Diarrhea diarrhea with discharge of watery stools.

水性流下 【shuǐ xìng liú xià】比喻湿邪所致的病变有向下趋势的特点。如腹泻、下肢倦怠或下肢浮肿等。

Water Is Flowing Down the pathological changes caused by dampness tend to develop downwards, just like water always flowing down. It may be manifested as diarrhea, lassitude or edema of the lower limbs, etc.

水针疗法 【shuǐ zhēn liáo fǎ】见穴位注射疗法。

Point Injection Therapy

水肿 【shuǐ zhǒng】(水胀、胕肿) 体内水湿潴留而全身浮肿的一种病证。多与肾、脾、肺、三焦、膀胱等脏腑功能失调有关。

Edema a condition of anasarca caused by the retention of fluid in the body, usually resulting from the dysfunction of the kidney, spleen, lung, triple energizer and bladder.

水渍疮 【shuǐ zì chuāng】因长时间浸入水中,加之局部摩擦而成的皮肤病。表现为局部皮肤肿胀、变白起皱,继而溃烂流水并有搔痒。

Paddy-Field Dermatitis dermatitis due to long—time soaking in the water with local abrasion; manifested as local swelling of the skin, whitened, wrinkled, followed by itching, erosion and oozing.

顺传 【shùn chuán】疾病按一般规律传变。如伤寒由表及里;温病由卫分传入气分等。

Disease Developing in Due Order the development of a disease in accordance with due order, for example, the exogenous febrile diseases develop from the superficies to the interior, or the seasonal febrile diseases develop from the weifen to the qifen.

顺证 【shùn zhèng】疾病按一般过程发展的表现。没有严重并发症,经过

Case with a Favourable Prognosis a disease which develops without

适当的治疗可逐渐痊愈。

瞤 【shùn】身体某一部分不自主跳动的症状。

数脉 【shuò mài】脉搏急速，每分钟超过90次以上，主热证。数而有力为实热，数而无力为虚热。

思伤脾 【sī shāng pí】思虑过度损伤脾胃，致脾运失常而产生食欲不振、消化不良、腹胀、大便溏等症状。

思则气结 【sī zé qì jié】由于思虑过度致脾气郁结，引起脾胃功能紊乱的病理。症见食欲不振、胸脘满闷、大便溏泄等。

嘶嗄 【sī shà】声音嘶哑。多因风热犯肺、津液受损所致。常见于急、慢性咽喉炎或喉癌及声带创伤等患者。

死舌痈 【sǐ shé yōng】指色白木痛的一种舌痈。由心火炽盛，胃中伏热熏蒸，化毒凝滞而成。

死胎 【sǐ tāi】即胎儿在子宫内死亡。

complication and can be cured readily after proper treatment.

Twitching an involuntary movement with slight spasmodic jerks of different parts of the body.

Fast Pulse a pulse condition with more than 90 beats per minute, indicating a heat-syndrome. The fast and strong pulse indicates sthenia-heat syndrome; while the fast and weak indicates asthenia-heat syndrome.

Anxiety Impairing the Spleen a condition of impairment of digestive function due to overanxiety injuring spleen and stomach, manifested as poor appetite, indigestion, flatulence, loose stools, etc.

Anxiety may Lead to Stagnation of Qi a morbid condition of functional disorder of the spleen and stomach due to anxiety; manifested as anorexia, fullness of the chest and epigastrium, loose stools or diarrhea, etc.

Hoarseness of Voice a morbid state caused by the attack of wind-heat to the lung and the consumption of body fluid, usually seen in acute and chronic laryngitis, laryngeal carcinoma or injury of vocal cords.

White-Colour Abscess of the Tongue a type of tongue abscess accompanied with numbness and pain, due to formation of pus resulting from the hyperactivity of heart-fire and the accumulation of heat in the stomach.

Dead Fetus fetus died in the uterus,

多因跌仆损伤胎体，或母体患热病，热毒伤胎，或母体素弱，病后胎元失养所致；也有胎儿脐带绕颈死者。

due to trauma, or damage of the fetus by heat when the mother is suffering from a febrile disease or under nourishment of the fetus resulting from debility of the mother, or suffocation of the fetus by twining of the umbilical cord, etc.

死胎不下 【sǐ tāi bù xià】胎儿死于母腹，不能自行娩出的病证。可发生于妊娠期及临产时，多因孕妇气血虚弱，子宫无力娩出胎儿或因瘀血阻滞所致。

Retention of Dead Fetus failure of expulsion of the nonviable fetus from the uterus during pregnancy and delivery; due to deficiency of qi and blood or the obstruction by blood stasis.

死血胁痛 【sǐ xuè xié tòng】指瘀血停留所致的胁痛。多由肝脾气滞，久病入络，血行瘀阻或跌仆闪挫，瘀血内停所致。症见胁肋刺痛，拒按，痛处固定不移，入夜痛甚，或见痞块、脉多沉涩等。

Hypochondriac Pain due to Blood Stasis a disorder due to accumulation of blood stasis in the body resulting from the stagnation of liver-qi, the obstruction of blood flow or trauma; manifested as localized stabbing pain over the hypochondria which is aggravated by pressure or at night, palpable mass, sunken and uneven pulse, etc.

四傍 【sì bàng】指心、肝、肺、肾四脏。根据五行的理论，五脏合五方，五脏中脾主中央，因此，将其他四脏称为四傍。

The Four nearby Zang-Organs referring to the heart, liver, lung and kidney. In accordance with the five-element theory, the five zang-organs match five locations (east, south, west, north and center), of which the spleen matches the center, and the others are considered as nearby zang-organs.

四海 【sì hǎi】指髓海、血海、气海和水谷之海。

Four Seas referring to the sea of marrows, the sea of blood, the sea of qi and the sea of water and cereals.

四极 【sì jí】即四肢。

Four Extremities

四末 【sì mò】1、指四肢，2、指手指和足趾。 **Four Distal Parts** 1. the four extremities 2. the fingers and toes.

四逆 【sì nì】四肢厥冷的症状。 **Cold Limbs** referrring to the cold sensation of the four extremities.

四气 【sì qì】(四性)中药所具有的寒、热、温、凉四种药性。 **Four Characters** referring to the nature of Chinese medicine concerning with its therapeutic effect, i. e., cold, hot, warm and cool.

四时 【sì shí】即春、夏、秋、冬四季。 **Four Seasons** a general term for spring, summer, autumn and winter.

四时不正之气 【sì shí bù zhèng zhī qì】即四季不正常气候，如冬天应寒反暖，春天应暖反寒。它往往能影响人体的适应性，降低机体的抗病能力。容易诱发各种疾病。 **Abnormal Weather in Four Seasons** the conditions, such as warm in winter while it should be cold and cold in spring while it should be warm, will often affect the adaptability of human body and decrease the body resistance, and will bring about various diseases.

四时之脉 【sì shí zhī mài】随四季气候变化而相应出现的脉象，如春季脉偏弦，冬季脉偏沉等。 **The Pulse Variations in the Four Seasons** the normal variation of the pulse condition of a healthy person occurring in different seasons, e. g., the pulse is likely to be wiry in spring and sunken in winter.

四维 【sì wéi】指四肢。 **Extremities**

四饮 【sì yǐn】痰饮、悬饮、溢饮、支饮等四种饮证的总称。 **Four Types of Water Retention** a collective term for phlegm retention, pleural effusion, anasarca and excessive fluid in the hypochondrium and epigastrium.

四诊 【sì zhěn】四种诊病方法。即望诊、闻诊、问诊和切诊。 **Four Diagnostic Methods** a joint term for inspection, auscultation and olfaction, interrogation, pulse feeling and palpation.

四诊合参 【sì zhěn hé cān】在辩证过程中，必须把通过望、闻、问、切等 **Comprehensive Analysis of the Data Gained by the Four Methods of Di-**

四种诊法所获得的材料,进行全面的分析综合,才能确切的判断病情,作出合理的诊断。

四肢拘急 【sì zhī jū jí】四肢肌肉拘挛,难以伸屈的一种症状。多因寒邪侵袭经脉或热灼阴液,使筋脉失养所致。

四肢麻木 【sì zhī má mù】即手足麻木,不知痛痒。多由气虚风痰侵入经络,营卫流通受阻或气血亏虚,经络失养引起。

四肢疲倦 【sì zhī pí juàn】简称肢倦。指四肢倦怠疲乏的症状。多由气血衰弱或脾虚湿邪内阻,四肢失养所致。

四肢无力 【sì zhī wú lì】指四肢软弱无力的症状。多见于痿、痹等证。

松皮癣 【sōng pí xuǎn】(白疕)患处皮肤损害如松皮状的一种皮肤病。多由风寒外袭,营卫失调或风热侵入毛孔,郁久化燥,使皮肤失养所致。症见癣形大小不一,上有白色皮屑,局

agnosis in differentiation of syndromes, a comprehensive analysis of the data gained by inspection, auscultation and olfaction, interrogation, pulse feeling and palpation must be made in order to judge the status of illness precisely and make a correct diagnosis.

Spasms of Limbs a morbid condition mostly caused by invasion of meridians by pathogenic cold or impairment of the yin fluid by intense heat, which impairs the nourishment of the muscular system.

Numbness of Limbs a morbid condition due to qi deficiency complicated by invasion of meridians and collaterals by pathogenic wind and phlegm, leading to the obstruction of the ying-wei system or deficiency of qi and blood which impairs the nourishment of meridians and collaterals.

Lassitude of Limbs a symptom mostly due to deficiency of qi and blood or retention of pathogenic dampness because of spleen deficiency, which impairs the nourishment of the limbs.

Myasthenia of Limbs a symptom which is mostly seen in Bi syndrome and Wei syndrome.

Psoriasis a skin disease in which the skin of the affected area is damaged and looks like pine skin, which is mostly caused by exogenous invasion of pathogenic wind and cold, causing

部搔痒，反复发作，经久不愈。类似银屑病。

送服 【sòng fú】服用丸剂的方法。根据丸剂的性质，可用温开水，淡盐水或清茶等送服。

搜风逐寒 【sōu fēng zhú hán】治疗风寒痰湿之邪留滞经络的方法。适用于中风、手足麻木日久不愈、腿臂局部疼痛或筋脉挛痛、屈伸不利等。

溲数 【sōu shuò】指小便频数、排尿次数增加。

粟疮 【sù chuāng】多由火邪内郁，外受风邪，风火相结，郁阻肌肤所致的疾病。症见遍身发疹如粟、色红作痒、搔之成疮、日久皮肤粗糙、厚如蛇皮。即丘疹性湿疹、痒疹。

disturbance of yingwei system or invasion of pathogenic wind and heat into skin pores, long term of qi stagnation turning into dryness, leading to poor nourishment of the skin, marked by kineas varying in size covered by silver white scales, local itching with repeated attacks, which is difficult to cure.

Taking Medicine with Water taking medicine with warm boiled water, slightly salty water or tea according to the nature of the pills which are taken.

Arresting Wind and Expelling Cold a therapeutic method to treat illness caused by retention of wind, cold and phlegm in the meridians, such as paralysis of the limbs as the sequela of apoplexy, local pain of the legs and arms or spasmodic pain of the muscles and limited movement.

Frequent Micturition freqent urine

Eczema Papulosum a skin disease usually caused by invasion of pathogenic fire and affection of of exopathic wind with both combined to accumulate in the superficial portion of the skin, marked by papules all over the body shaped like millets, red in color and itching in sensation, which may turn into ulceration after scratching, roughhess of skin a long time later which is as thick as that of the snake skin.

酸 【suān】酸味的药物。一般有收敛和固涩的作用,如山茱萸敛汗,五倍子涩肠止久泻。

酸甘化阴 【suān gān huà yīn】酸味和性味甘寒药同用以益阴的治法。适用于阴不济阳。症见失眠多梦、健忘、舌赤糜烂、脉细数,或脾阴不足、消化功能障碍等。

酸苦涌泄为阴 【suān kǔ yǒng xiè wéi yīn】酸味苦味药物有催吐、导泻的作用,其药性属阴。如胆矾(味酸能催吐)、大黄(味苦能泻下)均属阴。

酸咸无升 【suān xián wú shēng】酸味咸味药物的药性一般是向下向里的,没有升提的作用。

髓 【suǐ】奇恒之腑之一。包括脊髓和骨髓,由肾的精气和水谷精微所化生,有营养骨骼和脑的作用。

髓海 【suǐ hǎi】指脑。四海之一。脑是诸髓会聚的地方,故称。

Sour Taste referring to the drugs sour in taste which has the function of inducing astringency, such as Fructus Corni used to arrest sweating, Galla Chiensis to astringe the intestine to arrest long-standing diarrhea.

Nourishing Yin with Sour and Sweet Drugs a therapeutic method to promote the production of yin by using sour and sweet drugs in combination, indicated for syndromes with the failure of yin to keep yang well, marked by insomnia, dreaminess, forgetfulness, redness and erosion of the tongue, thready and fast pulse, or deficiency of the spleen-yin and its hypofunction in digestion.

Sour and Bitter Medicines Which Induce Vomiting And Diarrhea Are Attributive To Yin such as Chalcanthite (sour taste to induce vomiting) and Caulis Fibraureae (bitter taste to induce diarrhea) attributive to yin.

Sour and Satly Flavours with no Lifting Property drugs in sour and salty flavours have the property of being downward and inward, but no lifting.

Marrow one of the extraordinary organs, consisting of bone marrow and spinal cord formed by kidney essence and refined substance of foodstuff, having the function of nourishing the bone and tonifying the brain.

Reservoir (sea) of Marrow referring to the brain, one of the four

髓会 【suǐ huì】八会穴之一。即悬钟穴，骨髓的精气会聚的地方。

Influential Point of the Marrow the point where the essence of bone marrow meet, i. e., Xuanzhong (GB39).

髓涕 【suǐ tì】指脑漏症的鼻涕。

Marrow-Like Nasal Discharge incessant nasal discharge usually seen in sinusitis.

飧泄 【sūn xiè】(飧泻) 指泄泻完谷不化。因脾胃虚弱或风、湿、寒、热诸邪客犯肠胃所致。

Lienteric Diarrhea referring to diarrhea with undigested food, caused by deficiency of the spleen and stomach or invasion of intestine and stomach by pathogenic wind, dampness, cold and heat.

损伤瘀血 【sǔn shāng yū xuè】因外伤后血离经脉，停于肢体组织内所致。症状可因损伤部位不同、瘀血量之多少而异。如皮肤肿痛青紫、胸胁胀闷、身热、腹部瘀块、血瘕等。

Blood Stasis due to Injury a morbid condition caused by bleeding from the blood vessels and accumulated in the tissues of the limbs with different manifestations because of the different parts of injuries and the seriousness of the stasis, such as purplish green skin which is swelling and painful, distension and stuffiness of the chest and hypochondrium, fever, blood clot and blood mass in the abdomen.

缩脚流注 【suō jiǎo liú zhù】发于髂窝部肌肉深处的流注。患侧伸展受限，强伸则剧痛，可伴有发热、恶寒，患者多屈曲患腿以减轻疼痛。

Abscess of Iliac Fossa with Flexed Leg abscess deep in the muscles of iliac fossa which caused limitation of the leg of the affected side to extend. Any attempt to extend would cause severe pain accompanied by fever, and aversion to cold. Patients usually flex the affected leg to relieve the pain.

锁肛痔 【suǒ gāng zhì】肛门内外如竹节锁紧，形如海蜇、里急后重，粪便细而带扁，时流臭水的疾病。相当于肛管直肠癌。

Anorectal Carcinoma a morbid condition with the anus corrugated, shaped like jellyfish, tenesmus with the stool thready flat in shape, and with fetid watery discharge from time to time.

锁喉痈 【suǒ hóu yōng】生于喉结处的外痈。由外感风温，肺胃积热上壅所致。症见红肿绕喉、焮热疼痛、甚则肿延胸前、堵塞咽喉、汤水难下。即颈部蜂窝织炎。

Throat-Blocking Phlegmon phlegmon in the neck caused by invasion of exogenous wind and dampness, and upward invasion of the accumulated heat in the lung and stomach, characterized by redness and swelling around the throat, fever, pain, or even swelling which extends to the chest, obstruction of the throat and difficulty in swallowing.

锁口 【suǒ kǒu】指疮口不敛，周围坚硬的症证。多因疮疡溃后感受风热湿毒，或外用药物不当所致。

Boil with Indurated Edge a condition mostly due to ulcers affected by pathogenic wind, heat and dampness, or improper use of drugs externally.

锁子骨伤 【suǒ zǐ gǔ shāng】即锁骨骨折。多因跌、坠、撞、击所致。症见局部肿胀、疼痛、拒按，可摸得移位的骨折端，患侧上肢活动受限。

Fracture of the Clavicle a condition mostly caused by fall and contusion, marked by local swelling, pain, tenderness with the dislocated fractured part being easily felt, and limited movement of the upper limbs on the affected side.

溻皮疮 【tā pí chuāng】（胎溻皮疮）由孕母过食五辛炙煿等物，或父母患杨梅毒传染于胎儿所致的疾病。症见胎儿表皮呈片状脱落、肉色红润、如汤烫状，逐渐扩大，向四周迅速蔓延，甚则大部分皮脱或遍体无皮。

Exfoliative Dermatitis of Newborn a morbid condition due to the intake of hot spicy food of the pregnant mother or parents with syphilis, manifested by exfoliation by pieces with the fresh part red and moist, if like scald burn, it extends to the nearby areas rapidly, or even exfoliation occurring to the most part of the body

溻浴 【tā yù】外治法的一种。将药物煎成药液,洗浴、浸泡或湿敷患处。适用皮肤病、荨麻疹、关节炎等。

苔垢 【tāi gòu】舌苔污垢,常是消化不良或湿浊内停的反映。

苔滑 【tāi huá】舌苔湿润而光滑,常视其厚薄及颜色的不同而反映不同的病变。如苔薄白而滑,多为内有寒湿之邪。

苔润 【tāi rùn】舌苔湿润。湿润而薄白,为正常的舌苔;若湿润而厚腻则属病理性舌苔,多因湿邪过盛引起。

胎病 【tāi bìng】指婴儿癫痫。

胎不长 【tāi bù zhǎng】(胎痿不长)指胎儿生长的速度较正常缓慢。多因漏红伤胎;或孕妇素体虚弱;或有宿疾,气血不足,胎失滋养所致。

胎不正 【tāi bù zhèng】指胎位不正。妊娠后因气滞或临产惊恐,影响胞胎转运所致。

and even to the whole body.

Decoction Bath therapeutic method performed by soaking or bathing with decoction of medicinal herbs, or compress applied to the affected area, indicated for skin diseases, urticaria and arthritis.

Tongue Dirt tongue coating mixed with dirt, usually seen in dyspepsia, or retention of phlegm or dampness.

Moist and Glossy Fur a tongue coating whose thickness and color usually reflect different pathological changes, i. e. a thin whitish glossy coating is the sign of invasion by pathogenic cold and dampness.

Moist Fur thin whitish tongue coating with moderate moisture is mormal, but a moist and thick greasy coating usually indicates dampness syndromes.

Infantile Epilepsy epilepsy of infant.

Retardation of Growth of Fetus a morbid condition mostly caused by vaginal bleeding which impairs the growth of the fetus, or by the constitutional weakness of the pregnant mother, or the pregnant woman suffering from a chronic disease which leads to deficiency of qi and blood, and failure to nourish the fetus.

Abnormal Position of Fetus a morbid condition due to stagnation of qi during pregnancy or parturiet nervousness which impode the normal

胎赤【tāi chì】1、指新生儿头面肢体通红，状如涂丹。多因胎中感受热毒所致。2、指初生儿因秽液浸渍于眼眦中，使眼睑赤烂，至长大仍不愈。

胎动不安【tāi dòng bù ān】指妊娠期间，先感腰酸，腹部胀坠作痛，继有少量出血者。多由气虚、血虚、肾虚、血热、外伤等因素，致使冲任不固，不能摄血养胎所致。辩证分类：1、肾气不足证；2、气血虚弱证；3、血热证；4、外伤证。

胎动下血【tāi dòng xià xuè】孕妇有腹痛、胎动感，兼见阴道出血的病证。若流血量多，可致流产。

胎毒【tāi dú】1、妊娠期间母体的热毒遗留给胎儿，致使出生后的婴幼儿发生疮疖，痘疹等疾病。2、指先天性梅毒。

胎肥【tāi féi】婴儿生下遍身肌肉肥

turn of the fetus.

Infant with Red Skin (1) abnormal red skin of infant   a morbid state of the infant considered to be caused by exposure to heat toxin before birth. (2) exudative inflammation of eyelids in infants.

Threatened Abortion   a morbid condition first marked by lumbago, distending pain in the lower abdomen with a bearing-down sensation, then slight vaginal bleeding, mostly caused by deficiency of qi, blood and kidney, blood heat, and trauma, resulting in debility of thoroughfare and conception vessels and their failure in governing blood to nourish the fetus.

 Types of differentiation   1. syndrome due to destitution of kidney-qi   2. syndrome due to scarcity of qi and blood   3. syndrome due to blood heat   4. syndrome due to trauma.

Threatened Abortion with Vaginal Bleeding   a morbid condition in which the pregnant woman experiences abdominal pain and restless disturbance of the fetus, complicated by vaginal bleeding, if profuse, it would lead to abortion.

Fetal Toxicosis   (1) boils and eruptions of the newborn caused by heat toxin which is acquired from the mother before birth.   (2) Congenital syphilis.

Muscular Hypertrophy in Newborn

厚,满月后,渐渐消瘦,五心热,大便难、时时吐涎的疾病。 a morbid condition of corpulent newborn baby that becomes wasted a month after its birth, associated with symptoms of hot palms and soles, constipation and frequent salivation.

胎风 【tāi fēng】婴儿禀受先天不足,感受风邪或因断脐,疮痂未敛,以致风邪侵入,蕴结为热的疾病。症见壮热呕吐、精神不守、睡易惊醒、手足抽掣。 **Infantile Spasm** a morbid condition in babies due to congenital weak constitution, exposure to pathogenic wind or unhealing of the broken umbilicus leading to the invasion of pathogenic wind which turns into heat, marked by high fever, vomiting, restlessness and spasm of extremities.

胎风赤烂 【tāi fēng chì làn】新生儿或婴儿眼患赤烂症。多由胎儿禀受热毒所致。 **Infantile Blepharitis Marginalis** a morbid condition mostly due to exposure of the fetus to heat toxin.

胎寒 【tāi hán】婴儿出生百日内,腹痛肢冷、身起寒栗、时发战栗、曲足握拳、昼夜啼哭不止,甚或口噤不开的病证。 **Cold-Syndrome of Newborn** a morbid state of infants marked by abdominal pain huddling with cold extremities, shivering sometimes rigor, incessant drying, or lockjaw.

胎患内障 【tāi huàn nèi zhàng】(胎翳内障)胎儿产后睛珠混浊。相当于先天性白内障。由于孕妇患病,热结于内,影响胎儿所致。 **Congenital Cataract** a morbid condition in infants acquired before birth due to the pregnant woman's illness because of the accumulation of heat.

胎黄 【tāi huáng】指新生儿黄疸。多由娠母感受湿热,传于胞胎,或小儿先天元气不足,脾气虚弱,寒湿不化所致。辩证分类:1、湿热内蕴;2、脾虚湿郁;3、气血瘀积。 **Jaundice of Newborn** a condition due to damp-heat from the mother, or due to infantile congenital insufficiency, deficiency of spleen-qi leading to retention of cold-damp. Types differentiation 1. retention of damp-heat 2. deficiency of spleen resulting from damp 3. stagnation of qi and blood stasis.

胎疾 【tāi jí】(胎证、胎中病)指婴儿满月以内有病,也指小儿周岁以内有 **Diseases of Newborn** the disease that infants suffer within the first

病。多因胎禀不足或儿母妊娠时调摄失宜以及胎毒等引起。

胎漏 【tāi lòu】(胎前漏红) 指妊娠期间,阴道少量下血,时下时止者。病因及辩证分类同胎动不安。

胎气 【tāi qì】胎儿在母体内所受的精气,是胎儿脱离母体前后生长发育的重要物质。

胎热 【tāi rè】小儿生后目闭面赤,眼胞浮肿,遍体壮热,口气热,烦啼不已,溺赤便结的一种疾病。

胎疝 【tāi shàn】指新生儿阴囊肿大的病证。

胎水肿满 【tāi shuǐ zhǒng mǎn】妇女妊娠五、六个月以后,腹部较正常大,并伴有浮肿、胸膈满闷的病证。多因脾虚,运化失常,水湿停留,胞中蓄水,泛溢周身所致。

胎痫 【tāi xián】(胎搐) 婴儿百日内

month after their birth, mostly caused by congenital weak constitution or the poor nourishment of the mother during pregnancy as well as fetal toxicosis.

Vaginal Bleeding during Pregnancy referring to the slight intermitent vaginal bleeding during pregnancy whose causes and type of differentiations are the same as those of threatened abortion.

Original Qi of Fetus qi acquired from the mother, which is the material basis for the development of fetus before and after its birth.

Heat-Syndrome in Newborn a disorder of newborn marked by closed eyes, swollen eyelids, flushed face, high fever, hot breath, incessant crying, deep-colored urine and constipation.

Scrotal Swelling in Neonate a morbid condition of infant marked by swelling scrotum.

Overabundance of Amniotic Fluid a morbid condition marked by rapid expansion of the abdomen in the fifth or sixth month of pregnancy accompanied by edema, distending fullness in the chest and hypochondria, mostly caused by debility of the spleen, resulting in failure in transportation, retention of water and dampness in the uterus and even within the whole body.

Convulsion in Newborn a morbid

频发抽搐，身热面青，牙关紧闭，腰直身僵，睛斜目闭，多啼不乳的一种疾病。

胎元【tāi yuán】1、指子宫内的胚胎。2、母体中供养胎儿生长发育的物质。3、指胎盘。

胎自堕【tāi zì duò】妊娠早期胎失滋养而自行娩出的病证。多因气血虚损或肾虚冲任不固，胎失所养所致；亦可因跌仆或血热燔灼，胎有所伤引起。

太冲脉【tài chōng mài】冲脉的别称。它的功能正常对于调节月经、妊娠以及胎儿的发育很重要。

太息【tài xī】（叹气）以呼气为主的深呼吸。如见频频叹气，则可能是肝胆郁结，肺气不宣所致的症状。

太阳【tài yáng】1、即颞颥。2、位于体表阳经之一。3、穴位名称（经外奇穴）。

太阳病【tài yáng bìng】外邪侵袭太阳经所致的病变。临床上以头痛、颈项强急不舒、恶寒、发热、脉浮等为其特征。通常视其病邪所在部位又分为太阳经证和太阳腑证。

condition seen in infants during the first 100 days after its birth, accompanied by fever, cyanotic complexion, locked jaws, neck rigidity, deviated and closed eyes, incessant crying and difficulty in feeding.

1. **Embryo** 2. **Substances Acquired From the Mother Which Nourishes Fetus.** 3. **Placenta.**

Spontaneous Abortion a morbid state due to deficiency of qi and blood or debility of thoroughfare and conception vessels because of deficiency of the kidney, leading to the loss of power to nourish the embryo, or caused by traumatic injury and sprain or the impairment of fetus by blood heat.

Tai Chong Vessel another name for the thoroughfare vessel whose normal function would play an important role in regulating menstruation, pregnancy and the development of the fetus.

Sighing frequent sighing usually caused by stagnation of qi in the liver and gallbladder and obstruction of the lung-qi.

Taiyang (1) temporal arteries (2) one of the yang meridians in the superficial portion of the body (3) acupoint (EX-HN).

Taiyang Disease a morbid condition due to invasion of exopathic factors characterized by headache, pain of the neck, chills, fever, and floating pulse. It is usually classified into types such

太阳腑病 【tài yáng fǔ bìng】太阳经病邪不解内传膀胱所致的一种病变。临床上又视其病邪传入气分和血分的不同分为太阳蓄水证和太阳蓄血证两种。

太阳经病 【tài yáng jīng bìng】（太阳表证）发热恶寒同时存在，脉证均为邪在肌表的太阳病。根据其有汗与无汗而又可分为中风与伤寒。

太阳伤寒 【tài yáng shāng hán】外感风寒，寒邪束表，腠理闭塞所致的病证。症见发热、恶寒、无汗而喘、身痛、关节疼痛、脉浮紧等。

太阳头痛 【tài yáng tóu tòng】1、太阳病时出现的头痛。2、位于太阳经脉循行部位的头痛，表现为头痛上至巅顶、兼有项强、腰背痛。

as taiyang meridian syndrome and syndrome of taiyang fu-organs according to the position the invading pathogens.

Syndrome of Taiyang Fu-organs a syndrome in which the urinary bladder is attacked by the pathogen that causes the existing taiyang meridian syndrome, which is further classified clinically into taiyang syndrome of water retention and taiyang syndrome of blood retention according to qi or blood that is invaded.

Taiyang Meridian Syndrome a syndrome marked by the co-exisistance of fever and chills and a pulse that shows the pathogen exists in the superficial portion of the muscles which is furter classified into wind stroke and cold stroke according to if there is sweat or not.

Cold-Stroke Syndrome of Taiyang Meridian a syndrome due to invasion of exogenous pathogenic wind-cold, affecting the body superfices, resulting in closed pores, marked by fever, chills, abscence of sweating with shortness of breath, general pain, joint pain, and floating tense pulse.

Taiyang Headache (1) headache in the taiyang syndrome (2) headache in the area where the taiyang meridian passes with the top of the head involved, accompanied by stiff neck, backage and lumbago.

太阳与少阳合病　【tài yáng yǔ shào yáng hé bìng】太阳经与少阳经同时为病邪所侵,两经症状同时出现的一种病证。其证既有太阳病的头痛发热,又有少阳病的口苦咽干、目眩等。

Combined Syndrome of the Taiyang and Shaoyang Meridians　a morbid condition due to attack by pathogens simultaneously on the taiyang and shaoyang meridians with the simultaneous appearance of both meridian symptoms such as headache and fever or the taiyang meridian syndrome, and bitterness in the mouth and dry throat of the shaoyang meridian syndorme.

太阳与阳明合病　【tài yáng yǔ yáng míng hé bìng】太阳经与阳明经同时受累而出现两经证候的外感病。表现为头痛、项强（太阳病证）；身热、口渴、下利黄色粪水、肛门灼热（阳明病证）。

Combined Syndrome of Taiyang and Yangming Meridians　a morbid condition in which both taiyang and yangming meridians are attacked by the exopathic factors, marked by both meridians symptoms such as headache, rigidity of the neck (Taiyang meridian syndrome), fever, thirst, diarrhea with yellowish watery stool, hotness of the anus (Yanging meridian syndrome).

太阳中风　【tài yáng zhōng fēng】外感风寒病邪侵袭太阳经的病证。症见头项强痛、发热、恶风、自汗、脉浮缓等。

Attack of Taiyang Meridian by Wind　a morbid condition due to invasion of taiyang meridian by exogenous wind and cold, characterized by rigidity of the neck, fever, aversion to wind, spontaneous sweating, floating and slow pulse.

太阴　【tài yīn】经脉名称之一。位于三阴经的最外层。有阴气旺盛的意思。

Taiyin Meridian　one of the names for meridians, it exists on the exteriorest layer of the three yin meridians with the meaning of excessive yin-qi.

太阴病　【tài yīn bìng】以脾虚寒湿为主要病理变化的一种病证。多由三阳证治疗不当损伤脾阳,或风寒之邪

Taiyin Syndrome　a morbid condition mainly caused by hypofunction of the spleen and accumulation of cold

直接侵袭所引起。症见腹满呕吐、食欲不振、大便泄泻、时有腹痛、脉缓弱等。

and dampness, mostly due to the impairment of the spleen because of the improper treatment of three-yang syndrome, or directly caused by the invasion of pathogenic cold and dampness, marked by abdominal distension, vomiting, anorexia, diarrhea, occasional abdominal pain, soft and weak pulse.

太阴疽 【tài yīn jū】即肩胛部的疽。

太阴头痛 【tài yīn tóu tòng】由痰湿困脾，清阳不升所致的头痛。表现为头痛而重、疲乏、痰多、腹部胀满、脉沉缓等。

Taiyin Carbuncle referring to carbuncle on the scapular region.

Taiyin Headache headache due to retention of phlegm-dampness in the spleen (taiyin) which prevents the normal ascending of the clear yang-qi to the head, marked by pain and heavy feeling in the head, accompanied by overstrain, profuse expectoration, abdominal distension, deep and soft pulse.

瘫痪 【tān huàn】指四肢不用的疾患。多由肝肾亏虚，气血不足，复因邪气侵袭经络所致。常见于脑血管意外以及神经系统其他一些疾病。

Paralysis a morbid condition marked by weakness of the limbs, mostly caused by yin deficiency of the liver and kidney and qi deficiency, complicated by invasion of the meridian and collaterals by pathogenic factors, usually seen in cerebrovascular accident and other disease of the nervous system.

弹石脉 【tán shí mài】沉而坚实，有如用指弹石感的脉象。

Snap-on-Stone Pulse a moribund pulse which is deep solid yet forceful, resembling flicking a stone with finger tips.

弹针 【tán zhēn】针刺入穴位后用手指轻弹针柄部，使针体产生轻度震动的一种针刺手法。

Flicking the Needle an acupuncture technique whereby the handle of the inserted needle is gently flicked with

痰 【tán】脏腑病理变化的产物，包括呼吸道分泌的痰液。痰的形成多与肺、脾二脏功能失常有关，火热煎熬津液也可成痰。痰也是致病的因素之一，常可引起多种疾病，如喘咳、眩晕、胸痹、癫痫、惊风昏厥、瘰疬、骨及关节结核等。

痰包 【tán bāo】（匏舌、舌下痰包）即舌下囊肿。由痰火互结，留阻于舌下而成。症见结肿如匏瓜状、光滑柔软、色黄不痛、胀满舌下、妨碍饮食、语言。破后流出粘液如蛋清。

痰秘 【tán bì】因湿痰阻滞肠胃所致的便秘。症见大便秘结、胸胁痞闷、喘满、眩晕、头汗等。

痰喘 【tán chuǎn】痰浊壅肺引起的气喘。多由痰湿蕴肺，阻塞气道所致。症见呼吸急促、喘息有声、咳嗽、咯痰粘腻不爽、胸中满闷等。

Phlegm the product of the pathological changes in the zang-fu organs, including the sputum secreted in the respiratory tract, the formation of which is related to the functions of the lung and spleen, which can also be produced by the fire that drying the body fluid, and which, as one of the disease-causing factors, usually brings many diseases, such as asthma, dizziness syndrome, chest bi-syndrome, epilepsy, infantile convulsion. scrofula, bone and joint tuberculosis.

Sublingual Cyst a morbid condition due to phlegm-fire accumulated in the sublingual region, marked by a smooth and soft tumor beneath the tongue, which is yellow and painless, causing difficulty in eating and speaking with mucous substance discharge when it is broken.

Constipation due to Accumulation of Phlegm a morbid state accompanied by stuffiness in the hypochondrium, dyspnea, dizziness, sweating over the head.

Phlegm-dyspnea dyspnea due to phlegm and excessive fluid retention in the lung, mostly caused by phlegm-dampness in the lung obstructing the air passages, marked by shallow breathing in haste with breathing sound, cough, thick greasy sputum that is difficult to be expectorated,

痰多沫 【tán duō mò】吐泡沫痰。因脾肾阳虚，水湿不化所致。多见于老年患者。

痰呃 【tán è】因痰浊阻塞所致的呃逆。症见胸闷、呼吸不利、呃有痰声。

痰核 【tán hé】因脾胃不运，湿痰流聚而致皮下生核，大小不一、多少不等、无红无热、不硬不痛、推之可移、多生于颈项、下颔、四肢及背部。生于身体上部者多挟风热，生于下部多挟湿热。

痰火痉 【tán huǒ jìng】由于痰火壅盛所致的痉病。症见身热、手足振摇或搐搦、咳嗽多痰、脉洪数等。

痰火耳鸣 【tán huǒ ěr míng】指痰火上扰所致的耳鸣。

痰火扰心 【tán huǒ rǎo xīn】痰火上扰心神的病理。症见心烦、心悸、口苦、失眠、精神失常、狂躁、言语错乱、舌红苔黄腻、脉弦滑等。

fullness sensation in the chest.

Frothy Sputum a morbid state due to insufficiency of both the spleen and kidney, causing retention of body fluid, mostly seen in senile patients.

Hiccup due to Accumulation of Phlegm a morbid state marked by stiffness in the chest, difficult breathing, rale produced by the collection of sputum in the air passage during hiccup.

Subcutaneous Nodule nodules beneath the skin which vary in size and number, not hard, painless and movable on pushing, mostly seen in the neck, chin, limbs and back, usually caused by dysfunction of the spleen and stomach, and accumulation of phlegm-damp, with those seen in the upper part of the body mostly complicated by wind-heat, and those in the lower, by damp-heat.

Convulsive Seizure due to Phlegm-Fire a morbid condition marked by fever, tremor or convulsion of the hands and feet, productive cough, full and fast pulse.

Tinnitus due to Phlegm-Fire a morbid state due to up-stirring of the phlegm-fire.

Heart Disturbed by Phlegm-Fire a morbid state due to up-stirring of the heart by phlegm-fire, marked by dysphoria, palpitation, insomnia, amentia, mania, incoherent speech, redness of the tongue with yellowish greasy

痰火头痛 【tán huǒ tóu tòng】由痰火上逆所致的头痛。症见头痛脑鸣或一侧头痛、胸脘满闷、恶心、呕吐痰涎、心烦善怒、面红耳赤，口渴便秘、舌苔黄腻、脉洪滑数等。

Headache due to Phlegm-Fire headache due to upward adverse flow of phlegm-fire, accompanied by tinnitus cranii or migrane, fullness and stuffiness sensation in the chest and epigastrium, vomiting of sputum, dysphoria, irritability, flushed face and ears, thirst, constipation, yellowish greasy coating of the tongue, full slippery and fast pulse.

痰火眩晕 【tán huǒ xuàn yūn】因痰浊挟火，上蒙清阳所致的眩晕。症见眩晕、头目胀重、心烦口苦、恶心、泛吐痰涎、苔黄腻、脉弦滑等。

Dizziness due to Phlegm-Fire a morbid state due to phlegm-fire disturbing the head, accompanied by distension and heaviness in the head, dysphoria, bitterness in the mouth, nausea sialemesis, yellow greasy coating of the tongue, taut and slippery pulse.

痰火怔忡 【tán huǒ zhēng chōng】由痰火扰动所致的怔忡。见怔忡。

Severe Palpitation due to Phlegm-Fire a morbid condition due to the disturbing of phlegm fire, see "zheng zhong".

痰积 【tán jī】以痰多粘稠、咳咯难出、头晕目眩、胸闷隐痛、脉象弦滑等为主要临床表现的一种病证。多由痰浊凝滞胸膈所致。

Accumulation of Phlegm a morbid condition due to accumulation of phlegm in the chest, marked by profuse and viscid sputum which is difficult to be expectorated, dizziness, feeling of suppression and fullness of the chest with vague pain, taut and slippery pulse.

痰厥 【tán jué】厥证之一。指因痰盛气闭而引起的四肢厥冷，甚至昏厥的病证。

Phlegm Syncope suspension of consciousness and cold-limbs due to blockage of air-passage by profuse sputum.

痰厥头痛 【tán jué tóu tòng】由痰浊

Headache due to Adverse Rising of

痰 tan

上逆所致的头痛。症见头痛如裂、眩晕、身重、心神不安、语言颠倒、胸闷恶心、烦乱气促、泛吐痰涎或清水、四肢厥冷、脉弦滑等。

Phlegm a morbid condition marked by splitting pain in the head, dizziness, heaviness feeling of the body, restlessness, incoherent speech, stuffiness in the chest, nausea, dysphoria, shortness of breath, sialemesis or clear water, cold limbs, taut and slippery pulse.

痰疬 【tán lì】1、瘰疬的一种。多因脾失健运，痰聚而成。初起如梅李大，可遍及全身，久则渐红，后可破溃、溃后易敛。2、瘰疬生于项前足阳明胃经循行之处者。

Scrofula due to Accumulation of Phlegm 1. a type of scrofula due to hypofunction of the spleen and accumulation of phlegm, which are as large as plums and may appear all over the body, and which may turn red in the long run, then ulcerate and usually easy to heal. 2. scrofula in anterior neck where stomach meridian of foot-yangming passes.

痰迷心窍 【tán mí xīn qiào】指痰浊阻遏心神，引起意识障碍，症见神识模糊、喉中有痰声、胸闷，甚则昏迷不醒、苔白腻、脉滑等。

Mental Confusion due to Phlegm impairment of consciousness caused by invasion of phlegm to the heat, marked by confusion, sound of sputum in the throat, stuffiness in the chest, or even unconsciousness, whitish greasy coating of the tongue and slippery pulse.

痰粘稠 【tán nián chóu】痰液粘稠，常因风热犯肺所致。多见于外感风热的患者。

Thick Sputum a morbid state due to invasion of wind-heat to the lung, mostly seen in disease due to exogenous wind-heat.

痰疟 【tán nüè】指疟疾兼有郁痰者。症见寒热交作、热多寒少、头痛眩晕、呕吐痰涎、脉弦滑等。

Intermittent Fever due to Phlegm intermittent fever complicated by stagnation of phlegm, marked by alternating attack of chills and fever with the latter more frequent than the former, headache, dizziness, vom-

痰呕 【tán ǒu】（痰积呕吐、痰饮呕吐）以呕吐痰涎为主，伴见恶心、肠中漉漉有声、心悸、头晕眼花、舌苔腻等的一种疾病。因脾胃运化失常，聚湿成痰，留滞中脘所致。

痰痞 【tán pǐ】痰气凝结所致的痞证。多为水饮涎沫，凝聚成痰，气道壅滞引起。症见胸中或胃脘痞塞满闷、胁肋疼痛、呕逆、上腹部有寒冷感、按之有水声、或见发热、四肢麻木等。

痰癖 【tán pǐ】指水饮久停化痰，流移胁肋之间，以致有时胁痛的病证。

痰热阻肺 【tán rè zǔ fèi】指痰热壅阻于肺，发生喘咳的病理。症见发热、咳嗽、痰鸣、胸闷、咯黄稠痰或痰中带血，甚则胸痛、呼吸困难、舌红、苔黄、脉滑数。

痰湿 【tán shī】指因脾不健运，湿浊内停日久而产生的痰。症见痰多稀

...iting of sputum, taut and slippery pulse.

Vomiting due to Accumulation of Phlegm a morbid state chiefly marked by sialemesis accompanied by nausea, borborygmi, palpitation, dizziness, greasy coating of the tongue, caused by hypofunction of the spleen and stomach, causing the formation of sputum which accumulates in the middle abdomen.

Fullness Sensation due to Accumulation of Sputum a morbid condition due to accumulation of phlegm which is produced by retention of fluid and saliva, obstrucing the air passages, accompanied by pain in the hypochondrium, vomiting, hiccup, chill sensation in epigastrium, with water flowing sound heard on pressing, or fever, cold limbs.

Accumulation of Phlegm in Hypochondrium hypochondriac pain due to accumulation of phlegm in hypochondriac region which is produced by prolonged retention of fluid.

Accumulation of Phlegm and Heat in the Lung a morbid condition marked by fever, cough, rale, stuffiness in the chest, thick yellow sputum, or blood-stained expectoration, or even chest pain, dyspnea, redness of the tongue with yellowish coating, slippery and rapid pulse.

Phlegm-Dampness a morbid condition due to hypofunction of the spleen

白、胸闷、恶心、喘咳、食欲减退、舌胖苔滑腻等。and protracted retention of dampness, marked by profuse whitish watery sputum, stuffiness in the chest, nausea, dyspnea, cough, poor appetite, fatty tongue with slippery greasy coating.

痰湿不孕 【tán shī bù yùn】指妇人体质肥盛,恣食厚味,痰湿内生,影响冲任胞脉,难以摄精成孕。多伴有带下量多、月经不调。

Sterility due to Retention of Phlegm-Dampness a morbid condition caused by obese constitution resulted from habitual intake of oily greasy food which brings on retention of phlegm-damp in the interior, and impairs thoroughfare vessel (TV) and conception vessel (CV) and the uterine collaterals, mostly accompanied by profuse discharge of sticky leukorrhea and irregular menstruation.

痰湿内阻 【tán shī nèi zǔ】指由于脾运失常,聚湿成痰,痰湿之邪影响肺胃甚至冲任功能的一种病理。常可引起咳嗽痰多,月经不调等症。

Stagnation of Phlegm-Dampness a morbid condition due to hypofunction of the spleen resulting in accumulation of dampness which turns into sputum that causes damage to the lung and stomach or even to the function of thoroughfare vessel (TV) and conception vessel (CV), cough, abnormal menstruation may be developed.

痰湿头痛 【tán shī tóu tòng】由痰湿上蒙清窍所致的头痛。症见头部沉重、疼痛如裹、胸脘满闷、呕恶痰多、舌苔白腻、脉滑等。

Headache due to Phlegm-Dampness headache caused by the up-stirring of phlegm-dampness to the head, accompanied by heaviness and severe pain in the head, fullness and stuffiness sensation in the chest and epigastrium, vomiting, nausea, profuse sputum, whitish greasy coating of the tongue and slippery pulse.

痰湿阻肺 【tán shī zǔ fèi】痰湿壅阻于肺，使肺气不得宣降的病变。症见咳嗽、痰涎壅盛、痰白而稀、容易咯出、胸膈满闷、动则咳剧、气喘、舌苔白腻或白滑、脉濡缓等。

Accumulation of Phlegm-dampness in the Lung a morbid condition marked by cough with copious whitish thin sputum that is profuse but easily expectorated, fullness and stuffiness sensation in the chest, cough aggravated by exertion, dyspnea, whitish greasy coating of the tongue, soft and floating pulse.

痰稀白 【tán xī bái】痰液清稀色白，常因外感风寒，肺气失宣引起。亦见于脾肾阳虚患者。

Whitish Thin Sputum a morbid state usually caused by invasion of exogenous pathogenic cold-dampness, causing obstruction of the lung-qi, seen in patients with insufficiency of both the spleen and kidney.

痰哮 【tán xiāo】指由痰火内郁，风寒外束所致的哮证。症见气急喘促、喉中痰鸣、声如拽锯。

Asthma due to Stagnation of Profuse Phlegm a morbid condition marked by dyspnea with wheezing sound in the throat, which sounds like sawing.

痰泻 【tán xiè】（痰积泄泻）痰积于肺致肠胃功能失调所致的泄泻。症见时泻时止、或多或少、或下白胶如蛋白、头晕恶心、胸腹满闷、脉弦滑等。

Diarrhea due to Accumulation of Phlegm a morbid condition due to the functional disturbance of the intestines and stomach resulted from stagnation of phlegm in the lung marked by recurrent diarrhea with more or less pus discharged, dizziness, nausea, stuffiness sensation in the chest and abdomen, taut and slippery pulse.

痰饮 【tán yǐn】1、诸饮的总称。即体内过量水液停留或渗注于局部所致的疾病。多与肺、脾、肾功能失调有关。2、四饮之一。指饮邪留于肠胃的疾病，症见饮食减少、消瘦、肠鸣便溏、或伴有心悸短气、呕吐涎沫等。

Phlegm Retention (1) morbid conditions due to excessive retention of fluid or excudating fluid from a certain local area which is mostly resulted from dysfunction of the lung, spleen and kidney. (2) a morbid con-

痰饮咳嗽 【tán yǐn ké sòu】指因痰饮所致的咳嗽。症见咳嗽多痰、色白、或如泡沫。

痰饮胃脘痛 【tán yǐn wèi wǎn tòng】指痰饮停积中焦所致的胃脘痛。多由脾失健运，水湿凝聚，转成痰饮引起。症见胃痛食少、恶心烦闷、呕吐痰沫、脉弦滑，或伴见头晕目眩、心悸气短、腹中漉漉有声等。

痰饮眩晕 【tán yǐn xuàn yūn】因痰浊内停，上蒙清窍所致的眩晕。症见眩晕、头重、胸闷呕吐、痰多气促等。

痰壅遗精 【tán yōng yí jīng】因久思气结成痰，痰扰精室所致遗精。

痰滞恶阻 【tán zhì è zǔ】恶阻证型之一。平素脾胃虚弱，运化失常，聚湿成痰，孕后经血壅闭、冲脉之气上逆，痰饮随逆气上冲所致。症见恶心、呕

dition due to fluid retention in the stomach and intestines, marked by poor appetite, emaciation, borborygmus, loose stools, or accompanied by palpitation, shortness of breath, vomiting of forthy fluid.

Cough due to Retention of Phlegm a morbid state marked by productive cough with the sputum white in color like foams.

Stomachache due to Retention of Phlegm a morbid condition due to retention of fluid in the middle-energizer which turns into phlegm resulted from the dysfunction of the spleen, marked by abdominal pain, poor appetite, nausea, dysphoria, vomiting of frothy sputm, wiry and slippery pulse, or accompanied by dizziness, palpitation, shortness of breath, and gurgling sounds in the abdomen.

Dizziness due to Retention of Phlegm a morbid condition due to upward invasion of phlegm to the head, accompanied by heaviness in the head, stuffiness in the chest, vomiting, profuse sputum and dyspnea.

Emission due to Retention of Phlegm a morbid state due to stress and stagnation of qi which turns into phlegm, invading the seminal-fluid-storing area.

Morning Sickness due to Stagnation of Phlegm a morbid condition due to constitutional deficiency of the spleen and stomach, causing distur-

吐痰涎、胸满不食等。

bance in the transport and transformation and accumulation of dampness which turns into sputum, blocking blood meridian after pregnancy, leading to the upward adverse flow of qi in chong vessel (ChV), which brings sputum, marked by nausea, vomiting of sputum, fullness sensation in the chest, poor appetite.

痰中 【tán zhòng】由湿盛生痰，痰生热，热生风所致的类中风。症见猝然眩晕、发麻、昏倒不省人事、舌本强直、喉有痰声、四肢不举、脉象洪滑。

Apoplexy due to Phlegm a morbid condition due to excessive pathogenic dampness which turns into sputum that produces heat, bringing pathogenic wind, manifested by sudden dizziness, numbness, loss of consciousness, stiffness of the tongue, sputum-moving sound in throat, difficulty in raising the limbs, full and slippery pulse.

Stagnation of Phlegm in the Interior

痰浊内闭 【tán zhuó nèi bì】(痰闭) 1、泛指因痰湿之邪所致的闭证。2、指因痰迷心窍或痰火扰心所致的癫痫、狂躁等病变。

1. apoplectic attack which is believed to be caused by stagnation of phlegm. 2. mania and epilepsy due to stagnation of phlegm in the heart.

痰阻肺络 【tán zǔ fèi luò】由于肺受邪气侵袭，肺的调节水液代谢功能失常，致津液积聚成痰、阻滞于肺的病理。临床上常分痰热阻肺和痰湿阻肺。

Stagnation of Phlegm in the Lung a morbid condition due to invasion of pathogenic factors to the lung, causing its functional disturbance in metabolizing fluid, turning the accumulated fluid into sputum, blocking the lung, which is clinically classified as accumulation of phlegm-heat in the lung and accumulation of phlegm-dampness in the lung.

膻中 【tán zhōng】1、两乳间的正中部位。2、穴位名称。

Dan Zhong (1) a position of the body surface in the centre between

探吐 【tàn tù】用羽毛刺激咽部，引起呕吐，以排除上消化道毒物或食滞的方法。

汤液 【tāng yè】把药物加水煎成汤，去渣、取汁内服。汤液吸收快，作用易发挥，常用于新病、急病等。

溏泄 【táng xiè】指大便稀薄的泄泻。多因脾虚，感受寒湿所致。

糖哮 【táng xiāo】哮证的一种。指由食糖过多，酿湿生痰，痰气阻滞而引起的哮证。

烫火伤 【tàng huǒ shāng】指由于接触高温引起的灼伤，其中高温液体或蒸汽所致的叫火伤。

烫伤 【tàng shāng】高温液体或蒸气所引起的皮肤灼伤。

提插补泻 【tí chā bǔ xiè】针刺手法之一。针下得气后，先浅后深，重插轻提，提插幅度小，频率慢，操作时间短者为补法。先深后浅，轻插重提，提插幅度大，频率快，操作时间长者为泻法。

two breasts. (2) a name of an acupoint.

Inducing Vomiting causing vomiting by artificial stimulation of the throat with feather so as to get rid of the poisonous substance in the upper digestive tract or stagnation of food.

Decoction medicinal solution obtained by boiling the herbs with an appropriate amount of water for a period of time, to be taken after the herbs are removed, which can be easily absorbed and take effect very rapidly, usually used for new or acute diseases.

Loose Stool a morbid state mostly due to deficiency of the spleen and exposure to cold-dampness.

Sugar-Asthma asthma induced by excessive sugar intake, which turns dampness into sputum leading to stagnation of phlegm.

Scald and Burn burns caused by exposure to high temperature while scald by exposure to high-temperature fluid steam.

Scald skin conditions caused by high-temperature fluid or steam.

Reinforcing and Reducing by Lifting and Thrusting the Needle a manipulation of acupuncture, with the anticipated depth of insertion on the given acupoint divided into superficial, medium, and deep. Reinforcing is to insert the needle according to the superficial, medium and deep sequen-

体厥 【tǐ jué】指温疫阳亢已极，及全身冰冷的病证。见厥证。

Cold Feeling of the Whole Body a morbid condition marked by hyperactive yang due to epidemic dampness and cold feeling over the body.

体针疗法 【tǐ zhēn liáo fǎ】泛指用于针刺身体各部位经脉、穴位的针刺疗法。

Body Acupuncture a collective term for therapies by puncturing on the meridians and acupoints all over the body.

天癸 【tiān guǐ】1、指来源于肾精，促进人体生长、发育和生殖机能，维持妇女月经和胎孕所必须的物质。2、即月经。

Tian Gui (1) substance from the kidney essence which promotes the growth and development and reproductive function of the human body and helps menstruation and pregnancy in women.

天花 【tiān huā】（天痘、天行发斑疮、豌豆疮、百岁疮）一种病毒所致的烈性流行病。以全身发痘疮为特征，病程一般经过发热、见点、起胀、灌浆、收靥和结痂六个阶段。

Smallpox an epidemic disease caused by virus, manifested by small poxes all over the body with a course of six stages: fever, appearance of poxes, (which are) distended, perfusated, shrinked and incrusted.

天泡疮 【tiān pào chuāng】1、即脓疱疮。2、由心火脾湿内蕴所致的以皮疹为主的皮肤病。皮疹为水泡样，大小不一，界限清楚，根部红赤，成群发生，并伴有发热恶寒等全身症状。

Pemphigus (1) nong pao chuang (2) skin diseases caused by accumulation of heart-fire and spleen-dampness, chiefly manifested by skin rashes which are blister-like, vary in size with unclear margins and redness at the root part, and occur in groups, accompanied by systemic symptoms such as fever and chills.

天人相应 【tiān rén xiāng yìng】指人体组织结构、生理现象以及疾病同自

Correspondence between Man and Universe corresponding relations be-

然界的相互对应关系。

天庭 【tiān tíng】额部中央的部位。

天行赤眼 【tiān xíng chì yǎn】俗称红眼。由风热毒邪,时行病气所致的一种传染性较强,能造成广泛流行的眼疾。症见暴发眼睑、白睛红赤浮肿、痛痒交作、怕热羞明、眵泪粘稠,甚则黑睛生翳等。

天柱骨倒 【tiān zhù gǔ dǎo】见项软。

天柱骨折 【tiān zhù gǔ zhé】即颈椎骨折。

条剂 【tiáo jì】将药末附粘于纱布条上或单用药末加浆液搓成药条,插入伤口,用以化脓或腐蚀瘘管。

调服 【tiáo fú】方剂中的一些贵重的量少的药品,如犀角、羚羊角等,往往须另制成细末,取药汤少量,调入上述药末和匀服下,再服其余药。

调和肝脾 【tiáo hé gān pí】治疗肝气

tween the structure, physiological functions, pathological changes of the human body and the change of natural environments.

Forehead the part in the centre of the frontal part.

Actue Contagious Conjunctivitis a severe contagious disease by Chinese convention is referred to as "pink-eye disease", which is caused by invasion of wind-heat into the eye and is highly infectious and epidemic, marked by swelling of the eyelids, edema and hyperemia of bullbar conjunctiva, alternate attacks of pain and itching, dysphoria, photophobia, lacrimation with sticky discharge, or even nephelium of the black part of the eye.

Cervical Flaccidity see "flaccidity of neck".

Fracture of cervical vertibra

Medicated Roll a form of preparation made by medicating a stip of gauze or by rolling herb paste into a thread for inserting into the wound, or a supurative or eroded fistula.

(Medicinal Powder) to be Taken after Mixing with Liquid some rare drugs in a prescription such as Cornu Rhinocerotis, Cornu Saigae Tataricae, which are usually taken by individually grinding into powder and mixing evenly with a small amount of the decoction.

Regulating the Function of the Liver

犯脾，肝脾不和的方法。常用于症见胁胀或痛、肠鸣、大便稀薄、食欲不振、性情急躁、舌苔薄白、脉弦细等。

and Spleen a therapy for the derangement of the liver and spleen due to invasion in the chest and hypochondriac regions, increased borborygmi, loose stools, poor appetite, irritability, thin whitish coating of the tongue, wiry and thready pulse.

调和营卫 【tiáo hé yíng wèi】调整营卫失和，解除风邪的一种治疗方法。

Regulating Ying and Wei a treatment to rectify the unbalance between ying and wei and expelling wind.

调经 【tiáo jīng】治疗月经病的总称。包括月经不调、痛经、经闭、经量不正常等病证。临床上常按患者气血变化及寒热虚实不同进行处理，凡因月经病导致其他疾病者，一般以调经为主；而因其他疾病致月经不调者，则以治疗原发病为主。

Regulating Menstruation a collective term for the treatment of menstruation diseases such as irregular menstruation, dysmenorrhea amenorrhea and abnormality in the amount of the monthly blood. Different management methods are clinically adopted according the changes of the patient's qi and blood as well as whether it is due to cold, heat, deficiency or excess. Measures for regulating menstruation is taken for diseases caused by menstruation abnormalities, or vice versa, measures for treating the primary diseases be taken.

调身 【tiáo shēn】气功锻炼方法之一。即姿势和动作的锻炼。调身时要求能做到不宽不急，即不松垮，不紧张。

Regulation of the Body one of the training methods of qigong, which is concentrating on exercise of posture, the principle of "without overrelaxation and without overtension" should be obeyed.

调息 【tiáo xī】气功锻炼方法之一。即呼吸锻炼。调炼的方法为：一是下着安心，二是宽放身体，三是想气遍毛

Regulation of Breathing also called breathing exercise, one of the training methods of qigong with the character

孔出入,通同无障。要领为呼吸柔细深长。

调心 【tiáo xīn】是意念集中与运用的锻炼。

听声音 【tīng shēng yīn】闻诊之一。通过听觉器官了解患者语言、呼吸、咳嗽、呃逆、呻吟等的变化以帮助判断病情。

停经 【tíng jīng】月经周期建立后又停止来潮者,在妊娠期、哺乳期、绝经后的停经是生理现象,如因病引起的停经超过三个月以上者称闭经。

停饮胁痛 【tíng yǐn xié tòng】(痰饮胁痛)指由水饮停留胸胁所致的胁痛。症见胁肋疼痛或两胁走注疼痛、甚则漉漉有声、咳嗽气急、脉沉弦等。

停饮心悸 【tíng yǐn xīn jì】指由水饮内停,水气凌心所致的心悸。症见心悸,伴有胸脘痞满、头晕恶心、小便短少、苔白、脉弦等。

停饮眩晕 【tíng yǐn xuàn yūn】指因中阳不运,水饮内停所致的眩晕。症见

of deep, long, even and fine respiration which can be practised by calming mind, relaxation and by imagining qi passing through the pores of all body without disturbance.

Regulation of Mental Activity one of the training methods, which is concerning the concentration and application of the will.

Listening one of the ausculation and olfaction methods, to get to know the patient's condition better by listening to the patient's voice, breathing, coughing or groaning.

Amenorrhea refers to the case of no menstrual onset of a female who should have had menses as she had reached the adult age, excluding those physiological conditions before adolescence, in the period of pregnancy and lactation, and after menopause.

Hypochondriac Pain due to Fluid Retention a morbid condition marked by wandering pain in the hypochondriac regions, even accompanied with gurgling sounds, cough, dyspnea, deep and wiry pulse.

Palpitation due to Retention of Fluid a type of palpitation due to fluid retention, attacking the heart, accompanied by feeling of stuffiness and fullness in the chest and epigastrium, dizziness, nausea, oliguria, whitish coating of the tongue and taut pulse.

Dizziness due to Fluid Retention dizziness caused by dysfuntion of flu-

头目眩晕、怔忡心悸或脐下悸，呕吐涎沫等。id, marked by dizziness, accompanied by severe palpitation, or feeling throbbing below the umbilicus and vomiting of frothy fluid.

通腑泄热 【tōng fǔ xiè rè】（通泄）通泄大便以清除里热的治法。如用苦寒通便的药物，以清除在内的实热。

Removing Heat by Catharsis a therapy to relax the bowels to remove interior heat, e. g. by using drugs bitter and cold in nature so as to remove the interior heat of excess.

通剂 【tōng jì】具有通利壅滞功效的方剂。

Obstruction-Removing Prescription prescription used for the treatment of stasis or obstruction.

通经 【tōng jīng】治疗闭经（病理性闭经）使之通畅的方法。临床上常按虚实的不同，采用补益气血或行气活血以通经。前者适用于气血两虚引起的闭经；后者适用气滞血瘀引起的闭经。

Restoring Menstrual Flow a therapy to treat amenorrhea (pathological menorrhea), clinical measure for reinforcing qi and blood or promoting circulation of qi and blood is taken according to whether it is of deficiency or excess type, with the former measure applied for cases with amenorrthea due to deficiency in both qi and blood, and the latter for those due to stagnation of qi and blood stasis.

通可去滞 【tōng kě qù zhì】用通剂能够治疗气血壅阻或湿邪留滞等病证。

Removing Obstruction by Using Prescription with Dredging Effect stagnation of qi and blood or accumulation of pathogenic dampness can be removed by using prescription with dredging.

通脉 【tōng mài】用温散寒邪、通行阳气的药物，以振起脉搏的方法。适用于少阴病，阴寒盛于下，虚阳上浮。症见大便泄泻、四肢厥逆、面赤脉微等。

Invigorating Pulse-Beat a therapeutic method to invigorate the pulse beat by warming the flow of yang-qi, usually applied for shaoyin disease, excessive cold sensation of genitalia, upward floating of yang in deficiency condition, marked by diarrhea, cold

通阳 【tōng yáng】治疗因寒湿阻遏、痰凝瘀阻而致阳气不通的方法。通常采用祛邪药物结合具有温通作用的药物进行治疗。

通因通用 【tōng yīn tōng yòng】反治法之一。对某些本质属邪实的疾病。虽有如大便泄泻等通利的症状，仍应使用通利的方法，祛邪外出。

同病异治 【tóng bìng yì zhì】同一疾病，因个人体质、地点、时间、病机、类型等差异而采取不同的治疗方法。

童男 【tóng nán】天癸未至的男儿童。

童女 【tóng nǚ】天癸未至的女儿童。

瞳人干缺 【tóng rén gān quē】（瞳神缺陷）一般由瞳神缩小失治，黄仁与睛珠粘连所致。多属肝肾阴虚，虚火上炎。症见瞳神边缘如锯齿、似梅花、偏缺参差、失去正常之圆形。

瞳神 【tóng shén】（瞳、瞳仁、瞳子）包括瞳孔及其后方的晶体、玻璃体、

limbs, flushed face and faint pulse.

Activating Yang a therapy by using pathogenic-factor-removing drugs together with medicines of warm or hot nature to treat obstruction of yang-qi caused by accumulation of cold-dampness, phlegm, and blood stasis.

Treating Diarrhea with Purgatives one of the therapeutic methods contrary to the routine, to treat syndromes due to excessive factors with purgatives to eliminate factors out of the body, although there is diarrhea.

Treating the Same Disease with Different Methods one of the therapeutic principles in TCM, ie. treatment of the same disease should be varied with different conditions such as the patient's constitution, geographical localities climatic and seasonal changes, as well as manifestations and pathogenesis of the disease.

Virgin Boy referring to immature boys.

Vrigin Maid referring to immature girls.

Pupillary Metamorphosis due to Posterior Synechia a morbid condition due to deficiency of the liver-yin and kidney-yin, and flairing-up of fire of deficiency type, manifested by saw-tooth-like margins of the pupil, or pulm-blossom like, losing its normal shape.

Pupil referring to the pupil as well as the len in the posterior part, vitre-

视网膜等组织,是视觉和光感的重要部位。它配属于肾,而肝肾同源,故瞳神的疾病多与肝肾有关。

瞳神欹侧 【tóng shén qī cè】多因蟹睛致黄仁涌向破口与黑睛粘定,使瞳神变形移位,不得复原所引起;也有因先天或内眼手术所致。症见瞳神歪斜不正,亦有瞳神偏于黑睛边缘,甚至瞳神消失者。

瞳神散大 【tóng shén sàn dà】多由肝胆风火升扰或肝肾阴虚所致,外伤亦可引起。常见于绿风内障等。症见瞳神散大,展缩失灵。

瞳神缩小 【tóng shén suō xiǎo】多由肝胆火炽或肝肾阴亏、虚火上炎所致。症见瞳神缩小,甚者小如针孔,失去正常舒缩功能、抱轮红赤、羞明流泪、头目疼痛、视力下降。类似虹膜睫状体炎。

ous body and retina, which is the important part of sight and light sensation, and which belongs to the kidney and liver, thereby the disease of which are mostly related to the liver and kidney.

Pupillary Metamorphosis due to Anterior Synechia a morbid state due to the adhesion of the iris with the dark of the eye resulted from crab-like protruding eyes, or due to congenital factors or eye operations, marked by trismus, of the pupil, which might deviate to the margin of the dark of the eye, or even disappear.

Mydrasis a morbid state mostly caused by upward stirring of wind-fire in the liver, gallbladder, or deficiency of the liver-yin and kidney-yin, or even traumatic injuries, marked by dilatation of the pupil, causing its inability to functions normally, usually seen in glaucoma.

Myosis a morbid condition mostly caused by flaring of liver-gallbladder fire or deficiency of the liver-and-kidney-yin and flaring-up of fire of deficiency type, marked by contraction of pupil, or even as small as the eye of the needle, failure in performing its dilatating and contracting functions, ciliary hyperemia, photophobia, lacrimation, pain in the head and eyes and impaired eye-sight, resembling iridocyclitis.

痛风 【tòng fēng】指以疼痛较剧或游走性疼痛为主证的痹证。

痛经 【tòng jīng】指女子行经期间，或经来前后，小腹疼痛，或痛引腰骶，剧痛难忍，有的恶心呕吐，冷汗淋漓，以致昏厥者。多因气滞血瘀，寒湿凝滞，气血虚弱等致经络不通，胞脉失养所致。辩证分类：1、气滞血瘀证；2、寒湿凝滞证；3、肝经郁热证；4、气血虚弱证；5、肝肾不足证。

痛有定处 【tòng yǒu dìng chù】疼痛有相对固定的部位。多因瘀血内停所致。

头风 【tóu fēng】1、经久不愈时发时止的头痛。多因风寒或风热侵袭或痰瘀郁遏于头部经络所致。2、泛指头部感受风邪之症的总称。包括头痛、眩晕、口眼歪斜、头痒多屑等多种症候。

头风白屑 【tóu fēng bái xiè】又称白屑

Severe and Migratory Arthralgia bi syndrome marked by severe or wandering pain.

Dysmenorrhea referring to the periodic pain, intolerable in severe case, involving the lower abdomen or affecting the lumbosaceral region, sometimes accompanied by nausea, vomiting, cold sweat or even coma prior to, post or during the menstrual flow, mostly caused by stagnation of qi, blood stasis, accumulation of cold-dampness, deficiency of qi and blood, blocking the meridians and collaterals and failure in nourishing the uterus.

Types of differentiation 1. stagnation of qi and stasis of blood 2. retention of cold-damp 3. accumulation of heat in the liver meridian 4. insufficiency of qi and blood 5. yin deficiency of the liver and kidney.

Fixed Pain referring to pain which is relatively fixed, mostly caused by retention of blood stasis.

Wind Syndrome of Head 1. long-standing intermittent headache, mostly caused by wind-cold or invasion of wind-heat or retention of phlegm in meridians and collaterals of the head. 2. a general term for affections of the head by pathogenic wind, including headache, dizziness, facial paralysis and itching of the scalp with much scurf.

Seborrheic Dermatitis a morbid

风。症见头皮有弥漫而均匀的干燥白屑,抓时脱落,落后又生,甚痒,日久可引起毛发脱落。即今称为脂溢性皮炎。多由肌热当风,风邪侵入毛孔,郁久血燥,肌肤失养所致。

condition marked by dry silver-white scales diffused evenly over the scalp, decrustated by scratching, then appearing with the new ones, which are of severe itching, and with the hair falling off in the long run, mostly caused by invasion of pathogenic wind and heat dormant in between the skin and muscles, and long term qi stagnation turning into heat, causing dried blood and poor nourishment of the skin.

头汗 【tóu hàn】以头面局部多汗为特征的一种症状。可因水亏火旺或胃热上腾所致。

Perspiration on Forehead　a morbid state due to insufficiency of water and excess of fire, or up-stirring of stomach-heat.

头强 【tóu qiáng】指头项俯仰、转侧牵强的一种症状。多因血不养筋,风邪侵袭经络,或肝风内动所致。可见于痉病、惊厥、落枕等疾病。

Rigidity of the Nape　a morbid state marked by stiff neck with the head backward, and difficulty in turning, mostly due to failure of the blood to nourish the muscles, invasion of pathogenic wind into meridians and collaterals, or up-stirring of liver-wind, usually seen in convulsive disease, infantile convulsion, and neck sprain.

头热 【tóu rè】自觉头部发热的症状。多由阴虚火旺或肝风、肝阳上扰所致。

Feverish Sensation in the Head　a morbid state mostly caused by hyperactivity of fire due to yin deficiency, or up-stirring of liver-wind and liver-yang.

头软 【tóu ruǎn】(头项软) 表现为头项软弱,不能抬起的一种疾病。多因阳气不足或营养不良,脾气不升所致。

Flaccidity of Neck　a morbid state due to insufficiency of yang-qi or malnutrition, resulted from the failure of the spleen-qi to send up nutrients.

头痛 【tóu tòng】以头部(整个或局

Headache　a morbid condition usual-

部）疼痛为主症的病证。凡外感六淫或脏腑内伤均能引起。

头痛如劈 【tóu tòng rú pī】即头痛剧烈如刀劈。多因风寒侵入头部经络，或痰涎风火，郁遏经络，致气血壅滞引起。亦有头痛剧烈难忍，伴手足厥冷至肘膝关节以上者，多属病邪入脑的危重症状。

头项强痛 【tóu xiàng qiáng tòng】指头及颈项疼痛，伴后项部肌肉牵强不舒的症状。多因外感六淫，遏阻经脉所致。

头摇 【tóu yáo】头部不自主摇颤的一种症状。实证多由风火相煽，或阳明腑实，引动肝风所致；虚证则多因年老肝肾不足，或病后体虚，虚风内动所致。

头胀 【tóu zhàng】自觉头部胀重不适

ly caused by the six climatic conditions in excess as pathogenic factors or impairment of zang-fu organs.

Intense Headache as Splitting a morbid state marked by severe pain in the head like cutting, mostly caused by invasion of cold-dampness into the meridians and collaterals in the head, or accumulation of sputum and wind-fire in the meridians and collaterals, leading to stagnation of qi and blood, characterized by unbearable headache, accompanied by cold limbs involving the elbow and knee or even the upper, in severe cases.

Rigidity of Nape with Headache a morbid condition marked by pain of the nape and head accompanied by rigidity of the posterior part of the neck, mostly due to affection of the six climatic conditions in excess as pathogenic factors, blocking the meridians and collaterals.

Head Tremor a morbid condition marked by involuntary shaking of head with the excess syndrome mostly caused by fire and wind stirring each other, or excess in the yangming fu-organs, stirring the liver-wind, while with the deficiency syndrome mostly caused by hypofunction of the liver and kidney due to the old age, constitutional weakness after recovery from illness and stirring-up of endopathic wind of deficiency type.

Feeling of Fullness in the Head a

的症状。多因外感湿邪或肝火上逆，湿热内阻所致。

头重 【tóu zhòng】自觉头部重坠如裹的症状。多因外感湿邪或湿痰内阻所致。

头珠疔 【tóu zhū dīng】白色的鼻粘膜疔疮。

透斑 【tòu bān】使用清热凉血的药物，使斑点向外透达，以祛除病邪的治法。常用于温病热入营血致斑点隐隐之证。

透关射甲 【tòu guān shè jiǎ】食指掌面浅表小静脉从第一指节部位直到指甲端均有明显变化，是病情危重的表现。

透天凉 【tòu tiān liáng】古代针刺手法之一。属泻法，用于治疗热证。操作方法为：病人吸气时，随吸气将针慢慢刺入预定的深度，然后按压穴位周围皮肤，作多次轻捻针柄，病人觉局部或全身有凉感时，迅速向上稍行提针，再作同样捻转，再迅速稍行提针和捻转后迅速出针，不闭针孔。

morbid state mostly due to invasion of exogenous pathogenic dampness or upward adverse drive of the liver-fire and accumulation of damp-heat.

Heaviness in the Head a morbid state mostly caused by invasion of exogenous pathogenic dampness or accumulation of damp-phlegm.

Whitish Carbuncle of the Nasal Mucoma

Letting out of Skin Rashes a therapy for febrile diseases with indistinct maculation caused by invasion of pathogenic heat into the yin blood by applying drugs which possess the action of expelling heat from the blood.

Appearance of the Supperficial Veins Extending through the Three Passes toward the Finger Nail visible changes of the minor superficial veins of an infant's index finger from the proximal phalanx to the end of the finger-nail which is indicating a critical condition.

Cool-Producing Needling one of the ancient manipulation methods of needling which belongs to the reducing method, for the treatment of febrile diseases. Insert the needle slowly to the given depth while the patient is breathing out, and then, pressing the skin around the acupoint and twirl the needle gently. When the patient feels cool locally or systemically, rapidly lift the needle a little and repeat the same twirling. Lift and twirl it again in the same way and at last, withdraw the needle rapidly, and keep the hole open.

透邪 【tòu xié】(达邪) 使表邪透达外出的治法，多用于外感表证。
Expelling Pathogenic Factors from the Exterior a therapy to expel pathogenic factors from superficiality of the body for the treatment of febrile disease in early stage with exterior syndrome of wind-heat.

透泄 【tòu xiè】用辛凉药以透表邪，用苦味以清泄里热的一种治法。
Expelling Heat from the Exterior and Removing Heat from the Interior a therapeutic method of using diaphoretics pungent in flavour and cool in nature to eliminate pathogenic heat of the superfical portion of the body, together with drugs bitter in taste to remove pathogenic heat of the interior.

透针 【tòu zhēn】针刺入某一穴位后，将针尖刺抵相邻近的穴位或经脉的一种针法。多用于需要强刺激的患者。
Penetration Needling a needling method performed by piercing two or more adjoining meridians or points simultaneously in one insertion, usually used for a strong stimulation.

透疹 【tòu zhěn】透泄疹毒，使疹子容易发出的治法，一般采用辛凉透表的药物，使疹出不畅的患者顺利出疹，以免发生变证。
Promoting Eruption a therapeutic method for measles by using drugs pungent in flavour and cool in nature with the effect of dispelling pathogenic factors from the exterior portion of the body to promote eruption in order to prevent complications.

土不制水 【tǔ bù zhì shuǐ】脾脏虚弱不能运化水湿，引起机体水液代谢障碍的病理。常出现痰饮、浮肿等证。
Failure of Earth to Control Water a morbid condition due to hypofunction of the spleen (earth) to control water, leading to metabolic disturbance of body fluids, marked by spu-

土栗 【tǔ lì】（跟疽）因局部长期受压和磨擦，气血阻滞所致。生于足跟部，疮形如栗，色黄而亮，或可以化脓。

Infection of the Heel a morbid condition due to frequent squeezing or pressing frictions on certain local area, causing stagnation of qi and blood, usually seen on the heel with the carbuncles shaped like millets which are yellowish and bright, or supurative.

土生万物 【tǔ shēng wàn wù】五行中脾胃属土。因脾胃具有消化、吸收、为各脏腑组织器官的生长和机能活动提供营养物质的作用，故用以比喻脾胃这一生理特点。

Earth Produces Myriads of Things according to the theory of the five elements, the spleen and stomach correspond to earth, a figure of speech to show the physiological funtions of the spleen and stomach to digest food, absorb and supply the body with nutrients.

吐法 【tù fǎ】（涌吐、催吐法）即使用能引起呕吐的药物或其他能引起呕吐的物理刺激，使咽喉、胸膈和胃内的有害物质，随呕吐排出。此法孕妇禁用，体弱者慎用。

Emetic Therapy a therapeutic methods of using emetics or physical stimulation to induce vomiting for the removal of retained toxic substances in the throat, chest or stomach, which is prohibited to be used for pregnant women, and be cautious for patients of weak constitution.

吐粪 【tù fèn】（吐矢）呕吐物中混有粪便的症状。

Fecal Vomiting a disorder with feces in the vomitus.

吐纳法 【tǔ nà fǎ】利用深呼吸和控制意念，以进行保健和治病的一种方法。

Expiration and Inspiration a method to control the mind by breathing to keep fit or treating diseases.

吐弄舌 【tǔ nòng shé】舌体不正常的活动，时时伸舌于口外，旋即缩回或左右吐弄。常见于热性病心脾热盛的患儿。亦见于大脑发育不全的患儿。

Wagging Tongue tongue frequently sticking out and getting it back swiftly or wagging it, it is usually seen in the children with febrile disease when the central nervous system is involved

吐清水 【tǔ qīng shuǐ】指因脾胃虚寒，痰饮停积，宿食不化及虫扰等引起吐清水的症状。

吐乳 【tù rǔ】属小儿呕吐，即吐出乳液。多因哺乳不当，乳食停积或脾胃虚弱，运化功能障碍，胃失和降所致。

吐酸 【tù suān】酸水由胃中上泛，由口吐出的症状。脾胃虚寒，宿食不化，或胃有痰火等均可引起。

吐涎 【tù xián】口中有清稀的唾液吐出，多因胃寒或痰湿之邪困脾引起，也可见于中风患者。

吐血 【tù xuè】指血从口中吐出的症状，血可出自呼吸道及上消化道。多因郁怒、伤酒、伤食、劳倦等因素导致脏腑热盛，阴虚火旺或气虚脾寒引起。

兔唇 【tù chún】（兔缺）小儿生后，由于胚胎发育不全、上唇裂如兔唇。

推拿 【tuī ná】（按摩、按跷）1、是一种物理治疗方法，即通过推拿手法刺激患者体表的特定部位或穴位，运行患者的肢体，使症状得以缓解或消

or cerebral hypolasia.

Vomiting of Watery Fluid a morbid state due to insufficiency of the spleen-yang, retention of phlegm and indigestion or parasitic infestation.

Vomiting of Milk a morbid condition mostly caused by improper feeding, resulting in retention of milk or hypofuncition of the spleen and stomach, funcitonal disturbance in transport, and failure of descending of the stomach-qi.

Acid Regurgitation a symptom resulted from insufficiency of spleen-yang and indigestion, or phlegm-fire in the stomach.

Salivation a morbid state caused by cold in the stomach, or invasion of phlegm-dampness to the spleen. also seen in apoplexy.

Hematemesis a morbid state with the blood from the upper respiratory tract or the upper digestive tract, mostly caused by excessive heat in the zang-fu organs resulting from anger, excessive alcoholic indulgence, improper diet and overstrain, and hyperactivity of fire due to yin deficiency or deficiency of qi and cold in the spleen.

Harelip a moirbid state after birth due to aplasia of the embryo.

Massage Therapy 1. a kind of physical therapy used to relieve or eliminate symptoms and treat disease by stimulating position or acupoint on

推寻 【tuī xún】诊脉时适当移动指位，左右寻找，以了解脉搏变化的一种方法。

腿痛 【tuǐ tòng】指腿部肌肉关节疼痛。多因外感风寒湿热之邪，或跌仆、闪挫等致气血运行不畅所致。

癞疝 【tuí shàn】1、指寒湿引起的阴囊肿大。2、指妇女少腹肿的病证。3、指妇女阴户突出。

癞阴 【tuí yīn】指睾丸、阴茎疼痛的疾病。

退针 【tuì zhēn】将针刺入穴位后，逐渐由深至浅向外退出针体（以不拔出皮肤为度）的方法。

吞酸 【tūn suān】酸水自胃中上涌咽喉，随即咽下而不吐出口外的症状。多因肝气犯胃所致。

臀 【tún】位于腰下方，骶骨两侧的部分，相当于殿大肌突起部位。

臀痈 【tún yōng】生于臀部之痈。由膀胱湿热凝结而成。其症形大如盘，

除，以进行治病的一种疗法。2、正骨八法之一。

the surface of the body with manipulation, or by moving affected limbs. 2. one of the eight manipulation of bone setting.

Side to Side of the Fingers during Pulse Feeling　　one of the methods in pulse feeling.

Pain in the Leg　　referring to the pain in the muscles or joints of leg, mostly due to exposure to pathogenic wind, dampness, cold or heat, or traumatic injuries, contusion, blocking the circulation of qi and blood.

Tuishan　　(1) swelling of the scrotum due to cold-dampness　(2) swelling of lower abdomen in female　(3) projection of the vagina.

Pain in Testes or Penis　　referring to the morbid condition of the testes or penis.

Withdrawing of the Needle　　a manipulation by withdrawing the needle gradually from deep to superfical (not completely pulling out of the skin) when inserted into the acupoint.

Acid Swallow　　a symptom marked by regurgitation of acid fluid to the throat, then swallowing back, mostly caused by invasion of the liver-qi to the stomach.

Buttock　　the part which is below the waist and at the two sides of the sacral bone, or actually the protruding part of the greatest gluteal muscle.

Pyogenic Infection of the Buttock　　a morbid condition caused by accumula-

肿高根浅。因臀部肉厚，肿溃，收敛均较一般外痈迟缓。

tion of damp-heat in the urinary bladder, which is disc-like, severe swelling but not deep-rooted usually with a comparatively protracted course in ulcerating and healing because of the thick muscle.

托毒透脓法 【tuō dú tòu nóng fǎ】运用补益气血及解毒排脓的药物，扶助正气，以托毒外出的治法。适用于疮疡化脓未溃破，或已溃破而排脓不畅，邪盛而正气已虚者。

Pus Draining and Toxin Expelling a therapeutic method by using qi-blood-tonifying drugs and drugs for removing toxic substances and promoting pus discharging to strengthen the body resistance, which is usually applied for intact suppurative carbuncles, or ulcerated ones with difficulty in pus-discharge and excess of pathogenic factors with weak body resistance.

托疽 【tuō jū】生于膝旁阳关穴和阳陵泉穴的疽。属足少阳胆经的病变。患部肿痛灼热，继则穿溃流脓。

Arthritis of Needling Support suppurative inflammation on the lateral aspect of the knee at HsiyangKuan (GB33) and Yanglingch'uan (He-Seapoint, GB34), which is the pathological changes of gallbladder meridian of Foot-Shaoyang, GB, marked by swelling, pain, burning hotness, and then ulceration with pus discharging.

托盘疔 【tuō pán dīng】是手心毒之证情严重者。相当于手掌感染。

Palmar Pustule severe infection on the palm

脱肛 【tuō gāng】直肠或直肠粘膜脱出肛门的一种证候。多因气虚下陷或湿热下注大肠所致，多见于老人、小儿。

Prolapse of Rectum a morbid state marked by prolapse of rectum as well as its mucous membrane, mostly caused by prolapse of insufficiency qi or downward drive of damp-heat to the large intestine, mostly seen in senile patients or young children.

脱肛痔 【tuō gāng zhì】（盘肠痔）指

Hemorrhoid Complicated by Prolapse

直肠脱出或痔疮合并脱肛。多因患痔日久复感湿热外邪,久不痊愈,气虚失摄所致。

脱臼 【tuō jiù】(脱骱) 指组成关节的骨端因正常连接受到损害而离开其原来的解剖位置。一般为外伤引起。也有先天因素造成的。

脱疽 【tuō jū】(脱骨疽) 多因郁火毒邪蕴于脏腑,阴亏不能制火,或外感寒湿邪毒,营卫不调,气血凝滞所引起的疾病。发病缓慢,初起患趾色白、发凉、麻痛,日久趾红、转暗变黑,痛如火烧,筋骨腐烂,并蔓延至趾、脚面、小腿等处。多指血栓闭塞性脉管炎。辩证分类:1、寒湿阻络证;2、血脉瘀阻证;3、湿热毒盛证;4、气血两虚证。

of Rectum a morbid condition mostly caused by long-standing hemorrhoid complicated by affection of exogenous pathogenic damp-heat, causing difficuly in healing, insufficiency of qi and failure to absorb nutrients.

Dislocation also called luxation, referring to the condition in which bone joint dislocated from its normal anatomical position, usually caused by trauma, somtimes because of congenital factors.

Gangrene of Finger or Toe a morbid condition, mostly caused by accumulation of stagnated fire and toxic factors in zang-fu organs, and failure to eliminate fire due to deficiency of yin fluid or invasion of exogenous pathogenic cold-dampness, causing disharmony of Ying and wei and stagnation of qi and blood, marked by chronic onset, whiteness, cold and numbness of the limbs that are affected at the beginning, redness of toe, in the long run, which turns black with burning pain, putrefaction of the muscles which extends to the toes, the crus cerebri, and the leg, mostly seen in thromboangitis obliterans. Types of differentiation 1. blocking of the collaterals by pathogenic cold-dampness 2. blockage of the blood vessels 3. excess of toxic damp-heat 4. deficiency of both qi and blood.

脱气 【tuō qì】 1、虚劳病出现的阳气虚衰的证候。症见疾行则喘、手足逆冷、腹满、溏泄、食不消化、脉沉迟。2、指针刺失宜而致耗损正气。

Impairment of Qi (1) deficiency of yang-qi due to consumptive disease marked by shortness of breath during walking, cold extremities, abdominal distension, loose stools, dyspepsia, deep and soft pulse. (2) consumption of body resistance due to improper needling.

脱肉破䐃 【tuō ròu pò jiǒng】 指因内热炽盛,脾脏阴精亏损而出现的肌肉干瘪消瘦的病状。

Extreme Emaciation a morbid state caused by excessive interior heat, leading to deficiency of yin-essence in the spleen.

脱阳 【tuō yáng】 1、指阴寒内盛,阳气耗伤太过,以致神气不藏而出现幻觉、幻视、乱语或大汗淋漓等症状。2、指男子因性交而出现虚脱的症状。

Exhaustion of Yang (1) a morbid state caused by excess of severe pathogenic cold, leading to prostration of yang-qi and impairment of vital essence and energy, marked by visual hallucination, jargon, or profuse sweating. (2) collapse of the male due to exhaustion of yang-qi during or after sexual intercourse.

脱阴 【tuō yīn】 指由肝肾阴精过度损耗所致的视力严重减弱或丧失。可见于急性热病后期,慢性发热、虚劳及产后体弱等。

Exhaustion of Yin falling or loss of eyesight due to excessive consumption of yin essence of the liver and kidney, which may be found in patients with late acute febrile disease, chronic fever, consumption and postpartum weakness.

脱证 【tuō zhèng】 (脱) 由于阴阳气血严重耗损,脏腑功能衰竭所致的,以汗出如珠、四肢厥冷、口开目合、二便失禁、精神萎靡,甚至神昏、脉微欲绝为主要临床表现的证候。

Prostration Syndrome a morbid condition due to severe exhaustion of yin, yang, qi and blood, and functional failure of zang-fu organs, marked by profuse sweating, cold limbs, opening of mouth and closing of eyes, urinary and fecal incontinence, listlessness or even coma, small and indistinct pulse.

㖞僻不遂 【wāi pì bù suí】 指口眼歪斜、半身不遂的症状。多见于中风后遗症。

外吹 【wài chuī】产后发生的乳痈。

外感 【wài gǎn】即感受风、寒、暑、湿、燥、火、疫疠等外邪所致的疾病。

外感不得卧 【wài gǎn bù dé wò】外感病引起的失眠症状。

外感发热 【wài gǎn fā rè】因感受六淫或疫疠之气等外邪所引起的发热。据其热在表、在里或半表半里而有不同的临床表现。

外感头痛 【wài gǎn tóu tòng】因感受风、寒、湿、热等外邪所致的头痛。其特点是起病较急,头痛持续无间歇,多伴有其他外感症状,多属实证。

外感胃脘痛 【wài gǎn wèi wǎn tòng】因感受外邪所致的胃脘痛。以胃脘卒然暴痛为特征。寒邪犯胃时,多伴有恶寒肢冷、二便清利、口吐冷涎、脉浮紧或沉弦等。热邪犯胃时,多伴有口干舌燥、尿黄、脉数等。

Hemiplegia a morbid condition marked by deviation of the eyes and mouth, and hemiplegia, mostly seen in apoplexy sequel.

Postpartum mastitis

Affection by Exopathogen disease or morbid condition produced by and of the six external etiological factors (wind, cold, summer-heat, dampness, dryness, and fire) or other noxious factors.

Sleeplessness due to Exogenous Pathogenic Factor

Fever due to Exogenous Pathogenic Factor fever caused by any of the six external etiological factors as (wind, cold, summer-heat, dampness, dryness and fire) or other noxious factors with different manifestations by different conditions such as exterior heat, interior, or half exterior and half interior heat.

Headache due to Exogenous Pathogenic Factors headache caused by exogenous pathogenic factors such as wind, cold, dampness and heat, marked by sudden onset, persistent headache, accompanied by other symptoms of exopathic affection, mostly belonging to excess type.

Stomachache due to Exopathogen a morbid condition marked by sudden severe stomachache. When caused by invasion of cold, it is mostly accompanied by chills, cold limbs, loose stools and profuse clear urine, vomiting of

外感腰痛 【wài gǎn yāo tòng】因外邪侵袭经络所致的腰痛。表现以实证为多。

外寒 【wài hán】1、因外感寒邪,阳气不得宣泄所致的病状。症见恶寒、发热、头痛、无汗、身痛、脉浮紧等证。2、体表阳气不足,形寒怕冷的一种病状。

外踝疽 【wài huái jū】(脚拐毒)生于足踝处的疽。因寒湿下注,气血凝滞所致。

外科补法 【wài kē bǔ fǎ】用补益的药物,扶助正气,促进肉芽新生,使疮口早日愈合的一种治法。适用于慢性感染或溃疡后期,毒邪已去,气血虚衰,脓液清稀,疮口难愈者。

外科消法 【wài kē xiāo fǎ】(内消)运用内服药使疮疡消散的一种治法。

cold fluid, deep tense or deep taut pulse; when caused by invasion of heat, mostly accompanied by dryness of the lips and tongue, yellowish urine and rapid pulse.

Lumbago Caused by Exopathogen a morbid condition due to invasion of exogenous pathogenic factors to the channels and collaterals, mostly in the form of excess type.

Exopathic Cold (1) conditions caused by exogenous pathogenic cold, causing obstruction of yang-qi, marked by chills, fever, headache, abscence of sweat, pantalgia, floating and tense pulse. (2) chills and cold of extremities caused by yang deficiency.

Carbuncle on the Lateral Malleolus a morbid condition due to downward drive of cold-dampness and stagnation of qi and blood.

Tonification Therapy of External Diseases a therapeutic method by using tonifying drugs to strengthen the body resistance, promote the growth of new muscles and the early healing of the ulcerated carbuncles, which is usually applied for chronic infections or conditions in their anaphase of ulceration when the toxic factors removed, but still with deficiency of qi and blood, watery pus and difficulty to heal.

Resolution of Soft Tissue Inflammation by Taking Drugs treatment of ul-

外廉 【wài lián】外侧缘。

外伤 【wài shāng】1、扑击、跌仆所致的皮肤、软组织和骨关节的损伤。2、六淫外邪侵犯所引起的病证。与七情内伤相对而言。

外肾吊痛 【wài shèn diào tòng】阴囊肿胀坠痛的一种症状。常见于腹股沟疝。

外肾肿硬 【wài shèn zhǒng yìng】阴囊肿胀硬结的病证。

外湿 【wài shī】外感湿邪。如气候潮湿,久居湿地或涉水淋雨等感受外来湿邪。临床表现为头重、颈项酸痛、胸闷、四肢困倦、关节疼痛等。

外眼角 【wài yǎn jiǎo】(外眦)即上下眼睑在颞侧连结部。是足少阳经的起点处,有童子髎穴。

外因 【wài yīn】1、泛指各种外来的致病因素。2、古代三因分类法的一类病因,即风、寒、暑、湿、燥、火等六淫邪气。

外痈 【wài yōng】位于体表的化脓性感染。如蜂窝组织炎、急性皮肤脓肿等。

cers and carbuncles by elimination method with medications.

Lateral Aspect (as of a segment of extremities).

Trauma (1) trauma, contusion of the soft tissue and bone joints. (2) diseases caused by six pathogenic factors, opposite to those due to emotional disturbances.

Bearing-Down Pain of Scrotum a symptom of distension and bearing-down pain usually seen in the groin.

Indurated Swelling of Scrotum

Exopathic Dampness a morbid state due to damp climate, long-time dwelling in damp place, and catching cold in the water or rain, marked by heaviness in the head, aching pain of the neck, stuffiness in the chest, lassitude of limbs and joint pain.

Outer Canthus the both eyelids are at the temporal junction which is the starting point of shao yang meridian of Foot, and where there is the acu-point Tongziliao (GB 1).

Exogenous Pathogenic Factors (1) a collective term for all the exopathic factors (2) one of the three categories of etiologic factors, i. e., the six pathogenic factors (wind, cold, summer-heat, dampness, dryness, fire).

External Carbuncle suppurative infections on the body surface, such as cellulitis, acute skin abscess.

外证 【wài zhèng】指体表上有征象可见的外科疾病。如痈、疽、疔、疮、疖、瘤、瘰疬及灼伤等。

外治法 【wài zhì fǎ】（外取）泛指除口服药物以外，施于体表或从体外进行治疗的方法。如针灸、膏贴、熏洗、按摩等法。

外痔 【wài zhì】位于肛门齿线以下的痔疮。

弯针 【wān zhēn】针刺入人体后，针体发生弯曲的异常情况。多因病人肌肉突然收缩或体位改变或操作方法不当引起。可轻轻挪动，恢复原来体位，根据针弯曲的角度和方向，顺势将针徐徐拔出。切忌猛力抽拔或捻转。

顽疮 【wán chuāng】指经久不愈的疮疡。多因气血虚损，或气滞血瘀所致。

顽痰 【wán tán】指经久难愈的痰证。它常是某些顽固痰病的原因或表现，如哮喘反复发作、顽固性头痛等。

顽癣 【wán xuǎn】多因风、湿、热、

External Disease diseased conditions appeared on the body surface, such as carbuncle, deep-rooted carbuncle, furuncle, boil, tumor, scrofula as well as burn.

External Treatment collective term for all the external therapies except drug taken, such as acupuncture and moxibustion, external application, fumigating and bathing, as well as massage.

External Hemorrhoids hemorrhoids occurring below dentate line of the anus.

Bending of Needle (within the Tissue after Insertion) an abnormal condition caused by the sudden contraction of the patient's muscle or change of body position, or the improper manipulation, which can be corrected by gently returning to the original body position, withdrawing the needle slowly (not forcefully or by twirling) in a direction along with the bending.

Obstinate Pyogenic Sore of Skin referring to those which are difficult to heal, mostly caused by deficiency or stagnation of qi and blood.

Stubborn Phlegm referring to the phlegm syndrome which is difficult to be cured, and which is the cause or manifestation of some certain stubborn diseases, such as recurrent asthma, and stubborn headache.

Stubborn Tinea a morbid condition

虫四者为患，皮肤发痒，起粟米样红疹，表现落屑。病损互相融合，形成肥厚皮损，经久不愈，反复发作。见于神经性皮炎、慢性湿疹等。

mostly caused by pathogenic wind, dampness, heat and parasites, marked by itching, millet-like papules with scales falling off from their surface, impairment of the skin which becomes thick, because of the papule that form into groups, difficulty in healing with repeated attacks, mostly seen in neurodermatitis and chronic eczema.

顽症 【wán zhèng】经久难愈的病证。

Pertinacious Disease

丸 【wán】把药物研成细末，用蜜或水及赋形剂拌和后，制成圆形的药丸。服用方便，吸收较缓慢，药力较持久。

Pill a form of prepared drugs by mixing the ground drug powder with honey or water as well as excipient to make round-shaped pills which are convenient to take, absorbed gradually with longer-lasting effect.

腕骨折 【wàn gǔ zhé】腕骨因跌折、压轧而致骨折。伤处肿胀疼痛或腕缝错开、活动受限。

Carpal Bone Fracture fractured state marked by distending pain, dislocation of the wrist joint, and limited movement.

亡津 【wáng jīn】指津液严重耗损，常是伤津的进一步发展。多因热邪亢盛或误治所致。

Fluid Depletion a morbid state marked by severe consumption of body fluid, which is the further development of the inpairment of body fluid, mostly due to excessive pathogenic heat or erroneous treatment.

亡血 【wáng xuè】各种出血病证的总称。如吐血、衄血、便血、尿血等。

Hemorrhagia a collective term for syndrome with bleeding, such as hematemesis, bleeding from the eye, ear, nose, mouth or subcutaneous tissue, hemafecia, and hemauria.

亡血家 【wáng xuè jiā】即平素患有呕血、衄血、尿血、便血、崩漏等出血性疾病或外伤出血引起失血的病人。

Patient with Hemorrhagic Diathesis patients suffering from hemorrhagic diseases such as hematemesis, bleeding from the eye, ear, nose,

亡阳 【wáng yáng】 阳气衰竭的危重证候。多因大汗不止或剧烈吐泻等导致阳气严重耗损。症见大汗淋漓、汗出如珠、畏冷、精神萎靡、四肢厥冷、面色苍白、呼吸微弱、渴喜热饮、脉微欲绝或浮数无力等。

Yang Exhaustion critical case of exhaustion of yang-qi, mostly caused by incessant sweating, severe vomiting and diarrhea, marked by profuse and greasy perspiration, intolerance to cold, listlessness, cold limbs, pale complexion, weak breathing, thirst, predilection for hot drinks, indistinct pulse or floating, fast and weak pulse.

亡阴 【wáng yīn】阴液严重缺损的证候。多因高热、失血或剧烈呕吐、泄泻、出汗所致。症见身体干瘪、眼眶深陷、皮肤弹性减退、精神烦躁或昏迷、口干喜冷饮、唇舌干红、脉虚数或细数等。

Yin Depletion severe consumption of yin fluid due to high fever, bleeding or severe vomiting, diarrhea and sweating, marked by emaciation, deep hollowed eyes, decreased elasticity of the muscles, restlessness, or coma, delirium, dryness in the mouth with the preference for cold drinks, dry and reddish lips and tongue, week fast or thready fast pulse.

王烂疮 【wáng làn chuāng】由脏腑积热,蕴蒸肌肤,外受湿气所致的皮肤病。症见全身脓疮,逐渐增大蔓延、溃破流脓。即大疮性脓疮病。

Bullous Impetigo skin disease caused by accumulation of heat in the fu-organs, steaming the superficial portion of the skin, and exogenous pathogenic dampness, marked by pustulae all over the body which gradually increase in size, ulcerate with pus discharge.

望齿 【wàng chǐ】望诊内容之一。通过观察牙齿和牙龈的变化来帮助诊断的一种方法。因牙齿、牙龈与肾和胃有密切关系,通过观察它们的变化可以了解肾和胃的病变。

Observation of Teeth observation of the patient's teeth and gums to detect pathological changes of the kidney and stomach since they are closely related to each other.

望蛔虫证 【wàng huí chóng zhèng】通过面部望诊发现一些体征，作为诊断蛔虫病的参考。如面部白斑、巩膜蓝点，下唇颗粒等。

Observation of the Face for Signs of Ascariasis　signs of ascariasis obtained by observation of the face as a refference in making diagnosis, such as white patches on the face, blue spots on the sclera and granules on the lower lip.

望形态 【wàng xíng tài】望诊内容之一。观察患者的体形和动态。如肌肉、骨骼、皮肤、体位、姿态及活动情况等变化。

Observation of Physical Condition and Behaviour　one of the respect in observation on changes of, such as muscles, skeleton, skin, posture, mobility and strength.

望眼辨伤 【wàng yǎn biàn shāng】一种民间诊断方法，即通过观察球结膜血管的改变及瘀点所在，以帮助诊断受伤的部位和性质。

Observation of Eyes　a folk diagnostic method, i. e., to judge the position and nature of injuries by observing blood vessels of bulba conjunctiva and petechia.

望诊 【wàng zhěn】四诊之一。动用视觉，观察患者神色、动态、体表各部、舌质和舌苔、大小便和其他排泄物、分泌物等的变化，从而获取与疾病有关的资料。

Observation　one of the four methods of diagnosis, including observing the patient's mental state, facial expression, mobility, various parts of skin, tongue and coating, urine, stool and other excreta, and secretions to obtain the related messages of illness.

微黄苔 【wēi huáng tāi】舌苔呈微黄色且较薄，是外感风热的表现。

Mild Yellowish Fur　a mild yellowish thin coating of the tongue which is one of the manifestations of pathogenic wind-heat.

微火 【wēi huǒ】即文火。

Soft Fire

微脉 【wēi mài】细小无力，指感搏动微弱的一种脉象。多因阴阳气血均虚所致。常见于休克，虚脱的患者。

Indistinct Pulse　a weak pulse due to deficiency of yin, yang, qi and blood, usually seen in shock and collapse.

微者逆之 【wēi zhě nì zhī】对于病情轻的疾病，应采用逆治的方法。

Mild Illness Dealt with by Routine Treatment　a mild illness should be treated by routine treatment.

煨 【wēi】用湿纸、面糊或黄泥将药物

Roasting in Ashes　a process of

包好，放在火灰内，待外面的包裹物烧至焦黑，以吸去药物所含油质或增加药物的温性。

尾骶骨伤 【wěi dǐ gǔ shāng】伤后局部肿胀疼痛，压之痛剧，行走和坐受限，甚至不能平卧，翻身困难。

委中痈 【wěi zhōng yōng】（委中毒、曲鳅）生于膝腘窝委中穴部位之痈。多由胆经移热于膀胱经，或肾经气血阻滞而成；亦可因患肢破损、湿疹等感染诱发。

萎黄 【wěi huáng】身黄而不润泽的证候。多因脾胃虚弱，气血不足或兼有湿郁、虫积所致。

痿躄 【wěi bì】指双膝萎软无力。
痿厥 【wěi jué】指手足萎弱无力而不温。
痿证 【wěi zhèng】（痿）指肢体软弱无力，渐致肌肉萎缩而不能随意运动的病证，尤以下肢为甚。多因肺热伤津或湿热浸淫，或肝肾亏虚、精血不足，筋失濡养所致。

preparing Chinese drugs in which raw materials are wrapped in moistened paper, paste or mud and heated in smoldering cinder until the coating becomes charred and cracked so as to remove the oil from the drug and add its warm nature.

Fracture of Sacrum and Coccyx a condition marked by local swelling, pain, aggravated when pressed, and difficulty in walking, sitting-down, or even difficulty in lying on the back or turning over in bed.

Acute Pyogenic Infection of Popliteal Fossa an infection mostly caused by invasion of pathogenic heat to the urinary bladder from the gallbladder meridians, or stagnation of qi and blood in kidney meridians, or induced by injury of the affected limb and eczema.

Diminish and Yellowish Tinge of the Skin a morbid state mostly due to deficiency of the spleen and stomach, qi and blood or complicated by accumulation of pathogenic dampness and parasites.

Flaccidity of the Knees
Flaccidity with Cold Limbs

Flaccidity Syndrome a morbid condition marked by flaccidity of the limbs, gradually resulting in atrophy of the muscles and involuntary movement, mostly occurring to the lower limbs, caused by impairment of body fluid resulted from lung-heat, or invasion of pathogenic damp-heat, or deficiency of the liver and kidney, insufficiency of blood, leading to poor nourishment of muscles.

卫分证 【wèi fēn zhèng】外感风热病的初起阶段,病邪在表。症见发热、微恶风寒、口渴、苔薄白、舌边尖红、脉浮数等。其中以发热与恶寒并见为基本特征。

Weifen Syndrome the initial stage of an epidemic febrile disease with the pathogenic factors in the exterior, manifested by fever, slight aversion to wind and cold, thirst, redness of the tip and edge of the tongue with thin whitish coating, floating and fast pulse, among them it is chiefly characterized by the co-existance of fever and chills.

卫气 【wèi qì】人体阳气的一种。食物经脾胃消化吸收而生成卫气。具有护卫肌肤、抗御外邪、调节汗液的分泌,滋养腠理等功能。

Defensive Qi (Wei Qi) one type of yang-qi, the result of the digestion and absorption of food by the spleen and stomach, having the functions of protecting the integument and musculature against external pathogen, adjusting sweat secretion and mourishing the skin portion.

卫气不固 【wèi qì bù gù】(表气不固)卫气虚弱,抗病能力低下,外邪容易入侵的现象。发病时表现为自汗、怕风等。

Failure of Wei Qi to Protect the Body against Diseases a morbid state marked by spontaneous sweating and aversion to wind, caused by deficiency of the superficial qi, lowering the ability of the body to resist diseases, leading to the invasion of exopathic factors.

卫气同病 【wèi qì tóng bìng】外感表邪入里化热,气分已热盛而表寒仍未消除的病证。症见壮热、口渴、心烦、汗出、恶寒、身痛、舌苔薄白微黄等。

Syndrome of both Weifen and Qifen syndrome involving both weifen and qifen in epidemic febrile disease, in which pathogenic heat attacks the qifen (qi system) while the weifen syndrome still exists, manifested by high fever, thirst, dysphoria, sweating, aversion to cold, pantalgia, thin, whitish and slightly yellowish coating of the tongue.

卫气营血辨证 【wèi qì yíng xuè biàn zhèng】外感温热病的一种辩证方法。根据外感温热病的病理过程及其对人体卫气营血的损害分为四个阶段,以说明病变的深浅、轻重、性质及预后,从而为治疗提供依据。

Analysing and Differentiating the Development of an Epidemic Febrile Disease by Studying Condition of the Four Systems (Wei, Qi, Ying, Xue) one of the differentiating methods for epidemic febrile disease in which the disease is divided into four stages by its pathological course, and its damage caused to wei, qi, ying, xue of the body so as to explain its depth, severity, as well as prognosis and to supply basis for treatment.

卫强营弱 【wèi qiáng yíng ruò】指因阳气郁于肌表,内迫营阴而出汗的病理。症见发热而自汗。

Excess of Wei and Deficiency of Ying a morbid state due to stagnation of yang-qi in the superficial portion of the muscles, suppressing ying yin, marked by fever and spontaneous sweating.

卫弱营强 【wèi ruò yíng qiáng】指卫气虚弱,卫外不固致汗液自行溢出的病理。症见不发热而自汗。

Deficiency of Wei and Excess of Ying a morbid state caused by deficiency of wei and its failure to protect the body against diseases, marked by absence of fever, but spontaneous sweating.

卫营同病 【wèi yíng tóng bìng】即病从卫分传入营分而卫分证仍在的病理现象。临床表现既有发热、夜热甚、神志昏蒙、舌质红绛等营分症状,又有恶寒、咳嗽、舌苔薄白等卫分症状。

Syndrome of both Weifen and Yingfen a syndrome in which pathogenic heat attacks the yingfen (ying system) while the weifen syndrome still exists, manifested by not only the symptoms of yingfen, such as fever higher at night, loss of consciousness, dark red tongue, but also those of weifen, such as aversion to cold, cough, thin and whitish fur on the tongue.

未发病前服【wèi fā bìng qián fú】某些疾病应在症状发作前的适当时间服药, 如疟疾、癫痫等。

(Drug) Be taken Before the Onset of the Disease　　drugs should be taken at proper time before the onset for the disease such as malaria and epilepsy.

未老经断【wèi lǎo jīng duàn】未到停经年龄而出现闭经的病证。多因体质虚弱、产育过多、早婚等所致。

Premature Menopause　　a morbid condition due to constitutional weakness, grand multiparity and early marriage.

畏光【wèi guāng】患者怕见光亮, 遇光则涩痛不适, 不敢睁眼的症状。多因风火热邪上攻或阴虚血亏所致。

Photophobia　　a morbid state marked by fear of light of the eyes, indistinct pain or uncomfortable when exposure to light, difficulty in opening the eyes because of the light, mostly caused by upward drive of pathogenic wind, fire and heat, or deficiency of yin and blood.

胃【wèi】六腑之一。有受纳和消化食物的功能。中医学的胃与现代医学的胃概念大致相同,但有时则为胃肠的总称。

Stomach　　one of the six fu-organs, which has the functions of receiving and digesting food. The conception of "the stomach" in TCM is roughly the same as that in modern medicine with the exception that it sometimes serves as the collective term for "stomach and intestine".

胃病【wèi bìng】泛指胃的病变。由于饮食不节, 饥饱失调, 冷热不适; 或胃气虚弱, 胃阴不足影响胃的受纳和消化功能所致。常表现为脘腹胀满疼痛、呕吐恶心、嗳气纳减等症。

Diseases of the Stomach　　morbid conditions caused by improper diet, overeating of cold food, or deficiency of the stomach-qi, insufficiency of stomach-yin, causing impairment to the receiving and digesting functions

胃肠 【wèi cháng】胃和肠的总称。

胃寒 【wèi hán】脾胃阳虚的病理。症见呕吐清水、口淡喜热饮、便溏或泄泻、舌质胖、苔白润、脉沉迟等。

胃寒恶阻 【wèi hán è zǔ】妊娠后期脾胃虚寒，寒饮上逆所致。症见呕吐清水、倦怠畏寒、喜热饮。

胃火上升 【wèi huǒ shàng shēng】指胃热上炎而引起的口腔炎症的病理。症见口臭、牙龈肿痛、口腔溃疡或牙龈出血等。

胃家 【wèi jiā】泛指胃、大肠、小肠等。

胃家实 【wèi jiā shí】指热邪结于阳明，津液受损引起的胃肠实证。症见便秘、腹痛拒按、壮热、烦渴、大汗出、脉洪大。

胃气 【wèi qì】1、指胃的生理功能。2、

of the stomach, manifested by stuffiness and fullness sensation, and pain in the stomach, vomiting, nausea, belching and loss of appetite.

A Collective Term For Stomach And Intestines

Cold Syndrome of the Stomach a morbid condition due to deficiency of yang of the spleen and stomach, marked by watery vomits, whitish moist coating of the tongue with fatty proper, deep and slow pulse.

Morning Sickness due to Cold of the Stomach a morbid condition in the late period of pregnancy caused by cold by deficiency type of the spleen and stomach, and upward adverse flow of fluid, marked by watery vomits, lassitude, aversion to cold, predilection for hot drinks.

Flaring up of the Stomach-Fire referring to stomatitis caused by flaring up of the stomach-fire, marked by ozostomia, swelling and pain of the gum, stomatocace, or bleeding from the gum.

Gastrointestinal Tract referring to the stomach, large intestine and small intestine.

Excess Syndrome of the Stomach accumulation of pathogenic heat in yangming resulting in damage of fluid, marked by constipation, tenderness of the abdomen, high fever, polydripsia, profuse sweating, full and gigantic pulse.

The Stomach-Qi (1) the physiologi-

脾胃功能在脉象的反映,是构成正常脉象不可缺少的因素。

胃气不和 【wèi qì bù hé】指胃消化吸收功能失调的病理。多由胃阴不足,热邪犯胃或食滞胃脘所致。症见厌食或食后胃部胀闷、恶心、大便不正常等。

胃气不降 【wèi qì bù jiàng】指由于饮食不节、胃火冲逆或痰湿中阻致胃的通降功能障碍的病理。常见有饮食减退、胃部胀痛、嗳气呃逆、呕吐等症状。

胃气虚 【wèi qì xū】胃受纳和消化功能减弱所致的病证。症见上腹部胀闷、食欲减退、甚则呕吐、便溏、唇舌淡白等。

胃热 【wèi rè】指热邪犯胃或过食煎炒油炸食物致胃中燥热的证候。常见有口渴、口臭、食欲亢进、上腹部不适、小便少而黄、便秘、甚至口腔糜烂、牙龈肿痛等症状。

胃热恶阻 【wèi rè è zǔ】妊娠冲脉气

cal function of the stomach is one of the indispensable factor in constituting the normal pulse.

Disorder of the Stomach-Qi functional disturbance of the stomach in its digestion and absorption, mostly due to insufficiency of the stomach-yin, invasion of pathogenic heat to the stomach, or accumulation of food in the stomach, marked by anorexia, stuffiness in the stomach after eating, nausea, and abnormal bowel movement.

Failure of Descending of the Stomach-Qi dysfunction of the stomach in transporting food downward caused by improper diet, adverse rising of the stomach-fire or stagnation of phlegm-damp, marked by anorexia, distension and pain of the stomach, belching, hiccup, and vomiting.

Insufficiency of the Stomach-Qi weakened function of the stomach in receiving and digesting food, manifested by fullness and distension in the stomach, anorexia, or even vomiting, loose stool, pale lips and tongue.

Stomach-Heat impairment of the stomach by pathogenic heat or taking excessive heat-producing food, marked by thirst, halitosis, hyperexia, discomfort in the epigastrium, oliguria with yellowish urine, constipation, or even ulceration of the mouth, gingivitis.

Morning Sickness due to the Stomach-

盛,胃火上炎,胃气不降所致。症见恶心、呕吐、颜面潮红、口渴喜凉饮、便秘等。

胃热杀谷 【wèi rè shā gǔ】指胃受热邪影响引起消化功能亢进,多食易饥的病理。

胃热壅盛 【wèi rè yōng shèng】 1、胃中实热之邪壅盛,胃火上炎。症见烦渴引饮、口臭口烂、齿痛龈肿。2、温热病热结胃肠,则见高热便秘,腹痛,甚则出现神昏谵语、狂燥等症。

胃弱恶阻 【wèi ruò è zǔ】妊娠后胃气虚弱,气虚不运,胃失和降所致。症见恶闻食味、食入即吐、脘腹胀满等。

胃实 【wèi shí】指胃肠积热,热盛伤津,胃气壅滞不通所致的证候。症见脘腹胀痛、大便秘结、烦躁发热等。

Heat a morbid state after pregnancy caused by excess of qi in ChV, flaring up of stomach-fire and failure of the stomach-qi to descend, manifested by nausea, vomiting, flushed face, thirst with the preference for cool drinks, and constipation.

Polyphagia due to the Stomach-Heat hyperfunction of the stomach in digestion caused by invasion of heat to the stomach, marked by polyphagia.

Excessiveness of the Stomach-Heat (1) a morbid condition due to flaring up of the stomach-fire, marked by polydipsia and preference for cold drinks, halitosis, aphthous ulcer, toothache, gingivitis (2) accumulation of heat pathogen in the stomach and intestine, seen in epidemic febrile disease, marked by high fever, constipation, abdominal pain, or even coma, delirium, and restlessness.

Morning Sickness due to Weakness of the Stomach a morbid condition after pregnancy due to weakness of the stomach-qi, leading to dysfunction of the stomach in transporting food downward, marked by dislike of food, instant vomiting after food intake, distension and fullness in the abdomen.

Excess Syndrome of the Stomach a morbid condition due to consumption of body fluid and stagnation of the stomach-qi caused excessive heat accumulated in the stomach and intestine, marked by fullness and pain in epigastrium, constipation, dysphoria and fever.

胃脘 【wèi wǎn】胃的内腔。其体表部位相当于上腹部。

Gastric Cavity It's topographical region equals to that of the upper abdomen.

胃脘痛 【wèi wǎn tòng】(胃痛、胃心痛)指以胃脘部疼痛为主症的病证。常伴有痞闷或胀满、嗳气、泛酸、嘈杂、恶心呕吐等症。多因情志不畅、饮食不节、劳累受寒等引起。辩证分类：1、气滞证；2、胃寒证；3、胃热证；4、食滞证；5、瘀血证；6、阴虚证；7、虚寒证。

Epigastralgia a morbid condition accompanied by stuffiness or fullness and distension, beltching, acid regurgitation, discomfort sensation in the stomach, nausea, and vomiting, caused by emotional distress, improper diet, overstrain and invasion of cold. Types of differentiation 1. qi stagnation 2. asthenic cold in the stomach 3. asthenic heat in the stomach 4. food retention 5. blood stasis 6. deficiency of yin 7. cold of deficiency type.

胃虚 【wèi xū】通常是指胃气虚弱或胃阴不足的病证。

Deficiency Syndrome of the Stomach including insufficiency of stomach-qi and deficiency of stomach-yin.

胃阴 【wèi yīn】(胃汁)指胃中的津液，由水谷化生而来，是维持胃的生理功能不可缺少的物质，它和胃阳相互配合，以保持正常的消化功能。

Stomach-yin referring to the fluid in the stomach which is transformed from foodstuff, and is the indispensable substance in maintaining the normal physiological function of the stomach, ie, together with the stomach-yang, to maintain the normal function of digestion.

胃阴虚 【wèi yīn xū】(胃阴不足)指胃的阴液不足。多由火热之邪损耗胃的阴液所致。症见唇燥口干、喜喝水、饮食减少、大便干结、小便少、甚则干呕、呃逆、舌中深红而干、脉细数等。

Deficiency of the Stomach-Yin a morbid condition due to deficiency of fluid in the stomach caused by dryness of the mouth and lips, preference for cold drinks, anorexia, constipation, oliguria, even retching, hiccup,

胃胀 【wèi zhàng】指胃肠积热,热盛伤津,胃气壅滞不通或胃寒水谷不化所致的证候。症见脘腹胀痛、大便不通、烦躁发热等。

胃中燥矢 【wèi zhōng zào shǐ】指肠中大便燥结。多由胃肠实热内结,热盛伤津所致。

胃主腐熟 【wèi zhǔ fǔ shú】胃的功能之一。指胃能把饮食物进行初步消化的功能。

胃主降浊 【wèi zhǔ jiàng zhuó】胃的功能之一。即胃把消化的食物向下输送到肠道的功能。

胃主受纳 【wèi zhǔ shòu nà】胃的功能之一。胃有接受和容纳饮食物的功能。

温病 【wēn bìng】(温热病)1、多种外感急性热病的总称。以初起病较急,热象较盛,传变较快,容易伤阴等为特征。2、指伤寒病五种疾患之一。3、指春季发生的热性病。

dark red and dry tongue in the middle, thready and fast pulse.

Stomach Distension a morbid condition caused by accumulation of pathogenic heat in the stomach and intestines, which is excessive and consumes the body fluid, and stagnation of the stomach-qi, or due to stomach-cold and dyspepsia, marked by distension and pain in the stomach, difficulty in bowel movement, dysphoria and fever.

Dry Stool in the Intestinal Tract a morbid state mostly caused by accumulation of excessive heat in the stomach and intestines resulting in the consuming of the body fluid.

Stomach Function to Digest Food one of the functions of the stomach, which transforms food into chyme.

Stomach Serves to Transport the Digested Food downwards one of the functions of the stomach, by which the digested food is transported downwards to the intestines.

Stomach Serves to be a Storage one of the functions of the stomach, by which the food is received and stored in the stomach.

Seasonal Febrile Disease 1. a general term for acute febrile disease due to exogenous pathogens marked by acute onset, high fever, rapid progress and impairment of yin. 2. one of the five types of exogenous febrile disease. 3. febrile disease in spring.

温病派 【wēn bìng pài】 提倡和赞同温病学说的医家,自成一派,称为温病派。

School of Seasonal Febrile Disease a medical sect in which the members advocate or approve of the doctrine of seasonal febrile disease.

温病学 【wēi bìng xué】研究温热病的病因、病理和治疗的一门学科。

Science of Seasonal Febrile Disease science of theories on the etiology, pathology, treatment of seasonal febrile disease.

温病学说 【wēn bìng xué shuō】明清时期,在总结前人治疗伤寒病的基础上,通过长期的临床实践,对温热病的病因、病理和辨证治疗等有比较深刻的认识,逐步形成的比较系统完整的学说,称为温病学说。

Doctrine of Seasonal Febrile Disease during the periods of the Ming and Qing Dynasties, based on the experience of the predecessors in treating febrile disease, through long-term clinical practice, with more profound understanding of the etiology, pathology, differentiation and treatment of seasonal febrile disease, a systemic and comprehensive doctrine was gradually formed.

温补命门 【wēn bǔ mìng mén】用壮阳补火的药物,恢复脾肾阳气的方法。适用于命门火不足。症见五更泄泻、腹痛肠鸣、四肢冷、舌质淡、苔白、脉沉迟等。

Warming and Recuperating the Gate of Life a therapy for treating hypofunction of the spleen and kidney by the application of drugs of strengthening yang and fire, applicable to the case with insufficiency of fire in the gate of life, marked by diarrhea before dawn, abdominal pain and borborygmus, coldness of limbs, pale tongue with whitish coating, sunk and slow pulse.

温毒 【wēn dú】感受温邪热毒而引起的急性热病的统称。多发于冬春季节。临床以头面或咽喉肿痛、出血性斑疹、突然寒战高热、头痛、烦躁口渴、苔黄、舌红绛、脉洪数为特征。本病可见于流行性腮腺炎、头面丹毒、

Epidemic Heat-syndrome a general term for acute febrile diseases caused by virulent heat pathogen, occurring more frequently in winter and spring, marked by swelling and pain in the head, face and throat, hemorrhagic

猩红热、斑疹伤寒等。

skin eruption, sudden chill and high fever, headache, excessive thirst, yellow fur, bright red tongue, full and fast pulse, seen in epidemic mumps, erysipelas in the head and face, scarlet fever, typhus, etc.

温毒发斑 【wēn dú fā bān】由于温热之毒充斥身体各部分,影响营血运行透发于肌肤,而在皮肤上见到红或紫红色斑疹。

Skin Rashes Caused by Violent Heat-pathogen a morbid condition due to attack of virulent heat to all parts of the body, involving yingfen and xuefen marked by red or purplish red rashes over the skin.

温法 【wēn fǎ】(祛寒法)即使用温热药治疗寒证的方法,包括温中祛寒、温经祛寒、回阳救逆、甘温除热等。

Therapy by Warming one of the eight principal therapeutic methods, used for treating cold-syndromes with medicines of warm and hot nature; including warming the middle-energizer to dispel cold, expelling pathogenic cold by warming the meridians, recuperating depleted yang and rescuing the patient from collapse, relieving high fever with drugs of sweet flavor and warm nature.

温服 【wēn fú】汤剂煎好后,待不冷不热时服下,是目前汤剂的一般服法。

(Decoction) To be Taken Warm generally, a decoction is to be taken when it is neither too cold nor too hot.

温和灸 【wēn hé jiǔ】是将艾卷点燃的一端,与施灸部位的皮肤保持一寸左右的距离,使患者有温热而无灼痛感的一种灸法。

Mild Moxibustion a technique of suspended moxibustion whereby the lighted end of a moxa roll is held 1 cun (approximately 3.5cm) above the skin simply to produce a sensation of warmth, with no sensation of scorching pain.

温经祛寒 【wēn jīng qū hán】即温通经络,祛散寒邪的方法。适用于寒邪

Expelling Pathogenic Cold by Warming the Meridians a therapy for

凝滞经络，气血运行受阻，而见肢体关节疼痛、痛有定处，日轻夜重，或月经不调等症。 warming meridians to expell pathogenic cold. Used for treating blockade of the flow of qi and blood due to stagnation of pathogenic cold in the meridians, marked by arthralgia of limbs, spotted pain, light at daytime and severe at night, or irregular menstruation.

温麻 【wēn má】指感受温热、疫疠时行之气所致的麻疹病。症见壮热、烦渴、疹出稠密而色鲜红。 **Warm-Type Measles** measles caused by warm and heat pathogen or other infectious pathogens, marked by high fever, thirst, dense and scarlet measles.

温疟 【wēn nüè】疟疾之一。多因素有伏热，夏感疟邪或内有伏邪，至夏季感受暑热而发的一种疟疾。 **Pyrexial Malaria** a kind of malaria caused by latent heat, insidious pathogen in summer, summer-heat.

温脾 【wēn pí】用温中祛寒的方药，治疗脾胃虚寒的一种治法。 **Warming the Spleen** a method for treating the cold syndrome of the spleen by application of drugs for warming the middle-energizer to dispel cold.

温热 【wēn rè】1、病邪之一。指温邪或热邪。2、各种燥热病的统称。 **Warm-Heat** 1. one of the pathogenic factors, referring to warm pathogen or heat pathogen. 2. a gereral term for diseases caused by pathogenic dryness and heat.

温热痉 【wēn rè jìng】温热病邪侵袭经络所致的痉证。症见壮热、烦渴、汗出、神昏、四肢痉挛甚或角弓反张、脉洪数等。 **Convulsive Seizure Caused by Warm-Heat** convulsive syndrome caused by attacks of warm-heat pathogen on the meridians; marked by high fever, thirst, sweating, coma, spasm of limbs, or opisthotonos, full and fast pulse.

温肾 【wēn shèn】（补肾阳）治疗肾阳虚的方法。适用于肾阳不足。症见腰酸膝冷、软弱无力、阳萎、小便频数、清长、舌淡苔白、脉沉弱等。 **Warming the Kidney** a method for warming and recuperating kidney-yang, used for treating insufficiency of the kidney-yang, marked by weak-

温肾利水 【wēn shèn lì shuǐ】治疗肾阳虚水肿的方法。即使用温补肾阳辅以利水的药物,以治疗肾阳虚衰,气化不利,致水湿内停的病证。

Warming the Kidney to Promote Diuresis a method used in the treatment of edema due to hypofunction of the kidney, treating retention of the water within the body due to insufficiency of the kidney-yang and disturbance in qi transformation, by application of drugs with the action of warming and recuperating the kidney-yang together with diuretics.

温肾助阳 【wēn shèn zhù yáng】用具有温补肾阳的药物为主组成方剂,治疗肾阳虚衰的一种方法,适用于肾阳虚衰所引起的各种病证,如五更泄泻、腰酸肢冷等。

Warming the Kidney to Support Yang a method for treating insufficiency of kidney-yang by using a prescription mainly formed with drugs with the action of warming and recuperating kidney-yang, suitable for diseases due to insufficiency of kidney-yang, e. g. diarrhea before dawn, chronic nephritis and nephrosis.

温胃健中 【wēn wèi jiàn zhōng】是治疗胃气虚寒的一种方法。适用于上腹部隐痛而食后疼痛减轻、吐清水、大便泄泻、舌淡白、脉细等症。

Warming the Stomach and Strengthening the Middle Energizer a method for treating insufficiency of the stomach-qi with cold syndromes, used for treating dull pain in the upper part of the abdomen and pain relieved after meals, vomiting of watery fluid, diarrhea, pale tongue, thready pulse.

温下 【wēn xià】使用温性而有泻下作用的药物,治疗寒性积滞里实证的治法。适用于症见腹满而实、大便不通、

Purgation with Drugs of Warm Nature a method for treating cold-type constipation by administering purga-

手足凉、苔白腻、脉沉弦或沉迟者。tives of warm nature, applicable to the case manifested as abdominal distention, constipation, cold limbs, whitish and greasy fur, sunken and wiry pulse or sunken and slow pulse.

温邪 【wēn xié】各种温热病致病邪气的通称。如春温、暑温、冬温、湿温、秋燥等病因。

Warm-Pathogenic Factor a general term for various kinds of exopathic factors causing epidemic febrile diseases, e. g. spring-warm syndrome, summer fever, winter-warm syndrome, damp-warm syndrome, autumn-dryness disease.

温邪犯肺 【wēn xié fàn fèi】温热邪气侵犯肺脏的病理。症见发热、口干或咽喉充血肿痛、舌边尖红、脉浮数等。

Attack of Pathogenic Warm to the Lung pathologic manifestation due to the invasion of the lung by pathogenic warm, marked by fever, thirst, or redness and soreness of the throat, reddened tongue-edge, fast and floating pulse.

温血 【wēn xuè】治疗血分有寒的方法。1、温补血分。用甘温补气血的药物治疗气血虚弱引起的崩漏、吐血、舌质淡、脉虚无力等症；2、温化瘀血治疗因寒致瘀血内留的方法。

Warming the Blood a method for treating cold in the blood system. (1) tonifying the blood with drugs of warm nature; treating metrorrhagia and metrostaxis, hematemesis, pale tongue, weak and feeble pulse due to deficiency of qi and blood, by using drugs of sweet and warm nature to tonify the blood. (2) resolving blood stasis with drugs of warm nature, a method for treating blood stasis due to cold.

温阳 【wēn yáng】温通阳气的方法。包括回阳救逆和温中祛寒等。

Warming Yang a method of warming and activating yang-qi, including emergency treatment of collapse (depletion of yang) and warming the middle energizer for dispelling cold.

温阳利湿 【wēn yáng lì shī】（化气利水）。治阳气被水寒之邪阻遏而致小便不利的方法。常用温阳化气药与健脾利水药同用，使小便通畅。

Warming Yang for Diuresis a method for treating difficulty in urination due to cold-damp, by using drugs with the action of invigorating yang together with diuretics to promote diuresis.

温阳利水 【wēn yáng lì shuǐ】用温补脾肾的药物，扶助脾肾阳气的治法，以促进体内过剩水液从小便排出。

Warming Yang to Promote Diuresis a method of reinforcing yang-qi in the spleen and kidney by using drugs of warm nature to promote excretion of excess watery fluid from the body with the urine.

温养 【wēn yǎng】用温性有补益作用的药物，以补养正气的方法。

Warming and Nourishing a method for nourishing qi by using tonics of warm nature.

温疫 【wēn yì】（天行温疫）指各种热性流行性传染病或这些病的流行。

Infectious Epidemic Disease a general term for various kinds of infectious epidemic febrile diseases and their prevalence.

温针 【wēn zhēn】指针体刺入穴位后，在针柄或针体部，燃烧艾绒，使热通过针体传入体内，以达到温通经脉，行气活血作用的一种针法。

Acupuncture with the Needle Warmed by Burning Moxa one form of moxibustion, procedure that combines needling and moxibustion by attacking burning moxa stub to an already inserted needle and conducting heat to the body through the needle to promote flow of qi and circulation of blood by warming the meridians.

温中祛寒 【wēn zhōng qū hán】温法之一。治疗脾胃阳虚，阴寒内盛的方法。适用于脾胃虚寒。症见食不消化、呕吐清水、大便清稀、舌淡苔白、脉沉细等。

Warming the Middle Energizer to Dispel Cold one of the warming methods. a therapy for treating the internal cold syndrome due to hypofunction of the spleen and stomach, suitable for treating hypofunction and cold syndrome of the spleen and stomach, marked by indigestion, vom-

瘟黄 【wēn huáng】泛指伴有黄疸的烈性传染病。多因感受疫疠之气、湿热时毒所引起。症见高热神昏、身目呈深黄色、尿如柏汁、腹胀有水、胁痛、吐衄、便血或发斑疹、舌红绛、苔黄燥、脉弦洪等。

瘟痧 【wēn shā】由寒气郁伏,至春而发;或暑热凝滞至秋而发,互相传染的病证。症见恶寒发热或腹痛、头面肿胀或气急满闷、胸膈饱胀或下痢脓血等。

瘟疫 【wēn yì】(瘟) 感受疫疠之气所致的多种流行性急性传染病的总称。

文火 【wén huǒ】小而缓的火。
纹沉 【wén chén】食指掌面外侧浅表小静脉外观深沉。一般是病邪在里的表现。

iting watery fluids, watery stool, pale tongue with whitish coating, sunken and threadly pulse.

Fulminant Jaundice a general term for fulminating infectious diseases with jaundice, usually caused by epidemic pathogenic factors and pathogenic damp-heat, marked by coma due to high fever, dark yellow pigmentation of the body and eyes, dark yellow colored urine, distention of water in the abdomen, hypochondriac pain, hematemesis, hemafecia, or skin eruptions, deep-red tongue, dry, rough and yellowish fur, wiry and full pulse.

Epidemic Eruptive Disease an infectious disease occurring in spring due to cold latent in winter or occurring in autumn due to summer-heat in summer, marked by fever and chills, or abdominal pain, swelling of the head and face, or fullness of abdomen due to stagnation of qi, fullness of the chest and hypochondrium, or dysentery with pus and blood in the stool.

Infectious Epidemic Disease a general term for various kinds of acute infectious epidemic diseases caused by epidemic pathogenic factors.

Soft Fire soft and slow fire
Poor Visibitlity of the Superficial Venule of the Index finger a condition generally indicating that the pathogenic factor is located deeply in

纹浮 【wén fú】食指掌面外侧浅表小静脉浮现。一般是初感外邪病尚在表的征象。

Clear Appearance of the Superficial Venule of the Index Finger a condition indicating the primary stage of exposure to exogenous pathogenic factors with pathogenic factors still in the exterior.

纹滞 【wén zhì】食指掌面外侧浅表小静脉郁滞,血液回流不畅,通常是病邪稽留,营卫运行不畅所致。多属实证。

Congestion of the Superficial Venule of the Index Finger a condition indicative of excess syndrome usually caused by the retention of pathogenic factors and the disorder of circulation in ying and wei.

闻诊 【wén zhěn】四诊之一。通过听觉和嗅觉器官来了解患者语言、呼吸、咳嗽、呃逆、呻吟以及分泌物、排泄物的气味的变化,以判断病情。

Auscultation and Olfaction one of the diagnostic methods, consisting of listening (to the patient's voice, breathing, coughing, hicupping, moaning) and smelling (odor of the secretion and excretion) to ascertain the clinical status.

问耳目 【wèn ěr mù】十问内容之一。询问听力、视力的变化,有无耳鸣、耳痛、重听,眼睛有无痛痒及其伴随症状等。

Inquiring about Condition of Ears and Eyes one of the ten aspects in inquiring of the patient, including hearing acuity or any tinnitus and earache, visual acuity or any local itching, pain and other associated symptoms.

问二便 【wèn èr biàn】十问内容之一。通过了解大小便的变化,包括数量、性状、颜色、气味及伴随症状,以了解病情,协助诊断。

Inquiring about Defecation and Micturition one of the ten aspects in inquiring of the patient, including the amount, character, colour and smell of the urine and feces, as well as the associated symptoms, which is helpful to understand the progress of a disease and to establish a diagnosis.

问妇女 【wèn fù nǚ】根据妇女病理生

Inquiring about Female Condition

理特点，通过询问妇女的月经史、生育史及白带的变化等情况，以帮助判断病情。

问寒热 【wèn hán rè】十问内容之一。了解患者发热及恶寒情况，包括时间、规律、程度及其伴随症状，以辨别疾病的部位及正邪斗争的情况。

问汗 【wèn hàn】十问内容之一。通过了解患者出汗的情况，包括出汗的多少、时间、部位及伴随症状，以辨别病的虚实、表里、阴阳。

问起病 【wèn qǐ bìng】询问起病的时间、原因、经过、治疗情况以及主要症状和变化，以判断病情协助诊断。

问睡眠 【wèn shuì mián】十问内容之一。询问睡眠的变化，包括嗜睡失眠、多梦等情况，以帮助判断病情。如嗜睡多属阳虚阴盛或痰湿内阻等。

one of the contents in inquiring of the female patient, including menstrual history, delivery history, leucorrhea, etc., which is helpful to ascertain the clinical status.

Inquiring about Chillness and Fever one of the ten aspects in inquiring of the patient, including the time of occurrence, regularity and severity of chillness and fever, as well as the associated symptoms, which is helpful to determine the involved part of a disease and the condition of confliction between the healthy-qi and the pathogenic factor.

Inquiring about Perspiration one of the ten aspects in inquiring of the patient, including the amount, time and site of sweating as well as the associated symptoms, which is helpful to differentiate the disorder whether asthenic or sthenic, involving the superficies or the interior, attributive to yin or yang.

Inquiring about the Onset of Disease one of the contents in inquiring of the patient, which is helpful to establish a diagnosis, including the time of onset and its causative factor, the course of a disease, previous treatment as well as the changes of the principal symptoms.

Inquiring about Condition of Sleeping one of the ten aspects in inquiring of the patient, including sleepiness, insomnia, dreaminess, etc., which is helpful to understand the progress of a disease. For instance, the condition of sleepiness may be indicative of yang-insufficiency and yin-excess or stagnation of phlegm-dampness in the body.

问头身 【wèn tóu shēn】十问内容之一。1、了解头痛及眩晕的情况,包括时间、部位、持续时间、性质及伴随症状;2、了解身体疼痛的性质、部位及伴随症状。

Inquiring about the Condition of Head and Trunk one of the ten aspects in inquiring of the patient, including (1) the time of occurrence, site, duration and character of headache and dizziness as well as the associated symptoms; (2) the character and site of pain in the trunk as well as the associated symptoms.

问小儿 【wèn xiǎo ér】根据小儿病理生理特点,通过询问小儿父母的健康状况及小儿的喂养、发育等情况及既往史中的麻疹、水痘、天花的病史,以帮助判断病情和明确诊断。

inquiring about the Condition of a Child one of the contents in inquiring of a child patient, including the health condition of his parents, feeding habit, growth condition and past history esp. measles, chicken pox and small pox, which is helpful to establish a diagnosis.

问胸腹 【wèn xiōng fù】十问内容之一。通过询问胸腹的情况,有助于辨别脏腑的疾病。如两胁疼痛多属肝胆疾病等。

inquiring about the Condition of the Chest and Abdomen one of the ten aspects in inquiring of the patient, which is helpful to differentiate various visceral disorders, for instance, hypochondriac pain is usually indicative of the disorders of the liver or gallbladder.

问饮食口味 【wèn yǐn shí kǒu wèi】十问内容之一。通过询问患者饮食口味的情况,以了解脾胃的功能情况,判断病势的进退以及疾病的属性。

Inquiring about Taste for Food one of the ten aspects in inquiring of the patient, which is helpful to understand the functional condition of the spleen and stomach and to determine

问诊 【wèn zhěn】四诊之一。即询问患者的现病史、既往史、月经史、生育史、生活习惯、饮食嗜好以及年令、籍贯、职业、住址以及其他与病情有关情况。是判断病情、明确诊断的重要方法之一。

卧不安 【wò bù ān】不能安睡。饮食过饱或胃中有热等均可产生此证。

乌风内障 【wū fēng nèi zhàng】因阴虚火旺，内挟风痰所致的内眼病。症见瞳孔散大而混浊如浓雾,伴有眼珠疼痛及头痛，相当于青光眼。

乌癞 【wū lài】因恶风侵袭皮肤与血分之间,耗伤血液所致的以皮肤感觉异常为主症的疾病。初起时局部皮肤变黑,痒如虫行,继而出现手足麻木，丧失痛觉。类似疣型麻风。

乌痧 【wū shā】因痧毒结于脏腑，气血瘀滞所致的痧证。表现为全身胀痛难忍、面色黧黑、皮肤出现乌斑等。

Inquiring one of the four methods of physical examination for the diagnosis of diseases, i. e., to interrogate the patient about his present illness, past history, living and food habit, as well as age, native place, occupation, address and other related information.

Insomnia with Restlessness a condition caused by over eating, or retention of pathogenic heat in the stomach.

Glaucoma a condition caused by the hyperactivity of pathogenic fire due to yin-deficiency and the attack of wind-phlegm, marked by dilatat on and dull gray gleam of the pupil, accompanied with ocular pain and headache.

Blackish Dermatosis a disease with paraesthesia of the skin as the major symptom, caused by the consumption of blood due to attack of pathogenic wind involving the part between the skin and the xuefen; manifested as local blackish coloration and itching of the skin at onset, followed by numbness of the extremities and loss of pain sensation; similar to tuberculoid leprosy.

Eruptive Disease with Dark Purplish Rashes an eruptive disease caused by the stagnation of vital qi and blood due to accumulation of sha in the vis-

乌痧惊风 【wū shā jīng fēng】感受痧毒使经络阻滞，血行不畅所致的小儿惊风，并见全身发紫、烦躁不安。

Infantile Convulsion with Cyanosis infantile convulsion due to stagnation of meridian of flow and blood circulation, usually accompanied with cyanosis and irritability.

乌头类中毒 【wū tóu lèi zhòng dú】因服乌头、附子、天雄等类药物过量而引起的中毒。表现为口唇及四肢麻木、头晕、言语不清、视物模糊及心率加快等；重者出现心律不齐、血压下降、抽搐、昏迷、发绀、瞳孔散大及心跳呼吸停止。

Aconite Poisoning an intoxication by over dosage of aconite; manifested as numbness of the lips and extremities, dizziness, dysphasia, blurring of vision, tachycardia; and arrhythmia, hypotension, convulsion coma, cyanosis, dilated pupils, and cardiac and respiratory arrest in serious cases.

屋漏脉 【wū lòu mài】脉搏极其缓慢、节律不整、有不规则间歇的一种脉象。

Roof-Leaking Pulse a pulse condition characterized by very slow beats with irregular intervals.

无瘢痕灸 【wú bān hén jiǔ】不使灸处形成水泡、化脓及瘢痕的一种灸法。灸时艾柱放在皮肤上的时间较短，不致灼伤皮肤，故灸后不留痕迹。

Non-Scarring Moxibustion a method of moxibustion without the formation of local blister, pustule and scar. The moxa cone is applied on the skin for only a short time so that the skin is not cauterized.

无毒 【wú dú】无毒性的药物，即平性药。根据病情需要，在医师指导下，可以多服、久服。

No Toxicity referring to the drugs which are non-poisonous and can be taken frequently or in a larger dosage under the direction of physician.

无汗 【wú hàn】肌表腠理为暑湿所闭，或风寒束闭于表所致无汗出的一种症状。

Anhidrosis a symptom with absence of perspiration due to the hair follicles closed by summer-damp or due to wind attacking the superficies.

无名肿毒 【wú míng zhǒng dú】体表

Inflammation of Soft Tissues of Un-

骤发局部红肿的一种炎症症状。如蜂窝组织炎初起。

无痰干咳 【wú tán gān ké】意同干咳嗽。即咳嗽无痰。多因火郁,感受燥邪或肺阴不足所致。

无头疽 【wú tóu jū】位于筋骨或深部肌肉的化脓性感染。见于附骨疽、流注等多种疾病。

毋犯胃气 【wú fàn wèi qì】胃的消化功能,是人体得到营养物质,维持生理功能的保证,所以用药时,必须注意不要损害胃的功能。

毋实实 【wù shí shí】当病邪盛时,不能采用补的治法,以免使病邪更实。

毋虚虚 【wù xū xū】当正气虚的时候,不能采用攻伐的治法,以免使正气更虚。

蜈蚣咬伤 【wú gōng yǎo shāng】蜈蚣咬伤后,局部出现肿疼、发痒、周身麻木等症。

五败 【wǔ bài】指五脏严重损害,功能严重障碍 时的病理及临床表现。如严重水肿、腹胀、肚脐突出属脾败。

known Origin sudden onset of local redness and swelling after infection, such as the primary stage of phlegmon.

Nonproductive Cough a symptom usually caused by the stagnation of fire, the attack of dryness or the insufficiency of the lung-yin.

Deep Abscess suppurative infection of the bone or deep layer of muscle; seen in the cases of suppurative osteomyelitis and multiple abscess, etc.

Protecting the Stomach-qi a principle of drug application, i. e., the digestive function of the stomach should not be impaired, since it provides nourishments and maintains normal activities of the human body.

Sthenia-syndrome should not be Invigorated a principle of treatment that invigoration should not be applied when the pathogenic factor is hyperactive.

Asthenia-syndrome should not be Debilitated a principle of treatment that purgation should not be applied when the healthy-qi is deficient.

Centipede Bite injury by centipede manifested as local swelling, itching, numbness over the body, etc.

Serious Disorders of Five Viscera the morbid condition and clinical manifestations reflecting the severe damage and dysfunction of the five viscera, e. g., marked edema, flatulence and protrusion of the umbilicus

五崩 【wǔ bēng】指分泌物颜色不同的五种带下病。即白崩、赤崩、黄崩、青崩及黑崩。

五不男 【wǔ bù nán】古时指男性生殖器官先天性畸形或后天性功能失调所致不育的五种病证,即天、漏、犍、怯、变。

五不女 【wǔ bù nǚ】古时指女性生殖器官先天性畸形或后天性功能失调所致不育的五种病证,即螺、纹、鼓、角、脉。

五裁 【wǔ cái】人体对五味即酸、辛、咸、苦、甘应当有所节制,不宜过食,特别是身体有病时更应注意。如病在筋则应少吃或不吃酸味的食物。

五常 【wǔ cháng】水、火、土、金、水五类物质的正常运动。

五迟 【wǔ chí】小儿发育迟缓的五种表现。即立迟、行迟、发迟、齿迟及语迟。

symbolzie the serious disorder of the spleen.

Five Kinds of Leukorrhagia Leukorrhagia with secretions of five colours, i. e., profuse leucorrhea with whitish, reddish, yellowish, greenish and blackish discharge.

Five Kinds of Male Sterility in ancient times, referring to sterility caused by the congenital malformations or acquired dysfunction of the male genital organs, i. e., anorchism, habitual emission, castration, impotence and hermaphroditism.

Five Kinds of Female Sterility in ancient times, referring to sterility caused by the congenital malformations or acquired dysfunction of female genital organs, i. e., spiral lines on the vagina, atresia or stricture of the vagina, imperforated hymen, clitorism and primary amenorrhea.

Intake of Food of Five Tates in Moderation the food of five tastes, i. e., sour, acrid, salty, bitter and sweet, should be taken moderately, esp. for the diseased, for example, sour food should be limited for the patient with tendon disorder.

Motion of the Five Elements the normal motion of the five elements, i. e., wood, fire, earth, metal and water.

Five Kinds of Maldevelopment the five manifestations of growth tardiness in infants, i. e., tardiness of ability to stand, to walk and to speak, and of growth of the hair and the teeth.

五畜 【wǔ chù】五种牲畜。指牛、羊、猪、犬、鸡。
Five Kinds of Animals referring to the ox, sheep, pig, dog and chicken.

五喘恶候 【wǔ chuǎn è hòu】出现喘症即提示预后不良的五种疾病。即痘疮、惊风、虚肿、吐泻及下痢。为邪胜正衰，元气将脱的危象。
Dyspnea as a Critical Symptom in Five Diseases an unfavorable prognosis indicating that the pathogenic factor is hyperactive and the healthy qi is deficient, and the primordial qi is exhausted whenever dyspnea appears in the cases of smallpox, infantile convulsion, anasarca, vomiting with diarrhea and dysentery.

五疸 【wǔ dǎn】按《金匮要略》的叙述，有如下五种黄疸：即黄疸、谷疸、酒疸、女劳疸及黑疸。
Five Kinds of Jaundice a classification of jaundice according to the description in 《Synopsis of the Golden Chamber》, i. e., clinical jaundice, dietetic jaundice, overstrain jaundice and black jaundice.

五疔 【wǔ dīng】五种疔疮的合称。按颜色分类指青疔、赤疔、白疔、黑疔及黄疔；按脏腑分类，指心疔、肝疔、脾疔、肺疔及肾疔。
Five Kinds of Furuncle the classification of furuncle, i. e., green, red, white, black and yellow according to its colour; heart, liver, spleen, lung and kidney according to its involvement of viscera.

五夺 【wǔ duó】指气血津液严重耗损，禁用泻法的五种情况。即1、严重消瘦，身体极度衰弱；2、大出血后；3、大出汗后；4、严重泄泻后；5、分娩严重失血之后等。
Five Conditions of Body Exhaustion the serious disorders caused by the excessive consumption of qi, blood and body fluid, to which the purgatives are contraindicated, i. e., (1) cachexia; (2) massive hemorrhage; (3) profuse perspiration; (4) severe diarrhea and (5) severe loss of blood during delivery.

五度 【wǔ dù】即衡量神、气、血、形、志五者的有余与不足。
Determination of the Five Status an estimation for whether an excess or

insufficiency of the five status, i. e., spirit, qi, blood, body physique and mind.

五腑 【wǔ fǔ】（五中）即与五脏相合之腑。指小肠、大肠、胆、胃和膀胱。

Five Fu-organs referring to the small intestine, large intestine, gallbladder, stomach and urinary bladder, which match the five zang organs.

五疳 【wǔ gān】按五脏病变分类的五种疳证。即心疳、肝疳、脾疳、肺疳和肾疳。

Five Kinds of Infantile Malnutrition disorder of nutrition in children, classified by the pathological changes of the five viscera, i. e., heart-, liver-, spleen-, lung-, and kidney-malnutrition.

五更嗽 【wǔ gēng sòu】黎明前咳嗽发作或加重的病证。可因痰火、脾虚或食积所致。

Morning Cough paroxysms or aggravation of cough before dawn, resulting from phlegm-fire, spleen-asthenia, or dyspepsia.

五更泄 【wǔ gēng xiè】（晨泄、灌泻）于黎明前泄泻的病证。多因肾阳虚衰所致，亦有因食积、酒积、肝火而引起。

Morning Diarrhea a disease mostly caused by deficiency of kidney-yang, or by dyspepsia, alcoholism, and liver-fire.

五谷 【wǔ gǔ】五种谷类，如米、小豆、麦、大豆、黄粟。

Five Kinds of Cereal referring to rice, small bean, wheat, bean and millet.

五官 【wǔ guān】指鼻、眼、口、舌、耳五个器官，与五脏有密切关系。

Five Sense Organs the five sense organs, i. e., nose, eye, lip, tongue and ear, which bear a close relationship to the five viscera.

五软 【wǔ ruǎn】小儿发育不良所致动作缓弱的五种表现。即头软、项软、手脚软、肌肉软及口软。

Five Kinds of Flabbiness five manifestations of sluggish movement caused by underdevelopment in infants, i. e., flabbiness of head, of neck, of hands and feet, of muscles and of mouth.

五果 【wǔ guǒ】五种果类，如枣、杏、

Five Kinds of Fruits referring to

栗、李及桃。

五积 【wǔ jī】泛指胸腹部存在肿块的病证。

五精 【wǔ jīng】五脏所具有的精华物质，是五脏进行功能活动的物质基础。

五绝 【wǔ jué】五种卒死的情况。历代各家说法不一，如自缢、摧压、溺水、服毒、魇魅等。

五劳 【wǔ láo】1、心劳、肝劳、脾劳、肺劳及肾劳等五脏阴阳气血衰弱的疾病。2、指引起虚劳的五类致病因素。见五劳所伤。

五劳所伤 【wǔ láo suǒ shāng】指因劳逸不当，气、血、筋骨功能失调而引起的五类劳损。通常指久视伤血、久卧伤气、久坐伤肉、久立伤骨、久行伤筋。

五淋 【wǔ lín】五种不同病因和表现的淋证。一般指石淋、气淋、劳淋、膏淋及血淋。

date, apricot, chestnut, plum and peach.

Five Kinds of Masses generally referring to the disease with a mass in the abdomen.

Essence of the Five Viscera the essential substances stored in the five viscera, necessary for their functional activities.

Five Kinds of Sudden Death generally referring to hanging onself, death by crushing, drowning, sudden death with unknown cause, taking posion, etc.

Five Kinds of Impairment 1. diseases of the five zang organs i. e., the impairments of heart, liver, spleen, lung and kidney, resulting from the deficiency of yin, yang, qi and blood of the corresponding organ. 2. five kinds of pathogenic factors causing consumptive diseases.

Five Kinds of Impairments by Overstrain the functional disorders of qi, blood, tendon, muscle, and bone caused by overstrain, usually referring to impairment of blood by prolonged seeing, impairment of qi by prolonged lying, impairment of muscle by prolonged sitting, impairment of bone by prolonged standing, and impariment of tendon by prolonged walking.

Five Kinds of Stranguria the stranguria with different manifestations and etiologies, generally referring to those caused by urinary stone, by the disorder of qi, by overstrain, or those complicated with chyluria, or with hematuria.

五轮 【wǔ lún】眼科学的一种理论。即眼睛的五个部位，包括肉轮、血轮、气轮、风轮和水轮，用以说明眼与内脏的关系。

Five Wheels one of the ancient doctrines on ophthalmology, which divided the eye into five portions in accordance with the five zang organs, i. e., flesh-wheel (spleen), blood-wheel (vs. heart), qi-wheel (vs. lung), wind-wheel (vs. liver) and water-wheel (vs. kidney).

五脉 【wǔ mài】指五脏的脉象，即肝脉弦、心脉洪、脾脉缓、肺脉浮及肾脉沉。

Pulse Condition of the Five Zang-organs the five kinds of pulse condition corresponding to the characteristics of the five zang-organs, i. e., the liver-pulse is wiry, the heart-pulse is bounding (full), the spleen-pulse is even and soft, the lung-pulse is floating, and the kidney-pulse is sunken.

五色 【wǔ sè】即青、黄、赤、白、黑五种颜色。与五脏有一定的关系，常用五色的变化来帮助了解病情，但必须与其他临床资料结合起来，不能硬套。

Five Colours referring to the colours of green, red, yellow, white and black, which match the five zang organs. The observation of the colours is helpful for establishing a diagnosis if it is combined with other clinical data.

五色带下 【wǔ sè dài xià】阴道分泌物呈多种颜色的带下病。多因湿热蕴结下焦，积瘀成毒，损伤冲任带脉所致。

Leucorrhagia with Varicoloured Discharge profuse leucorrhagia caused by the impairment of TV, CV and BV resulting from the retention of pathogenic dampness-heat in the lower-energizer.

五色痢 【wǔ sè lì】粪便有多种颜色的痢疾。

Dysentery with Multicoloured Stool.

五色五味所入 【wǔ sè wǔ wèi suǒ rù】古人据五行学说，将药物五色五味的

Attribution of the Five Colours and the Five Tastes the attribution of five

五行所属与脏腑经络相配。如色青、味酸属木，入足厥阴肝、足少阳胆。此属归经学说的内容之一。

五色诊 【wǔ sè zhěn】望诊内容之一。根据患者面部出现青、黄、赤、白、黑等色泽的变化来进行分析病情和诊断的方法。

五色主病 【wǔ sè zhǔ bìng】青、赤、黄、白、黑五种病色所主的病证。1、以五色配五脏，认为五色与五脏疾病有关，即青主肝病，赤主心病，黄主脾病，白主肺病，黑主肾病。2、以五色来辨别疾病的性质，即青主风、主惊、主寒、主痛；赤主热；黄主湿；白主血虚、主寒；黑主痛、主血瘀、主劳伤等。

五善 【wǔ shàn】表示疮疡疾病预后良好的五种证候。即起居饮食如常，大小便通调，脓色鲜而不臭及脓溃肿消，精神良好、语声清朗，身体壮健等。

colours and five tastes matched with the viscera and meridians based on the theory of five elements, e. g., the blue colour and sour taste attribute to wood and match the liver meridian of foot Jueyin as well as the gallbladder meridian of foot Shaoyang.

Inspection of the Five Colours of Complexion a method of examination for the analysis and diagnosis of a disease according to the colour changes of the complexion, i. e., green, yellow, red, white, and black.

Five Colours as References for Diagnosis 1. based on the viewpoint of the five colours matching with the five viscera, it is said that green colour symbolizes liver disease, red symbolizes heart, yellow symbolizes spleen, white symbolizes lung, and black symbolizes kidney. 2. The nature of disease may be differentiated by means of the five colours such as, green colour may be traced to wind, to frightening, to cold, to pain; red to heat; yellow to dampness; white to blood deficiency, to cold; black to pain, to blood stasis, to overstrain, etc.

Five Favourable Conditions conditions with favourable prognosis in pyogonic infections of skin, including regular life with normal appetite; normal urination and defecation, bright-coloured pus without smell, well drainage of the pus with subsidence

五声 【wǔ shēng】指呼、笑、歌、哭、呻（呻吟）等五类声音。

五十动 【wǔ shí dòng】古代诊脉常规。古代诊脉至少要观察脉搏跳动五十次，以辨别脉搏的变化。

五实 【wǔ shí】五脏均受实热闭阻的综合证候。

五水 【wǔ shuǐ】即心水、肝水、脾水、肺水及肾水。一般认为是水肿病因五脏受水气的影响而出现的不同症状。

五体 【wǔ tǐ】机体的五种组织，即筋、脉、肉、皮、骨等。

五味 【wǔ wèi】指中药的辛、甘、酸、苦、咸五种味道。

五味偏嗜 【wǔ wèi piān shì】长期偏食五味的某一味，或某类食物，对人体可能产生不良反应或致病。

五味所合 【wǔ wèi suǒ hé】五味与五脏相配属，即心与苦味、肺与辛味、肝与酸味、脾与甘味、肾与咸味。

of swelling, spiritedness and clear speech, and good health.

Five Sounds the five kinds of sound, shouting, laughing, singing, crying and moaning.

Fifty Beats a routine examination of pulse condition in ancient times, i. e., to feel the pulse for at least fifty beats in order to discriminate the changes of the pulse.

Sthenia-syndrome of Five Zang-Organs the morbid condition and clinical manifestations due to stagnation of sthenic heat in the five zang-organs.

Five Kinds of Edema referring to heart-edema, liver-edema, spleen-edema, lung-edema and kidney-edema, symptoms vary with the different organs affected by the retention of fluid.

Body Constituents the five tissues of the body, i. e., tendon, vessel, muscle, skin and bone.

Five Tastes referring to the tastes of traditional Chinese medicines, i. e., acrid, sweet, sour, bitter and salty.

Food Partiality a partiality for particular taste (sour, bitter, sweet, acrid or salty) or particular kind of food, which may have side effect on the human body and become a pathogenic factor.

What the Five Kinds of Tastes Match with the five kinds of tastes match with the five viscera, i. e., the heart with bitter, the lung with

五味所禁 【wǔ wèi suǒ jìn】(五禁) 五脏发生病变时对五味的禁忌,如肝病禁辛、心病禁咸、脾病禁酸、肾病禁甘、肺病禁苦。

五味所伤 【wǔ wèi suǒ shāng】由于过份的嗜好五味,以致伤害人体的皮、肉、筋骨、脉等。

五味所入 【wǔ wèi suǒ rù】由于五味与五脏有一定的配属关系,不同药味对某些脏腑有选择性,如酸入肝,酸味药物可以对肝脏病变起治疗或药引的作用。

五泄 【wǔ xiè】 五种泄泻的总称。即飧泄、溏泄、鹜泄、濡泄、滑泄。

五心烦热 【wǔ xīn fán rè】指两手足心及心胸等部位有烦热感的证候。多由阴虚火旺,或病后虚热未清,以及火热内郁等引起,是虚劳及劳瘵等病的常见症状。

acrid, the liver with sour, the spleen with sweet, and the kidney with salty.

To what the Five Kinds of Tastes are Contraindicated the five kinds of tastes are contraindicated to certain diseases of viscera, e. g., the acrid taste is contraindicated to the diseases of liver; the salty taste, to heart diseases; the sour taste, to spleen diseases; the acrid taste, to kidney diseases; the bitter taste, to lung diseases.

What the Five Kinds of Tastes Impair over-eating of the food with the five tastes may impair the skin, muscle, tendon, bone and vessel.

What the Five Kinds of Tastes Attribute to since the five kinds of tastes are attributive to the five viscera, various tastes of the drugs act selectively to certain viscera, e. g., the drugs of sour taste may treat hepatic diseases or act as a guide to the liver.

Five Kinds of Diarrhea referring to diarrhea with stools containing indigested food, with loose stools, with stools like duck-feces, with watery stools and with incontinence of feces.

Feverish Sensation of Five Centers referring to the feverish sensation over the palms, soles and the chest; a common symptom of consumptive diseases usually caused by the deficiency of yin and the hyperactivity of pathogenic fire, by the remnants of

五行学说 【wǔ xíng xué shuō】中国古代哲学理论。阐明五行（水、火、土、金、木）的物质属性及其相互关系。中医学用它来说明脏腑器官的属性、相互之间的关系、生理现象和病理变化，并用以指导疾病的诊断和治疗。

五虚 【wǔ xū】《素问》描述的五种危重证候。即脉细、皮寒、气少、大小便滑泄及饮食不入，表示五脏俱虚，预后不良。

五液 【wǔ yè】即汗、涕、泪、涎、唾等五种分泌液的合称。

五宜 【wǔ yí】五脏有病时，各有所相适宜的药物，以利于病的治疗。如肺病宜吃黄黍、鸡肉、桃、葱等。

五瘿 【wǔ yǐng】按颈部肿块的性状与病因的不同而分的五种瘿病。即石

asthenic heat during convalescence, or by the retention of fire-heat.

Five-Element Theory a theory on philosophy in ancient China, classifying the material characters and the mutual relationships of the five elements (wood, fire, earth, metal and water). These five elements are considered as the essential constituents of the material universe and their motion is in accordance with certain rules (generation, restriction, etc.). In TCM, the five-element theory is chiefly used for explaining the properties of viscera of the human body, their mutual relations, physiological phenomena and pathological changes. It is also served as a guide for dignosing and treating diseases.

Asthenia of the Five Zang-Organs the five critical conditions described in Plain Questions, indicating asthenia of the five viscera and poor prognosis, i. e., small pulse, cold skin, shortness of breath, incontinence of urine and feces, and loss of appetite.

Five Kinds of Secretions including the sweat, nasal discharge, tears, serous saliva and mucous saliva.

Foods Suitable for the Five Zang-Organs a dietetic therapy for visceral diseases, e. g., glutinous millet, chicken meat, peach, scallion, etc. are said to be beneficial to lung diseases.

Five Kinds of Goiter the cervical masses classified according to its

瘿、肉瘿、筋瘿、血瘿及气瘿的合称。

五硬 【wǔ yìng】身体有五个部位活动不灵的病证。一般指头颈手足等处。多为肝受风邪或禀赋不足、真阳太虚所致。

五有余 【wǔ yǒu yú】五脏有余，即五脏邪气有余，属五脏的实证。

五运六气 【wǔ yùn liù qì】五运即木、火、土、金、水的运行。六气是指风、寒、暑、湿、燥、火六气的变化。在中医学中，五运六气这一理论主要被应用于解释气候变化与疾病发生的关系。

五脏 【wǔ zàng】是心、肝、脾、肺、肾五个脏器的合称。它虽然有一定的解剖概念，但不能与解剖学中的各脏器完全等同，而应把它看作是一个功能的单位。

五脏痹 【wǔ zàng bì】痹证迁延不愈，复感风寒湿邪，侵入五脏而出现的病证即肝痹、心痹、肾痹、脾痹和肺痹。

character and etiology, such as indurated goiter, toxic goiter, vasculated goiter, blood goiter and qi-goiter.

Five Cases of Stiffness stiffness of five parts of the body, mostly seen in the neck, hands and feet; usually caused by the attack of pathogenic wind on the liver, or congenital insufficiency.

Hyperactivity of Pathogens in the Five Zang-Organs referring to the sthenia-syndrome of the five viscera.

Five Elements' Motion and Six Kinds of Weather an ancient theory dealing with the motion of the five elements (wood, fire, earth, metal and water), and the changes of six kinds of weather (wind, cold, summer-heat, dampness, dryness, fire). In TCM, it is chiefly applied to interpret the relationship between the weather changes and the development of diseases.

Five Viscera (Zang-Organs) a joint-name for the heart, liver, spleen, lung and kidney, each of them is considered as a functional unit. The terms for five viscera in TCM do not completely match those used in western medicine.

Bi-Syndrome Involving the Five Zang Organs impairments of the five zang organs in a patient suffering from long-term bi — syndrome and being attacked by wind, cold and dampness i. e., liver, heart, kidney,

五脏化液 【wǔ zàng huà yè】即心为汗、肺为涕、肝为泪、脾为涎,肾为唾。五液分泌的异常能反映五脏的状况。

Secretions Derived from the Five Zang Organs the five kinds of secretions derived from the five zang-organs, i. e., the sweat from the heart, the nasal discharge from the lung, the tears from the liver, the serous saliva from the spleen, and the mucous saliva from the kidney. The disorders of these secretions may reflect the conditions of the five zang organs.

五脏六腑咳 【wǔ zàng liù fǔ ké】一般指五脏六腑疾病影响到肺引起的咳嗽;另一方面久咳亦可影响脏腑的功能。

Cough due to Disorders of the Five Zang Organs and Six Fu Organs generally, the disorders of other organs will involve the lung and cough ensues. Moreover, cough of long duration will also affect the function of other organs.

五脏所藏 【wǔ zàng suǒ cáng】即心藏神、肝藏魂、脾藏意、肺藏魄、肾藏志。它说明人的精神活动是以五脏精气为物质基础的,五脏功能紊乱能影响精神状态。

What the Five Zang Organs Store the heart, liver, spleen, lung and kidney store up the spirit, soul, ideas, inferior spirit and will respectively. This implies that the essence of the five zang organs serves as the material basis of the mental activities and the functional disorders of the five zang organs are responsible for mental impairments.

五脏所恶 【wǔ zàng suǒ wù】(五恶)五脏生理特点之一。即心恶热、肺恶寒、肝恶风、脾恶湿、肾恶燥。

What the Five Zang Organs are Adverse to one of the physiological characteristics of the five zang organs, i. e., the heart is adverse to heat, the lung to cold, the liver to wind, the spleen to dampness, and the kidney to dryness.

五脏所主 【wǔ zàng suǒ zhǔ】指五脏

What the Five Zang Organs Dominate

与其他器官的联系。如心主脉、肺主皮、肝主筋、肾主骨、脾主肉等。

a term implicating the relationship between the five zang organs and other tissues i. e. , the heart, liver, spleen, lung and kidney dominate the vessel, tendon, muscle, skin and bone respectively.

五志化火 【wǔ zhì huà huǒ】指喜、怒、忧、思、恐等五种精神活动失调，使气机紊乱、脏腑阴液亏损而出现的病理性功能亢进的现象。

Fire-Syndrome Caused by the Disorders of Five Emotion a condition of pathological hyperfunction due to disorders of qi and consumption of yin-fluid of the viscera which results from emotional upsets, i. e. , over joy, anger, melancholy, anxiety, terror, etc.

五志过极 【wǔ zhì guò jí】指喜、怒、忧、思、恐等各种精神活动过度，它往往可以引起脏腑功能失调，导致疾病的发生。

Overacting of the Five Emotional Activities states of hyperactivities of the five emotions, i. e. , over joy, anger, melancholy, anxiety and terror, which may lead to functional disorders of the viscera and cause trouble.

五种恶候 【wǔ zhǒng è hòu】肿病的五种逆证。即五心肿、人中肿、舌肿、膝胫肿及阴茎肿。

Five Edematous Cases with Unfavourable Prognosis the serious condition including edema of the five centers, edema over the renzhong point, edema of the tongue, edema from the knee to the foot, and edema of the penis.

五走 【wǔ zǒu】五味所走的部位或脏器。如酸走筋、咸走骨等；酸先走肝、苦先走心等。

What Part the Five Tastes Match the specific action on various tissues and viscera exerted by the diets and drugs with the five tastes, e. g. , sour taste acts on the tendons, salty taste acts on the bones, etc. and sour taste affects the liver first, bitter affects the heart first, etc.

武火 【wǔ huǒ】大而猛的火。

物偶入睛 【wù ǒu rù jīng】细小异物飞溅入眼。可引起眼沙涩刺痛、羞明流泪、白睛红赤或黑睛生翳等。

误下 【wù xià】不能用泻下法治疗的疾病，误有泻下法。属误治之一。

恶风 【wù fēng】即怕风。多因外邪伤卫所致。

恶寒 【wù hán】即怕冷。由于感受外邪引起，或因阳虚、痰饮、郁火所致。

恶热 【wù rè】即怕热，是外感热病反映于外的一种证候。亦可见于某些内伤疾患，如饮食不当，热邪内积于胃，阴虚而阳气浮越于表等。

恶食 【wù shí】即厌恶饮食。多因饮食所伤，宿食不化所致；亦可因脾胃气虚，运化失职所致。

鹜溏 【wù táng】指泄泻便如鸭粪。多由脾气虚，大肠有寒而致。

吸促 【xī cù】吸气浅短。是呼吸困难的表现之一。常因肺气大虚所致。

Hot Fire fire, which is strong, usually used for making decoction.

Foreign Body Entering the Eye a condition manifested as pain, photophobia, lacrimation, conjunctival conjestion, or even nebula.

Erroneous Application of Purgatives an erroneous treatment applied to the disease which is contraindicated to purgation.

Aversion to Wind a symptom due to impairment of weifen by exogenous factor.

Aversion to Cold a symptom due to attack of exogenous pathogens or due to yang deficiency, phlegm retention, or accumulation of fire.

Aversion to Heat a symptom seen in febrile diseases caused by exogenous pathogens which involves the interior; also seen in the disorders of viscera, such as retention of heat in the stomach due to improper diet, yin deficiency of their qi.

Anorexia a symptom usually due to improper diet and retention of indigestive food, or to dysfunction of the spleen and stomach resulting from the deficiency of their qi.

Buck-Stool Diarrhea diarrhea with duck-stool-like discharge, which is caused by deficiency of spleen-qi and accumulation of pathogenic cold in the large intestine.

Shallow Inspiration one of the manifestations of dyspnea usually

吸而微数 【xī ér wēi shuò】吸气短促。多因邪气壅塞中焦，肺气不降所致。

吸入 【xī rù】吸入药物的烟或蒸气以治疗疾病的一种治法。

吸远 【xī yuǎn】吸气深而困难。是呼吸困难表现之一。因元气衰竭，肾不纳气所致。

息 【xī】1、即呼吸的古称。2、同瘜。3、与熄通。4、即止、结、留滞的意思。

息粗 【xī cū】指呼吸气粗而沉重，多属实证、痰证等。

息贲 【xī bēn】古病名。为五积之一，多为痰热壅阻，肺气郁结所致的右胁下包块，常伴见呼吸急促、胸背痛、咯血、发热、恶寒、咳嗽等。

息高 【xī gāo】指严重呼吸困难、喘促、息短、张口抬肩的证候。多为元气虚脱、肺气将绝的危候。

息微 【xī wēi】呼吸浅表，气息微弱，多见于虚证。

caused by marked deficiency of lung-qi.

Short and Rapid Inspiration　a disorder caused by the retention of pathogenic factors in the middle energizer leading to the failure of descending of the lung-qi.

Inhalation　a treatment by inhaling the smoke or steam of medicines.

Deep and Difficult Inspiration　one of the manifestations of dyspnea due to exhaustion of primordial-qi and the failure of the kidney to store qi.

Xi　1. a term syn with respiration in ancient times　2. syn with polyp　3. to put out a fire　4. stop, stay, stasis.

Raucous Breathing　a symptom of noisy and heavy respiration, usually seen in sthenia-syndrome, phlegm-syndrome, etc.

Lumps Located at Right Hypochondrium　a disorder due to retention of phlegm and heat, and stagnation of lung-qi, usually accompanied with rapid respiration, chest pain, backache, hemoptysis, fever, chilliness, cough, etc.

Severe Dyspnea　a critical condition due to exhaustion of primordial qi and lung qi, characterized by rapid and short respiration, breathing with mouth opening and shoulder elevating.

Weak Breathing　a symptom of shallow and weak respiration, which is usually seen in asthenia syndrome.

息肉痔 【xī ròu zhì】相当于大肠息肉。大便时突出肛门，常有鲜血及粘液随粪便排出。由湿热下迫大肠，经络阻滞，瘀血浊气凝聚而成。

Rectal Polyp a protruding growth from the mucosa of rectum visible outside the anus during defecation, usually accompanied with bloody and mucous discharge; caused by the attack of damp-heat to the large intestine leading to the blockage of meridians with retention of blood stasis and damp pathogen.

溪谷 【xī gǔ】1、肌肉纹理间的缝隙或凹陷部分。2、泛指经络穴位。

Groove 1. the spaces between the strips of muscles 2. locations of acupints and paths of meridians in general.

熄风 【xī fēng】平息内风的方法。适用于内脏病变致晕眩、震颤、抽搐、小儿惊风和癫痫等病证。一般可分为滋阴熄风、平肝熄风、泻火熄风、和血熄风等。

Calming Wind Syndrome a treatment for endogenous wind syndrome, applicable to the patient suffering from visceral disorders, manifested as dizziness, tremor, convulsion, epilepsy, etc. accomplished by nourishing yin, by calming the liver, by expelling the fire, and by regulating the blood.

膝盖损断 【xī gài sǔn duàn】因跌扑所致的膝盖骨折。局部肿痛及压痛、皮下瘀血，膝关节活动受限。

Fracture of Patella breaking of the patella due to trauma, marked by local swelling, pain and tenderness, bruise, and limitation of the movement of the knee joint.

膝 【xī】大、小腿交接部分，前人称为筋之府。

Knee articulation of the thigh and leg, it is also called "house of tendons" in ancient times.

膝痛 【xī tòng】指膝部肌肉、经脉及骨节间作痛。多因肝肾虚，风寒湿气外袭所致。

Arthralgia of Knee a disorder usually due to asthenia of the liver and kidney and exposure to the wind, cold and dampness pathogens.

席疮 【xí chuāng】（印疮、褥疮）久着席褥，受压迫部位出现坏死溃烂性疮疡。

Decubitus an ulceration caused by prolonged local pressure in a patient who had to lie too still in bed for a

洗 【xǐ】用水洗去药物表面附着的泥沙或其他不洁物。

喜热饮 【xǐ rè yǐn】喜欢喝热水或热的流质饮食。通常是寒性病的表现之一。

喜冷饮 【xǐ lěng yǐn】喜欢喝冷的流质食物和水，通常是热性病的表现。

喜按 【xǐ àn】疼痛部位因按压而减轻，患者常喜按压。多属虚证。

喜伤心 【xǐ shāng xīn】喜乐过极损伤心神而致失眠、心悸等症状。

喜则气缓 【xǐ zé qì huǎn】指狂喜暴乐，损伤心神的病理。症见心悸、失眠、甚至精神失常等。

细脉 【xì mài】细而软、状如丝线的一种脉象。多因气血两虚所致。

虾游脉 【xiā yóu mài】搏动隐隐约约，一搏即逝的脉象。

虾蟆瘟 【xiā má wēn】指以胁项红肿为主要症状的一种疾病。多由感受温热邪毒所致。见大头瘟。

下病上取 【xià bìng shàng qǔ】疾病的

long period of time.

Washing a method of processing medicinal herbs by cleaning with water, to get rid of the mud, sand and other dirts attached to the surface of the crude herb.

Desire for Hot Drinks a manifestation of cold syndrome in general.

Desire for Cold Drinks a manifestation of heat syndrome in general.

Desire for Pressure a sign indicative of asthenia-syndrome, elicited by pressure over the affected part when the pain is relieved.

Over Joy Impairing the Heart (the mental system) a condition of emotional disorder manifested as insomnia, palpitation, etc.

Over Joy may Lead to the Sluggishness of Qi a morbid condition of impairment of spiritual activity resulting form over joy, manifested as palpitation, insomnia, or even amentia.

Small Pulse a pulse condition characterized by small, soft and thready beats, which is usually caused by the deficiency of qi and blood.

Shrimp-swimming Pulse a pulse condition characterized by indistinct, weak beats with long intervals.

Epidemic Disease with Redness and Swelling of Cheeks a disease usually caused by the attack of virulent heat.

**Treating the Disease in the Lower Por-

症状表现偏于下部者,针刺上部的穴位,或用药物从上部治疗的方法。如有部分小便不利的患者,与肺气不宣有关,用宣通肺气的方法达到利尿的目的。

tion by Managing the Upper Portion a treatment for the disease affecting the lower portion by acupuncture to the points in the upper portion or application of drugs acting on the upper portion. For instance, dysuria may be treated by releasing the stagnated lung-qi to promote diuresis.

下法 【xià fǎ】(泻下) 运用泻下、攻逐、润下的药物以通导大便、消除积滞、荡涤实热、攻逐水饮的治法。一般分为寒下、温下、润下等。

Purgation a treatment for eliminating the indigested food, sthenic heat and fluid by the application of potent or mild purgatives, generally classified into purgation with drugs of cold nature, that with drugs of warm nature and that with drugs of lubricant nature.

下发背 【xià fā bèi】位于腰部命门部位的有头疽。

Carbuncle of the Lumbar Region carbuncle located at the mingmen (gate of life) point.

下丹田 【xià dān tián】是三丹田中最重要的一处。其部位有定在脐下一寸三分、二寸、脐下二寸四分、脐下一寸五分及腹部以下如会阴等不同部位者。

Lower Dantian the most important area in Dan Tian, locating 1.3 Cun, 2 Cun, 2.4Cun, 1.5Cun inferior to the umbilicus or area below abdomen such as Huiyin according to different opinions.

下疳 【xià gān】发于外生殖器的梅毒性皮肤粘膜损害。初起时皮损如豆粒大 硬结,不痛亦不溃破,为硬性下疳;初起如小疮,渐行破溃者,则为软性下疳。

Chancre the primary sore of syphilis; a painless, indurated papule occurring at the site of entry of the infection over the external genitals, called also hard chancre; while that ulcerates later called soft chancre.

下汲肾阴 【xià jí shèn yīn】心火过亢,引起命门火旺,而致耗损肾阴的病理。

Kidney-yin Consumed by Sthenic Heart Fire a morbid condition of consumption of kidney-yin due to hyperactivity of fire from the gate of life which is produced by the sthenia of

下焦 【xià jiao】三焦下部,即脐以下部分,从生理功能上说,它包括了大肠、小肠、肾及膀胱。

下焦主出 【xià jiāo zhǔ chū】下焦的主要功能是通过二便排出废物。

下焦如渎 【xià jiāo rú dú】喻下焦的功能特点。因下焦的主要功能是将废物(尿液、粪便)排出体外。

下厥上冒 【xià jué shàng mào】指脾胃功能失常,升降失调所致的胃气上冒头部的病理。症见头昏花、恶心、呕吐等。

下厥上竭 【xià jué shàng jié】指阳亡于下,阴竭于上的病理。因少阴病误用汗法所致的危重证候。

下利 【xià lì】指腹泻的症状。

下利清谷 【xià lì qīng gǔ】是以腹泻粪便清稀,杂有不消化食物为特征的证候。多因脾肾阳虚所致。常伴有恶寒肢冷、神倦、脉微等症状。

heart fire.

Lower Energizer the lower portion of the triple energizer corresponding to the body cavity below the level of the umbilicus. Functionally, it includes the small and large intestines, kidney and bladder.

Lower Energizer Administers Excretion one of the functions of the lower energizer, by which the waste products are excreted through feces and urine.

Lower Energizer is Analogized to a Sluice a metaphor for the functional characteristics of the lower energizer. As comparable with a sluice, the lower energizer excretes the waste products as urine and feces.

Dizziness due to Abnormal Rising of Qi a morbid condition of abnormal rising of stomach-qi which is caused by the dysfunction of the spleen and stomach, manifested as dizziness, nausea, vomiting, etc.

Loss of Yang in the Lower Part and Exhaustion of Yin in the Upper Part a critical condition occurring in shaoyin disease which is treated erroneously by diaphoretic method.

Diarrhea a symptom with abnormal frequency and liquidity of fecal discharges.

Watery Diarrhea with Indigested Food in the Stool diarrhea caused by the deficiency of spleen-yang and kidney yang, usually accompanied with

下品 【xià pǐn】古代认为多毒而不能久服的药物,一般多用来祛邪,破积聚或泻下等,称为下品。

下迫 【xià pò】表现为大便或小便便意急迫而又排出不畅的症状。

下泉 【xià quán】即小便。

下窍 【xià qiào】指尿道口和肛门。

下损及上 【xià sǔn jí shàng】指五脏虚损而产生的衰弱性的疾病,由下部发展到上部的病理过程,自肾损开始而损及肝、脾、心、肺。

下脘 【xià wǎn】1、指胃脘下口幽门部。2、穴位名称。

下消 【xià xiāo】以多尿、小便如膏脂样为特征的消渴病。

下者举之 【xià zhě jǔ zhī】指属气虚下陷的疾病,应采用补气升提的方法治疗。如子宫脱垂属中气下陷的,一般多采用补中益气的药物,以升举中

chilliness, cold extremities, lassitude, weak pulse, etc.

Low Grade of Medicines one of the classifications of the traditional Chinese medicines in ancient times, referring to the potent and poisonous medicines which should not be used frequently, such as those for expelling pathogens, removing stasis and purging.

Tenesmus a symptom of ineffectual and painful straining in defecation or urination.

Lower Stream urine.

Lower Orifice referring to the external urethral orifice and the anus.

Debilitated Diseases in the Lower Part Involving the Upper the pathological process of debilitated diseases due to asthenia of five zang organs, which extends from the lower part to the upper part of the body, i. e., the involvement of the liver, spleen, heart and lung by primary asthenia of the kidney.

Xiawan 1. Lower part of gastric cavity, corresponding to the surface position of pylorus 2. Xiawan, a name of acupoint.

Diabetes Involving the Lower Energizer diabetes characterized by polyuria and chyluria.

Illness with Collapse of Middle Energizer-Qi should be Treated with Lifting-up Method a therapeutic principle for treating disease with col-

气。

下注疮 【xià zhù chuāng】位于小腿的渗出性皮肤病。患部肿胀，皮损处常有渗液淋漓不断，缠绵难愈。相当于小腿部的湿疹。多由外受风湿毒邪，荣卫凝滞所致。

夏令麻疹 【xià lìng má zhěn】夏暑季节出现的麻疹，咳嗽轻、麻疹密，与冬春季发病者不尽相同。

夏季热 【xià jì rè】多见于2—5岁之体弱儿童。夏季发病，入夏之后，长期发热，伴有口渴、多饮、多尿，无汗或少汗。随气温降低或在阴凉环境下能自行缓解。辨证分类：1、暑伤肺胃 2、上盛下虚。

夏洪 【xià hóng】夏季的脉象可偏于洪大，这是脉象随气候变化而发生相应变化的一种生理现象。因夏季阳气旺盛，所以脉搏也相对的洪大。

先天 【xiān tiān】1、来源于双亲之精，对个体的生长、发育起着重要的作用。2、出生前。

lapse of middle energizer-qi, e. g., uterine prolapse should be treated with drugs of strengthening the middle energizer and benefiting qi in order to lift up the middle energizer-qi.

Eczema of Shank an exudative dermatosis located at the shank, appearing as swelling, oozing, and with a protracted course, usually caused by stagnation of rongwei due to the attack of exogenous wind and wetness pathogens.

Summer Measles measles occurring in summer, marked by dense rashes and mild cough as compared with that occurring in winter and spring.

Summer Fever illness of weak children of 2-5 years old in summer, marked by persistent fever, polydipsia, polyuria, anhidrosis or scanty sweat usually automatically relieved in lower temperature or in the shade. Differential types: 1. impairment of the lung and stomach by the attack of summer-heat. 2. excess in the upper and deficiency in the lower.

Wave like (pulse) in Summer a physiological phenomenon that the normal pulse condition varies with the seasonal variations. Because the yang-qi in summer is properous, the pulse tends to be full and large.

Innateness. 1. the substance derived from the essence of the parents, which is neccessary for the growth of an individual. 2. the prenatal stage.

先攻后补 【xiān gōng hòu bǔ】病人具有用攻下法的适应症,但使用攻下法之后出现虚弱的症状,此时应根据具体情况使用补益的方法。这种先用攻下后用补益的方法称先攻后补。

Therapy Beginning with Elimination of Pathogenic Factors by Restoration of Healthy Qi a treatment suited for the patient becoming debilitated after the application of purgatives. In such case, tonics should be employed after the purgative therapy.

先别阴阳 【xiān bié yīn yáng】运用四诊的方法观察疾病时,首先应分清疾病的阴阳属性。这是辨证论治的基本原则。

Distinguish First Whether Yin or Yang a basic principle for the differential diagnosis of disease which is accomplished by the four methods of physical examination in clinical practice.

痫病 【xián bìng】大发作时,突然昏倒、不省人事、两目斜视、四肢抽搐、口吐涎沫、或有吼声、醒后如常人。小发作时,仅有突然呆木、面色苍白、或两目凝视、头向前倾,短时间即恢复正常。辨证分类:1、风痰闭阻证 2、痰火内闭证 3、肝肾亏虚证 4、心脾两虚证。

Epilepsy In severe case, manifested as sudden faint, coma, strabismus of eyes, tic of limbs, vomiting of saliva and froth, or roaring, and returned to normal after regaining consciousness. In mild case, manifested only as sudden dementia, pale face, or staring of eyes, forward bending of the head, and returned to normal in a short time. Differential types 1. a syndrome due to retention of wind-phlegm 2. a syndrome due to retention of phlegm fire 3. a syndrome due to deficiency of the liver and kidney 4. a syndrome due to deficiency of the heart and spleen.

先补后攻 【xiān bǔ hòu gōng】对体质虚弱又有实邪需用攻下的方法治疗,因体弱难以承受,宜先用补益法。这种先用补益后用攻伐的方法称先补后攻。

Therapy Beginning with the Restoration of Healthy Qi Followed by the Elimination of Pathogenic Factors a treatment suited for a debilitated patient when the pathogenic factor is sthenic. In such case, the patient is unendurable to the purgatives, and

先兆子痫 【xiān zhào zǐ xián】妊娠二十四周后,出现高血压、水肿、蛋白尿,并伴有头痛、眩晕、呕吐等证候。因妊娠后阴虚加重,肝阳上亢,或阴损及阳,脾肾阳虚,或肝郁化热所致。

Preeclampsia a condition characterized by hypertention, edema and proteinuria and accompanied with headache, dizziness and vomiting, occurring after the 24th week of gestation; caused by yin deficiency aggravated by pregnancy leading to hyperactivivy of liver-yang, or impairment of yin involving yang leading to deficiency of spleen-yang and kidney-yang, or heat pathogen produced by stagnation of liver-qi.

先兆流产 【xiān zhào liú chǎn】妊娠期出现腹痛、腰酸下坠、阴道少量流血而子宫颈口未开者。

Threatened Abortion a condition during pregnancy, manifested as abdominal pain, bearing-down sensation over the loins and slight vaginal bleeding in the absence of cervical dilatation.

咸味涌泄为阴 【xián wèi yǒng xiè yīn】咸味药有催吐、润下的作用,它的药性属阴。如盐汤(吐食积)、芒硝(能润下大便)均属阴。

Salty Medicines with Emetic and Purgative Effects Are Attributive to Yin the yin-yang attribution of medicines in accordance with their tastes and actions, e. g., salt water with emetic effect and Natrir Sulfas with mild purgative effect attribute to yin.

咸寒增液 【xián hán zēng yè】使用咸寒而有润下作用的药物,治疗温病日久,肝肾阴伤,或阴虚便秘的一种方法。

Increasing the Production of Body Fluid with Drugs of Salty Taste and Cold Nature a treatment for impairment of liver-yin and kidney-yin during a prolonged seasonal febrile disease, or constipation due to yin-deficiency, by the application of demul-

咸 【xián】咸味药物一般有软坚和润下的作用，如海藻软坚散结，芒硝咸寒润燥等。

弦脉 【xián mài】脉体直而长，有紧张感，如指按琴弦上的一种脉象。多见于高血压、肝胆疾病及痛证的患者。

呃乳 【xiàn rǔ】吐乳直出而不停留的一种疾病，为胃气上逆所致。

相乘 【xiāng chéng】五行学说术语。借木、火、土、金、水五种物质之间互相过分制约和排斥的反常变化，来说明一脏偏克，导致另一脏偏虚的病理。如肝气过亢可乘袭脾胃，称为木乘土。

相反 【xiāng fǎn】指两种药物同用可能产生毒性或副作用。如乌头反半夏。

相克 【xiāng kè】五行学说术语。借木、火、土、金、水五种物质之间互相制约和排斥的关系，来说明脏腑之间相互制约的生理现象。其次序是木克土、土克水、水克火、火克金、金克木。

相生 【xiāng shēng】五行中互相资生、

cent cathartics of salty taste and cold nature.

Salty (Drugs) the drugs of salty taste which possess the action of softening masses (e. g., Sargassum) or keeping the bowels loose (e. g., Natri Sulfas).

Wiry Pulse a pulse condition which is straight, long and tense, with a feeling of pressing over a string, usually seen in patients suffering from hypertension, liver and gallbladder diseases and painful disorders.

Milk Regurgitation mild vomiting after feeding, caused by upward and adverse flow of stomach-qi.

Subjugation in Five Elements an abnormal excessive checking relationship between the five elements (wood, fire, earth, metal and water), e. g., if the liver (wood) is redundant in qi, it will encroach on the spleen (earth) instead of merely checking it, and is referred to as "wood subjugates earth".

Mutual Addition toxicity or side effect produced by simultaneours use of two drugs, such as Radix Aconiti Praeparata and Rhizoma Pinelliae.

Restriction or Checking Relation in Five Elements the five elements interact in the following sequence - water, fire, metal, wood and earth - in which each element is considered to restrict the subsequent one.

Generation (in the Five Elements)

互相促进的关系，在木、火、土、金、水的循环中，依次的顺序为相生。即木生火、火生土、土生金、金生水、水生木。

the promotion of growth among the five elements. The five-element cycle is arranged in the order of wood, fire, earth, metal and water. One element generates the other clockwise and sequentially, i. e., wood generates fire, fire generates earth, earth generates metal, metal generates water and water generates wood.

相使 【xiāng shǐ】两种以上药物同用，一种药物为主，其余药起辅助作用，以提高药效，如款冬花以杏仁为使。

Enhancement of Effect by another Medicine the effect of the major drug being enhanced by other subsidiary drugs, such as Semen Armeniacae Amarum increases the effect of Flos Farfarae.

相恶 【xiāng wù】两种药物同用，一种药物能减弱另一种药物性能，如黄芩能减弱生姜的温性，称为生姜恶黄芩。

Mutual Inhibition the effect of a drug being inhibited by another, such as the warm nature of Rhizoma zingiberis Recens is decreased by Radiz Scutellariae.

相畏 【xiāng wèi】两种药物同用时，一种药物受到另一种药物的抑制，其毒性或功效被减低，甚至完全丧失功效。

Incompatibility the effect and toxicity of a drug being inhibited by another.

相须 【xiāng xū】将两种性能相类似的药物同用，能起相互增强作用的效能，如知母和黄柏同用。

Mutual Promotion increase of effect to each other when two drugs of similar nature are used simultaneously, such as Rhizoma Anemarrhenae and Cortex Phellodendri.

相侮 【xiāng wǔ】一种病理现象。指五行中反方向的相克，即反克，是五行中失去正常协调的一种表现，如木被土所克。

Reversal Restriction (in the five elements) a morbid condition in which one element fails to restrict the other in the normal, regular order but in reverse order. For instance, wood is restricted by earth.

相火 【xiàng huǒ】 与君火相对而言。二火相互配合，以温养脏腑，推动脏腑功能活动，一般认为相火的根源发自命门，而寄于肝、胆、三焦等脏腑内。

Ministerial Fire a kind of physiological fire which, in cooperation with the king fire, warms and nourishes the viscera and promotes their functional activities. It is believed that ministerial fire originates from the life gate and is stored in the liver, gall-bladder, and the tri-energizer.

相火妄动 【xiàng huǒ wàng dòng】 指肝肾阴虚而出现肝火上炎和肾脏虚火内灼的病理。症见眩晕头痛、视物不明、耳鸣耳聋、易怒、五心烦热, 性欲亢进、遗精早泄等。

Ministerial Fire Upsetting in the Body a morbid condition of flaming up of liver-fire and burning of asthenic fire of the kidney caused by deficiency of both liver-yin and kidney-yin; manifested as dizziness, headache, blurring of vision, tinnitus, deafness, irritabiltiy, dreamfulness, feverish sensation of the palms, soles and chest, excessive libido, noctural emission, precocious ejaculation, etc.

项强 【xiàng qiáng】 指颈项肌肉筋脉牵强引痛。多因感受风寒湿邪侵袭太阳经脉，经脉不舒所致。亦可因失血伤津，筋脉失养所致。

Stiffness of Neck muscular rigidity and pain over the neck, due to stagnation of taiyang meridian qi resulting from the attack of cold-dampness pathogen, or due to malnutrition of muscles resulting from hemorrhage and consumption of body fluid.

项软 【xiàng ruǎn】（天柱骨倒）指项颈软弱无力。多因肾气精髓衰耗所致。可见于小儿体虚、老年或久病阳气衰惫的患者。

Flaccidity of Neck a disorder due to consumption of kidney-qi and essence-marrow; seen in the debilitated infants, and the patient with chronic disease and the aged whose yang-qi is exhausted.

项背强 【xiàng bèi qiáng】 指后项背脊间肌肉筋脉牵强板滞不适。多由风寒湿邪乘袭足太阳经或津液亏耗, 气血凝滞, 脉络失养或因外伤所致。

Stiffness of Neck and Back a disorder resulting from the attack of wind, cold and dampness pathogens to the Foot-taiyang meridians, or

哮病 【xiào bìng】以发作时喉中哮鸣有声,呼吸急促,甚则张口抬肩,不能平卧,口唇指甲紫绀为主症的病证。多因饮食不当,情志失调,劳累过度,或气候突变等引起。辨证分类:分发作期和缓解期,前者包括冷哮、热哮和虚哮,后者包括肺虚、脾虚和肾虚。

哮喘 【xiāo chuǎn】是哮证气与喘证的合称。指以呼吸急促或喘鸣有声、呼吸困难为特征的一种疾病。多因外邪侵袭、痰浊内盛,肺气不得宣肃;或肺肾虚弱,气失摄纳所致。

消补兼施 【xiāo bǔ jiān shī】消法和补法同时并用的治法。常用于虚实并见病证。如脾胃虚弱而有食物不消化、胃部及腹部胀闷、大便稀烂、舌苔黄

from the damage of vessels by the consumption of body fluid, by the stagnation of qi and blood or by injury.

Bronchial Wheezing a morbid condition marked by asthmatic breathing with wheezing sound in the throat, or even with opening mouth and raising shoulders, having difficulty lying down and with cyanosis of the lips and finger nails during attack, mostly due to improper diet, emotional disturbance, overstrain, or sudden change of the weather. Types of differentiation, two types: asthma during attacks and asthma during remission stage, the former including asthma due to cold, asthma due to heat, and asthma due to deficiency; the latter including deficiency of the lung, deficiency of the spleen and deficiency of the kidney.

Asthma and Dyspnea a disease characterized by recurrent attacks of dyspnea with bronchial wheezing; due to failure of dispersing and descending of lung-qi resulting from the attack of exogenous pathogens and the stagnation of phlegm-dampness, or to the disorder of inspiration resulting from asthenia of the lung and kidney.

Dispersion and Invigoration Therapies it is applied simultaneously in a treatment for the case with coexistence of asthenia and sthenia syn-

腻、脉弱无力等。

drome, e. g., asthenia of the spleen and stomach accompanied with retention of indigested food, manifested as epigastric and abdominal fullness, discharge of loose stool, yellowish and greasy fur on the tongue, weak pulse, etc.

消导 【xiāo dǎo】用健脾理气和助消化的药物,消除食滞,恢复脾胃运化功能的治法。适用于食积停滞、腹胀胸闷、时有腹痛、大便泄泻、嗳腐吞酸、苔厚黄腻、脉滑等。

Promoting Digestion a treatment for dyspepsia and restoring the functions of the spleen and stomach by means of digestives and drugs for strengthening the spleen and regulating qi; applicable to the case manifested as indigestion, flatulence, feeling of oppression over the chest, abdominal pain, diarrhea, acid regurgitation, yellowish and thick greasy fur on the tongue, smooth pulse, etc.

消法 【xiāo fǎ】消除气郁、血瘀、痰湿、食积等实邪的一种治法。

Dispelling Therapy a treatment for dispelling sthenic pathogenic factors, such as stagnated qi, blood stasis, phlegm-dampness, indigested foods, etc.

消谷善饥 【xiāo gǔ shàn jī】食欲亢进,食下不久,即感饥饿的证候。多由胃热炽盛,胃阴亏耗所致。是消渴病的主症之一。

Polyorexia one of the chief symptoms of diabetes due to hyperactivity of stomach-fire and consumption of the stomach-yin.

消瘅 【xiāo dàn】1、即消渴 2、以肌肉消瘦为特征的一种病证。因肝、心、肾三经阴虚内热所致。

Xiaodan. 1. diabetes. 2. a disorder characterized by emaciation, due to yin-deficiency and retention of heat pathogen in the liver, heart, and kidney meridians.

消渴 【xiāo kě】口渴多饮,多食善饥,小便量多,形体消瘦。后期或见烦渴、头痛、恶心、腹痛、呼吸短促等严重症状,甚则发生昏迷厥逆危象。辨证

Diabetes a disease characterized by polyphagia, polydipsia, polyuria and emaciation; and at the advanced stage, marked by thirst, headache,

分类：1、燥热伤津证 2、胃热津亏证 3、气阴两虚证 4、阴阳两虚证 5、阴虚阳浮证。

nausea, abdominal pain, shortness of breath, or even coma and cold limbs. Types of differentiation 1. a syndrome due to impairment of body fluid by dryness-heat 2. a syndrome due to consumption of body fluid by stomach-heat 3. an asthenia syndrome of qi and yin 4. an asthenia-syndrome of yin and yang 5. a syndrome of floating of yang due to yin deficiency.

消痞 【xiāo pǐ】（化痞）消法之一。治疗痞积、痞满的方法。

Eliminating Mass and Relieving Fullness a therapy for the treatment of mass and fullness of the chest by oral use of medicines.

消痞化积 【xiāo pǐ huà jī】用行气化瘀、消滞软坚的药物，以消除胸腹闷满或腹腔肿块的一种方法。如胁下肿块或小儿疳积等病，均可采用此法。

Relieving Distension and Eliminating Mass a treatment for fullness of the chest and abdomen or abdominal mass, such as hypochondriac mass, infantile malnutrition, etc, with drugs of activating qi, eliminating blood stasis and softening induration, and digestives.

消食导滞 【xiāo shí dǎo zhì】（消食化滞、消导）消法之一。是消除食滞，恢复脾胃功能的一种治法。常用于食积停滞、胸脘痞满、腹胀时痛、嗳腐吞酸、恶食，或泄泻、苔黄腻、脉滑。

Relieving Dyspepsia a treatment for indigestion and restoring the functions of the spleen and stomach, applicable to the case manifested as feeling of fullness in the chest and epigastrium, abdominal flatulence and pain, acid regurgitation, anorexia, diarrhea, yellowish and greasy fur on the tongue, smooth pulse, etc.

消痰 【xiāo tán】攻伐浊痰留滞的治法。适用于痰饮伏于肺脏或痰浊积聚的病证。本法多用能损伤正气，体弱的患者慎用。

Dissipating Phlegm a treatment for dissipating the accumulation of phlegm, applicable to the case with retention of phlegm in the lung or accumulation of phlegm-dampness. Frequent use of this treatment should be avoided, esp. to the debilitated patient since the healthy qi may be damaged.

消痰平喘 【xiāo tán píng chuǎn】治疗痰多气逆的方法。适用于痰饮内伏肺脏所致的肺气上逆。症见喘咳痰多、胸闷、食欲减退、舌苔粘腻、脉滑等。

Eliminating Sputum to Relieve Asthma a treatment for profuse expectoration and adverse rising of qi, applicable to the case with accumulation of sputum in the lung with adverse rising of lung-qi, manifested as asthma, productive cough, oppressive feeling over the chest, poor appetite, greasy fur on the tongue, smooth pulse, etc.

消痰软坚 【xiāo tán ruǎn jiān】用具有化痰软坚散结的药物治疗痰浊结聚或瘰疬等病证的方法。

Eliminating Phlegm and Softening Indurated Mass a treatment for accumulation of phlegm or scrofula by the application of drugs of eliminating the phlegm and softening the indurated mass.

小便不利 【xiǎo biàn bù lì】指小便量减少,排出困难。多因水湿失运,气化不利或津血耗损所致,常与肺、脾、肾、三焦及膀胱的功能障碍有关。

Dysuria dysuria in micturition due to hypofunction of qi, retention of dampness or consumption of body fluid and blood, usually referrable to the dysfunctions of the lung, spleen, kidney, triple energizer and bladder.

小便不禁 【xiǎo biàn bù jìn】(小便失禁、失溲)即小便不能随意控制而自行排出的病证。本证以虚寒为多,亦有属实热者,前者多因肾元不足下焦虚寒所致,后者常由膀胱火邪妄动或肝经郁热内结引起。

Incontinence of Urine involuntary passage of urine, most of which appear as asthenia cold syndrome and are attributable to deficiency of kidney-qi and asthenia-cold of the lower energizer; some appear as sthenia-heat syndrome, and are attributable to the stirring of fire pathogen in the bladder or retention of heat pathogen in the liver meridian.

小便淋沥 【xiǎo biàn lín lì】指排尿次

Stranguria frequent, slow and diffi-

数多，量少而不畅，滴沥不尽的证候。本症多由肾气不固，脾肾两虚所致，亦可因下焦湿热引起。

小便黄赤 【xiǎo biàn huáng chì】（溺赤）即小便色黄，甚至呈红色。本症多由内热和湿热蕴结所致，亦有因虚热引起者。

小便频数 【xiǎo biàn pín shuò】多由外邪侵袭，脏腑功能失调或虚损所致。膀胱湿热，肝气郁结，中气虚弱，肾阳衰弱，肾阴不足等可出现本症状。

小便涩痛 【xiǎo biàn sè tòng】指小便排出不畅、疼痛的症状。多由湿热流注膀胱所致。常见于泌尿系感染、结石等疾病。

小产 【xiǎo chǎn】（半产）胎儿三个月以上未足月而产。多因气血虚弱、肾虚、血热、外伤等损伤冲任脉，不能摄血养胎所致。

小肠 【xiǎo cháng】六腑之一。上接幽门下连大肠，包括十二指肠、回肠、空肠。它有进一步消化吸收食物的作用。

cult urination; usually caused by the deficiency of kidney qi or the asthenia of the spleen and kidney, and also by the stagnation of dampness-heat in the lower energizer.

Deep-Coloured Urine discharge of darkened urine mostly caused by the retention of heat pathogen and dampness-heat, or occassionally by asthenia-heat.

Frequent Micturition a symptom due to attack of exogenous pathogenic factors and dysfunction or debitlity of the internal organs, such as damp-heat in the bladder, stagnation of liver-qi, deficiency of middle energizer qi, weakness of kidney-yang, insufficiency of kidney-yin, etc.

Stranguria slow and painful urination due to attack of the bladder by damp-heat pathogen, usually seen in urinary infection and stones, etc.

Abortion the premature expulsion from the uterus of the fetus over three months, due to failure of nourishing the fetus resulting from impairment of thoroughfare and conception vessels by the deficiency of qi and blood, kidney-asthenia, blood-heat or trauma.

Small Intestine one of the six fu organs, connecting the pyloric opening of the stomach and the large intestine, including duodenum, ileum and jejunum, where the food is further digested and absorbed.

小肠病 【xiǎo cháng bìng】泛指小肠功能失调引起的病证。多因饮食不节，损伤脾胃，累及小肠或心火下移所致。属虚寒证者，表现为少腹隐痛、肠鸣、大便稀烂、小便频数而不畅；属实热证者，表现为腹胀心烦、小便短赤、口舌生疮等。

Disorder of the Small Intestine generally referring to the disease due to functional disorder of the small intestine, resulting from the impairment of the spleen and stomach by immoderate diet involving the small intestine, or due to attack of heart-fire. The disease of asthenia-cold type is marked by dull pain of the lower abdomen, increased borborygmus, loose stools, frequent but difficult micturition; while the sthenia-heat type is marked by abdominal distention, restlessness, oliguria with reddish urine and aphthae.

小肠咳 【xiǎo cháng ké】咳嗽时伴有放屁的一种病证。

Small Intestinal Cough a disorder characterized by cough accompanied with breaking wind.

小肠疝 【xiǎo cháng shàn】由于小肠虚，风冷之邪入侵所致的病证。症见小腹冷痛，牵引睾丸及腰背部。

Small Intestinal Pain a disorder due to attack of wind and cold pathogens to the asthenic small intestine, manifested as coldness and pain in the lower abdomen referring to the testes, loins and back.

小肠实热 【xiǎo cháng shí rè】热邪郁积小肠所致的病证。症见心烦、耳鸣、咽痛、口舌生疮、小便短赤、腹胀、苔黄、脉滑数等。

Stheniaheat in the Small Intestine a disorder due to accumulation of pathogenic heat in the small intestine; manifested as restlessness, tinnitus, sorethroat, aphthae, scanty dark urine, abdominal flatulence, yellowish fur on the tongue, fast and smooth pulse, etc.

小肠虚寒 【xiǎo cháng xū hán】寒邪侵袭小肠或小肠功能衰弱所致的病证。证见小腹隐痛、肠鸣泄泻、小便频数、排出不畅、舌淡、苔白、脉缓

Asthenia Cold of the Small Intestine a disorder due to cold pathogen attacking the small intestine or hypofunction of the small intestine; mani-

弱等。

小肠胀【xiǎo cháng zhàng】由于小肠受寒，气机不畅所致的病证。症见少腹胀满、牵引腰部作痛。

小肠主受盛【xiǎo cháng zhǔ shòu shèng】小肠的功能之一。小肠有承受来自胃中的、经过初步消化的食物并将其进一步消化、吸收的作用。

小毒【xiǎo dú】毒性轻微的药物，虽然对身体损害不大，但也不能多服久服。

小儿暴惊【xiǎo ér bào jīng】小儿突然受惊后，致气怯痰逆，精神闷乱而引起惊叫啼哭的病证。

小儿发痧【xiǎo ér fā shā】小儿因寒邪外束、气血内郁而引起的痧证。表现为似寒非寒、似热非热、四肢急倦、腹痛纳呆、表情痛苦。

小儿虫吐【xiǎo ér chóng tù】常因小儿胃肠功能失调，或发高热或驱虫不当，致蛔虫上窜，从口吐出的一种病证。

fested as dull aching over the lower abdomen, increased borborygmus, diarrhea, frequent urination and difficulty in micturition, pale tongue with whitish fur, slow and weak pulse, etc.

Flatulence of the Small Intestine   a disorder caused by the attack of cold pathogen to the small intestine leading to its dysfuntion; manifested as distention of the lower abdomen with pain referring to the loins.

Small Intestine Controls Reception   one of the functions of the small intestine, by which the digested food from the stomach is received for further digestion and absorption.

Mild Toxicity   referring to the drugs which are slightly poisonous and should not be taken frequently or in a large dosage.

Sudden Fright in Children   a condition of crying in fear due to disorder of qi and attack of phlegm after being frightened suddenly in children.

Eruptive Diseases in Children   eruptive diseases caused by the attack of cold pathogen from the exterior and stagnation of qi and blood in the interior; manifested as chilly and feverish feeling but not really chill and fever, lassitude, abdominal pain, anorexia, painful expression, etc.

Worm Vomiting in Children   a symptom due to irritability of the roundworms resulting from the functional disorder of the stomach and in-

小儿卒利 【xiǎo ér cù lì】指小儿由于肠胃虚弱,暴受冷热之气而引起的突然泄泻。

小儿表热 【xiǎo ér biǎo rè】小儿由外感风邪引起的发热。其病位在表,多伴有鼻塞、流涕、喷嚏、咳嗽等表证。根据其偏寒或偏热,可分为风寒表证和风热表证两大类。

小儿疳眼 【xiǎo ér gān yǎn】(疳眼)继发于小儿疳积的眼病。因脾胃亏损,精血不足,目失濡养,肝热上攻所致。表现为眼部干涩羞明,黑睛生翳,溃破后形成蟹睛或旋螺突起;严重者可致眼球枯萎失明。相当于角膜软化症。

小儿感冒 【xiǎo ér gǎn mào】以发热恶寒、鼻塞流涕、喷嚏等症为主,多兼咳嗽,可伴呕吐、腹泻或高热惊厥。辨证分类:1、风寒证 2、风热证 3、暑湿证 4、兼证可见夹痰、夹食、夹惊。

testines, improper application of ascaricides and high fever.

Abrupt Onset of Diarrhea in Children a condition due to impairment of the asthenic intestines and stomach by the sudden attack of cold and heat pathogens.

Superficial Heat Syndrome in Children fever in children caused by the attack of exogenous wind pathogen, usually accompanied with manifestations of superficies-syndrome, such as stuffy nose, nasal discharge, sneezing and cough, etc. It is classified into superficies-syndrome of wind-cold and of wind-heat according to predomination of cold or heat.

Eye Disease Secondary to Infantile Malnutrition infantile malnutrition with involvement of the eyes, caused by asthenia of the spleen and stomach, insufficiency of essence and blood and the attack of liver-fire; manifested as xerophthalmia, photophobia, formation of nebula on the cornea, and prolapse of the iris or projecting staphyloma after the perforation of cornea, bullar atrophy and blindness may ensue in the serious case. Corresponding to keratomalacia.

Common Cold in Children a morbid condition manifested as high fever and aversion to cold, nasal obstruction and nasal discharge, sneezing, etc., and accompanied with cough, vomiting, diarrhea or high fever and con-

小儿寒吐 【xiǎo ér hán tù】小儿因脾胃虚寒而引起的呕吐。表现为朝食暮吐或暮食朝吐，吐出物多为无臭味的未消化食物，伴有腹部隐痛，大便稀溏或四肢厥冷等症状。

小儿惊吐 【xiǎo ér jīng tù】（惊膈吐）小儿受惊后，肝胃不和而引起呕吐的病证。表现为呕吐清稀涎液、面色发青、烦躁不安、低热、不思饮食等，严重者可伴有手足轻度抽搐。

小儿脚挛 【xiǎo ér jiǎo luán】小儿脚趾挛缩不能伸展的一种症状。由于其母怀孕时脏腑有积冷，感受风邪，使胎儿生后，肾气不足，气血营养不能供给所致。

小儿客忤 【xiǎo ér kè wǔ】小儿受惊后出现的一种证候。除常见啼哭、面色改变外，尚可出现吐泻、腹痛、瘈疭等症状。

小儿咳逆 【xiǎo ér ké nì】小儿因哺乳

vulsion. Differential types: 1. a wind-cold syndrome 2. a wind-heat syndrome 3. a summe-heat dampness syndrome 4. a syndrome accompanied with phlegm, indigestion and convulsion.

Cold-type Vomiting in Children　a type of vomiting due to asthenia-cold of the spleen and stomach; manifested as vomiting of odorless, indigested foods which have been retained in the stomach for hours; accompanied with dull abdominal pain, loose stools or cold limbs, etc.

Vomiting in Children Induced by Frightening　a symptom caused by the functional incoordination of the spleen and stomach; manifested as vomiting of watery fluid, bluish complexion, restlessness, low fever, poor appetite, and twitchings of hands and feet in the serious case.

Spasm of Toes in Infants　inability to extend the toes in infants, due to deficiency of kidney-qi and undernourishment by qi and blood after birth resulting from the exposure to wind pathogen in the maternal body whose internal organs are subject to the damage of pathogenic cold.

Epileptoid Attack in Children Induced by Terror　a syndrome in childern after getting fright, marked by crying, change of complexion, vomiting, abdominal pain and convulsion.

Choking Cough in Children　a

时乳汁溢入气管,引起呛咳的一种症状。

小儿咳嗽 【xiǎo ér ké sòu】咳嗽为主要症状,多继发于感冒之后,常因气候变化而发作。痰多的患儿,喉间可闻痰鸣声。好发于冬春季节。辨证分类:1、风寒证 2、风热证 3、痰热证 4、痰湿证 5、气虚证 6、阴虚证

小儿实热 【xiǎo ér shí rè】小儿由于实证引起的发热。常见于外感风邪的表证和饮食内伤的里证。表证实热表现为发热、头痛等。

小儿羸瘦 【xiǎo ér léi shòu】由于小儿脾胃嫩弱,常因喂养不当而损伤脾胃,影响气血生化,肌肤失于营养而致体虚瘦弱的证候。

小儿暑温 【xiǎo ér shǔ wēn】(流行性乙型脑炎)发病大多急骤,初起发热无汗,头痛呕吐,颈项抵抗感或强直,嗜睡或烦躁不安,偶有惊厥。发病后持续高热,嗜睡,昏迷,惊厥。起病

symptom due to milk entering the trachea during feeding.

Cough in Children a morbid condition marked by cough, secondary to common cold, usually occurring with climatical changes. Rales can be heard in the throat of children with accumulation of sputum. It usually occurs in spring and winter. Differential types 1. a wind-cold syndrome 2. a wind-heat syndrome 3. a phlegm-heat syndrome 4. a phlegm-dampness syndrome 5. an asthenia-qi syndrome 6. an asthenia-yin syndrome.

Sthenia-Heat Syndrome in Children-Fever a condition resulting from sthenia-syndrome, which may be caused by the attack of exogenous wind pathogen and manifested as superficial sthenia-heat syndrome, consisting of fever, headache, etc; and may be caused by the internal damage by improper diet and manifested as interior sthenia-heat syndrome.

Emaciation in Children a condition characterized by general debility, resulting from malnutrition. This tends to occur in children because their spleen and stomach are tender and easily impaired by improper feeding.

Summer Fever in Children referring to epidemic encephalitis B, a morbid condition marked by abrupt and acute onset, fever and anhidrosis, headache and vomiting, stiffness of

急暴者,可突然出现闭证、脱证。病程至二周左右,一般可逐渐向愈,但部分重症患儿可有不规则发热、意识障碍、失语、吞咽困难、肢体瘫痪等恢复期症状,本病多发于盛夏季节。辨证分类:1、邪在卫气 2、邪在气营 3、邪在营血 4、正虚邪恋。

neck, sleepiness or restlessness, and occassional convulsion, at the onset of the disease; and persistent high fever, sleepiness, coma and convulsion after the invasion of the disease. In the acute and serious case, sthenia-type coma and prostration syndrome may appear. The disease usually lasts about 2 weeks and can be gradually recovered. But in some serious child patients, convalescent symptoms, such as irregular fever, disorder of consciousness, aphasia, dysphasia, acroparalysis may appear. The disease often occurs in summer. Differential types 1. pathogens in weiqi 2. pathogens in qi and ying 3. pathogens in ying and blood 4. deficiency of healthy qi and sthenia of pathogens.

小儿水肿 【xiǎo ér shuǐ zhǒng】(急慢性肾炎及肾病综合症)阳水:浮肿多由眼睑开始,逐渐遍及全身,而以上身肿为甚,皮肤光亮。浮肿时尿量明显减少,甚至尿闭。部分患儿出现肉眼血尿。常伴有血压增高。阴水:病程长,反复不愈,全身明显浮肿,呈凹陷性,浮肿最明显处为眼睑,下肢及阴囊,而以腰以下肿为甚,皮肤苍白,甚至伴有腹水、胸水、脉沉无力。发病年龄多数在2—7岁之间。辨证分类:1、常证:风水相搏;湿热内蕴;脾虚湿困;脾肾阳虚。2、变证:水气上凌;邪犯心肝;水毒内闭。

Edema in Children acute and chronic nephritis or nephrotic syndrome. Yang-type edema: edema usually appears in the eyelids at first, and then gradually over the body, esp. severe in the upper part if the body, with bright colored skin; oliguria or even anuresis; hematuria in some child patients; often accompanied with hypertension. Yin-type edema: long course and slow recovery; marked by obvious pitting edema all over the body, most obvious at the eyelids, lower limbs and scrotum, esp severe below the waist, pale skin, and even accompanied with ascites, hydrothorax and sunken and weak pulse. It mostly occurs in children of 2-7 years old. Differential types 1. mild case: conflict between wind and water; retention of dampness-heat in the interior; water retention due to hypofunction of the spleen; insufficiency of both the spleen and the kidney. 2. deteriorated case: upward flowing of the retained fluid in the body; attack of pathogenic factors on the heart and liver; noxious water disease in the interior.

小儿哮喘【xiǎo ér xiāo chuǎn】（吼病）发作前常有喷嚏、咳嗽等先兆症状，或夜间突然发作。发作时喉间哮鸣，呼吸困难，咯痰不爽。甚则不能平卧、烦躁不安等。或有诱发因素，如气候转变、受凉，或接触某些过敏物质等。辨证分类：1、发作期：寒性哮喘；热性哮喘；外寒内热；虚实夹杂。2、缓解期：肺气虚；脾气虚；肾气虚。

Asthma in Children a common respiratory disease in children, marked by presymptoms such as sneezing and cough, or abrupt occurring at night; manifested as bronchial wheezing, dyspnea, difficulty in expectoration; or even being unable to lie in horizontal position and restlessness, etc; or induced by climatical changes, cold, or exposure to allergic substances. Differential types 1. stage of attack: asthma of cold type; asthma of heat type; cold in the exterior and heat in the interior; mixed asthenia and sthenia. 2. remission stage: deficiency of lung—qi, spleen—qi and kindey—qi.

小儿泄泻【xiǎo ér xiè xiè】大便次数增多，每日3—5次，或多达10次以上，呈淡黄色，如蛋花汤样，或色褐而臭，可有大量粘液。或伴有恶心、呕吐、腹痛、发热、口渴等症。辨证分类：1、常证：伤食泻；湿热泻；风寒泻；脾虚泻；脾肾阳虚泻。2、变证：

Diarrhea in Children it is marked by abnormal frequency and liquidity of fecal discharges, yellowish in colour and watery, or dark-coloured and stinking, with some mucus, 3-5 times or even 10 times a day; or accompanied with nausea, vomiting, abdomi-

伤阴；伤阳。

nal pain, fever and thirst, etc. Differential types 1. mild case: diarrhea due to improper diet; due to wind-cold pathogens; due to dampness-heat pathogens; due to hypofunction of the spleen; due to deficiency of spleen-yang and kidney-yang respectively. 2. deteriorated case: impairment of yin or yang.

小儿虚热 【xiǎo ér xū rè】多由于小儿脾胃虚弱，气血不足，阴虚阳亢所致的一种病证。表现为颜面潮红，时而㿠白、唇红口干、手足心热、乍凉乍温。大便干燥或溏泻，小便短黄或频数清长等。亦可见于某些危重疾病，因汗出太过、吐泻过久或发热持续时间过长所致。

Asthenia-heat Syndrome in Children　　a syndrome caused by asthenia of the spleen and stomach, insufficiency of qi and blood, deficiency of yin and domination of yang, also seen in the serious cases after profuse sweating, persistent vomiting and diarrhea, and continuous high fever; characterized by reddish or pale cheek, reddish lips, thirst, feverish sensation over the palms and soles, cold or warm feeling, constipation or diarrhea, oliguria with yellowish urine or frequent micturition with watery urine, etc.

小方 【xiǎo fāng】方剂组成形式之一。小方的组成药味少、分量轻、药性缓和，适用于邪气轻浅，病情较轻，无兼证者。

Small Prescription　　a prescription composed of medicines of relatively small number, smaller dosage and milder effect, suited for the disease due to pathogens of lesser virulency, and the disease of lesser severity and without complication.

小腹 【xiǎo fù】腹部脐下部分。

Lower Abdomen　　the portion of abdomen below the umbilicus.

小腹疽 【xiǎo fù jū】（腹痈）即生于脐下腹部的痈。多由七情火郁所致。

Carbuncle over the Lower Abdomen　　a disorder usually caused by emotional upsets with stagnation of fire pathogen.

小 xiao

小腹痛 【xiǎo fù tòng】（少腹痛）指下腹部疼痛。多因膀胱湿热，大肠燥结，肾虚或其它疾病（如疝气、痛经、带下、淋证等）所致。

Pain in the Lower Abdomen a symptom caused by the accumulation of dampness-heat pathogen in the bladder, dryness of the large intestine, asthenia of kidney, or secondary to other diseases such as hernia, menorrhalgia, leucorrhea, stranguria, etc.

小腹满 【xiǎo fù mǎn】（少腹满）由冷结膀胱所致。症见上腹胀满，按之疼痛、四肢厥冷。亦可由癃闭、淋证等多种疾病引起。

Distention of the Lower Abdomen a symptom manifested as distention of the lower abdomen, tenderness and cold limbs, caused by stagnation of pathogenic cold in the bladder, or retention of urine, stranguria, etc.

小夹板 【xiǎo jiā bǎn】四肢骨折时用作固定骨折部位的薄板，用柳木、杉木或胶合板等按肢体的长短制成。

Small Splint a piece of wood for the fixation of fractured bones of the limbs, made of willow, China fir or plywood in various size according to the length of the limb.

小户嫁痛 【xiǎo hù jià tòng】泛指妇女阴道口疼痛。多由肝经郁热、脾虚聚湿、致湿热下注引起；或由性交所致。

Vaginodynia pain in the vagina, mostly due to pathogenic heat in the liver meridian or accumulation of dampness pathogen as a result of spleen-asthenia leading to the local attack of dampness-heat pathogen, or due to sexual intercourse.

小逆 【xiǎo nì】在治疗上出了较小的差错。

A Fault of Treatment

小结胸 【xiǎo jié xiōng】《伤寒论》中的一个证型。因痰热互结所致。症见胃脘部硬满、压痛、舌苔黄微腻、脉浮滑等。

Mild Syndorme Resulting from Pathogens Accumulated in the Thorax a syndrome recorded in Treatise on Exogenous Febrile Diseases, which is caused by the phlegm and heat pathogens blended together in the thorax; manifested as epigastric distention, tenderness, yellowish and

小伤寒 【xiǎo shāng hán】感受风寒所致的一种四时感冒。症见头痛恶寒、鼻塞流涕、喷嚏、发热不明显、舌苔薄白而润等。

小舌 【xiǎo shé】指悬雍垂。因其在口腔内，形似舌，故称为小舌。

小溪 【xiǎo xī】肌肉纹理间小的凹陷。

小腿转筋 【xiǎo tuǐ zhuǎn jīn】即腓肠肌痉挛。多由气血不足，风冷或寒湿侵袭所致；亦可由于剧烈吐泻，津液亏损，或久病伤阴引起。

小心 【xiǎo xīn】1、指心包络。2、指命门。3、穴位名称。

小中风 【xiǎo zhòng fēng】以阵发性头晕眼花为特征的一种病证。

协热下利 【xié rè xià lì】指外热夹里寒所引起的泄泻。本病多由外邪未解，误用下法，脾胃之阳受损所致。症见形寒身热、腹泻不止、上腹部有痞硬不适感等。

thin greasy fur on the tongue, floating and smooth pulse, etc.

Mild Form of Common Cold a disease due to wind and cold pathogens, manifested as headache, chilliness, nasal obstruction, rhinorrhea, sneezing, low grade fever, and thin, whitish and moist fur on the tongue.

Small Tongue referring to uvula. It is so called beacused it is located in the oral cavity and resembles the tongue in shape.

Small Groove the small spaces between the strips of musles.

Spasm of the Calf cramps of the gastrocnemius muscle, usually caused by the deficiency of qi and blood and the attack of wind-cold pathogen or cold-dampness pathogen, also by severe vomiting and diarrhea leading to dehydration, or by impairment of yin by prolonged illness.

Small Heart 1. the envelope of the heart (pericardium) 2. referring to the gate of life 3. a name of acupoint.

Mild Apopletoid Attack a disorder characterized by intermittent dizziness.

Diarrhea due to Exogenous Heat Pathogen a disease, complicated by pathogenic cold in the interior, a disorder caused by the misuse of purgatives leading to the damage of stomach-yang and spleen-yang while the exogenous heat pathogens are not

邪 【xié】（邪气）泛指各种致病因素及其病理损害，如六淫等。

Pathogenic Factor various pathogenic factors and the pathological damages caused by them, e. g., the six pathogenic factors (wind, coldness, summer heat, damp, dryness, fire).

邪害空窍 【xié hài kōng qiào】 指致病因素侵害口、鼻、耳、目等器官所发生的病证。

Pathogens Involving the Orifices of the Head the disorders due to the involvement of the mouth, nose, ear, eye, etc. by the pathogenic agents.

邪恋心包 【xié liàn xīn bāo】 侵袭心包的邪气留恋不去的病理，症见持续昏迷、惊厥等。

Pathogens Lingering in Pericardium a morbid condition manifested as perisstent coma and convulsion.

邪留三焦 【xié liú sān jiāo】 1、湿热之邪留恋三焦气分的病理。症见咳嗽、胸闷、腹胀、便溏、小便不利等。2、病邪困扰三焦，引起水液代谢障碍所致的病证，症见胸胁胀闷、小便不利、下腹部有窘迫感。

Retention of Pathogens in Triple Energizer 1. a morbid condition due to retention of dampness-heat pathogen in the qifen (stage) of triple energizer; manifested as cough, feeling of oppression over the chest, flatulence, loose stools, dysuria, etc. 2. a disorder of metabolism of body fluid due to retention of pathogens in the triple energizer; manifested as sensation of fullness or oppression over the chest, hypochondrium and lower abdomen, dysuria, etc.

邪气盛则实 【xié qì shèng zé shí】 在疾病过程中，致病因素强盛，机体抗病能力较强，二者激烈斗争，出现功能亢盛的表现。常见有高热、烦燥、腹痛拒按、大便秘结、小便短赤、脉滑数有力等症。

Domination of Pathogens is Considered as Sthenia-Syndrome manifestation of hyperfunction of the body during the process of a disease, in which the relatively strong body resistance fights against the sthenic pathogenic factors violently; manifest-

邪之所凑，其气必虚 【xié zhī suǒ còu, qí qì bì xū】致病因素之所以侵入机体并造成病理损害，主要是机体抗病能力低下的缘故。

胁 【xié】侧胸部。该部为肝经所过。

胁肋疽 【xié lèi ju】生于胁肋部的疽。多由肝气郁滞，痰火壅滞肝胆二经，气血为毒邪所阻滞引起。

胁肋胀痛 【xié lèi zhàng tòng】指一侧或两侧胁肋胀痛。多由气郁、痰凝、脉络阻滞所致。

胁痛 【xié tòng】指胁肋一侧或两侧疼痛。多因肝胆湿热，肝气郁结，痰瘀停着，致肝胆经络气血运行不畅或肝阴不足，肝经失养引起。

胁下痞鞕 【xié xià pǐ yìng】指胁部满

ed as high fever, irritability, abdominal pain and tenderness, constipation, oliguria with deep-coloured urine, smooth and fast, strong pulse, etc.

Whenever the Body is Exposed to the Pathogens, Deficiency of Qi must be Present a theory of pathogenesis signifying that whenever the pathogenic agent can invade into the body and caused disease, the body resistance is lowering.

Lateral Side of the Thorax a region where the liver meridian passes.

Purulent Infection of Hypochondrium Suppurative inflammation over the hypochondriac region, caused by the stagnation of liver-qi and accumulation of phlegm-fire in the liver meridian and gallbladder meridian leading to stagnation of qi and blood.

Distending Pain over Hypochondrium a symptom caused by the stagnation of qi and phlegm and the obstruction of collaterals.

Hypochondriac Pain a symptom due to sluggishness of qi and blood flow in the meridians of the liver and gallbladder resulting from the accumulation of dampness-heat pathogen in the liver and gallbladder, the stagnation of liver-qi, and the retention of phlegm and blood stasis, or due to insufficiency of liver-yin resulting in the failure to nourish the liver meridian.

Fullness and Rigidity over

闷、按之坚硬的证候。通常与痰浊、瘀血凝聚有关,常兼见寒热、呕吐等症。

Hypochondrium a symptom due to retention of phlegm-dampness or blood stasis, usually accompanied with fever, chilliness, vomiting, etc.

胁痈 【xié yōng】发于腋下,胸之两侧的痈疽。多由七情所伤、郁怒、肝火所致。

Carbuncle on Hypochondrium a condition due to stagnation of anger and hyperactivity of liver-fire resulting from emotional upsets.

斜飞脉 【xié fēi mài】桡动脉的位置斜向桡骨茎突背侧处,是一种生理性变异的脉位。

Ectopic Radial Pulse radial pulse palpable on the posterior part of the radius resulting from the radial artery located away from its normal position.

泻剂 【xiè jì】用具有泻下作用的药物如大黄、芒硝等组成的方剂。

Prescription with Purgative Effect a precription composed of purgatives such as Radix et Rhei, Natri sulfas, etc.

泻可去闭 【xiè kě qu bì】用泻剂治疗里实证,如胃家实所引起的腹胀与大便秘结。

Purgative may Relieve Sthenia-Syndrome application of purgatives to treat sthenia-syndrome in the interior, such as abdominal flatulence and constipation due to sthenia-syndrome of the stomach and intestines.

泄泻 【xiè xiè】大便稀薄或如水样,次数增多。急性暴泻,起病突然,病程短。慢性久泻,起病缓慢,病程较长,反复发作,时轻时重。辨证分类 1、寒湿证 2、湿热证 3、食滞证 4、肝郁证 5、脾虚证 6、肾虚证。

Diarrhea a disease marked by abnormal frequency and liquidity of fecal discharges; in the acute case, characterized by abrupt onset and short course of disease; in the chronic case, characterized by slow onset, long course of disease, recurrent occurring, sometimes mild and sometimes severe. Differential types 1. cold-dampness syndrome 2. dampness-heat syndrome 3. indigestion syndrome 4. syndrome of stagnation of the liver-qi 5. syndrome of deficiency of the spleen 6. syndrome of deficiency of the kidney.

泻肝 【xiè gān】（清肝泻火）用苦寒药物以清泄肝火的方法。常用于肝的实火上升者。症见头痛眩晕、耳聋耳鸣，甚则吐血、急躁易怒、便秘、苔黄、脉弦数等。

Clearing away the Liver-Fire a treatment for the elimination of liver-fire by the application of drugs of bitter taste and cold nature, applicable to the case with abnormal rising of the sthenic liver-fire manifested as headache, dizziness, deafness, tinnitus, flushed face, congestion of the conjunctiva, dry mouth with bitter taste, hypochondriac pain, hematemesis, irritability, constipation, yellowish fur on the tongue, wiry and fast pulse, etc.

泻肺 【xiè fèi】（泻白）是清泻肺内热邪的方法。适用于肺内蕴热。症见咳嗽气喘、发热不退而傍晚加剧、舌红苔黄、脉细数等。

Purging the Sthenic Lung-Qi a treatment for eliminating the heat pathogen in the lung, applicable to the case with retention of heat pathogen in the lung, manifested as cough, shortness of breath, continuous fever which is higher in the evening, reddish tongue with yellowish fur, small and fast pulse, etc.

泻火熄风 【xiè huǒ xī fēng】（清热熄风）用苦寒清热泻火和镇痉熄风药，治疗热极生风的方法。适用于热性病热邪极盛。症见高热、四肢抽搐、两目上翻、项强、甚则角弓反张、神志昏迷、舌红苔黄、脉弦数有力等。

Purging Fire Pathogen to Stop the Wind-Syndrome a treatment for wind-syndrome due to hyperactivity of heat pathogen, applicable to the case with overabundance of heat pathogen in febrile diseases, manifested as high fever, convulsion, upward staring of the eyes, stiffness of neck or even opisthotonos, coma, reddish tongue with yellowish fur, wiry and fast, vigorous pulse, etc.

泻下禁例 【xiè xià jìn lì】禁用泻法的

**Cases for which Purgatives are Con-

蟹心　xie xin

病例。如无胃肠积滞、津血亏损、产后、病后、老人、孕妇等。

traindicated　referring to the case such as absence of gastrointestinal stasis, consumption of body fluid and blood, the puperperant, during convalescence, the aged, pregnancy, etc.

蟹睛　【xiè jīng】（损翳、蟹睛疼痛外障）多属肝有郁热，上冲于目，以致黑睛翳溃或外伤所致。症见黑睛破损，黄仁从破口突出如珠，形似蟹睛，周围绕以白翳，目痛剧烈，羞明泪出，相当于虹膜脱出，愈后留瘢痕。

Perforation of Cornea with Prolapse of Iiris　a condition due to attack of the pathogenic heat accumulated in the liver to the eye, or due to injury; marked by ulceration of the cornea surrounded by nebula, accompanied with intense pain, photophobia and lacrimation.

心包络　【xīn bāo luò】脏腑之一。位于心的外围，具有保护心脏的功能，也与中枢神经系统的一些功能有关。如热入心包，可出现神昏谵语。

Pericardium　the envelope of the heart, serving as the protector of the heart. It is considered that some functions of the central nervous system have relation to the pericardium. If heat pathogen attacks pericardium, symptoms as delirium may appear.

心痹　【xīn bì】因心气痹阻引起以胸闷为主症的病证。表现为胸闷气喘、心悸心痛、咽干、叹气及烦躁易惊等。

Cardiac Bi-Syndrome　a syndrome with feeling of oppression over the chest as the major symptom, caused by the stagnation of heart-qi; accompanied with dyspnea. palpitation, precordial pain, dry throat, sighing, irritability, timidness, etc.

心病　【xīn bìng】泛指心脏功能失调而产生的各种病证。常表现为胸闷、胸痛、气短乏力、心悸怔忡、失眠健忘、精神恍惚、善惊易悲等。

Heart Disease　a general term for various diseases by the dysfunction of the heart; usually manifested as feeling of oppression over the chest, chest pain, shortness of breath, tiredness, palpitation, insomnia, amnesia, restlessness and fidgety, timidness, sentimentality, etc.

心动悸　【xīn dòng jì】自觉心脏剧烈跳

Severe Palpitation　violent beatin

动、悸动不安的一种症状。

心烦 【xīn fán】即心胸烦闷不安。多由内热（包括实热和虚热）引起。

心疳 【xīn gān】（惊疳）因乳食失调，心经郁热所致的疳证。表现为发热、颊赤面黄、口舌生疮、烦躁、口渴饮冷、小便赤涩、盗汗、磨牙、易惊等。

心汗 【xīn hàn】心前区局部多汗的症状。多因忧思惊恐伤及心脾所致。

心合脉 【xīn hé mài】五脏和五体相合。心的生理功能和脉有密切的关系，心主血，血行脉中，心通过脉来实现血液循环的功能。

心合小肠 【xīn hé xiǎo cháng】脏腑相合之一。指心和小肠之间的相互关联和影响。它们通过经络互相络属，在生理上互相协调，在病理上互相影响。

心火上炎 【xīn huǒ shàng yán】肾阴亏虚，不能上滋心阴，致心火独亢；或

and palpitating of the heart which is noted by the patient subjectively.

Feeling of Oppression over the Chest a symptom due to disturbance of the endogenous pathogenic heat, including sthenic heat and asthenic heat.

Infantile Malnutrition due to Disorder of Heart infantile malnutrition due to improper feeding and retention of pathogenic heat in the heart meridian; manifested as fever, flushed cheek, sallow complexion, aphthae, restlessness, thirst with desire for cold drinks, scanty dark urine, night sweat, teeth grinding and liability to be frightened, etc.

Perspiration over the Precordial Region a sign caused by the impairment of the heart and spleen resulting from sorrow and terror.

Heart is Connected with the Vessels the close relationship between the heart and the blood vessels. The vessels serve as the passages of blood; through which the heart exerts its effect on controlling the blood.

The Heart is Connected with the Small Intestine the paired relationship between the heart and the small intestine which are connected with each other by the network of meridian. They cooperate in functioning and involve each other when diseased.

Flaring-up of Heart-Fire a morbid condition due to hyperactivity of

心阴不足，虚火上升所致的病证。症见口舌生疮、心烦、失眠等。

heart-fire resulting from deficiency of kidney-yin and inability to nourish heart-yin; or due to deficiency of heart-yin leading to the rising up of asthenic fire; manifested as aphthae, restlessness, insomnia, etc.

心火内炽 【xīn huǒ nèi chì】心火过盛的病理。症见心烦失眠、心悸不安，甚则狂躁谵语、喜笑不休等。

Hyperactivity of Heart-Fire in the Interior a morbid condition manifested as insomnia, palpitation or even mania, delirium, frequent guffaw, etc.

心开窍于舌 【xīn kāi qiào yú shé】指舌为心之外候，又称舌为"心之苗"。舌司味觉和表达语言的功能，有赖于心的生理功能正常。心的生理功能异常，可导致味觉的改变和舌强语塞等病理现象。因此，从舌的形态、色泽变化可以察知气血的盛衰和判断心的生理功能情况。

Tongue is the Orifice to the Heart the functions of taste and speech of the tongue depend on the normal physiological function of the heart. The abnormal physilological function of the heart may lead to change of taste, stiff tongue and loss of speech. Thus, the hyperactivity or deficiency of qi and blood and the physiological function of the heart can be reflected in the changes in forms and colours of the tongue.

心悸 【xīn jì】自觉心跳，悸动不安的一种症状。多由气虚、血虚、停饮或气滞血瘀所致。

Palpitation unduly rapid action of the heart which is noted by the patient, usually caused by the deficiency of qi and blood, fluid retention in the body, qi-sluggishness and blood stasis.

心咳 【xīn ké】（心经咳嗽）指咳嗽时伴有胸痛的病证。甚则有咽喉肿痛、异物阻塞感等症。

Cough due to Involvement of Heart Meridian a disorder characterized by cough and chest pain, or even accompanied with sorethroat, feeling of foreign body in the throat, etc.

心劳 【xīn láo】因心血耗损所致的病证。主要表现为心烦失眠、心悸易惊。

Heart-Strain a disorder caused by consumption of heart-blood, chiefly manifested as irritability,

心脾两虚 【xīn pí liǎng xū】心脾两脏气血虚弱的病理。症见心悸、怔忡、失眠、多梦、健忘、食欲减退、大便稀溏、倦怠乏力或便血、皮下出血、月经过多,舌淡、脉细弱等。

Asthenia of both Heart and Spleen a morbid condition of the deficiency of qi and blood of the heart and spleen; manifested as palpitation, insomnia, dreaminess, amnesia, poor appetite, loose stools, fatigue, hematochezia, subcutaneous bleeding, menorrhagia, pale tongue, small and weak pulse, etc.

心、其华在面 【xīn, qí huá zài miàn】指心主血脉的功能可以表现于面部,通过望面部的色泽了解人体血气的盛衰变化。

Complexion Reflects the Condition of the Heart observation of the complexion may be helpful for the estimation of the hyperactivity or deficiency of the blood and qi which, in turn, indicates the function of the heart.

心气 【xīn qì】泛指心的功能活动,此外中医学认为精神活动也与心气有关。

Heart-Qi generally referring to the function of the cardiovascular system. In addition, it is considered to be also related to mental activities.

心气不固 【xīn qì bù gù】指心气虚弱不能收敛的病理。症见健忘易惊、心悸、自汗或动则汗出等。

Weakness of Heart-Qi a morbid condition of deficiency of heart-qi with failure of holding itself; manifested as amnesia, timidness, palpitation, spontaneous perspiration, and perspiration when moving, etc.

心气不宁 【xīn qì bù níng】泛指心神不安、心悸易惊、心烦不寐等症状。多因劳神过度、或心血不足、或因惊恐损及心气所致。

Disorder of Heart-Qi a morbid condition manifested as restlessness, palpitation, timidness, insomnia, etc; often caused by impairment of heart-qi resulting from mental overstrain, insufficiency of heart-blood, and terror, etc.

心气盛 【xīn qì shèng】心的病理性功

Sthenia of Heart-Qi a morbid state

能亢进。症见精神过度兴奋、心烦失眠、甚则出现狂躁等。of hyperfunction of the heart; manifested as over excitation, restlessness, insomnia, even mania, etc.

心气虚 【xīn qì xū】（心气不足）心脏功能低下的病理。症见心悸、气短乏力、胸闷不舒、自汗、脉细弱或结代等。

Deficiency of Heart-Qi a morbid state of hypofunction of the heart; manifested as palpitation, shortness of breath, fatigue, feeling of oppression over the chest, spontaneous perspiration, weak and small pulse or irregular pulse, etc.

心气虚不得卧 【xīn qì xū bù dé wò】因心气虚引起以失眠为主症的病证。表现为夜卧不安、睡后易醒、心悸、疲倦乏力、喜热恶冷、脉迟或无力。

Insomnia due to Deficiency to Heart-Qi a disorder manifested as sleeplessness, wakefulness, palpitation, lassitude, aversion to cold and inclination to heat, and slow or weak pulse.

心热 【xīn rè】（心气热）泛指心的各种热性病，因心藏神故心气亢盛常伴有神志方面的改变。症见心中烦热、睡眠不宁、喜笑不休、小便赤，甚至神昏谵语，舌红脉数等。

Heart-Heat referring to various heat syndromes of the heart due to hyperactivity of the heart-qi, manifested as restlessness, insomnia, mental confusion, deep-coloured urine, even delirium, red tongue, fast pulse, etc.

心疝 【xīn shàn】因心经受寒而致的一种病证。表现为腹痛并有腹皮隆起、自觉有气自脐上冲于心。

Heart-Meridian Colic a morbid condition caused by the pathogenic cold involving the heart meridian, manifested as abdominal pain with visible mass, a subjective feelng of gas rushing up from the navel to the thorax.

心肾相交 【xīn shèn xiàng jiāo】脏腑相关理论之一。心属火、藏神、肾属水、藏精。两脏互相作用，互相制约，以维持正常的生理活动，肾中真阳上升，能温养心火，心火能制肾水泛滥而助真阳；肾水又能制心火，使不致过亢而益心阴，这种关系也称水火相

Harmorny of the Heart and Kidney the heart dominates fire, houses the mind and belongs to yang. The kidney dominates water, houses the water and belongs to yin. The relationship between the heart and kidney, therefore, concerns the balance be-

济。

tween yin and yang, ascending and descending. Under normal physiological conditions, heart yang descends, together with the kidney yang, to warm kidney yin and kidney water. In contrast, kidney yin accends, together with heart yin, to moisten heart yang and prevent it from becoming hyperactive. This relationship mutual communi-cation and restriction is called "harmony of heart and kidney." When water and fire are in harmony, a relative balance between above and below, yin and yang, is maintained, ensuring the normal physiological function of the heart and kidney.

心神烦乱 【xīn shén fán luàn】指心烦不安、意识错乱。本症多由热邪（实热或虚热）内扰心神引起。

Mental Confusion a symptom mostly resulting from heat factors (sthenic or asthenic heat), interfering the mind.

心痛 【xīn tòng】1、指心绞痛 2、指胃脘痛。

Cardialgia 1. angina pectoris 2. epigastric pain.

心痛彻背 【xīn tòng chè bèi】胸痛牵连至背部的一种症状。

Chest Pain Involving the Back a symptom manifested as the chest pain affecting the back.

心恶热 【xīn wù rè】心为火脏，热邪易影响心的生理功能，故称为心恶热。如高热患者易出现神志不清、谵语、狂躁等热伤神明的症状。或出现津血耗伤或迫血妄行，热伤血脉的症状。

Heart Hates Heat one of the physiological characteristics of the heart. Its functions are easily affected by the pathogenic heat. For instance, the cases with high fever have such symptoms of impairment of mental activity as unconsciousness, delirium and restlessness, or symptoms of consumption of both the body fluid and blood, of the attack of pathogenic

心系 【xīn xì】指心脏与其他脏器相联系的脉络。

心下悸 【xīn xià jì】①指自觉近膻中处悸动不适②指心悸。

心下痞痛 【xīn xià pǐ tòng】（心下痛）胃脘部胀满、疼痛的一种症状。

心下痞满 【xīn xià pǐ mǎn】胃脘部胀满，按之柔软而不痛的一种症状。

心下支结 【xīn xià zhī jié】指胃脘部自觉有物梗阻而烦闷不舒。可见于外感和杂病的多种疾病。

心虚 【xīn xū】①泛指心之阴、阳、气、血不足的各种病证②同心气虚。

心虚胆怯 【xīn xū dǎn qiè】指心中空虚，容易恐惧的一种证候。多因心血不足，心气衰弱所致。

心血 【xīn xuè】即心所主的血。心血不仅能营养周身各部分组织，也是神志活动的物质基础之一。

心血虚 【xīn xuè xū】（心血不足）多由失血，过度劳神，或血的生化之源不足所致。症见头晕、面色苍白、心悸、心烦、失眠、多梦、健忘、脉细

heat to the blood vessels.

Heart Vessels the large blood vessels connecting directly with the heart, by which the heart connects with other organs.

Epigastric Throbbing 1. pulsation over the tanzhong region 2. palpitation.

Distention and Pain over the Epigastric Region

Epigastric Fullness a feeling of distention over the epigastric region, softness on palpation but no tenderness.

Obstruction and Fullness of Epigastric Region a subjective feeling of obstruction over the epigastric region, seen in the cases with exogenous diseases or internal diseases.

Heart-Asthenia 1. referring to the various diseases due to deficiency of yin, yang, qi and blood of the heart. 2. deficiency of the heart-qi.

Timidness due to Heart-Asthenia a syndrome due to insufficiency of the heart blood and qi, marked by uneasiness or timidness.

Heart-Blood the blood controlled by the heart, which is the nutrient for all the body tissues and organs, also one of the basic materials for mental activities.

Deficiency of Heart-Blood a morbid condition due to loss of blood, overtaxing or insufficiency of production of blood, manifested as dizziness,

弱等。

心血虚不得卧 【xīn xuè xū bù dé wò】由于用心过度，心血虚耗而心神不宁。表现为夜卧则惊、五心烦热、口燥舌干、脉细数。

心阳 【xīn yáng】心的阳气，也是心脏功能的体现。心阳不足可出现寒象，如四肢厥冷、脉微欲绝等。

心阳虚 【xīn yáng xu】①阳虚之体、由误汗、误下、或劳心过度致心悸，气短，自汗，形寒肢冷，口淡，舌质淡，苔白润，脉迟弱等。②心气虚。

心移热于小肠 【xīn yí rè yú xiǎo cháng】心与小肠互为表里，病变时可互相影响。心有热可下移于小肠。症见心烦，口舌生疮，尿少，尿痛，尿血等。

pallor, palpitation, restlessness, insomnia, dreamfulness, amnesia, weak and small pulse.

Sleeplessness due to Deficiency of the Heart Blood a morbid condition related to emotional distress caused by over-mental work and deficiency and consumption of the heart blood, manifested by fear in the sleep, dysphoria with feverish sensation in the chest, palms and soles, dry mouth and tongue, weak and fast pulse.

Heart Yang yang-qi of the heart is also reflection of the heart function, so cold syndrome sometimes appear in the insufficiency of heart-yang such as cold limbs, feeble and weak pulse.

Deficiency of Heart-Yang 1. yang deficiency due to erroneous administration of diaphoretics and purgations or over-exertion of the heart resulting in palpitation, shortness of breath, spontaneous perspiration, chill and cold in extremities, tastelessness of mouth, pale tongue with white and moist coat, weak and slow pulse. 2. deficiency of the heart-qi.

Transmission of Pathogenic Heat of the Heart to the Small Intestine the heart and small intestine are interior-exteriorly related, which may lead to their coordination in some of their functions when there is any pathological change. The heat in the heart may transmit the small intestine, manifested by irritability, ulceration of the mouth and tongue, scanty urine with pain, hematuria.

心阴 【xīn yīn】是心脏的阴液,为营血的组成部分,在生理和病理上与心血密切相关,并和肺阴、肾阴等的消长盈亏有关。

Heart-Yin referring to yin-fluid of the heart, component part of ying-blood, closely related to the heart-blood in physiology and pathology and also related to the sufficiency and insufficiency of the lung-yin and kidney-yin.

心阴虚 【xīn yīn xū】(心阴不足)指劳神过度或久病,热病耗伤心阴所致。症见心烦、失眠、心悸、低热、盗汗、口干、脉细数等。

Deficiency of the Heart-Yin a morbid condition due to over-exertion of emotion or chronic illness, febrile illness exausting the heart-yin, manifested by restlessness, insomnia, palpitation, low-graded fever, spontaneous perspiration, dry mouth, fine and fast pulse.

心营过耗 【xīn yíng guò hào】指心阴耗损太过,热性病久热伤阴或虚损病阴虚火旺均能大量消耗血液中营养物质。症见夜热、心烦、容易出汗、舌质深红、脉细数等。

Over-exhaustion of the Heart-Ying referring to over exhaustion of the heart-yin, impairment of yin due to prolonged heat in febrile or deficiency of yin accompanied with flamming up of pathogenic fire due to deficiency and impairment syndrome which give rise to large consumption of nutritious materials in the blood, manifested as fever during the night, restlessness, freguent sweating, deep red colour of the tongue proper, fine and fast pulse.

心者,君主之官 【xīn zhě, jūn zhǔ zhī guān】中医学认为心是五脏之主,有调节脏腑生理功能的重要作用。故以君主喻其对人体的重要性。

The Heart, the Monarch in tradtional Chinese medicine, the heart is supposed to be the chief of the five zang organs, it plays an important role in adjusting physiological functions of the five zang, and therefor is

心中憺憺大动 【xīn zhōng dǎn dǎn dà dòng】心跳剧烈，心神不宁的一种症状。多因阴虚水亏、虚火内扰，心神不能自主所致。

心主神明 【xīn zhǔ shén míng】心的重要功能之一。中医学认为，意识、思维等高极中枢活动，是由心所主持的。

心主汗 【xīn zhǔ hàn】中医学认为汗和血是同源的，心和血又有密切的关系，临床上许多汗症与心有关。

心主言 【xīn zhǔ yán】心的生理功能之一。言语是表达思维意识的一种重要形式，受心神的主宰和控制，如心受病邪侵犯时，出现谵语等症状。

心主血脉 【xīn zhǔ xuè mài】心的生理功能之一。心主持血液运行，是血液循环的原动力。

compared to be monarch to show its importance to the body.

Violent Palpitation with Empty Sensation a morbid condition of violent heart beat and emotional distress usually due to insufficiency of water as a result of yin-deficiency, stirring up of emdopathic wind of deficiency type and failure of controlling mental activities.

The Heart Is in Charge of Mental Activities one of the key functions of the heart. In traditional Chineses medicine, consciousness, thinking and high — level nerve central activities are supposed to be governed by the heart.

The Heart Controls Sweat in traditional Chinese medicine, sweat and blood are homologous, the heart and blood are closely related. Clinically many sweat syndromes are connected with the heart.

The Heart Governs Speech one of the physiological functions. Speech is an important form of expressing thinking and consciousness and governed and controlled by the spirit in the heart. When heart is invaded by pathogenic factor, delirium may appear.

The Heart Governs the Blood Circulation one of the physiological functions of the heart. The heart takes charge of the blood circulation and is original motive power of the

辛【xīn】辛味的药物。一般有疏散和行气的作用,如荆芥疏散风寒、砂仁行气等。

辛甘发散为阳【xīn gān fā sàn wéi yáng】辛味甘味药有发散的作用,其药性属阳,如防风桂枝的性味辛甘、能发散解肌表。

辛甘化阳【xīn gān huà yáng】辛味、甘味药同用,以扶助阳气的治法。适用于脾肾等阳虚的病证。

辛寒生津【xīn hán shēng jīn】用性味辛寒的药物清胃热生津液的方法。常用于胃火炽盛、胃阴不足者,症见口中有秽气、舌苔焦黄、脉大而虚等。

辛开苦泄【xīn kāi kǔ xiè】①用辛味

blood circulation.

Pungent pungent for dispelling wind and heat and promoting flow of qi, such as schizonepeta used to promote flow of qi.

Drugs of Sweet Taste and Pungent Flavour which Induce Persipiration are Attributive to Yang drugs pungent in flavour and sweet in taste with the action of inducing perspiration pertain to yang, e. g. pungent flavour and sweet taste of ledebouriella root and cinnamom twig exert the action of inducing sweat and expelling pathogenic factors from muscles and skin.

Reinforcing Yang with Drugs Pungent in Flavour and Sweet in Taste a therapeutic method to combine pungent drugs with sweet drugs to reinforce yang-qi, which is indicated for the syndrome of deficiency of the spleen-yang and kidney-yang.

Promoting the Production of Body Fluid with Drugs of Pungent Flavour and Cold Property a therapeutic method of removing stomach-heat and promoting the production of body fluid with drugs of pungent flavour and cold property, usually used to treat morbid condition of excessiveness of stomach-heat and insufficiency of stomach-yin marked by halitosis, aphthous ulcer, sallow coat on the tongue, large and feeble pulse.

**Pungent Drugs for Disperison and Bit-

药发散表邪,用苦味药清泄里热。② 因痰湿热阻滞而出现痞闷胀满,用辛味药行气散结,用苦寒药泄热。

ter Drugs for Purgation (1) administering pungent drugs to disperse exopathogen and bitter drugs to relieve endopathic heat. (2) using pungent drugs with the action of promoting flow of qi and dispersing accumulation of pathogen and bitter drugs with the action of relieving heat to treat epigastric distress and fullness caused by accumulation of phlegm-heat and phlegm-dampness.

辛凉解表 【xīn liáng jiě biǎo】具有疏风解热作用的药物,治疗风热表症或温病初起的治法。适用于恶寒轻而发热较重,有汗的风热表证。

Relieving the Exterior Syndrome with Drugs Pungent in Flavour and Cool in Property a therapeutic method of using drugs with action of scattering wind and dispersing exopathogen to treat exterior syndrome of wind-heat or onset of seasonal febrile disease, indicated for exterior syndrome marked by slight chill, with high fever and presence of perspiration.

辛凉清气 【xīn liáng qīng qì】用辛寒的药物,清气分之热邪的方法。常用于温热病邪入气分,症见高热、不恶寒、口渴、大汗出、舌红苔黄、脉洪大等。

Removing Heat from Qi with Drugs of Pungent flavour and Cool Nature a therapeutic method of using drugs of pungent flavour and cold property to clear away pathogenic heat from qi system. Usually used to treat morbid condition of pathogenic heat invading qi system, marked by high fever, absence of chill, thirst, profuse sweating, red tongue with yellowish coating, full and large pulse.

辛温解表 【xīn wēn jiě biǎo】用辛温发散的药物治疗风寒之邪在表的一种治疗方法。一般用于恶寒重而发热

Relieving the Exerior Syndrome with Drugs Pungent in Flavour and Warm in Property a therapeutic

较轻,全身酸痛,无汗的风寒表证。上半身浮肿、较重的早期水肿等。method of administering drugs of pungent flavour and warm property with the action of inducing perspiration to treat exterior pathogenic wind-cold, usually used for exterior syndrome of wind-cold marked by aversion to cold with slight fever, pantalgia and absence of sweat, general edema in the upper part of the body, early stage of watery distention.

新感 【xīn gǎn】即感受病邪后很快发病的温病。

New Affection immediate onset of the epidemic febrile disease after invasion by the exopathogen.

新感温病 【xīn gǎn wēn bìng】感受外邪,随感随发,初起有恶风或恶寒表证的温病,与伏气温病相对而言。

Epidemic Febrile Disease Occuring Immediately after the Attack of Exopathogen epidemic febrile disease characterized by immediate onset after invasion by exopathogen and exterior syndrome marked by aversion to wind or cold at the onset, opposite to epidemic febrile disease occurring after incubation.

馨饪之邪 【xīn rèn zhī xié】饮食不当可成为致病之邪,如过食馨香厚味的饮食,可引起伤食病。

Pathogenic Factors due to Improper Diet improper diet may become pathogenic factors leading to disease, immoderately eating (and drinking) rich food may cause syndrome of impairment by overeating.

囟门 【xìn mén】指婴儿未完全骨化的颅骨所剩下的空隙。

Fontanel referring to the remaining gap due to incomplete ossified cranial bone in infant.

囟陷 【xìn xiàn】指囟门下陷。婴儿在半岁内,前囟微下陷属正常生理状态。如因婴儿禀赋不足或因久病元气亏虚脾气不能上充,致囟门下陷则为病理状态,往往伴有面色萎黄、神疲

Sunken Fontanel in Infant referring to the sunken point of fontanel. Slight sinking in front fontanel in infant within six months is attributable to normal physiological state. If

气短、食少便溏、四肢不温等症状。

sunken fontanel in infant is caused by congenital deficiency or by impairment of primordial qi and the spleen-qi failing to send up nutrients due to chronic disease, it is believed to be pathogenic state, often accompanied with sallow complexion, mental fatigue, shortness of breath, anoreixa, watery stool, cold limbs.

囟填 【xìn tián】囟门肿起如堆。因热者,柔软红色;因寒者,牢韧坚硬。

Bulging of Fontanel in Infant swelling fontanel, which is soft and red in case with fever; firm and hard in case with cold.

腥臭气 【xīng chòu qì】指病者的痰液、汗液、白带、粪便等分泌物或排泄物所产生的特殊腥臭气味。

Fish Stench referring to special smell from secretion or excreta in patient's sputum, sweat, leukorrhea, feces.

行迟 【xíng chí】小儿周岁以后,甚至二、三岁仍不能行走者。

Retaudation of Walking in Children referring to young children who can not walk after one year old, even after two or three years old.

行经腹痛 【xíng jīng fù tòng】(痛经)指在月经期间或行经前后出现下腹疼痛,甚则剧痛难忍,且常伴有腰痛的一种病变。气滞、血瘀、寒湿凝滞、肝肾亏损等均可导致本病。

Dysmenorrhea referring to morbid condition with pain in the lower abdomen during or around menstruation, in severe cases too painful to be tolerated, usually accompanied with lumbago, which may be brought about by stagnancy of qi, blood stasis, stagnation of cold-dampness, deficiency of the liver-yin and kidney-yin.

行气 【xíng qì】(通气、化气、利气)是治疗由于气滞而产生的胸腹胀闷疼痛的方法。

Promoting Flow of Qi a therapeutic method of treating distending or dull pain caused by stagnation of qi.

行气活血 【xíng qì huó xuè】治疗气滞血瘀的方法。临床上常以理气药和活

Promoting Flow of Qi and Blood Circulation a therapeutic method of

血祛瘀药同用，治疗心、腹、胁等部位的疼痛、时发时止、月经不调、跌扑损伤、产后恶露不行等属于气滞血瘀的病证。

行针 【xíng zhēn】进针后用各种方法运行针体，以达到得气、补泻目的的各种方法。

形肥经少 【xíng féi jīng shǎo】妇女身体肥胖，月经量逐渐减少，色淡质稀或夹带下等。多因素体脾虚，影响水谷之精微化生为血，湿痰凝于经隧所致。

形体 【xíng tǐ】指人体身形和体质。对形体的观察有助于辨证论治。

形气 【xíng qì】指身形体质和脏腑组织的功能。在正常情况下，形与气互相协调的任何一方出现偏盛偏虚，都

treating stagnation of qi and blood stasis, usually used clinically in combination with drugs with action of activating blood and removing stagnations to treat pains attacking the heart, abdomen and ribs and syndrome of stagnancy of qi and blood stasis manifested as menoxenia, injuries from falls, fractures, contusions and strains, postnatal retaining of lochia.

Needle Transmission various ways of manipulating the needle to induce needle sensation and reinforce the body resistance following needle insertion.

Reduced Menstrual Discharge due to Obesity women's fat body, reduction of menstrual discharge in reddish and thin colour mixed with morbid leukorrhea, usually caused by disturbance in transmiting food essence to the blood and stagnation of damp-phlegm in pathway due to deficiency of the spleen related to general debility.

Configuration and Constitution of a Human Body referring to physical appearance and constitution. Observation of configuration and constitution of a human body is helpful to differentiation and treatment of common syndromes.

Physical Appearance and Qi referring to configuration and constitution of a human body and function of zang

是病态。

形气相失 【xíng qì xiāng shī】病人的身形体质与正气或病情发展不平衡。如某些痰饮病患者身体虽然肥胖，但动则心悸、气喘、汗出，这就是形盛气虚，这类形气不相称的病证，预后较差。

形气相得 【xíng qì xiāng dé】指病人的形体与正气或病情发展相平衡，通常以此作为判断疾病预后良好的依据之一。如身形状实，其气也盛，这些病人即使病情较重，预后仍较好。

形脏 【xíng zàng】①胃、大肠、小肠及膀胱四个腑。②指头角、耳目、口齿、胸中四处。

醒脾 【xǐng pí】指用芳香健脾药健运脾气以治疗脾为湿困，运化无力的病证。

— fu tissue. In normal condition, physical appearance and qi are coordinated. Extreme excess and extreme deficiency in either side is supposed to be pathogenic condition.

Physical Appearance and Qi Lacking in Balance the patient's configuration and constitution and qi are not well balanced in their development. Some patients with phlegm retention, though very fat, suffer from palpitation, marked by dyspnea, perspiration on slight exertion, the syndrome by excess of physical appearance and deficiciency of qi and lacking in balance resulting in poor prognosis.

Physical Appearance and Qi in Balance the patient's configuration and contitution are well balanced in their development, usually as a proof for the judgement of favorable prognosis. Some patients are strong in physical appearance and also excessive in qi, therefore they still have favorable prognosis even if their conditions are more severe.

Substantial Organs (1) four fu organs including the stomach, large intestine, small intestine and gall-bladder. (2) referring to fur organs including the head, ear and eyes. mouth teeth, and chest.

Enlivening the Spleen a therapeutic method of administering drugs with fragrant odour to invigorate and acti-

性能 【xìng néng】即药物的性质作用，如四气、五味和升、降、浮、沉等。

Property and Action the action of drugs such as the four properties, the five tastes, the ascending, descending, floating and sinking actions.

胸骨伤 【xiōng gǔ shāng】包括胸肋部的肋骨伤折。多因跌打压撞所致。局部疼痛、呼吸短促，尤于深呼吸或咳嗽时疼痛加剧，严重者可以出现咯血、呼吸困难、气胸、血胸等。

Fracture of Rib including the fracture in the chest and ribs, usually caused by fall, contusion, stabbing and knocking accompanied by local pain, shortness of breath, especially aggravated during deep breath and cough, in severe cases accompanied by hemoptysis, breath in difficulty pneumothorax, blood stasis in the chest.

胸痹 【xiōng bì】一般指以胸膺部窒塞疼痛为主的病证。①指痰浊，瘀血等阴邪凝结，胸阳失宣，气机闭阻，脉络不通所致，甚则痛引彻背、常伴喘息、不得平卧等。②即胃痹。

Obstruction of Qi in the Chest generally denoting a morbid condition marked by choking pain in the front chest. (1) often referring to the stagnation of such yin pathogens as thick phlegm and blood stasis, failure of facilitating function of chest-yang, interference with functional activities of qi and obstruction of meridians manifested as fullness or pain in the chest, pain in case of severity, pain over the whole back, often accompanied with asthma, difficulty in lying flat. (2) obstruction of qi in the stomach.

胸痞 【xiōng pǐ】指胸中满闷而不痛的症状。多由湿浊上壅，痰凝气滞，胸阳遏郁所致。

Feeling of Stuffiness in the Chest referring to a syndrome with a feeling of fullness and stuffiness in the chest but without pain, generally caused by stagnation of dampness pathogen in the chest leading to blockage of ascending flow of qi, and subsequent obstruction of the chest-yang.

胸满 【xiōng mǎn】指胸部胀满的症状。因风寒、热壅、停饮、气滞、瘀血等所致。

Feeling of Fullness in the Chest referring to symptom characterized by distention and fullness feeling in the chest, caused by wind-cold, stagnation of heat, obstruction of qi and blood stasis.

胸痛 【xiōng tòng】指胸部正中或偏侧疼痛的自觉症状。温热犯肺，寒痰壅塞，水饮留积胸胁，心阳不足，心血瘀阻，或肝火上犯等均可引起。

Pain in the Chest referring to Subjective Symptoms of pain occurring in the middle or to the lateral, usually resulting from invasion of heat into the lung, stagnation of cold-phlegm, accumulation of excessive fluid in the chest, deficiency of the chest-yang, stagnancy of the heart-blood; or ascending invasion of the liver-fire.

胸围 【xiōng wéi】胸部与在乳头相平部位的周围长度，一般用来测量胸廓大小和取穴标准。

Circumference of the Chest the surrounding length of the position where the chest is in line with the nipple, usually serving as measurement of thoracic size and standard of acupoints.

胸胁苦满 【xiōng xié kǔ mǎn】指胸胁部闷满不舒的症状。因肝胆经气机失调，胆火内郁于胸膈所致。

Feeling of Fullness and Discomfort in the Chest and Hypochondrium referring to symptom characterized by fullness and discomfort in the chest and hypochondrium, which is caused by disorder of qi in the meridians of the liver and gallbladder, and stagnation of the gallbladder-fire in the chest.

胸下结硬 【xiōng xià jié yìng】指胸膈

Distension, Pain and Rigidity in the

间有胀满、疼痛、硬块样的感觉。多由痰湿与邪热相蕴结所致。

Upper Abdomen denoting the feeling of distension, fullness, pain and rigidity in the chest, which is generally caused by accumulation of phlegm-dampness and heat pathogen.

胸中痞鞕 【xiōng zhōng pǐ yìng】指胸中痞塞硬满自觉有物堵住的症状。多由痰涎阻隔，寒邪上壅所致。

Feeling of Stuffiness and Choking in Chest referring to the symptom characterized by stuffiness choking and subjective obstruction sensation in the chest, which usually caused by dampness and phlegm stagnated in the middle portion of the body involving the chest, cold pathogen ascending and obstructing flow of qi.

胸中烦热 【xiōng zhōng fán rè】指胸中烦闷觉热。多属内热；或因外感余热未清；或心火亢盛所致。

Irritable Feverish Sensation in the Chest referring to irritability and hot sensation in the chest, mainly attributable to interior heat; or caused by residual heat of exopathy; or by hyperactivity of the heart-fire.

胸膺 【xiōng yīng】即前胸部。

The Front Part of the Chest

胸中之府 【xiōng zhōng zhī fǔ】即背部。

The Seat of the Chest referring to the back.

休息痢 【xiū xī lì】积年累月，屡止屡发，经久不愈的痢疾。多因治疗失宜，或气血不足，脾肾虚弱，湿热伏于肠胃所致。

Chronic Dysentery with Frequent Relapse dysentery wth remissions and exacebations and refractory to treatment for a prolonged duration, or insufficiency of qi and blood, deficiency of the spleen and kidney leading to accumulation of damp-heat in the gastrointestine.

嗅气味 【xiù qì wèi】闻诊内容之一。通过嗅觉了解病人排泄物和分泌物气味的变化，以帮助分析病情。

Smelling the Odour a part of ausculation and olfaction, through which the changes of patient's excreta and secretion can be learned and it is

虚秘 【xū bì】则于正虚不运而致的便秘。多因气虚、阳虚，或年老体弱、精血不足，以及产后血虚津少所致。

虚痢 【xū lì】指痢疾之属于虚者。多因痢久不愈或虚人患痢所致。除下利脓血外，兼见困倦、谷食难化、腹痛等。

虚喘 【xū chuǎn】指气喘由于正气虚者。多因禀赋素弱、久喘或病后真元耗损致肺气虚弱，肾不纳气所致。以喘促而气短难续、动则加剧、声音低微、舌淡脉弱为特点。

虚痓 【xū cè】因气血虚极不能养筋或大失血所致的痓病。症见四肢搐搦、头目昏花、自汗、神疲、气短、舌质淡、脉细弦等。

favourable to the analysis of patient's condition.

Constipation of Insufficiency Type referring to constipation due to insufficiency of genuine qi which caused dysfunction of the spleen and stomach, mostly caused by deficiency of qi, deficiency of yang, or debility because of old age, insufficiency of essence and blood, as well as deficiency of the blood and loss of body fluid after childbirth.

Dysentery of Deficiency Type referring to dysentery in debilitated patient and dysentery of prolonged duration marked by purulent bloody stools, lassitude, indigestion, and abdominal pain.

Asthma of Insufficiency Type referring to asthma resulting from insufficiency of healthy qi, mostly caused by chronic asthma due to general debility or weakness of the lung-qi and failure of the kidney in receiving air after illness due to over consumption of healthy qi, characterized by shortness of breath and dyspnea upon exertion, weak voice, pale tongue and weak pulse.

Tetany due to Deficiency of Qi and Blood a convulsive disease resulting from inability to nourish the tendons and muscles because of extreme deficiency of qi and blood or from heavy loss of blood, marked by convulsion of the extremities, blurred vi-

虚烦 【xū fán】指阴虚内热，虚火内扰而见心中烦乱不宁，似胀不胀、悒悒闷闷、夜寐不宁。多见于外感热病，经汗、吐、下后余热不清者或后期阴津耗伤，亦可见于劳心思虑过度者。

虚风内动 【xū fēng nèi dòng】由于阴虚、血虚内生的风证。多见于失液、失血或久病伤阴后，由津亏血枯，血不养筋，阴不潜阳而肝风内窜所致，症见眩晕、震颤、抽搐、甚则昏迷等。

虚火 【xū huǒ】①真阴亏损引起的热性证候。症见低热或午后潮热、手足心灼热、口干、盗汗、舌嫩红或深红、脉虚数等。②阴盛格阳引起的假热症状。

sion, spontaneous perspiration, general debility, shortness of breath, pale colour of tongue proper, small and thready pulse.

Fidgeting due to Deficiency referring to interior heat due to deficiency of yin and interference of fire of deficiency type in the interior characterized by restlessness, poor appetite with faint distension and stuffiness in the stomach, sleeplessness, mostly seen in febrile disease of exopathy in which remnant heat is not cleared up after sweating, vomitting and purging or impairment of body fluid in the advanced stage, sometimes seen in case with over anxiency.

Stirring-Up of Endopathic Wind of Deficiency Type a wind syndrome showing deficiency of yin and blood, mostly due to impairment of fluid and blood or mostly due to endopathic stirring of the liver-wind resulting from impairment of fluid and deficiency of the blood, poor nourishment of tendons and muscles, hyperactivity of the liver-yang following loss of fluid and blood or impairment of yin because of prolonged illness.

Fire of Deficiency Type (1) a morbid condition showing heat syndrome due to impairment of yin, marked by low fever, hot sensaton in palms and soles, dry mouth, night sweat, light or deep reddish tongue, feeble and fast pulse. (2) a morbid condition showing pseudo-heat symptoms due to excess of yin which keeps yang outside.

虚火上炎 【xū huǒ shàng yán】由于肾阴亏损,水不制火上升的病理。症见咽干、咽痛、头昏目眩、心烦不眠、手足心热、舌质嫩红、脉细数等。

Flaring Up of Fire of Deficiency Type   a morbid condition showing flarring-up of the fire of deficiency type, resulting from deficiency of the kidney-yin and failure of water to control fire, marked by dry throat, sore throat, blurred vision, irritability and sleeplessness, hot sensation in palms and soles, light reddish coating on the tongue, thready and fast pulse.

虚寒 【xū hán】正气虚兼内寒的证候。症见面黄少华、食欲不振、怕冷、口淡不渴、精神不振、身倦乏力、小便清长、大便稀烂或泄泻清水、舌淡苔白、脉沉迟无力等。

Cold of Insufficiency Type   a morbid condition resulting from insufficiency of qi with endogenous cold, marked by pale complexion, loss of appetite, aversion to cold, tastelessness, absence of thirst, listlessness, fatigue debility, polyuria with watery urine, loose stools, tongue with whitish coating, deep, slow and weak pulse.

虚寒洞泄 【xū hán dòng xiè】通常是指肾阳虚衰,命门火衰,致脾阳不足,不能腐熟水谷而引起的泄泻。

Diarrhea due to Cold of Insufficiency Type   generally referring to diarrhea resulting from insufficiency of the spleen-yang, disability to thoroughly decompose water and grain, due to deficiency and exhaustion of the kidney-yang and decline of fire of the life gate.

虚黄 【xū huáng】多因疸病日久或脾虚血亏,不能营养肌肤所致。症见肌肤萎黄、口淡、怔忡、脚软、微寒发热、小便浊涩、食少便溏、舌淡、脉细弱等。

Sallow Complexion of Insufficiency Type   a morbid condition resulting from prolonged jaundice or hypofunction of the spleen with deficiency of blood and poor nourishment of complexion, marked by sallow and withered skin, tastelessness in the mouth, violent palpitation, weakness of the legs, slight chill with fever, turbid and scanty urine, appetite, loose stools, pale tongue, thready and weak pulse.

虚家 【xū jiā】指平素体质虚弱的人。

Debilitated Patient referring to patient suffering from general debility.

虚劳 【xū láo】(虚损) 由于气血不足，脏腑虚损所致的多种疾病。以及相互传染的骨蒸，传尸。

Consumptive Disease referring to various disease caused by insufficiency of qi and blood and impairment of zang and fu organs as well as infections hectic fever due to yin-deficiency and tuberculosis.

虚劳腰痛 【xū láo yāo tòng】指因劳伤于肾，肾气不足气化失常而致的腰痛。症见腰痛牵引少腹、小便不利、脉沉等。

Lumbago due to Consumption denoting lumbago resulting from consumption impairing the kidney, insufficiency of the kidney-qi and interruption of activities of qi, marked by lumbago affecting lower abdomen, difficulty of urination, deep pulse, etc.

虚劳盗汗 【xū láo dào hàn】由脏腑虚损导致的阴阳气血失调而引起的盗汗证。

Night Sweat due to Consumption a night sweat state resulting from deficiency and impairment of zang and fu organs with imbalance of the relationship between qi and blood and that between yin and yang.

虚积痢 【xū jī lì】指脾胃虚弱而致积滞的痢疾。小儿饮食不节或过食肥甘，胃肠积滞，积滞过久而致。症见腹痛而软、喜按、里急后重、腹泻日夜无度。

Dysentery of Deficiency Type referring to dysentery caused by deficiency of the spleen and stomach, for infants usually by improper diet or over-eating of greasy and sweet food resulting in accumulation of food in the stomach and intestine for a long time,

虚脉 【xū mài】①脉象之一,脉软无力,寻按呈空虚感。②实热证用刺络泻血,以泄其热。③指充盈度不足的络脉。

Feeble Pulse (1) one of the conditions showing soft and weak pulse, hollow sensation by searching. (2) heat syndrome of excess type to be dealt with by blood-letting puncture to purging away heat through bleeding. (3) referring to collateral branch of the large meridian which is not sufficient.

虚疟 【xū nüè】疟疾的一种类型。多因正虚体弱,又感疟邪;或因久疟不愈,使元气亏耗所致。症见寒热不甚、饮食减少、自汗、乏力、脉虚软等。

Asthenia-Type Malaria one kind of intermittent fever, mostly caused by deficiency of qi and general debility, invasion by pathogenic factors of intermittent fever, or by prolonged intermittent fever leading to impairment of primodial qi, marked by moderate chills and fever, poor appetite, spontaneous persperation; weakness and fatigue, feeble and soft pulse.

虚热 【xū rè】阴、阳、气、血不足而引起的发热,常有阴虚、阳虚、气虚、血虚之分。

Fever of Deficiency Type fever caused by deficiency of yin, yang, qi and blood, often classified into deficiency of yin, deficiency of yang, deficiency of qi and deficiency of blood.

虚痞 【xū pǐ】指由脾胃心肾虚衰,阴阳气血亏损引起的痞证。症状以空腹时脘腹痞闷为特征,常兼见纳呆、气短、便溏、食入不化、腹胀喜暖畏寒等。

Stuffy Sensation of Deficiency Type stuffy sensation caused by deficiency and exhaustion of the spleen and stomach, heart and kidney and impairment of yin, yang, qi and blood, characterized by epigastric and abdominal distension and stuffiness when stomach is empty, often accompanied with loss of appetite, shortness of breath, loose stools, indigeston, abdominal distension, preference for warmth and aversion to cold.

虚热经行先期 【xū rè jīng xíng xiān qī】是经行先期证型之一。因阴血不足,虚热内扰冲任所致。症见经期提前、经量较少、血色鲜红、质稠粘、并有颧红、手足心发热等。

Advanced Menstruation due to Heat of Deficiency Type one of advanced menstruation syndromes due to insufficiency of yin-blood, deficient heat involving the chong and ren meridians interiorly, marked by menstruation ahead of the time with the amount less than usual, bright red in colour, and property mucoid, accompanied by red cheek, hot sensaton in the palms and soles.

虚实 【xū shí】八纲中两个相对的概念。是指机体抵抗力强弱和病邪盛衰的表现。虚,通常指正气亏损,抵抗力弱;实,通常指邪气亢盛,正邪斗争剧烈。

Deficiency and Excess two opposite concepts of the eight principal syndromes, referring to the manifestation of the adequacy of the bodily resistance to disease and the virulence of pathogens. Deficiency, referring to impairment of vital qi resulting in weak resistance; excess, generally referring to rampancy of pathogens and intense struggle between the normal and the abnormal.

虚痫 【xū xián】遇劳即发的痫病。常发于郁闷之人。多因病后体虚,或复得感六淫,气血痰积所致。

Epilepsy of Deficiency Type attack of epilepsy after overfatigue often occurring in depressed patients mostly due to bodily debility after illness, or repeated affection of six pathogens and accumulation of qi, blood and phlegm.

虚痰 【xū tán】①泛指由于元气虚引起的痰证。②即寒痰。

Phlegm Syndrome of Deficiency Type (1) generally denoting phlegm syndrome due to deficiency of primordial qi. (2) cold phlegm syndrome.

虚陷 【xū xiàn】多见于有头疽收口期。因脾胃虚弱气血亏耗所致，症见疮口腐肉虽脱，但新肉不生，经久不敛，身有寒热，相当于脓毒血证。

虚邪 【xū xié】致病邪气的通称。因邪气往往乘虚而入侵人体，故名。

虚阳上浮 【xū yáng shàng fú】1、由于肾阳衰微，阴盛于下，致微弱的阳气浮越于上的病理。2、指精血亏损、阳无所附，浮越于上的病理。

虚胀 【xū zhàng】腹胀满而属虚证者。多因脾肾阳虚或肝肾阴虚所致。症见神疲纳呆、畏寒肢冷、舌淡脉细、或形体消瘦、面色黧黑、烦躁衄血、舌绛脉细。

Deficiency Type of Inward Penetration of Pyogenic Agent   a morbid condition seen in the healing stage of boils, caused by deficiency and weaked by poor growth of the granulation tissue in spite of sloughing off of the necrotic tissue and a delay in the wound healing, accompanied by fever and chills, which is equivalent to pyemia.

Debilitating Pathogenic Factors   a general term for pathogens, which usually invade the human body when it is debilitated.

Upward Floating of Asthenic Yang   (1) pathological changes marked by upward floating of asthenic yang due to declination of the kidney in the lower portion of the body. (2) referring to pathogenical changes marked by upward floating of yang due to consumption of essence and blood, the foundation upon which yang-qi depends in order to remain stable.

Distension of Deficiency Type   deficiency syndrome with abdominal distension and fullness, mostly due to deficiency of the spleen-yang and kidney-yang or deficiency of the liver-yin and kidney-yin, marked by mental fatigue, loss of appetite, aversion to cold, coldness of limbs, pale tongue, thready pulse, or emaciation, brown complexion, irritability, nosebleeds, deep redness of tongue proper, thready pulse.

虚者补其母 【xū zhě bǔ qí mǔ】运用五行相生和五脏母子关系的理论,治疗五脏的虚弱性疾病。如肾为肝母,治疗肝的虚证,除补肝外还要结合补肾。

Treating the Asthenia-Syndrome of the Child-Organ by means of Reinforcing the Mother-Organ a method of treating deficiency syndromes of five zang-organs by applying theory of generation in five elements, inter-promotions of five elements and the theory of relationship between mother organ and child organ in five zang-organs, for instance, in the case of deficient liver, is kidney as supposed to be mother of the liver, should be tonified in combination with the kidney.

虚者补之 【xū zhě bǔ zhī】(衰者补之)即属于正气虚衰的疾病,一般宜用补益的方法治疗。

Illness of Deficiency Type should be Treated by Tonifying Method illness that is attributable to deficiency and exhaustion of primordial qi generally advisable to be treated with tonifying method.

虚证 【xū zhèng】由于正气不足,抗邪能力低下,或各种生理功能衰退所产生的证候。临床可分阴虚、阳虚、气虚、血虚或阴阳两虚、气血两虚等。

Syndrome of Deficiency a morbid condition showing deficiency of healthy qi, lowered body resistance, and declining of function, it is classified clinically as yin—deficiency, yang—deficiency, qi—deficiency, blood-deficiency, or deficiency of both yin and yang, deficiency of both qi and blood.

虚坐努责 【xū zuò nǔ zé】指时时欲大便,但登厕努挣而少有粪便排出之症。比里急后重更甚。多因久痢伤及阴血所致。

Fruitless Defecation referring to frequent bowel movements but with each attempt in vain, more severe than tenesmus, which is often due to prolonged dysentery impairing yin-blood.

虚中夹实 【xū zhōng jiá shí】指虚弱的病体夹有实邪,但以虚为主的一种

Deficiency Complicated with Excess dominant deficiency syndromes

病理现象。

蓄血 【xù xuè】1、指外感热病，邪热入里与血相搏，而致瘀热蓄结于内的病证。症见小腹胀痛，甚则出现精神神经症状。2、多种瘀血证的总称。

蓄血发黄 【xù xuè fā huáng】多因瘀热内蓄，胆汁外溢所致。症见身黄、少腹硬、小便自利、其人如狂、脉沉结等。

宣痹通阳 【xuān bì tōng yáng】宣散痹阻、温通阳气的治法。通常用于治疗因阳气痹阻所致的病证。

宣肺 【xuān fèi】（宣白）宣通肺气的方法。适用于肺气不利。症见咳嗽、气喘、痰多等。

宣剂 【xuān jì】用宣开散郁药物组成，具有解除壅塞功效的方剂。

complicated with excess symptoms.

Syndrome of Blood Retention 1. a symptom complex of febrile disease of exopathy caused by accumulation of sludged blood in the interior as a result of an internal invasion of the pathogenic heat to combine with the blood, marked by distension and pain in the lower part of the abdomen, or mental disorders in severe cases (2) general term of multimorbid states of blood stasis.

Jaundice due to Accumulation of Stagnant Blood syndrome often caused by accumulation of stagnant heat and out-flow of bile, marked by sallow skin, hypogastric fullness, incontinence of urine, mania, deep and slow pulse, etc.

Activating Yang by Removing Obstruction of Qi and Blood Circulation a therapeutic method of clearing away obstruction, warming and promoting yang-qi, which is usually indicated for syndrome caused by obstruction of yang-qi.

Promoting the Dispersing Function of the Lung a therapeutic method of smoothing circulation of the lung-qi, indicated for functional disturbance of the lung-qi, manifested as cough, asthma, expectoration, etc.

Dispersing Prescription a prescription with composition of drugs that have dispersing action, indicated for removing stagnancy and obstruction.

宣肺化痰 【xuān fèi huà tán】化痰法之一。是治疗外感风寒痰多的方法。适用于风寒外束肺气不宣。症见咳嗽、痰多、鼻塞喉痒、舌苔薄白等。

宣可去壅 【xuān kě qù yōng】用宣散之药,去除壅郁之证。

宣通水道 【xuān tōng shuǐ dào】开肺气而利水湿的治法。适用于肺气不利水湿潴留。症见咳嗽气喘,或有发热恶寒浮肿在上半身和面部,小便不利、苔白、脉浮滑等。

痃癖 【xuán pǐ】是脐腹部或胁肋部患有癖块的泛称。因饮食不节,脾胃受伤,寒痰结聚,气血凝滞而致。常伴有消瘦、食少、疲乏等症状。

Ventilating the Lung and Resolving Phlegm one of the methods to resolve the phlegm, and treat affection which is caused by exopathogenic wind-cold, indicated for wind and cold restricting the lungs with the result of impaired circulation of lung qi, marked by cough with expecteration, stuffiness of nose, discomfort in the throat, thin and whitish coating on the tongue.

Dispersion Is Able To Remove Obstruction a therapeutic method for removing stagnancy and obstruction by using drugs that have dispersing action.

Promoting Diuresis by Activaton Dispersing Function of the Lung a therapeutic method of clearing the lung-qi and promoting diuresis indicated for disturbance of lung-qi and retention of dampness, marked by cough and asthma, complicated by fever and chill, edema in upper part of the body and in face, disturbance of urination with the amount scanty and colour deep yellow, whitish coating on the tongue, floating and slippery pulse.

Mass Beside Umbilicus a general name for the masses on the sides of umbilicus or hypochondrium, due to accumulaton of cold-phlegm and stagnacy of qi and blood as a result of impairment of the spleen and stomach which is related to improper diet, of-

旋耳疮 【xuán ěr chuāng】耳后折缝间皮肤渐红，久则流水、湿烂作痒，甚则折缝裂开如被刀割状。多由胆经、脾经湿热上蒸，或耳道流脓延及外耳所致。

Intertrigo Behind the Ear an infection of the skin behind the ear characterized by redness ulceration with discharge and itching sensation, even with the folding line splitting open as if it were cut with knife mostly caused by upward spreading of damp-heat in gall bladder meridian and spleen meridian, or purulent discharge from auditory meatus.

旋螺突起 【xuán luó tū qǐ】(螺盖翳) 黑珠高起如螺，色青白或带黑。类似角膜葡萄肿。

Staphyloma of Cornea cornea protruding just like a snail, whitish bluish, or dark colour, which is similar to staphyloma of cornea.

悬癖 【xuán pǐ】胁下有癖气如弦索状扛起，咳嗽或唾涎时则牵悬胁下而痛。常由悬饮证久延不愈所致。

Stringlike Mass in Hypochondriac Region mass at the right hypochondrium like a string manifested as hypochondrial pain on cough or swallow, often caused by prolonged fluid retention in the hypochondrium.

悬痈风 【xuán qí fēng】悬雍垂红肿，胀硬下垂，白膜裹满，下端尖头处生血泡，色红、舌伸缩不利，疼痛异常。因肝肾二经痰热火毒蕴结；过食辛辣厚味，肺胃积热上熏咽喉所致。

Hematoma on Uvula red, swelling, distending and hard uvula which is hanging down and coated with tunica, the redlish blood blister on the lower and of the uvula with extreme pain and disturbance of tongue movement, which is due to accumulation of phlegm-heat and fire-toxin in the meridians of both liver and kidney; or due to over-eating food with hot and pungent flavor resulting in accumulation of heat in the spleen and stomach upwardly stifling the throat.

悬饮 【xuán yǐn】因饮邪停留于胸胁

Pleural Effusion a morbid condi-

所致的饮证。症见咳唾胸胁引痛,转侧及呼吸时加重,多有恶寒发热,脉沉弦。类似渗出性胸膜炎。辨证分类:1、邪郁少阳证 2、饮停胸胁证 3、络脉不和证。

tion due to fluid retention in the hypochondrium, manifested by cough with pain of hypochondrium, which is worsened on turning round and breathing; mostly accompanied by chills, fever, deep and thready pulse. Types of differentiation 1. accumulation of pathogenic factors in shaoyang meridian 2. fluid retention in the hypochondrium 3. disharmony of collaterals and vessels.

悬痈 【xuán yōng】①生于任脉经会阴穴部位的痈,由湿热下注所致。常经久难愈久而成瘘。②指悬壅垂所生的痈肿。

Acute Pyogenic Infection of Perineum 1. an inflammatiory lesion at the point of perineum where ren meridian runs accross, resulting from lngering of noxious dampness, often lasting long course to fail to heal and consequently forming fistula; 2. referring to abscess of uvula.

悬壅垂 【xuán yōng chuí】(悬壅)悬于软腭中央的小块圆的、可摆动的组织。

Uvula a round and swaying issure which hangs in the centre of soft palate.

眩晕 【xuàn yūn】(眩冒、头眩、冒眩)指眼花头眩的证候。感受外邪及气血脏腑受伤,均可引起,但以风火、湿痰及心脾血虚,肾精不足等为最常见。

Vertigo dizziness and dimness of the eyesight, which may be brought about by invasion of exopathogens or impairment of qi and blood, zang and fu, but generally related to wind-fire, damp-phlegm, as well as blood-deficiency of the heart and spleen and insufficiency of kidney essence.

眩仆 【xuàn pū】指因眩晕而仆倒症状。

Falling due to Faint a symptom characterized by faint and falling.

穴位埋线疗法 【xué wèi mái xiàn liáo fǎ】用肠线埋于穴处的一种治疗方法。可用于治疗哮喘、溃疡病等。

Catgut Implantaton at Acupoint Therapy a therapy of imbedding catgut in the point for treating asthma, gastric and duodenal ulcer.

穴位封闭疗法 【xué wèi fēng bì liáo fǎ】用具有麻醉、镇静作用的药物注射入穴位的一种治疗方法。

穴位注射疗法 【xué wèi zhù shè liáo fǎ】将药液注射入穴位的一种治疗方法。

穴位刺激结扎疗法 【xué wèi cì jī jié zhā liáo fǎ】用器械刺激并结扎穴位的皮下组织的一种治疗方法。多用于治疗小儿麻痹后遗证。

血 【xuè】由饮食物的精华通过气化作用而成的一种物质,它循环运行于脉道以奉养全身。

血崩 【xuè bēng】指不在经期内突然阴道大量流血。多发于青春期及更年期妇女。常因血热、血虚、肝肾阴虚、血瘀等致冲任不固所引起。

血崩腹痛 【xuè bēng fù tòng】患血崩而兼见腹痛。血瘀者腹痛拒按,血块下后则痛减;血虚者腹隐痛而喜按。

Acupoint Block Therapy   a therapy of injecting anaesthetic into acupuncture points.

Acupoint Drug Injection Therapy   a therapy of injecting liquid medicine into the acupoint.

Point-Stimulation and Point-Suture Therapy   a therapy to apply mechanical stimulation to the patient and, then, to suture (the acupuncture) the hypodermis at the acupoint, often indicated for sequelea of Poliomyelitis.

Blood   a kind of material transformed from the essence of food produced through functional activity of qi, which circulates through the blood vessels and nourishes the body tissues.

Metrorrhagia   copious vaginal bleeding between menstural periods, gererally occuring in women at the time of adolescence and climacterium, it is often caused by blood-heat, blood-deficiency, deficiency of the liver-yin and kidney-yin, and blood stasis that altogether lead to weakness of the thoroughfare and conception vessels.

Metrorrhagia with Abdominal Pain   a syndrome of metrorrhagia complicated by abdominal pain, or abdominal tenderness in case of blood stasis that is relieved with the blood mass removed; predilection for pressure in case of abdominal vague pain with de-

血崩昏暗 【xuè bēng hūn àn】因血崩失血过多,心肝失养,出现头晕眼黑、突然昏倒不省人事的证候。

血痹 【xuè bì】 1、因气血虚弱邪入血分的痹证。由于当风睡卧或因劳汗出,风邪乘虚而入,使气血闭阻不通所致的病证。症见肢体不仁、肢节疼痛、脉微涩、尺脉小紧等。2、指风痹,游走无定处者。

血不归经 【xuè bù guī jīng】血液不按经脉运行而溢于脉外。临床多见于因气虚、气逆、血瘀、火热等原因引起的崩漏、吐血、便血、尿血及皮下出血等。

血不循经 【xuè bù xún jīng】即血不按经脉运行。见血不归经。

血不养筋 【xuè bù yǎng jīn】肝血不足而出现筋脉拘急或肢体麻木的病理,临床上可见于贫血及失血患者。

ficiency of the blood.

Faintness due to Metrorrhagia a syndrome characterized by dizziness and blurred vision, sudden faintness and loss of consciousness which are caused by failure to nourish the heart and liver as a result of over-bleeding.

Blood-Bi a morbid condition due to deficiency of qi and blood and invasion of pathogens into blood system, or due to obstruction of qi and blood as a result of invasion of wind-pathogens which is related to exposure to wind during sleeping or perspiration during work, with symptoms of numbness and joint pain, weak and hesitant pulse with palpation at curegionbit small and tight.

(2) wind-bi with chief manifestations of migratory pain of the limbs.

Escape of Blood from Vessels and Meridians the pathological manifestations in which the blood does not circulate in the blood vessels but escapes out of them, clinically seen in such syndromes as metrorrhagia and metrostaxis, hematemesis, hemafecia, hematuria and subcutaneours hemorrhage which are due to qi-deficiency, reversed flow of qi, stagnancy of blood, fire-heat, etc.

Failure of Blood to Circulate in the Vessels

Failure of Blood to Nourish Tendon and Muscle a pathogenic manifestation characterized by spasm of the tendons and muscle becsuse of insufficiency of the liver-blood, clinically often seen in patients with anemia and blood loss.

血分热毒 【xuè fèn rè dú】1、热邪深陷血分的病证。症见高热神昏、皮肤斑疹、吐血、便血、舌质深绛及紫绛等。2、指外科某些急性、多发性化脓性感染伴有高热、神昏、舌质红绛等症。

Noxious Heat in the Blood System 1. invasion of pathogenc heat into the blood system marked by high fever, coma, skin eruption, hematemesis, hemafecia, dark red or maroon tongue proper. 2. referring to some surgical acute, multiple and purulent infections accompanied by high fever, coma, red and maroon tongue proper.

血分证 【xuè fèn zhèng】热病最深重的阶段。多从营分传来,以伤阴、动风、动血、耗血为特征。症见高热、夜间热甚、神昏谵语、抽搐、出血、斑疹、舌深紫或绛、脉细数等。

Syndrome of the Xue Fen (Blood System) a critial stage of epidemic febrile disease usually transmitted from the nutrient (ying) system, characterized by impairment of yin, stirring up of the wind and bleeding, with symptoms of high fever which is aggravated at night, coma, delirium, convulsion, hematemesis, dark red or maroon tongue, thready and fast pulse.

血分瘀热 【xuè fèn yú rè】1、指热邪瘀积于血分。2、瘀血滞留,郁而化热或热邪深陷营血分,阻滞血络而夹瘀,均可致热互结。

Pathogenic Heat Accumulated in the Xue Fen (Blood System) 1. referring pathogenic heat accumulating in the blood system. 2. protracted blood stasis, stagnation converted into heat or deep peneptration pathogenic factor into nutrious (ying) and blood systems, blockage of blood in collaterals mixed with stagnancy responsible for stagnation of heat and blood stasis.

血风疮 【xuè fēng chuāng】由肝经血

Itching Eruptions due to Wind-Heat in

热,脾经湿热,肺经风热交感所致而成的皮肤病。症见全身皮疹如粟米状,瘙痒抓破时流水,逐渐蔓延成片,病久瘙痒倍增,且伴有心烦失眠、咽干不渴、大便燥结等。

血疳疮 【xuè gān chuāng】由风热闭塞腠理而成。皮肤出疹如粟,或红斑成片,色暗红如紫疥,瘙痒脱屑,甚则延及全身。即玫瑰糠疹。

血攻痔 【xuè gōng zhì】即出血较多的内痔。

血蛊 【xuè gǔ】(血鼓,血臌)本病多因气血瘀滞,影响水湿运化所致。症见腹部膨大、腹壁静脉怒张、大便色黑、小便短赤,或见衄血、吐血、脉芤涩等。可见于门脉性肝硬变、血吸虫性肝硬变等病。

血海 【xuè hǎi】1、指冲脉。四海之一。是十二经脉所汇聚的地方。2、指肝脏。3、经穴名之一。

Blood a kind of skin disease due to blood-heat in liver meridian, dampheat in spleen meridian and wind-heat in lung meridian marked by general skin eruption like grain of rice, watery discharge with scratching gradually spreading all over the skin of the body, rapidly growing itching sensation during long course, accompanied by irritability, isomnia, dry throat without thirst, dry stools.

Pityriasis Rosea caused by blockage of texture and interspace by pathogenic wind-heat, with symptoms of skin eruption, erythema in spatches with colour dark red just like purpura, itching sensation with desqamation, spreading over the skin all over the body, that is pityriasis rosea.

Internal Hemorrhoids with massive bleeding

Tymponitis due to Blood Stasis a morbid condition gererally caused by stagnation of qi and blood interrupting the transportation of water in the body, marked by abdominal distention, varicosis, melena, scanty and dark urine, or epistaxis, hematemesis, hesitant pulse, usually seen in protal cirrhosis or schistosomial cirrhosis of the liver.

Reservoir of Blood 1. referring to thoroughfare vessel, one of the four reservoirs, the crossing where the twelve merdians all run through.

2. referring to the liver.　3. one of acupoints.

血寒经行后期　【xuè hán jīng xíng hòu qī】经行后期证型之一，多因寒邪袭入胞宫，血为寒凝所致。症见月经周期错后、经量减少、夹有瘀块、小腹冷痛、得热经行通畅等。

Retarded Menstruation due to Blood-Cold　delayed menstruation due to attack of pathogenic cold in the uterus and stagnancy of boold because of cold, marked by delayed menstruation, reduction of the amount of menstrual flow, complicated by stagnated masses, cold pain in lower part of abdomen, normal menstrual flow on hot compress.

血寒月经过少　【xuè hán yuè jīng guò shǎo】经来血量过少、色淡质稀、伴有形寒畏冷、小腹冷痛、喜得温热等。多因素体阳虚，阴寒内行，化气生血功能不足，冲任血少所致。

Hypomenorrhea due to Blood-Cold　abnormal scanty menstruation, thin blood with light colour, accompanied by chill and cold in extremities, aversion to cold, cold-pain in lower abdomen, and preference for warmth, which is usually due to general debility and deficiency of yang, internal production of yin-cold, insufficiency in metabolic functions and in promoting generation of blood, insufficient blood in TV (thoroughfare vessel) and CV (conception vessel).

血汗　【xuè hàn】（红汗）指汗出色淡红如血。

Hematohidrosis　referring to perspiration which is light red just like blood.

血会　【xuè huì】八会之一。即膈俞穴，血的精华均会于此。

Influential Point to Blood　one of the eight influential point, i. e. acupoint geshu (B17) where essence of blood converges.

血积　【xuè jī】由气逆血郁，凝结成积，或外伤瘀血内蓄所致的一种病证。症见面色萎黄，脘腹或胁肋部有肿块不移、时觉疼痛、便秘、黑便等。

Accumulation of Extravasted Blood　a morbid condition resulting from reversed flow of qi and stagnancy of blood or trauma with blood stasis

血箭 【xuè jiàn】皮肤出现红斑及毛孔出血,甚至血射如箭的一种病证。多由心经火盛、迫血妄行所致。

血箭痔 【xuè jiàn zhì】伴有大量出血的内痔。

血瘕 【xuè jiǎ】少腹有积气包块、急痛、阴道内有冷感或见背痛、腰痛的一种病证。多因月经期间邪气与瘀血结聚,阻于经络而成。

血厥 【xuè jué】1、指因失血过多,暴怒气逆,血郁于上而引起的昏厥重证。2、参见郁冒条。

血枯经闭 【xuè kū jīng bì】停经三个月以上,伴面色㿠白无华、消瘦、饮食减少或午后潮热、口干、大便干结、尿黄等的一种病证。本病多因阴血亏损,血海空虚,或热邪灼烁阴液,冲任空虚所致。

marked by withered and yellowish complexion, epigastric and hypochondric mass. which is unmovable and painful sometimes, constipation, dark stools.

Hematohidrosis presence of erythema on the skin and bleeding from sweat pore like a shooting arrow, usually caused by excessive fire in the heart-meridian leading to the blood flowing out of the vessels.

Internal Hemorrhoids with Massive Bleeding internal hemorrhoids accompanied by massive bleeding.

Blood Jia a morbid condition marked by accumulated qi and masses in the hypogastrium accompanied with sharp pain, cold sensation in vagina, or backache and lumbago, usually due to accumulation of pathogenic qi and blood stasis during menstruation and subsequent blockage of meridians and collaterals.

Syncope due to Excessive Bleeding a severe syndrome of faintness caused by over-bleeding, or converted flow of qi related to violent anger, ascending blood stagnancy. (2) see list of oppressive feeling and dizziness.

Amenorrhea due to Blood Depletion a morbid condition happening three months later after amenorrhea, accompanied by pale and withered complexion, emaciation, poor appetite, or afternoon fever, dry mouth, dry stools, yellowish urine, which is generally caused by impairment of yin-blood, deficiency of sea of blood, or by pathogenic heat burning yin-fluid and deficiency of TV and CV.

血亏经闭 【xuè kuī jīng bì】阴血亏损所致的闭经。多因久病失血而致阴虚血亏，冲任空虚引起。症见月经日渐减少，渐致停闭，且多伴面色萎黄、纳呆、形体消瘦、皮肤干燥等。

Amenorrhea due to Deficiency of Blood amenorrhea resulting from deficiency and impairment of yin-blood, involving causes such chronic course with loss of blood responsible for deficiency of yin and blood, and hollow and deficiency of TV and CV, manifested as progressive scanty menstruation coming to its stand, often accompanied by withered complexion, loss of appetite, emaciation, dryness of skin, etc.

血疬 【xuè lì】瘰疬的一种，即瘰疬核块红肿疼痛者。

Inflamed Scrofula one kind of scrofulae, i. e. lymphadenitis scrofula which is red, swelling and painful.

血痢 【xuè lì】（赤痢）因热毒盛于血分伤及肠络所致的下痢。实证可见泻下血色鲜红、腹痛、里急后重、舌苔黄腻、脉滑数有力等。虚证可见泻下血色晦暗，面色苍白，脉弱。

Dysentery with Blood Stool a kind of dysentery caused by excessiveness of heat-toxin in blood system impairing intestine-collateral, in excess syndrome manifested as bright red colour of stool, abdominal pain, tenesmus, yellowish and greasy coating on the tongue, slipery, fast and forceful pulse, while in deficiency syndrome dark grey colour of blood stool, withered and yellowish complexion, weak pulse.

血淋 【xuè lín】淋证之一。主症为小便涩痛有血。可因血虚、血冷、血热、血瘀所致。

Stranguria Complicated by Hematuria one of the stranguria with main symptoms of painful and dribbling urination with bloody urine, often due to blood-deficiency, blood-cold, blood-

血瘤 【xuè liú】因血结气滞,经络不通,复受外邪所搏而致。瘤体皮色紫红,软硬间杂,隐约若有红丝缠绕,偶有擦破则血流不止、常发于唇、颈、四肢。

血轮 【xuè lún】即眼眦,配属于心。它的病变与心和小肠有关。

血尿 【xuè niào】血样尿或尿中有凝血块,但无尿痛。多因肾阴不足,心经火旺,下移小肠;或脾肾两亏,血失统摄所致。

血热疮 【xuè rè chuāng】由风热闭塞腠理而成。皮疹呈丘疹状,剧痒。类似玫瑰糠疹。

血热滑胎 【xuè rè huá tāi】孕妇素体阳盛,有滑胎病史,怀孕后因热伏冲任,迫血妄行,损伤胎元而引起的习惯性流产。症见小腹作痛、心烦不宁、口渴喜凉饮,甚则阴道流血,以致胎动欲坠。

heat, blood stasis.

Angioma condition due to stagnation of blood and obstruction of qi resulting in blockage of meridians and collaterals and invasion by exopathogen, with its outlayer purple and red in colour, mixture of softness and firmness in proper, faintly visible red thread twining aruond, persistant bleeding from broken point, often occuring on lip, neck and four extremities.

Blood Wheel orbiculus attributable to the heart, whose pathogenic changes are related to the heart and small intestine.

Hematuria bloody urine or bloody masses in urine but without urodynia, often caused ny insufficiency of kidney-yin and hyperactivity of fire in the heart meridian transfering downward to the small intestine; or by deficiency of both spleen and kidney, which results in their failure to control the blood.

Sore due to Blood-Heat a skin disease due to blockage of texture and interspace by wind-heat, papulae on the affected part with severe itching, which is similar to pityriasis rosea.

Habitual Abortion due to Blood-Heat habitual abortion occuring in pregnant woman who has the history of habitual abortion with hyperactivity of yang in the body, and whose fetus is impaired after pregnance because of accumulation of heat in the TV and CV with bleeding, marked by pain in the lower abdomen, restlessness, thirst with fondness of cool drink, even bleeding from the vagina to cause continuous moving of the fetus with inclination of abortion.

血热月经过多【xuè rè yuè jīng guò duō】月经周期正常但经来时间延长,经量增多。多因血热内扰,热伤冲任、迫血妄行所致。属实热者,血色深红或紫,稠粘或有臭秽气味,面红口干,烦燥不安;虚弱者,多有午后手足心热、舌红、苔少。

Menorrhagia due to Blood-Heat regular intervals between menstruation circles but prolonged bleeding time and profuse menstruation, which is usually caused by internal interference of blood-heat impairing TV and CV with the result of blood disorder, which is attributable to excess heat syndrome with symptoms of dark red or purple colour, thick and sticky quality, sometimes accompanied with fish-stench, flushed face and dry mouth, irritability and restlessness; in the case of weakness which is often with hot sensation in palms and soles, red tongue with scanty coating.

血疝【xuè shàn】 1、指小腹内瘀血结痛。症见腹硬满有形、疼痛、甚或黑便、月经不调。2、指阴囊外伤后形成的血肿。3、在少腹两旁脓血夹杂的疝证。

Hernial Pain due to Blood Stasis
1. referring to swelling and pain in the lower abdomen due to accuumulation of stagnant blood, marked by formative fullness and firmness, pain, even dark stool, disorder of menstruation.   2. referring to hematoma of the scrotum caused by trauma.
3. referring to bloody and purulent hernial on both sides of the lower abdomen.

血室【xuè shì】1、肝脏。2、子宫。3、冲脉。

Blood Room   1. the liver   2. the uterus   3. the thoroughfare vessel

血栓痔 【xuè shuān zhì】（葡萄痔）是由内热血燥，或便时用力过度，或强力负重，以致损伤血络，积瘀而成。症见肛门左右如乳头突出、色青紫、剧痛，亦有化脓破溃成漏者。

血随气陷 【xuè suí qì xiàn】气虚下陷导致出血的病理。症见精神不振、肢体倦怠、出血量多或连续不断、面色苍白、舌淡、脉沉细无力等。多见于功能性子宫出血及某些便血患者。

血脱 【xuè tuō】（脱血）指因禀赋不足，或思虑、劳倦、房室、酒食所伤，或慢性出血后，真阴亏损，血海空虚所致的一种病证。症见面白无华、头晕目花、四肢清冷、脉空虚等。

血为气母 【xuè wèi qì mǔ】说明气血之间的关系。血是气的物质基础，气的正常功能有赖于血的滋养。

血心痛 【xuè xīn tòng】（死血心痛、

(TV).

Thrombotic Hemorrhoid impairment of superficial venules with accumulation of extravasted blood due to internal heat and dry blood, or overexertion during bowel movement, or bearing a heavy load with over-exertion, marked by breast-like protuberance around anal region whose colour is dark purple, accompanied with severe pain, even development of fistula after disbrosis forms.

Bleeding Resulting from Exhaustion of Qi pathogenical changes of profuse or incessant bleeding due to deficiency and sinking of qi, marked by listlessness, lassitude, profuse or incessant bleeding, pale complexion, pale tongue, sunken, feeble and thready pulse, usually seen in patients with functional uterine bleeding and hemafecia.

Blood Prostration a morbid condition marked by pale complexion, vertigo, cold limbs, feeble pulse caused by impairment of genuine yin and exhaustion of blood as a result of anxiety and worry, intemperance in sexual life, improper diet or chronic bleeding.

Blood Being Mother of Qi denoting the relationship between qi and blood, blood is the material basis of qi while the normal function of qi is dependent on the nourishment of blood.

Epigastric Pain due to Blood Stasis

蓄血心痛）由于瘀血引起的胃脘痛。多因跌扑损伤；或嗜好热酒、热食，瘀血留于胃中所致。

血虚 【xuè xū】指血分亏损而出现虚弱症状的病理。常由于失血过多、思虑过度、寄生虫或脏腑虚损、不能化生精微所致。临床表现为面白、唇色淡白、头晕眼花、心悸、失眠、手足发麻、脉细无力等症。

血虚痹 【xuè xū bì】血虚不能濡养四肢或兼感风寒湿邪所致的痹证。症见皮肤麻木不仁、活动时肢节疼痛、多见芤脉。

血虚不孕 【xuè xū bù yùn】由于素体脾胃虚弱，或久病，失血伤阴，致阴血不足，冲任空虚，不能养精成孕所引起的不孕证。常伴有身体虚弱、面色萎黄、疲乏无力等症。

epigastric pain resulting from blood stasis, usually caused by traumatic injury, or blood stagnated in the stomach as a result of addiction for hot alcohol or hot food.

Deficiency of Blood a pathological changes showing weakness with impairment of (xuefen) blood system, usually caused by massive bleeding over-anxiety, parasitic diseases or damage of the internal organs resulting in failure to produce vital essence, clinically characterized by pale complexion, pale lips, giddiness, palpitation, insomnia, numbness of the extremities, thready and feeble pulse.

Arthropathy due to Deficiency of Blood a morbid condition due to deficiency of blood responsible for the failure to nourish the limbs or complicated by attack of pathogenic wind, cold or dampness, marked by numbness, joint pain on moving the limbs, usually accompanied by hollow pulse.

Sterility due to Deficiency of Blood a sterility syndrome in which insuficiency yin-blood, hollowness of TV and CV result in the failure to nourish vital essence and pregnancy as a result of deficiency and weakness of the spleen and stomach, or loss of blood and impairment of yin related to chronic disease, often accompanied by general debility, withhered and yellowish complexion, lassitude and weakness.

血虚耳聋 【xuè xū ěr lóng】由肝肾精血亏损，耳窍失养引起的耳聋。症见腰膝酸软、耳鸣盗汗、唇红颧赤、头晕目眩、耳聋渐甚。

Deafness due to Deficiency of Blood a morbid state caused by malnourishment of the ear due to impairment of essence and blood in the liver and kidney, manifested as soreness and weakness of the loins and legs, tinitus, night sweat, red lips and flushed cheek, blurred vision, progressive deafness.

血虚发热 【xuè xū fā rè】血虚而致的一种虚热。多由失血后阴血亏虚，阴阳失调所致。症见肌热面红、燥渴、甚则烦躁、睡卧不安、脉洪大而虚、重按无力等。

Fever due to Deficiency of Blood a deficient fever caused by deficiency of blood, as a result of loss of blood leading to deficiency of yin-blood and disorders of yin and yang with symptoms of flushed face, thirst or even restlessness, insomnia, full but feeble pulse which is weaken by palpation with force.

血虚腹痛 【xuè xū fù tòng】因失血过多或思虑过度，耗伤阴血，经脉涩滞所致的腹痛。症见腹部微痛、痛无定处、饥劳则痛甚、面色萎黄、疲乏无力、脉细涩或细数等。

Abdominal Pain due to Deficiency of Blood abdominal pain due to exhaustion and impairment of yin-blood, obstruction and stagnancy in the meridians as a result of massive bleeding or over anxiety, marked by slight pain in the abdomen which is wandering and become aggravated on anger and exertion, withered and yellowish complexion, fatigue and weakness, thready and hesitant or thready and fast pulse.

血虚滑胎 【xuè xū huá tāi】滑胎证型之一，孕妇平素血虚，有滑胎病史，怀孕后阴血益虚，胎失滋养，症见面色淡黄、神疲乏力、或有浮肿、腰酸腹痛，甚则阴道流血、胎动欲坠。

Threatened Abortion due to Deficiency of Blood one of the abortion syndromes, occuring in pregnant women in a state of blood-deficiency, with a history of abortion, and malnourishment of embryo after pregnancy as a result of deficiency of yin-blood, marked by yellowish complexion, lassitude and fatigue, or edema, soreness in the loins and pain in the abdomen, even vaginal bleeding, threatening abortion.

血虚经行后期 【xuè xū jīng xíng hòu qī】因血虚冲任不足,血海不充,胞宫不能按时满溢所致的一种月经病。症见月经周期延后、经量减少、色淡质稀,伴面色萎黄、头晕心悸、舌质淡、脉细等。

Delayed Menstruation due to Deficiency of Blood a morbid sate marked by delayed circle of menstruation, which is scanty in amount, pale in colour and thin in quality, accompanied with withered and yellowish complexion, dizziness and palpitation, pale coating on the tongue, thready pulse, resulting from insufficiency of TV and CV, insufficiency of blood sea with the result of irregular overflowing of blood in uterus.

血虚生风 【xuè xū shēng fēng】由于失血、贫血、致使血不养筋的病理。症见眩晕、抽搐、震颤等。

Endopathic Wind due to Blood Deficiency a pathological change caused by failure of blood to nourish tendens and muscles resulting from impairment of blood and anemia, marked by blurred vision, convulsion, tremor.

血虚头痛 【xuè xū tóu tòng】由血虚不能上荣所致的头痛。症见眉尖及头抽痛、头隐隐作痛、头晕眼花、面色㿠白、易惊、心悸等。

Headache due to Deficiency of Blood a condition resulting from deficiency of blood with the result of difficulty of blood to flow upward, marked by drawing pain on eyebrow or forehead, vague pain in the head, dizziness and blurred vision, pallar, irritability, palpitation.

血虚手脚麻木 【xuè xū shǒu jiǎo má mù】指因血虚,四肢失去营血的滋养而引起的麻木、不痛痒的症状。

Numbness of Limbs due to Deficiency of Blood a symptom showing numbness and painlessness due to

血虚心悸 【xuè xū xīn jì】由心血不足，心失所养所致。症见心悸，面色不华、唇与指甲苍白、四肢无力、眩晕失眠、舌质淡、脉细弱等。

血虚痿 【xuè xū wěi】由产后或失血，血虚不能养筋所致的痿证。症见手足痿弱无力、运动障碍，伴有面色萎黄、脉多细弱。

血虚眩晕 【xuè xū xuàn yūn】由阴血亏损所致的眩晕。多因失血、热病灼伤营血、或心脾两虚等引起。眩晕伴有五心烦热、不寐盗汗、形体消瘦、舌质红、脉细者，属阴虚；如伴见面色㿠白、神疲乏力、心悸纳少者，属心脾两虚。

血虚腰痛 【xuè xū yāo tòng】腰痛的一种。多因失血过多及素患血虚，筋脉失养所致。

failure of nourishment by blood.

Palpitation due to Deficiency of Blood a condition marked by palpitation, dim complexion, pale lips and nails, weakness of extremities, blurred vision, insomnia, pale coating on the tongue, thready and feeble pulse, resulting from insufficiency of heart blood with the heart suffering from malnourishment.

Flaccidity of Limbs due to Deficiency of Blood a postpartum syndrome result of deficiency of blood related to impairment of blood, manifested as weak extremities, difficulty of movement, accompanied by withered and yellowish complexion, thready and feeble pulse.

Dizziness due to Deficiency of Blood a morbid condition of consumption of yin-blood, usually related to impairment of blood, febrile disease burning ying-blood, or deficiency of both heart and spleen. in case that pertains to yin deficiency accompanied by dysphoria with feverish sensation in the chest, palms and soles, night sweat, emaciation, red fur on the tongue, thready pulse, in case that pertains to deficiency of both heart and spleen with pallor, fatigue and weakness, palpitation, poor appetite.

Lumbage due to Deficiency of Blood one kind of lumbago, usually caused by over bleeding, or bodily deficiency of blood with the result of malnourishment of tenden and meridians.

血虚月经过少 【xuè xū yuè jīng guò shǎo】因素体虚弱或久病阴血亏损，或脾胃损伤，生化之源不足，致血海不充引起的月经过少。症见月经量过少、色淡红，伴有面色萎黄、头晕心悸、小腹隐痛等。

Hypomenorrhea due to Deficiency of Blood a morbid state of scanty menstruation due to insufficiency of blood, resulting from general weakness or impairment of yin-blood related to chronic disease, or damage of the spleen and stomach, insufficiency of the resource of growth and development, marked by scanty menstruation which is light red in colour, accompanied by withered and yellowish complexion, dizziness and palpitation, vague pain in the lower abdomen.

血虚自汗 【xuè xū zì hàn】因血虚引起的自汗证。多由血虚气弱，肌表不固所致。

Spontaneous Sweating due to Deficiency of Blood spontaneous sweating syndrome caused by deficiency of blood, resulting from deficiency of blood and weakness of qi with failure to strengthen superficial resistance.

血瘿 【xuè yīng】多因肝火暴盛，逼血沸腾，复被外邪所搏而致，症见颈生瘿块，皮色紫红，上有交叉露现的赤脉红丝。相当于颈部血管瘤。

Hemangioma of the Neck boiling blood forced by violently predominant liver-fire, and attacked by exopathogenic factor, manifested as the thryroid mass which is purple and red in colour, complexed with interlacing blood vessels visible in the overlying skin, equivalent to cervical hemangioma.

血瘀 【xuè yū】血流瘀滞或离经之血凝结不化的病证。多因气滞、气虚、血寒、血热或跌打损伤所致。

Blood Stasis a morbid state of sluggish flow of blood or stagnancy of blood out of vessels, usually caused by stagnancy of qi, deficiency of qi, blood-cold, blood-heat, or trauma.

血瘀崩漏 【xuè yū bēng lòu】因瘀血

Metrorrhagia due to Blood Stasis

停滞引起的子宫出血不止。多因瘀血不去，新血不得归经引起。症见阴道流血、淋沥不止，或突然大量流血、色紫黑、有血块、下腹部疼痛拒按、血块下后痛减等。

profuse uterine bleeding due to accumulation of blood stasis in uterus, usually caused by retention of blood stasis in the uterus follwed by escape of fresh blood from vessels, with such symptoms as uterine bleeding, metrostaxis, or sudden profuse bleeding with its color purple and dark complicated with bloody masses, abdominal pain and tenderness which can be relieved after bloody masses are removed.

血瘀经行后期 【xuè yū jīng xíng hòu qī】因气滞寒凝瘀血内阻冲任，血行不畅，经行不得按时下达所引起的一种月经病。症见经期错后、经量涩少、血色紫黯夹有血块、小腹胀痛拒按、血块去后则感舒适。

Retarded Menstruation due to Blood Stasis a morbid state resulting from blockage of blood-flow and irregular menstuation circle which are involved in stagnancy of qi and accumulation of cold, internal obstruction of TV and CV by blood stasis, marked by delayed menstruation, which is scanty in amount, purple and dark in color, mixed with bloody masses, abdominal distention and tenderness which can be relieved as bloody masses removed.

血瘀不孕 【xuè xū bù yùn】指婚后育龄妇女三年以上不受孕伴有月经错后、痛经、经行涩滞不畅血块多等。多因肝郁气滞，瘀血内阻冲任胞宫，不能摄精受孕所致。

Sterility due to Blood Stasis referring to women who are not pregnant for over three years after marrige, accompanied by delayed menstruation, abdominal pain during mensturation, impeded menstruation flow, profuse bloody masses, usually caused by stagnancy of the liver leading to stagnancy of qi flow, blood stasis obstructing internally TV and CV and fetus, which are responsible for dis-

血瘀痛经 【xuè yū tòng jīng】经前或经行时小腹刺痛拒按的病证。多因瘀血内阻,冲任胞脉血行不畅血滞胞中所致。症见经来涩滞不畅夹有瘀块,血块下后经来通畅,腹痛可缓解。

Dysmenorrihea due to Blood Stasis a morbid state of stabbing pain and tenderness in the lower abdomen prior to or during menstruation, usually caused by internal obstruction of blood stasis, blocked flow of blood in TV and CV and in uterus leading to stagnancy of blood in uterus, marked by impeded menstruation flow with bloody masses, smooth flow of blood after bloody masses are discharged, and subsequent relieving of abdominal pain.

血瘀痿 【xuè yū wěi】由产后恶露未尽,瘀血流于腰膝,或跌扑损伤,瘀血不消所致的痿证。症见四肢痿软、不能运动、疼痛、脉涩等。

Flaccidity of Limbs due to Blood Stasis a syndrome of flaccidity of limbs due to prolonged postpartum lochia, blood stasis reaching lumbago and kness, or traumatic injury with persistant blood stasis, marked by soreness and weakness of limbs, disability of movement, pain, hesitant pulse.

血证 【xuè zhèng】指各种出血性病证。包括呕血、吐血、咳血、咯血、鼻衄、肌衄、舌衄、尿血、便血等。

Bleeding Syndrome blood trouble referring to various bleeding syndromes, including hematemesis, hemoptysis, bleeding from muscle, nose and tongue, hematuria, hemafecia, etc.

血痔 【xuè zhì】是指便血明显的内痔。

Bleeding Internal Hemorrhoids referring to internal hemorrhoids with evident hemafecia.

血痣 【xuè zhì】多为先天性或肝经怒火郁结而成。好发于面、颈、躯干等处。初起痣色鲜红或呈紫红,境界分明,渐大如豆,高出皮肤,表面光滑,触破时流鲜血。

Vascular Nevus usually congenital defect or caused by accumulation of fire in liver-meridian, inclined to occur on the face, neck, trunk, which is bright red or maroon in color, well

血滞腹痛 【xuè zhì fù tòng】(瘀血腹痛) 多因七情所伤，肝失条达，以致气血郁滞所致。症见腹痛，痛处固定，触痛拒按，或腹痛经久不愈、舌质紫暗、脉濇等。可见于胰腺炎、肠粘连、宫外孕等疾病。

Abdominal Pain due to Blood Stasis a morbid condition due to impairment of the seven emotions, with disregulation of the liver leading to stagnancy of qi and blood, manifested as abdominal pain which is fixed and tender; or abdominal pain which is persistant and chronic, maroon coating on the tongue, hesitant pulse, often seen in such disease as pancreatits, intestinal adhesion, ectopic pregnancy, etc.

血滞经闭 【xuè zhì jīng bì】因情志不畅，气郁血滞，冲任阻闭，经血不能下达胞宫所致的闭经。症见面色紫暗、下腹疼痛拒按，或痛连两肋。

Amenorrhea due to Blood Stasis a morbid condition caused by emotional troubles, stagnancy of qi and blood, blockage of TV and CV which are responsible for absence of blood in the uterus, manifested as dark purple complexion, abdominal pain and tenderness, or pain spreading to both ribs.

血肿 【xuè zhǒng】指水肿因于血瘀为主者，多因瘀血留滞，水湿不化所致的浮肿。症见四肢浮肿、皮肉间有红丝血痕，或妇女先停经后见全身水肿、小腹胀痛拒按、小便清长等。

Edema due to Blood Stasis usually referring to cases caused by blood stasis resulting from stagnancy of blood stasis and accumulation of water-dampness, marked by edema in the extremities, red threat-like bloody trace seen inside, or general edema in women after menstruation, abdominal distension, pain and tenderness, polyuria with watery urine, etc.

循经传 【xún jīng chuán】指外感热病顺六经的次序传变，一般是由表入

Orderly Transmission of the Disease transmission of a disease due to ex-

里，由阳及阴。

熏蒸 【xūn zhēng】 利用药物煮沸后产生的蒸汽或药物燃烧时产生的烟以薰蒸肌体的方法，用于治疗关节肿痛活动障碍或某些皮肤病等。

压垫 【yā diàn】 在骨折复位后，辅助夹板作外固定的用具。为了使夹板更适合肢体外形及固定需要，可用纸、棉花、纱布等制成各种不同形式的压垫，如平垫、塔形垫、梯形垫、分骨垫等。

牙 【yá】 是埋于颌部的骨质构造，为咀嚼食物的器官。牙的生长及病变常与肾的功能有关。

牙疔 【yá dīng】 位于牙龈的疔疮。

牙疳 【yá gān】 表现为齿龈红肿疼痛，糜烂而流出腐臭血水的一种病证。

牙痛 【yá tòng】 （齿痛）多因龋齿所致，也有因风火、风寒、虚火所引起。

牙龈 【yá yín】 指牙床周围组织，分

opathogens from one meridian to another, generally from the superficies into the interior, from yang into yin.

Fumigation and Steaming a therapeutic method of using the steam of hot decoction (vapour of steaming drug) or the smoke of burning drug to heat the body, indicated for swelling and painful joints with difficulty in moving or some skin disease.

Pressure Pad a stool used as assistant of splints for the immobilization after reduction of fracture in order to make splints more suitable for the bodily external form and for the fixation of fractrue, pads made of paper, cotton and gauze can be used in different ways such as pressure pad, flat pad, tower-shaped pad, ladder-shaped pad, bone-seperating pad, etc.

Tooth Substance of bone imbedded in the jaw, and organ for chewing food, the growth and pathological changes often related to the function of the kiney.

Pustule of the Gum pustule occuring on the gum.

Ulcerative Gingivitis a morbid syndrome marked by painful swelling of the gum, resulting in ulceration with stinking discharge of bloody fluid.

Toothache usually caused by dental caries, sometimes caused by wind-fire, wind-cold and asthenia-fire.

Gum referring to the tissue around

上龈、下龈。胃、大肠经分别布于上下牙龈,故牙龈的病变常与胃和大肠有关。

牙宣 【yá xuān】牙龈日渐萎缩,牙根宣露,并伴有牙血、溢脓的一种病证。多因胃经积热与风寒之邪相搏,热不得宣而致,可见于慢性牙周炎。

牙痈 【yá yōng】指因阳明胃经火毒郁而不宣,上攻于牙龈所致的病证。症见齿龈红肿疼痛,甚则肿连腮颊或发寒热、便秘等。

咽 【yān】(咽嗌)鼻咽部、口咽部和喉咽部。通过咽部、鼻腔和喉连接,口腔与食道连接。

咽喉 【yān hóu】1、指口咽部。2、咽和喉的总称。

咽门 【yān mén】即咽之入门,下连食道和气管。

盐哮 【yán xiāo】指食过多咸味饮食引起的哮证。由饮食酸咸太过,痰湿结聚,一遇风寒,则气郁痰壅而发。

dental bed, classified as upper gum and lower gum, over which distribute the meridians of the stomach and large intestine which therefore are connected with the pathological changes of gums.

Gingival Atrophy　　a condition in which the gum becomes astrophic, resulting in exposure of the teeth root with frequent ooze of bloody fluid or pus, usually cuased by accumulated heat in the stomach meridian fighting pathogenic wind-cold with the result of failure to relieve heat stagnancy, seen in chronic periodontitis.

Toothache　　a morbid state in which stagnancy of fire-toxins in the stomach of Yangming meridian attacks upwardly the gums, manifested as painful and swollen gums, even involving cheeks, or with chill and fever, constipation, etc.

Pharynx　　including nasal pharynx, oral pharynx and laryngeal pharynx, through pharynx nasal cavity connecting with laryngeal, oral cavity with esophagus.

Throat　　1. referring to oral pharynx 2. collective term for both pharynx and larynx.

Laryngopharynx　　referring to the door of pharynx, joining downwardly with esophagus an trachea.

Salt Asthma　　asthma induced by overeating salty food, resulting from too much intake off sour and salty foods leading to accumulation of phlegm-dampness which gives rise to stagnancy of qi and accumulation of phlegm on exposure to wind-cold.

颜 【yán】1、指面部正中部分。2、指两眉之间的部位。3、指额部中央部分。

Face 1. referring to central part of the face. 2. referring to position between eyebrown. 3. referring to central part in the forehead.

眼 【yǎn】五官之一,为肝之窍。眼的功能与全身脏腑经络的功能有关。而与肝的关系尤为密切,肝的病变可以反映在眼上,眼的疾病常从肝论治。

Eye specific body opening of the liver, the function of the eye is related to the function of meridian and collaterals in zang and fu organs all over the body, especially to the liver. The pathological changes in the liver can be reflected from the eye while eye disease can be analysed an differentiated from the liver.

眼系 【yǎn xì】眼球内连于脑的脉络。相当于视神经及有关的脉管。

Ocular Connections the meridian and collateral connecting the eyeball with the brain, equal to ocular nerves or related meridian and vessel.

眼胞痰核 【yǎn bāo tán hé】多由脾胃蕴热与痰湿相结,阻滞经络而发。症见胞睑皮里肉外长一核状硬结,疼痛不明显。相当于睑板腺囊肿。

Chalazion usually attacking when the accmulated heat in the spleen and stomach combine with phlegm-dampness and leads to blockage of meridian and collateral, marked by outward growth in the lid which is a hard, circumscribed nodule, equal to meibomian cyst.

眼弦赤烂 【yǎn xián chì làn】(眼缘赤烂、烂弦风)即眼缘炎。多由脾胃蕴积湿热,复受风邪,风与湿热相搏,结于眼缘而发。症见眼缘红赤溃烂、痒痛并作,可致睫毛脱落,甚至睑缘变形。

Marginal Blepharits usually attacking when damp-heat is accumulated in the spleen and stomach complicated repeated exposure to pathogenic wind to result in fight between wind and damp-heat, marked by redness and ulceration of eyelid

眼偷针 【yǎn tōu zhēn】（针眼）症见胞睑边缘长小疖，初起形如麦粒，有轻微痛痒，继而出现红肿，多由风热或脾胃热毒所致。相当于麦粒肿。

眼珠 【yǎn zhū】即眼球。为视觉器官，位于眼眶内，呈球形。

眼珠牵斜 【yǎn zhū qiān xié】眼珠偏于一侧，或偏向上方。多由风痰内阻，筋脉挛急牵引；或因脾气虚弱，目系弛缓，眼珠运转失于平衡所致。

罨 【yǎn】用湿润的棉织布盖在患部的一种外治法。

验方 【yàn fāng】（经验方）经过实践验证有效的方剂。

厌食 【yàn shí】指长期食欲不振，而无其他疾病者。伴有面色少华，形体偏瘦等症。多因喂养不当，过食生冷，甘甜厚味、零食及偏食等引起。辨证分类：1、脾胃不和 2、脾胃气虚 3、脾胃阴虚。

margin which is aching and itching to make eyelashes come off, even make eyelid margin out of shape.

Hordeolum marked by small sores eveloping over eyelid margin whcih are shaped-like wheat grain, at onset accompanied by slight pain and itching, and then followed by red swelling, usually caused by wind-heat or heat-toxins in the spleen and stomach, similar to hordeolum.

Eyeball the organ of sight, lying in the orbit shaped-like a ball.

Strabismus deviation of eyeball in the lateral or upward direction, usually caused by interior blockage by wind-phlegm and traction of spasms of the tendons, muscles and skin or deficiency of spleen-qi with the result of relaxation of ocular connections and imbalance of eyeball movement.

Compress a superficial measure of local application of soaked cloth.

Proved Prescription experienced prescription, which is proved effective through practice but not yet listed in medical works and prescriptions.

Anorexia a morbid state marked by long-standing poor appetite but with no other illness, accompanied by pallor complexion and emaciation, mostly caused by improper feeding, over intake of cold or raw food, or overeating of greasy oily food, between meal nibbles or pica. Types of differentiation 1. disharmony of the

羊水 【yáng shuǐ】妊娠期子宫羊膜腔内的液体。有保护胎儿的作用。

羊水过多 【yáng shuǐ guò duō】足月妊娠时，羊水量超过二千毫升。

羊痫风 【yáng xián fēng】癫痫病的俗称。见痫证。

羊须疮 【yáng xū chuāng】因脾胃湿热郁于肌肤，复感风邪而成。下颏部出现小如粟米，大如黄豆的红色丘疹，热痒微痛，破流黄水，浸淫成片。

阳 【yáng】与阴相对的一类事物或性质。凡是运动的、外在的、上升的、温热的、明亮的、功能的、亢进的都属于阳。中医学广泛应用这一术语解释人体的生理、病理现象和指导对疾病的诊断、治疗。例如把疾病的表证、热证、实证归属于阳。

阳斑 【yáng bān】（阳证发斑）即发斑

spleen and stomach 2. deficiency of the spleen and stomach-qi 3. deficiency of the spleen — yin and stomach-yin.

Amnionic Fluid fluid in amnionic cavity during pregnancy with a protectant role for fetus.

Polyhydramnios amniotic fluid exceeding two thousand ml. at delivery of fetus on expected term.

The Popular Name of Epilepsy

Sycosis a skin disease resulting from stagnancy of damp-heat in the spleen and stomach depressing skin, and repeated attack by pathogenic wind, marked by red maculae in the mandible which are like either granule or legumes in size with itching and slight pain on exposure to heat, yellowish discharge when broken which can spread and affect surounding area.

Yang one aspect of matters or natures that is opposite to yin. matters and phenomena, which are dynamic, external, ascending, hot and warm, brilliant, functional, hyperactive, belong to yang. The term is widely applied in TCM to explain phenomema of physiology and pathology in the human body and to guide diagnosis and treatment of diseases, e.g. superficies, interior and excess syndromes being yang.

Yang Macule also called a macule

属实热性质者。多因外感热病，热郁阳明所致。

阳病 【yáng bìng】 1、指三阳经的病变。2、实证、热证的统称。

Yang Disease 1. referring to pathogenic changes of three yang meridians. 2. collective term for excessive and febrile syndromes.

阳病治阴 【yáng bìng zhì yīn】阴阳学说在治疗上的运用。1、属阳热亢盛的疾病，常耗伤阴津，治宜甘寒生津保存阴液；2、疾病的症状在阳经，可针刺阴经的穴位治疗。

Treating Yin for Yang Disease an application of yin-yang theory on the treatment. 1. disease with exessiveness of yang-heat may impair yin fluid, it is advisable to treat them by promoting the production of body fluid to nourish yin with drugs sweet in taste and cold in nature. 2. disease with symptoms of yang meridian may be treated by acupuncture of a yin meridian.

阳常有余，阴常不足 【yáng cháng yǒu yú, yīn cháng bù zú】这是古代医学家朱丹溪提出的一种观点。人体阴精易受致病因子的耗损呈现不足，由于阴精不足，易于出现虚火，故称为阳常有余。

Yang Is often Overabundant while Yin Is often Deficient this is a theory formulated by ancient physician, Zhu Danxi. The essence and blood are easily consumed by pathogenic factor and so tend to be deficient, as a result, deficient fire is apt to be present. Therefore yang is often overabundant.

阳化气，阴成形 【yáng huà qì, yīn chéng xíng】阳是机体进行生命活动的原动力。阴是构成机体有形成分的物质。

Yang Forms Vital Qi and Yin Shapes up the Body yang is dynamic power of living activity in the boy, while yin is formed materials of bodily constitution.

阳黄 【yáng huáng】黄疸病的一种。多因感受外邪，湿热之邪侵及肝胆，胆热液泄所致。症见急性发病、巩膜及

Yang Jaundice one kind of jaundice disease usually caused by affection of exopathogenic factor, invasion of the

皮肤黄染鲜明呈橘黄色为特征,伴有发热、口渴、食欲不振、大便秘结、尿黄如浓茶、腹胀胁痛、舌红、苔黄腻、脉弦数等。

阳结 【yáng jié】1、指胃肠邪实所致的便秘。2、脉象名。

阳痉 【yáng jìng】1、指刚痉。2、指痉病无四肢厥冷者。多因风热邪盛所致。

阳绝 【yáng jué】脉搏仅在寸部可触及,而关、尺两部不能察觉到脉动的一种脉象。

阳厥 【yáng jué】1、指突受刺激过度而出现善怒发狂的疾病。2、见热厥。

阳络伤则血外溢 【yáng luò shāng zé xuè wài yì】指在上部、属表的络脉损伤,引起咯血、鼻出血等证的病理。

阳明 【yáng míng】经脉名称之一,包括足阳明胃经和手阳明大肠经。本经

liver and gallbladder by pathogenic damp-heat followed by the biliary fever and purgation of fluid, manifested as acute onset, bright yellow coloration of the eyes and skin, accompanied by fever, thirst, poor appetite, constipation, yellow urine like strong tea, abdominal distension and hypochondrial pain, red tongue with yellowish and greasy coating, thready and fast pulse.

Yang-Type Constipation 1. referring to constipation caused by excess of pathogenic heat in the stomach and intestine. 2. those with uneven pulse.

Yang-Type Convulsion 1. referring to convulsion. 2. referring to the case of convulsion with cold limbs, usually caused by excess of pathogenic wind and heat.

Disappearance of Yang Pulse a condition with pulse beat only palpable at cun location but imperceptible at guan and chi locations.

Yang-Type Syncope 1. mania induced by sudden emotional upset. 2. see the list of heat—type syncope.

Injury of Yang Collateral Causing Hemorrhages externally referring to injury of collateral lying in the upper and superficial parts of the body, marked by hemoptysis, epistaxis, etc.

Yangming one of the terms of meridans, including the stomach meridian

多血多气，阳气最盛。 of foot yangming and the large intestine meridian of hand yangming which are filled with sufficient blood and qi and especially with excessive yang-qi, developing on the foundation of yin-qi in taiyang and shaoyang merdians.

阳明病 【yáng míng bìng】六经病的一种。指外感病过程中阳热亢盛的阶段，属里实热证。以身热汗多、不恶寒反恶热为特征。一般分为经证（或经病）与腑证（或腑病）。见阳明经病及阳明腑病。 **Yangming Disease** one kind of the six merdian diseases, referring to the stage of hyperactivity of yang heat in the course of exopathogenic disease, which pertains to interior heat syndrome of excess type, and characterized by fever, profuse sweating, aversion to hot, generally classified into syndrome of meridian and syndrome of fu-organ as seen in the item of meridian disease of yangming meridian and fu-organ disease of yangming meridian.

阳明经病 【yáng míng jīng bìng】（阳明经证）指无形之邪热盛于胃经所致的一种阳明病。症见身大热、大汗出、口大渴、脉洪大等。 **Yangming Meridian Disease** a syndrome caused by excessiveness of pathogenic heat invading stomach meridian, manifested as high fever, profuse sweating, extreme thirst and full pulse.

阳明腑病 【yáng míng fǔ bìng】（阳明腑证）阳明病的一种证型，是有形之燥实结于胃腑所致。症见壮热或日晡潮热、手足濈然汗出、腹满痛或绕脐痛、大便秘结、谵语、脉沉实等。 **Yangming Fu-Orgarn Disease** one syndrome of yangming disease, caused by excessive heat accumulating in the stomach, manifested as strong heat, hectic fever, sweating in the hand and feet, abdominal fullness and pain or pain around umbilicus, comstipation, delirium, sunken and solid pulse.

阳明头痛 【yáng míng tóu tòng】1、指 **Yangming Headache** 1. referring to

伤寒阳明病头痛。症见头痛，身热、不恶寒而恶热。2、头痛在阳明经脉循行部位。痛在额前，常痛连目珠。

the headache of febrile yangming disease, marked by headache, fever, chill with fever, aversion to hot. 2. headache occuring on the points where yangming meridian circulates, usually felt in the forehead and often involving eyeball.

阳明与少阳合病 【yáng míng yǔ shǎo yáng hé bìng】即阳明和少阳两经合病，除出现阳明病的身热、不恶寒，又有少阳病的口苦、咽干、目眩等外，必见下利。

Diseases Involving the Yangming and Shaoyang Meridians simultaneously the simultaneous occurrence of yangming and shaoyang diseases, diarrhea is inevitable in addition to fever and without chills attributable to yangming disease and bitter taste, dry throat, blurred vision.

阳气 【yáng qì】与阴气相对，就功能与形态来说，阳气指功能，就脏腑功能来说，指六腑之气；就人体生理活动与病理变化来说，凡属于外表的、向上的、亢盛的、增强的、轻清的均为阳气。

Yang-Qi it is the opposite of yin-qi. As for the function and form, it denotes the former, as for the function of zang-fu organ, it refers to the qi in the six fu organs; while concerning the physiological activities and pathological changes in the body, all those which are exterior, upward, hyperactivity, strengthening and clear are considered as yang-qi.

阳窍 【yáng qiào】即七窍。指耳、目、口、鼻。

Yang Orifices i. e. seven orifices, referring to ears, eyes. mouth, and nose.

阳杀阴藏【yáng shā yīn cáng】基于阴阳双方互相依存这一规律，阳气肃杀收束，阴气则封垫潜藏。

Yin Becomes Deficient when Yang is Weakened on the basis of the concept of interdependence between yin and yang, yin-qi declines whenever yang-qi debilitated.

阳生阴长 【yáng shēng yīn zhǎng】阴阳双方互相依存，只有阳气生化正常，阴气才能不断滋长。

Yin Grows while Yang Is Generating on the basis of the basis of the concept of the interdependence between

阳生于阴 【yáng shēng yú yīn】阳来源于阴。人体的功能活动必须依附于阴所代表的精血津液等物质为基础。

阳胜则热 【yáng shèng zé rè】阳气偏胜,则可产生热性的病变。

阳胜则阴病 【yáng shèng zé yīn bìng】阳热偏盛,必消耗阴液,而出现各种伤津、伤阴的病证。如发热、口干、便秘等。

阳盛 【yáng shèng】(阳热亢盛)一般指邪热盛,而人体正气亦盛的病理。表现壮热、无汗、气粗、烦躁、口干等症。

阳盛格阴 【yáng shèng gé yīn】指热极似寒的一种反常表现。病的本质属热,因邪伏于里,阳气被抑不能外达。出现四肢厥冷、脉沉伏等假寒症状。

阳盛阴伤 【yáng shèng yīn shāng】阳热过盛而致耗伤阴津的病理。

yin and yang, yin grows normally whenever yang generates properly.

Yang Is Originated from Yin yang comes from yin. Functional activities in the human body must depend on the essence, blood, thin fluid that belong to yin.

An Excess of Yang Brings about Heat Syndrome febrile pathological changes may develope when yang-qi is excessive.

An Excess of Yang Leads to Deficiency of Yin when yang-heat is intensified, yin-fluid would be exhausted, and then various syndromes of impairment of body fluid or yin would result, such as fever, dry tongue, constipation, etc.

Excess of Yang generally referring to the pathological changes in which overactivity of pathogenic heat and that of vital qi, manifested as strong heat, absence of sweat, shortness of breath, restlessness, dry tonuge.

Yin Is Kept superficially by Excess of Yang in the Interior a morbid state due to extreme heat inside the body but with manifestations of pseudo-cold syndrome, the disease pertains to heat syndrome by essence, but, as pathogens are hidden interiorly and yang-qi is restrained, exhibits as false heat marked by cold limbs, sunken and hidden pulse.

An Excess of Yang Leads to Consumption of Yin Fluid a morbid state

阳盛则外热 【yáng shèng zé wài rè】人体感受外邪之后，卫外的阳气盛于体表与邪气相争，引起发热的病理。

阳暑 【yáng shǔ】因盛夏季节在烈日下劳动或长途奔走，感受暑热所致的伤暑证，症见头痛、高热、烦躁、大汗、脉洪数等。

阳水 【yáng shuǐ】由肺气失宣，三焦壅滞，不能通调水道下输膀胱所致的实热型水肿。症见恶寒发热、咳嗽咽痛、面部先肿、小便赤涩、大便秘、腹胀满、苔腻脉数等。

阳损及阴 【yáng sǔn jí yīn】阳气不足而影响阴精化生不足。如长期胃肠道消化吸收功能障碍导致形体消瘦。

阳痿 【yáng wěi】（阴痿）指男子未到性功能衰退时期，出现阴茎不能勃

due to overexcess of yang-heat with the result of consumption and exhaustion of yin fluid.

Excess of Yang Induces Exterior Heat after affection by exogenous pathogens, yang-qi outside wei-system is confronted with pathogenic qi in the superficial, which results in fever.

Yang Summer-Heat Syndrome a disease due to attack of summer-heat during working or walking in the hot summer, manifested as headache, high fever, irritability, profuse sweating, full and fast pulse.

Yang-Type Edema a type of edema caused by dysfunction of the lung and stagnancy of the triple energizers leading to the failure of the lung to play a clearing and descending role in the fluid passages and gallbladder, with manifestation of chill and fever, cough with sore throat, edema starting in the face, dark and astringent urine, constipation, abdominal fullness and distension, greasy coating on the tongue and fast pulse.

Deficiency of Yang Affecting Yin insufficiency of yang-qi affects the production of yin-essence, for example, long-termed functional disturbance of gastric-intestinal tract in digestion and absorption may result in emaciation.

Impotence a sexual disorder showing soft and flabby penis, debili-

起，或举而不坚、不久的病证。多因房劳过度，命门火衰所致；亦有因肝肾虚火，心脾受损，或湿热下注所致。ty of penis erection before declining stage of sexual function, usually caused by frequent sexual life leading to decline of the fire of the life gate; or by flaring up of asthenic fire in the liver an kidney leading to the impairment of the heart and spleen; or by downward flow of damp-heat.

阳邪 【yáng xié】1、指六淫病邪中的风、燥、暑、火等四种邪气，因其致病多表现为阳热症候，易伤阴津，故名。2、指侵犯阳经的邪气。

Yang Factors 1. referring to four of the six pathogenic factors including wind, dryness, summer-heat, fire which usually bring about yang-heat syndrome and is apt to impair yin-fluid and so termed yang factors. 2. referring to pathogenic qi that invades yang meridians.

阳虚 【yáng xū】阳气不足，或机能衰退的证候。阳虚则生内寒，症见神疲无力、少气懒言、畏寒肢冷、自汗、面色淡白、小便清长、大便稀溏、舌质淡嫩、脉虚大或沉细等。

Insufficiency of Yang a morbid state due to insufficiency of yang qi, decline of function, marked by fatigue, debility, intolerance of cold, spontaneous perspiration, pallor, watery urine, loose stools, pale and tender tongue, feeble and large or sunken and thready pulse.

阳虚发热 【yáng xū fā rè】1、指肾阳虚衰火不归源而致的虚热病。2、指劳倦内伤，脾胃气虚而致的虚热。

Fever due to Yang Insufficiency 1. referring to asthenia fever syndrome caused by deficiency and weakness of yang qi in the kidney with fire failing to return to the source. 2. referring to the asthenic fever caused by internal impairment resulting from over strain with deficiency of the spleen and stomach-qi.

阳虚水泛 【yáng xū shuǐ fàn】脾肾功能低下，机体水液运行障碍而泛溢于脏腑与躯体之间形成水肿或痰饮等

Overflow of Water due to Deficiency of Yang pathological changes showing edema or phlegm retention caused

阳虚头痛 【yáng xū tóu tòng】指由于阳气不足,清阳不能上升于头所致的头痛。症见头痛隐隐、畏寒肢冷、体倦乏力、食欲不振、舌淡脉微细或浮数无力等。

Headache due to Yang Deficiency denoting the headache caused by insufficiency of yang-qi with clear yang failing to go ascendingly, manifested as vague headache, intolerance of cold, cold limbs, general fatigue, poor appetite, pale tongue, weak and thready or floating, fast and weak pulse.

阳虚湿阻 【yáng xū shī zǔ】指脾肾阳虚,温运失职,致水湿内停的一种病变。常引起浮肿、小便不利、泄泻、肢体疲乏、便溏等症状。

Stagnation of Dampness due to Insufficiency of Yang a pathological change showing internal stagnation of damp caused by deficiency of the spleen yang and kidney yang with the result of dysfunction in warming and transporting nutrients and water, manifested as edema, dyspepsia, diarrhea, lassitued, loose stools.

阳虚恶寒 【yáng xū wù hán】因阳气虚弱不能温养分肉,充皮毛所致。症见恶寒踡卧、自汗、脉沉细等。

Chillness due to Yang Insufficiency a condition caused by disability to warm and nourish muscle and to replenish skin resulting from weakness of yang qi, marked by aversion to cold, spontaneous perspiration, sunken and thready pulse.

阳虚眩晕 【yáng xū xuàn yūn】因阳气不足,清阳不能升达头部所致的眩晕。症见头晕或头痛,或眩晕欲倒、耳鸣耳聋、怕冷、气短、自汗、手足冷、脉沉细等。

Dizziness due to Deficiency of Yang a morbid state caused by insufficiency of yang qi with the result of disability of fresh yang qi to rise to the head, marked by dizziness or headache, or blurred vision with ten-

阳虚阴盛 【yáng xū yīn shèng】由于肾阳虚，不能温养脏腑，出现阴寒内盛症候，症见形寒肢冷、水肿、泄泻、脉沉微等。

Excess of Yin due to Yang Insufficiency a morbid condition showing internal excess of yin-cold resulting from deficiency of kidney-yang with the result of failure to warm and nourish zang-fu organ, manifested as chill and cold in extremities, watery edema, diarrhea, sunken and weak pulse.

阳虚则外寒 【yáng xū zé wài hán】机体阳气虚弱，脏腑功能低下而产生的外寒的病证，症见面色㿠白、畏寒、肢冷等证的病理。

Insufficiency of Yang Brings about Cold Syndrome a morbid state of cold syndrome resulting from weakness of yang-qi and hypofunction of zang-fu organ with manifestations of pallor complexion, intolerance of cold, cold limbs.

阳虚自汗 【yáng xū zì hàn】由于阳虚表疏，腠理不密，故汗液易泄，症见畏寒、汗出觉冷、倦怠、脉细等。

Spontaneous Perspiration due to Yang Deficiency inclination to sweating caused by loose texture and interspace of the skin, muscle as a result of yang deficiency, manifested as intolerance of cold, cold sensation after perspiration. lassitude, thready pulse, etc.

阳脏 【yáng zàng】1、患者的阳盛体质。2、五脏中指心、肝二脏属阳。

Yang Organ 1. those with constitution of yang hyperactivity. 2. the liver and heart of the five zang organs belong to the category of yang.

阳证 【yáng zhèng】八纲中的表证、热证、实证。症见发热恶寒、面赤头痛、身热喜凉、狂躁不安、口唇燥裂、烦渴引饮、语声粗壮、呼吸气粗、大便秘结或臭秽、腹痛拒按、小便短赤、舌

Yang Syndrome the superficices, heat and excessive syndromes, classified according to the diagnostic principle of the eight principal syndromes, marked by fever, aversion to

红、苔黄燥及脉浮洪数有力等。

cold, flushed face, headache, feverish body with preferance of the cool, violent restlessness, dry and splitting limps, extreme thirst and desire for drinking, deep and resonant voice, constipation with unbearable stink, abdominal pain and tenderness dark and scanty urine, red tongue with yellow and dry coating, floating, full, fast and forceful pulse.

阳证似阴 【yáng zhèng sì yīn】指热病发展到极期，所出现的一种假象，即疾病属阳证，反见四肢厥冷、脉沉伏等类似阴证的症状。可见于热性病发展到严重阶段而出现的一种假象。

Yang Syndrome Appearing as Yin Syndrome a false phenomenon occurring at the extreme stage of febrile disease, i. e. a case of yang nature with some manifestations of yin syndrome such as cold limbs, sunken and deep pulse, often seen in febrile diseases developing to severe stage.

阳中之阳 【yáng zhōng zhī yáng】任何事物都可以分为阴阳两方面，属于阳的事物又可分为两方面，其中分属于阳的一方称为阳中之阳。

The Yang Aspect of Yang everything may be divided into two aspects, yin and yang. An object belonging to the yang category may, in turn, be subdivided into two parts. Its yang part is called "yang aspect of yang."

阳中之阴 【yáng zhōng zhī yīn】任何事物都可以分为阴阳两方面，属于阳的事物又可分为两方面，其中分属阴的一方面称阳中之阴。

The Yin Aspect of Yang everything may be devided into two aspects-yin and yang. An object belonging to the yang category may, in turn, be subdivided into two parts. Its yin part is called "yin aspect of yang".

扬刺 【yáng cì】古代针刺手法之一。在患处正中浅刺一针，左右上下各浅刺一针，刺时浮扬于浅表。用于治疗范围较大，病位较浅的寒痹。

Centro-Square Needling an ancient acupunctrue method of inserting superficially one needle at the center of the affected area and anoth-

杨梅疮 【yáng méi chuāng】(棉花疮、雷疮)梅毒的皮肤损害。

疡医 【yáng yī】周代官方卫生机构分科医生的一种。是治疗肿疡、溃疡、金疮、折伤等外科疾病的医生。

养肝 【yǎng gān】(柔肝、养血柔肝)使用养血滋阴的药物,以治疗肝阴不足的方法。适用于肝阴虚者。症见视力减退、夜盲、时有头晕耳鸣、睡眠不佳、多梦、口干少津、脉细弱等。

养心安神 【yǎng xīn ān shén】治疗阴虚心神不安的方法。常用于心血亏损。症见心悸易惊、健忘失眠、精神恍惚、多梦遗精、大便干燥或便秘、口舌生疮、舌红少苔、脉细数等。

养血解表 【yǎng xuè jiě biǎo】使用养

er four needles around it in a square shape, indicated for cases of relatively widespread and superficial cold arthralgia.

Skin Damagement Caused by Syphilis

Surgeon one of the specialities of medicine in Chou Dynasty, who attended to surgical diseases such as incised wounds, fractures, local infections, ulcers.

Nourishing the Liver also termed soothing the liver, nourishing the blood and soothing the liver. A method of administrating drugs with action of nourishing blood and yin for the treatment of insufficiency of liver yin marked by diminution of vision, night bliness, occasional dizziness and tinnitus, insomnia with excessive dreaming in the sleep, dry mouth with reduced salva, thready and weak pulse.

Nourishing the Heart to Calm the Mind a method to treat restlessness due to yin deficiency, usually indicated for the uneasiness of the mind due to deficiency of the blood in the heart, manifested by palpitation with easy panic, amnesia, insomnia, impairment of consciousness, dreamfulness, spermatorrhea, dry stools or constipation, ulceration of the mouth and tongue, red tongue with scanty coating, thready and fast pulse.

Enriching Blood and Inducing Di-

血药和解表药组方,用于治疗阴血亏虚之感冒,以达到既能补养阴血不足,又能解除表邪的目的。

养血润燥 【yǎng xuè rùn zào】治疗血虚便秘的方法。症见面色苍白、头眩心惊、大便干结或便秘、舌质淡嫩、脉细数等。

养阴解表 【yǎng yīn jiě biǎo】(滋阴解表)是治疗素体阴虚而患外感表证的一种方法,其处方常由养阴药与解表药组成。

养阴润燥 【yǎng yīn rùn zào】治疗燥伤肺胃阴分的方法。适用于肺胃阴液不足。症见咽干口渴、午后身热、或干咳少痰、舌红、脉细数等。

养阴清肺 【yǎng yīn qíng fèi】治疗肺热阴虚的方法。适用于阴虚咽喉痛、白喉、劳伤咳嗽、干咳、少痰、偶见血丝。午后低热、盗汗、胸闷隐痛、口干、舌红、脉细数等。

aphoresis   a composition of blood-nourishing drugs and disphoretics, indicated for the cold due to deficiency of yin-blood for the purpose of nourishing insufficiency of yin-blood and removing pathogenic factor from the exterior.

Enriching the Blood and Moistening Dryness   a method to treat constipation due to deficiency of blood, with manifestation of pallor, vertigo, trembling constipation, pale and tender coating on the tongue, thready and fast pulse.

Nourishing Yin and Relieving Superficies-syndrome   a method to treat affection due to exopathgen with superficies-syndrome caused by yin deficiency related to general debility, the prescription for it made up of yin-nourishing drugs and drugs for the treatment of exterior syndrome.

Nourishing Yin to Moisten Dryness   a method to treat impairment of yin-fluid in the lung and stomach, indicated for insufficiency of yin-fluid in the lung and stomach with manifestation of dry throat, thirst, feverish body in the afternoon, or dry and nonproductive cough, red tongue, thready and fast pulse.

Nourishing Yin to Clear away the Lung-heat   a method to treat yin deficiency due to the heat in the lung, indicated for sore throat of yin deficiency type, diphtheria, cough caused by internal injury related to overstrain, dry and nonproductive cough, with occasional bloody sputum, low fever in the afternoon, night sweat, stuffiness in the chest with vague pain, dry mouth, red tongue, thready and fast pluse.

痒风 【yǎng fēng】皮肤无原发损害而遍身瘙痒、夜间尤甚、常因搔抓至皮破血流而见抓痕、血痂、色素沉着及革化等。即皮肤瘙痒证。为湿热蕴于肌肤，不得疏泄所致。

Pruritus general itching over the body without original injury on the skin, as is severe at night, often the lesion becomes broken with bleeding when scraching, marked by scratch mark, blood scabs, pigmentation and sclerosis, resulting form accumulation of heat in muscle and skin.

夭疽 【yāo jū】生于耳后乳突后部位的痈疽。常由胆经郁血凝结所致。因该处位于头部，邪毒容易扩散而引起多种凶险的症状。

Carbuncle on the Left Mastoid Region carbuncle on the posterior part of mastoid process behind the ear, often caused by stagnancy of blood in bladder meridian, as the lesion lies on the head, pathogenic toxin may easily spread to cause various dangerous symptoms.

腰背痛 【yāo bèi tòng】指腰及脊背部牵引作痛。多因肾气虚弱、风湿之邪乘袭经络所致。

Pain along Spinal Column referring to the drawing pain in the back and spinal column, usually caused by weakness of kidney-qi followed by attack of meridians by pathogenic wind-dampness.

腰尻痛 【yāo kāo tòng】指腰脊连及尾骶部疼痛。尻部系肝、肾经与督脉所循。腰尻痛多由肾脏虚亏所致。

Lumbosacral Pain referring to the pain involving lumbosacral portion and caudal portion where the meridians of liver and kidney and governor vessel run, usually resulting from deficiency of the kidney.

腰骨损断 【yāo gǔ sǔn duàn】腰骨因

Fracture of the Lumbar Vertebra

跌打、坠撞所伤。局部肿胀、疼痛、畸形、活动受限、严重者损及脊髓，出现下肢麻痹及瘫痪。

injury of lumber vertebra caused by trauma, with symptoms of swelling of local lesion, pain, deformity, limited movement, sometimes so severe as to injure spinal cord with the result of paralytic lower extremities or paralysis.

腰脊痛 【yāo jí tòng】指腰椎及其周围疼痛。腰部外伤、瘀血停滞，或肾虚内热均可引起。

Pain along the Spinal Column referring to the pain in and around lumbar vetebra, for which surgical injury, stagnation of blood stasis or internal heat due to kindey-deficiency may be responsible.

腰酸 【yāo suān】指腰部酸楚不适感。多因房劳肾虚所致。

Soreness of the Waist referring to the soreness and discomfort in the lumbar portion, usually caused by kidney-deficiency as a result o frequent sexual life.

腰痛 【yāo tòng】指腰部一侧或两侧疼痛或痛连脊椎的病证。凡因劳累过度，肾气亏损或因感受外邪，外伤等致腰部经络受阻，气血运行不畅，均可发生腰痛。

Lumbago a morbid condition referring to the pain on either or both sides of the waist or pain involving spinal cord, caused by over exertion, with impairment of kindey-qi or affection of exopathogens, or trauma which give rise to obstruction of the meridian and collateral in lumber and blockage of flow of qi and blood in them.

摇针 【yáo zhēn】将针刺入人体以后，一手固定穴位，一手摇动针体的一种针刺手法。

Shaking the Needle an acupuncture method of shaking the needle with one hand while fixing the acupoint with the other hand after inserting the needle into the body.

药艾条 【yào ài tiáo】指艾绒中掺有药末的艾条。常用于治疗风湿性关节炎等疾病。

Medicinal Moxa Stick referring to moxa stick in which medicinal powder is penetrating through the moxa, usually indicated for the treatment of rheumatic arthritis and others.

药膏 【yào gāo】供敷贴用膏剂。
Herb Paste　ointment for external use.

药罐 【yào guàn】即将竹罐放在配制好的中药煎剂中,煎沸后取出,待稍凉再进行拔罐的方法。
Medicinal Cupping　a cupping method in which a bamboo cup is placed in the prescribed medicinal herbs over decoction, taken out after the decoction is boiling, and used for cupping after slightly cooled.

药筒拔法 【yào tǒng bá fǎ】外治法的一种。根据证情选药,再与竹筒同煮,乘竹筒热,急将竹筒口合疮上,吸取脓液毒水。一般用于吸引疮疡的脓毒外出或毒蛇咬伤后吸引毒水外出。
Medicinal Cupping for Pus Drainage　a method for external treatment, choose herbs according to the syndrome, boil herbs together with bamboo cup and then cover the opening of hot bamboo cup over the boil lesion to drain the pus poisonous fluid in it, usually indicated for suppurative infection on body surface with its poisoning pus flowing out or injury caused by poisoning snake.

药线引流 【yào xiàn yǐn liú】外治法的一种。用吸水性较强的纸,搓成纸捻,外粘或内裹药粉。插入窦道或漏管中,引流去腐,促其疮口愈合。
Drainage with Medicated Thread　a method for external treatment, select water-absorbing paper, roll it with medicinal powder inside or outside, and then insert it into sinus or fistula to drain out slough and serev the healing.

药熨 【yào yùn】外治法的一种。其操作方法有二:一种是将药煮好后,用棉织物浸在药汁中,稍拧干,趁热敷在治疗的部位;另一种是将药用锅炒热后,用棉织物包裹后熨敷治疗的部位。
Press with Medicinal Pad　a method for external treatment, used in ways: one is to decoct herbs first, and then soak cotton cloth in the decoction for a while, twist the cloth slightly and press it on the lesion when it is hot; the other is to heat the herbs by frying first, use cotton cloth to wrap the

噎膈 【yē gé】(噎塞、鬲咽、隔噎) 指吞咽食物时,自觉胸骨后有梗噎难下之感,久则饮食难入,甚则食入即吐的病证。多因忧思气结,痰气交阻,或酒色过度,肾阴亏损;或阴虚火旺,瘀热交阻所致。辨证分类1、痰气交阻证2、瘀血内结证3、津亏热结证4、气虚阳微证。

夜盲 【yè máng】(鸡盲、雀目) 指在夜间或黑暗处视物不清的一种疾病。多由脾胃虚弱,导致肝血亏虚或肾阴不足引起。

夜嗽 【yè sòu】 指夜间咳嗽连声、白天则缓解的一种证候。或兼有口苦胁痛、食欲不振等。多由肾阴亏损,虚火上炎所致。

夜啼 【yè tí】 婴儿日间安静,入夜多啼,甚至通宵难入睡,天明渐转静。为小儿神气未充,心火上乘所致。

hot herbs, and then press the parcel on the lesion for the treatment.

Dysphagia a disease marked by feeling of obstruction during swallowing or even instant vomiting after food intake, which is mostly caused by accumulation of phlegm and obstruction of phlegm and qi due to emotional upsets or caused by consumption of the kidney-yin due to alcholic indulgence or hypersexuality, or caused by overabundance of fire due to yin deficiency and obstruction of accumulated heat. Types of differentiation 1. obstruction of accumulated phlegm and qi. 2. accumulation of blood stasis interior. 3. consumption of the body fluid due to heat retention. 4. exhaustion of yang and qi.

Night Blindness referring to blurring of vision at night or in darkness, it is often caused by insufficiency of liver-blood or kidney-yin due to the hypofunction of the spleen and stomach.

Nocturnal Cough a symptom marked by persistent coughing at night but relieved at daytime, it is accompanied with bitter taste in the mouth, hypochondriac pain, poor appetite, etc. mostly due to consumption of the kidney-yin.

Morbid Night Crying of Babies a disorder in infants marked by calmness at daytime, crying at night, or even insomnia the whole night, but

液道 【yè dào】即体内津液升降的道路。

液燥生风 【yè zào shēng fēng】由于阴液亏损，筋脉失养，虚风内动的病理。常见眩晕、抽搐、震颤等症。

腋痛 【yè tòng】即腋部疼痛。风寒、燥热外邪伤肺，或郁怒伤肝、积热熏肺、肾火上冲均可引起。

腋痈 【yè yōng】指生于腋部的痈，其病因症状及辨证分类用颈痈。

一逆 【yī nì】治疗上出了一次差错。

移指 【yí zhǐ】诊脉方法之一。即适当移动食指、中指及无名指的位置，以进一步了解寸、关、尺三部脉象的变化。

遗毒 【yí dú】指胎儿感染父母梅疮遗毒所致的疾病。表现为婴儿出生后周身皮肤红赤、脓血淋漓、腐烂成斑、皮肉坏损。即先天性梅毒。

calmed down at daybreak, usually due to mental unerdevelopment of flaring up of the heart-fire.

Fluid Passage the passage through which the body fluid circulates up and down.

Wind Syndrome due to Fluid Consumption a morbid condition of malnutrition of muscles and tendons due to consumption of yin-fluid, often resulting in wind-syndrome, such as dizziness, convulsion, tremor, etc.

Armpit Pain a symptom due to impairment of the lung by wind-cold, dryness-heat pathogens, etc. or due to impairment of the liver by anger or attack on the lung by the accmulated heat or upward rushing of kidney-fire.

Armpit Carbuncle referring to the carbuncle in the armpit, its cause, symptoms and differential typing are the same as those of cervical carbuncle.

Error an error in the treatment.

Finger Shifting a method for pulse feeling by changing the positions of the three palpating fingers to get further information of the changes of pulse conditions of cun, guan and chi regions.

Congenital Syphilis referring to syphilis acquired in uterus, marked by general skin lesion at birth time, redness and erosion with purulent and bloody discharge.

遗精 【yí jīng】指不因性交而精液自行泄出的病证,有梦遗和滑精之分。多因心肾不交、肾气不固、相火炽盛或湿热下注等引起。

遗尿 【yí niào】(遗溺)指睡眠中小便遗出。多见于小儿。因下元虚冷,肾气不固,或脾肺气虚,不能约束水道所致。辨证分类:1、肾气不足 2、脾肺气虚 3、肝经湿热

以毒攻毒 【yǐ dú gōng dú】使用有毒性的药物治疗某些毒邪所致的疾病的一种治法。包括外用和内服,但这类药有较大的毒性和副作用,故使用时应注意用量和用法。

异病同治 【yì bìng tóng zhì】不同的疾病,若病机相同,可用同一种方法治疗。如脱肛、泄泻、子宫下垂等,若均属脾虚中气下陷所致,则都可用补中益气的方法治疗。

Seminal Emission involuntary discharge of semen, mostly due to imbalance between heart-yang and kidney-yin, deficiency of kidney-qi, overabundance of ministerial fire, or downwards attack of dampness-heat.

Enuresis involuntary discharge of urine in children when sleeping at night, caused by asthenia-cold of the lower energizer, deficiency of kidney-qi, or failure voluntary control of urination due to qi deficiency both in the spleen and lung. Types of differentiation 1. deficiency of the kidney-qi. 2. deficiency of the spleen-qi and lung-qi. 3. damp-heat of the live meridian.

Treating the Toxifying Disease with Poisonous Agents a treatment for some diseases due to virulent pathogens by topical or oral use of poisinous drugs. The dosage and the method of application should be carfully chosen since the drugs have significant toxicity and side effects.

Treating Different Diseases with the Same Therapeutic Principle a therapeutic principle in which same therapy is applied to treat the different diseases with the same pathogenesis, e. g., prolapse of rectum, diarrhea, uterine prolapse can be treated by the therapy of reinforcing the middle energizer and invigorating qi if the pathogeneses of these diseases are asthenia of the spleen and collapse of

异气 【yì qì】(疫疠之气) 指具有强烈传染性的病邪。一般认为它的产生与气候的反常有关。

疫疠 【yì lì】指某些具有强烈传染性的、可造成大流行的疾病。

疫疟 【yì nüè】指能引起流行、病情较严重的疟疾。症见寒热往来,壮热多汗、口渴胸闷,甚则神昏等。

疫疔 【yì dīng】因感染疫毒而发的一种疔疮。多见于从事畜牧业及皮毛制革工作者。好发于头面、颈项及手臂等部位。相当于皮肤炭疽。

疫痢 【yì lì】(疫毒痢) 传染性强而病情严重的痢疾。症见发病急骤、高热头痛、烦躁口渴、腹痛剧烈、下脓血便或血水、舌红绛、苔黄燥、脉滑数;重者可见昏迷、痉厥、呼吸急促、四肢厥冷。类似中毒性菌痢。

疫喉痧 【yì hóu shā】因时行疫疠邪毒入侵咽喉所致的传染病。常发于冬春季节。症见咽喉红肿疼痛,喉核溃烂,上覆白腐假膜,易拭去,疼痛剧如刀割,吞咽困难,寒热大作,全身痧点隐隐,呈遍体猩红及分散小丘疹,痧

the middle energizer qi.

Epidemic Pathogenic Factor referring to the pathogenic factors which cause epidemic diseases, generally considered as a result of climatic abnormality.

Pestilence a virulent infectious disease which tends to be epidemic.

Endemic Malaria referring to malaria widely prevalent and with serious symptoms, manifested as alternate episodes of chills and high fever, profuse sweating, thirst, feeling of oppression over the chest, or even coma, etc.

Cutaneous Anthrax an infectious disease usually involving the skin of the head, neck and arms, it mostly found in the workers engaged in the animal husblandry tannery.

Fulminant Dysentery dysentery which is highly infective and serious, manifested as sudden onset, high fever, headache, irritability, thirst, intense abdominal pain, dischare of purulent and bloody stool or bloody fluid, crimson tongue with yellowish and dry fur, smooth and fast pulse, in serious case, as coma, convulsion, dyspnea and cold limbs.

Scarlet Fever an infectious disease usually occurring in winter and spring, which is due to attack of epidemic pestilent pathogen on the throat, marked by membranous pharyngo-tonsillitis, knife-cutting-

退后皮肤有糖皮样脱屑现象。like pain, difficulty in swallowing, occurrence of chills and fever, diffuse scarlet erythema of the body with pinpoint papular eruptions which subside with fine scaling desquamation.

疫疹 【yì zhěn】一种传染性较强,多兼发热的出疹性传染病。由于感受疫疠之邪,热毒内盛,外发于肌肤所致。症见鲜红或紫黑色皮疹、发热恶寒、头痛,甚则烦躁谵语、舌起芒刺、脉数等。

Epidemic Eruptive Disease a highly infectious disease caused by the retention of virulent heat inside the body involving the superficies after the exposure to the epidemic pathogen; manifested as brigh red or dark purplish eruptions, fever, chilliness, headache, or even irritability and delirium, thick and rough fur on the tongue, fast pulse, etc.

益气养血 【yì qì yǎng xuè】补气药和补血药并用治法。适用于气血俱虚。症见面色苍白或萎黄、心悸怔肿、食欲不振、气短懒言、四肢倦怠、头晕目眩、舌质淡苔白、脉细弱。

Invigorating Qi and Nourishing Blood a treatment for deficiency of both qi and blood with qi-tonics and hematics, which is applicable to the syndrome marked by pale or sallow complexion, palpitation, poor appetite, shortness of breath, fatigue, dizziness, pale tongue with whitish fur, small and weak pulse or feeble, large and weak pulse, etc.

益气生津 【yì qì shēng jīn】用益气生津的药物,治疗气津两虚的方法。常用于气津两虚。症见汗出过多、倦怠气短、口干渴、舌质红干少津、脉虚数者。

Supplementing Qi and Promoting the Production of Body Fluid a treatment for deficiency of both qi and blood with drugs for supplementing qi and promoting the production of body fluid, which is applicable to the case manifested as profuse sweating, fatigue, shortness of breath, thirst, reddish and dry tongue, feeble and fast pulse, etc.

益气健脾 【yì qì jiàn pí】用具有补脾 **Replenishing Qi to Invigorate the**

益气作用的药物，治疗脾胃虚弱的一种治法。适用于脾胃虚弱所致的食欲不振、泄泻、呕吐等病证。

益气解表 【yì qì jiě biǎo】（补气解表）补气和解表药合用，以治疗平素气虚又有外感表证的一种治法。

意守 【yì shǒu】是指在气功锻炼中，在身心安静的情况下，把意念放在身体内外某一部位或某一处。

益胃 【yì wèi】治疗胃虚的方法。1、使用甘温的药物，温中补虚，治胃气虚寒；2、用滋养胃阴的药物，治胃阴不足。

嗌 【yì】即食管的上口，为饮食水谷进入食管的通道。

溢乳 【yì rǔ】指婴儿饮乳过多而致乳汁溢出。

溢饮 【yì yǐn】四饮之一。多因脾虚不运，或饮邪泛滥于体表肌肤所致。症

Spleen a treatment for the hypofunction of the spleen and stomach by using prescriptions composed of drugs with the action of invigorating the spleen and qi, which is applicable to the disorders, such as anorexia, diarrhea, vomiting, etc.

Supplementing Qi and Expelling Superficial Pathogenic Factors a treatment for superficies-syndrome which caused by exogenous pathogens resulting from deficiency of qi by the combined use of drugs for invigorating qi and for expelling superficial pathogens.

Concentrating Will during Practising Qi Gong concentrating will on a certain part of the body or outside the body, under the static state of the body and mind.

Reinforcing the Stomach a treatment for stomach-asthenia: 1. treating asthenia-cold of stomach-qi with drugs of sweet and warm nature to warm the middle energizer and invigorate the asthenic sate. 2. treating insufficiency of stomach-yin with drugs for nourishing stomach-yin.

Laryngopharynx part of pharynx which is continuous inferiorly with the esopagus.

Milk Vomiting a condition in infants which is caused by over-feeding.

Anassrca one of the four boy retention mostly due to hypofunction of

见肢体疼痛沉重、浮肿或伴有喘咳。

溢血 【yì xuě】指血液不循经脉流行，溢出体外，表现为咳血、咯血、吐血、衄血等上窍的出血。

翳 【yì】1、引起黑睛混浊的外障眼病。如凝脂翳、宿翳等。2、晶体混浊之目障。如圆翳、震惊翳等。

因人制宜 【yīn rén zhì yí】在治疗上要根据病人的具体情况，如病人的生理、病理特点及病人的体质，所处环境等来考虑治疗方法，使能切合病情变化。

因地制宜 【yīn dì zhì yí】由于地区气候环境等因素的不同，对人体产生一定的影响，治疗时应根据地区的特点，来制定适宜的治疗方法。如南方炎热多雨地区，往往出现湿热证候，治疗时应考虑气候变化的特点。

因时制宜【yīn shí zhì yí】人体生活在自然界，四季的气候变化对人体产生一定的影响，治疗时应考虑气候变化的特点。

the spleen; manifested as general edema, pain and heaviness of limbs, or accompanied with cough.

Hemorrhage the escape of blood from the meridians visible outside the body, hemoptysis, hematemesis, epistaxis, etc.

Yi 1. Nebula a slight corneal opacity or scar, such as suppurative keratitis, keratoleukoma, etc. 2. Cataract. an opacity of the crystalline lens of the eye with interference of vision.

Treating the Disease according to the Individual Condition a therapeutic principle that the treatment should be chosen according to the physiological and pathological characteristics of the patient and also his physique and environment.

Treating the Disease according to the Environment a therapeutic principle that the treatment should be chosen according to the environment, since the human body may be affected by the environmental variations. For instance, the method of removing heat and dampness is usually applied in the southern area because of its hot and rainy weather.

Treating the Disease according to the Climate a therapeutic principle that the treatment should be chosen according to the climate, since the human body may be affected by the climatic variations of the four seasons.

阴 【yīn】与阳相对的一类事物或性质。凡是沉静的、内在的、下降的、寒冷的、晦暗的、物质的、抑制的、衰减的、都属阴。中医学广泛应用这一术语解释人体的生理、病理现象和指导对疾病的诊断、治疗。例如把疾病的里证、寒证、虚证归属于阴。

Yin a philosophical term in ancient China, referring to the things or characters opposite to yang. The condition which appears as inert, internal, downward, cold, dim, material, inhibitive and declining is attributive to yin. In TCM, it is widely used for interpreting the physiological and pathological phenomena of the human body, and for directing the diagnosis and treatment of the diseases, for instance, interior syndrome, cold-syndrome and asthenia syndrome are all ascribed to yin.

阴刺 【yīn cì】古代刺法之一。指治疗寒厥时左右配穴针刺的方法。如下膝寒厥，可针刺两足内踝后少阴经穴。

Yin Puncture an ancient acupuncture method for cold limbs by puncturing the corresponding points of both sides, e.g., coldness of the lower limbs may be treated by puncturing the points of shaoyin meridian of both sides behind the medial malleoli.

阴汗 【yīn hàn】1、即冷汗，指阳衰阴盛所致的汗证。2、指外生殖器及其附近局部多汗。

Yin Perspiration 1. night sweat due to deficiency of yang and overabundance of yin. 2. polyhidrosis around the external genitals.

阴狐疝 【yīn hú shàn】(狐疝)症见阴囊时大时小，腹胀作痛。多由肝气失于疏泄所致。即腹股沟疝。

Inguinal Hernia a condition due to disorder of the liver-qi, manifested as intermittent swelling of the scrotum and distending pain in the abdomen.

阴户 【yīn hù】又名产门。即阴道口。

Yin House vaginal orice.

阴户肿痛 【yīn hù zhǒng tòng】指妇女外阴部肿胀作痛的病证，伴有腹部坠胀不适，或小便涩滞，或带下淋漓等。多因郁怒伤肝，肝郁气滞犯脾，湿热下注所致。

Vulvitis (Swelling and Pain of Vulva) a disorder accompanied with bearing-down sensation over the lower abdomen, or dysuria, or leucorrhagia; mostly due to impairment of the liver by stagnated anger, stagnation of liver-qi attacking the spleen, and retention of dampness-heat.

阴黄 【yīn huáng】 1、黄疸病两大类型之一。多因脾阳不振，寒湿内蕴或过服寒凉所致；亦可因阳黄日久转化而致。以巩膜及皮肤黄染，色泽晦暗不鲜明为特征，并见神疲乏力、胁部隐痛、腹胀、食欲减退、小便短黄、大便稀烂、舌质淡、苔腻、脉沉细迟等。2、黄疸二十八候之一。3、三十六黄之一。

Yin Jaundice 1. one of the two major types of jaundice, which is often caused by the dysfunction of spleen-yang, retention of cold-dampness excessive intake of food in cold nature, or resulting from the development of yang jaundice; it is characterize by yellow tinged sclera and skin with dim and lusterless appearance, and accompanied with lassitude, dull hypochondriac pain, abdominal flatulence, poor appetite, oliguria, loose stools, pale tongue with greasy fur, sunken and small, slow pulse, etc. 2. one of the twenty-eight syndromes of jaundice. 3. one of the thirty—six types of jaundice.

阴火 【yīn huǒ】 饮食劳倦，喜怒忧思所生之火，起于下焦，属心火。

Yin Fire a fire attributed to heart-fire originating from the lower energizer, caused by improper diet, overstrain, emotional upsets.

阴结 【yīn jié】 1、指虚秘。凡脾阳虚衰，传送失常，或精血亏耗，大肠干燥所致的大便闭结，均称阴结。2、证名、即冷秘。3、脉象名。

Yin Constipaiton 1. asthenia-type constipation, a type of constipation due to dysfunction of the spleen resulting from the deficiency of spleen-yang or dehydration of large intestine resulting from the consumption of essence and blood. 2. cold-type constipation. 3. a term for pulse condition.

阴竭阳脱 【yīn jié yáng tuō】指属阴的生命物质基础的枯竭，则属阳的生命活动随之消失的病理。如大量的失血导致气脱。症见面色苍白，口开目合，

Exhaustion of Yin and Collapse of Yang a morbid state of the cessation of life activities (which are attributive to yin) resulting from the

汗出如油，脉微欲绝等。

exhaustion of essential substances (which are attributive to yang). For instance, profuse bleeding leads to collapse of qi, manifested as pale complexion, mouth open and eyes closed, profuse oil—like sweating, faint and impalpable pulse, etc.

阴绝 【yīn jué】脉搏只在尺部能触及，而寸、关两部不能触及。是阴气偏绝的表现。

Disappearance of Yin-Pulse a pulse condition that can be felt only at the chi region, and impalpable at the cun and guan regions, indicating the exhaustion of yin-qi.

阴冷 【yīn lěng】（阴寒）自觉前阴寒冷。多因肾阳虚衰，寒气凝结所致，也可因肝经湿热引起。

Cold Feeling of External Genitals a condition mostly caused by the retention of coldness resulting from the deficiency of kidney-yang, and also by the accumulation of dampness-heat in the liver meridian.

阴络伤则血内溢 【yīn luò shāng zé xuè nèi yì】指下部、属里的络脉损伤引起便血的病理。多因大肠湿热下注，伤及血络，或脾虚不摄，血不循经所致。

Damage of Yin Collaterals Results in Bleeding from the Lower Part of the Body a morbid condition due do damage of the collaterals of the internal and lower part of the body, manifested as bloody stools, mostly caused by impairment of blood collaterals resulting from the downward flow of dampness-heat in the large intestine, or the failure of blood to circulate within vessels resulting from asthenia of the spleen.

阴平阳秘 【yīng píng jáng bì】阴精充沛，阳气固密，阴阳双方彼此保持协调，平衡，这是人体保持健康，进行正常生命活动的基本条件。

Yin and Yang in Equilibrium yin and yang are regulated and adjusted continuously, so as to keep in equilibrium in healthy persons. This is an essential factor in carrying on the normal life activities.

阴气 【yīn qì】1、与阳气相对。就功能与形态来说,阴气指形态;就脏腑机能来说,指五脏之气;就人体生理活动与病理变化来说,凡属于内在的、向下的、抑制的、减弱的、重浊的均为阴气。2、同阴器。即外生殖器。

阴窍 【yīn qiào】通常指尿道口和肛门。

阴热 【yīn rè】通常指阴虚发热;或急性病后期阴津消耗而产生的发热。

阴疝 【yīn shàn】因寒邪侵袭肝经而致睾丸急痛、肿胀的病证。

阴生于阳 【yīng shēng yǔ yáng】根据阴阳互相依存的道理,阴以阳的存在为自己存在的前提,即阴来源于阳。也就是就人体的一切有形物质必须通过人体的功能活动而产生。

阴胜则阳病。 【yīn shèng zé yáng bìng】指阴胜的病变必然损伤人体的阳气,导致阳气衰减。出现畏寒、四肢不温、舌淡、脉迟等症。

阴盛 【yīn shèng】即阴寒偏盛的病理,一般表现为生理功能衰退,往往与阳衰并存。

Yin Qi 1. It is opposite to yang-qi. As for the function and morphology, yin-qi refers to morphology. As for the functions of the zang and fu organs, it refers to the qi of the five viscera. As for the physiological activities and pathological changes, it refers to those which are internal, downward, inhibitive, declinging, turbid, etc. 2. external genitals.

Yin Orifice referring to the external urethral orifice and the anus.

Yin Fever referring to the fever due to yin-deficiency, or that results from the consumption of yin-fluid during the advanced stage of an acute febrile disease.

Yin-Type Testalgia pain and swelling in the testicle, due to the attack of coldness in the liver meridian.

Yin Originates form Yang according to the interdependence between yin and yang, the production of all the tangible materials must depend upon the physiological functions of the body.

An Excess of Yin Leads to Deficiency of Yang a morbid condition with overabundance of yin-cold leads to the hypofunction of yang-qi, manifested as aversion to cold, cold limbs, pale tongue, slow pulse, etc.

Excess of Yin a morbid condition of overabundance of yin-cold, generally manifested as declination of various physiological functions, usually ac-

阴盛格阳 【yīn shèng gé yáng】指体内阴寒内盛,阳气被拒于外而出现真寒假热的证候。表现为身虽热,反喜盖衣被,口虽渴而饮水不多或喜热饮,脉虽大但按之无力等症。

Excessive Yin Repelling Yang a syndrome of real cold false heat, in which yang is kept externally by yin-excess in the interior; manifested as fever but desire for being covered up, thirst but disinclinaltion for drinks or inclination for hot drinks, large and weak pulse, etc.

阴盛阳虚 【yīn shèng yáng xū】指阴寒内盛,导致阳气虚衰的病理。常见有畏寒、肢冷、泄泻、水肿、舌质淡等症。

Overabundant Yin and Deficiency Yang a morbid state of overabundance of yin-cold in the interior leading to the deficiency of yang-qi; manifested as aversion to cold, limbs, diarrhea, edema, pale tongue, etc.

阴盛则寒 【yīn shèng zé hán】指因阴邪所致疾病性质而言。即阴寒偏盛,阳气偏衰,导致寒证的病理。表现为脏腑功能衰退,出现水肿、痰饮等寒性病证。

Excess of Yin May Lead to Cold a morbid state of overabundauce of yin-cold and deficiency of yang-qi leading to cold syndrome; manifested as hypofunction of viscera, such as edema, phlegm-retention syndrome, etc.

阴虱疮 【yīn shī chuāng】是阴虱寄生所致的皮肤病。生于阴毛际,初起红色或淡红色丘疹,奇痒,搔破感染成疮。

Eruption around the Pubic Region due to Lice Bite a rash appearing as red or pink papule with intolerable itching, maybe complicated by infection after scratched.

阴蚀 【yīn shí】外阴部溃烂的疾病。多因情志郁火,损伤肝脾,湿热下注所致。症见外阴溃烂,或痒或痛,肿胀等,多伴有赤白带下,小便淋漓等。

Erotion of Vulva a disorder due to retention of pathogenic fire from emotional upsets impairing the liver and spleen, leading to downward flow of pathogenic dampness-heat; manifested as erosion of the vulva, itching, pain and swelling, usually accompanied with reddish and whitish vaginal discharge and stranguria.

阴暑 【yīn shǔ】因暑季纳凉,寒袭肌

Yin Summer-Heat Syndrome a type

肤，或饮冷不节，寒凉伤脏所致的伤暑。症见发热头痛、无汗恶寒、肢体酸痛、或呕吐、泻利、腹痛等。

of summer-heat syndrome, due to attack of the superficies by cold pathogen, immoderate intake of cold drinks leading to the impairment of viscera; manifested as fever, headache, anhidrosis, aversion to cold, general aching, or vomiting, diarrhea, abdominal pain, etc.

阴水 【yīn shuǐ】水肿两大类型之一。由脾肾阳虚，不能运化水湿所致。症见面浮足肿、按之凹陷、胸闷食减、肢冷神疲、便溏尿少、身重腰酸、舌胖苔白、脉沉迟弱等虚寒证候。

Yin-Type Edema one of the two major types of edema due to retention of fluid in the body resulting from the deficiency of spleen-yang and kidney-yang; manifested as asthenia-cold syndrome such as pitted edema of face and feet, feeling of oppression over the chest, poor appetite, cold limbs, listlessness, loose stools, oliguria, lumbago, corpulent tongue with whitish fur, sunken and solw, weak pulse, etc.

阴损及阳 【yīn sǔn jí yáng】阴精亏损导致阳气化生不足的病理。如长期慢性出血使机体生理功能衰退。

Deficiency of Yin Affecting Yang a morbid state in which the consumption of yin-essence results in the deficiency of yang-qi, e. g., chronic bleeding may lead to hypofunction of the body.

阴缩 【yīn suō】指前阴内缩的证候。包括男子阴茎、阴囊内缩及妇人阴道内缩，多因寒入厥阴或阳明热邪陷入厥阴所致。

Shrindage of the External Genitals a syndrome of the shrinkage of the external genitals such as penis, scrotum or vagina, mostly due to attack of coldness to jueyin or invasion of heat from yangming to jueyin.

阴挺 【yīn tǐng】（阴痉、阴菌）相当于子宫脱垂、阴道壁膨出等病。多因气虚下陷或肾气不足所致。

Vaginal Hernia a disorder caused by the deficiency of middle energizer qi or insufficiency of kidney-qi, seen in hysteroptosis, rectocele, cystocele,

阴头痛 【yīn tóu yōng】即龟头痛。症见龟头紫肿疼痛。

阴脱 【yīn tuō】1、指妇女阴户开而不闭,肿痛或小便淋漓。多因分娩损伤胞络,或房劳过度所致。2、见阴挺。

阴痫 【yīn xián】1、属于虚寒的痫症。由阳痫频发,体质转虚,或攻下太过,元气受伤所致。症见发作时肢体偏冷,手足不抽搐,其脉多沉。2、指小儿慢惊风。

阴邪 【yīn xié】1、指六淫中寒、湿等致病因素,常影响机体的气化功能。2、指侵犯阴经的致病因素。

阴虚 【yīn xū】阴液不足,津血亏损的证候。常见低热、手足心热、午后潮热、消瘦盗汗、唇红口干、小便黄短、舌质红、少苔或无苔、脉细数无力等症。

阴虚喘 【yīn xū chuǎn】指阴虚阳浮而

etc.

Infection of Glans Penis a disorder marked by swelling and pain of the glans penis.

Vaginal Hernai 1. a condition manifested as dilatation of the vaginal orifice with local swelling and pain, or even stranguria, due to impairment of bao collaterals during labour, or excessive sexual intercourse. 2. Atonia of Vagina

Yin Epilepsy 1. a type of epilepsy due to debilitation by repeated attack of epilepsy of yang-type, or the damage of primordial qi by excessive intake of purgative; manifested as cold limbs and sunken pulse, but no crying, no spasms of the extremities during the seizure. 2. referring to chronic infantile convulsion.

Yin Pathogens 1. the pathogenic factors of yin nature, such as cold and dampness, which often affect the activity and the circulation of qi. 2. the pathogenic factors attacking the yin meridians.

Yin-Deficiency a syndrome due to insufficiency of yin-fluid and consumption of body fluid and blood; manifested as low fever, warm palms and soles, afternoon fever, emaciation, night sweat, red lips, dry mouth, oliguria with yellowish urine, red tongue with little coating, small, fast and weak pulse, etc.

Dyspnea due to Yin-Deficiency a

致的气喘。多因阴血亏损虚耗,阳气失于依附,直冲清道而成。症见气喘发作时有气从脐下冲上,可伴有潮热、盗汗等。

disorder caused by the attack of the floating yang-qi on the air passage resulting from the consumption of yin-blood or kidney-yin; manifested as feeling of gas rushing up from the lower abdomen during dyspnea, accompanied with hectic fever and night sweat, etc.

阴虚盗汗 【yīn xū dào hàn】由于阴虚热扰,心液外泄而出现夜眠时汗出的症候,常兼见烦热口干、疲乏、脉细数等。

Night Sweat due to Yin-Deficiency a syndrome caused by the escape of heart-fluid resulting from fever due to yin-deficiency, usually accompanied with restlessness, fever, dry mouth, fatigue, small and fast pulse, etc.

阴虚发热 【yīn xū fā rè】指机体精血阴液耗损过度所致的虚热病证。主要表现为潮热、夜间发热并常有盗汗、口干、舌质红、脉细数等症。

Fever due to Yin-Deficiency heat-syndrome of asthenia-type due to excessive consumption of essence, blood, and yin-fluid, it is characterized by hectic fever and night fever, and usually accompanied with night sweat, dry mouth, reddish tongue, small and fast pulse, etc.

阴虚肺燥 【yīn xū fèi zào】由于阴虚内热、灼伤肺阴引起肺燥的病证。症见干咳无痰、或痰中带血、咽痛嘶哑、舌嫩红苔少、脉细数等。

Lung-Dryness due to Yin-Deficiency a morbid condition due to impairment of lung-yin by the heat originated from yin-deficiency; manifested as dry cough or coughing with blood sputum, sorethroat, hoarseness of voice, red and tender tongue without fur, small and fast pulse, etc.

阴虚咳嗽 【yīn xū ké sòu】因阴虚津少、肺阴不足,肺气上逆所致的咳嗽。症见干咳、少痰或无痰、或痰中带血丝、咽干口燥、形体消瘦、神疲乏力、食欲减退,午后潮热、心烦失眠、夜寐盗汗、舌质红、苔少而干、脉细数

Cough due to Yin-Deficiency a morbid state caused by the insufficiency of lung-yin and adverse rising of lung-qi resulting from yin-deficiency and consumption of body fluid; manifested as nonproductive cough or

等。

cough with blood-tinged sputum, dry throat and mouth, emaciation, fatigue, poor appetite, afternoon fever, restlessness, insomnia, night sweat, red tongue with a little dry fur, small and fast pulse, etc.

阴虚喉痹　【yīn xū hóu bì】因阴虚，虚火上炎所致的喉痹。症见咽部不适，微痛、干痒、灼热、异物感等。

Sorethroat due to Yin-Deficiency　a condition caused by flaring up of the asthenic fire resulting from yin-deficiency, manifested as mild pain, itching, burning and irritating sensation over the throat, etc.

阴虚火旺　【yīn xū huǒ wàn】由于阴精亏损所导致的虚火亢盛的病理。症见烦躁易怒、两颧潮红、口干咽痛、性欲亢进等。

Deficiency of Yin Leads to Hyperactivity of Fire　a morbid state of hyperactivity of asthenic fire caused by the consumption of yin-essence; manifested as irritability, flushed cheeks, dry mouth, sore throat, hypersexuality, etc.

阴虚头痛　【yīn xū tóu tòng】由阴虚火动所致的头痛病证。症见头痛而兼心烦内热、面红、失眠、舌红、脉细数等。

Headache due to Yin-Deficiency　a disorder caused by hyperactivity of fire resulting from the deficiency of yin; manifested as headache, and accompanied with restlessness, feverish sensation inside the body, flushed face, insomnia, red tongue, small and fast pulse, etc.

阴虚痿　【yīn xū wěi】由久病或房欲不节，肝肾不足，阴虚火旺，伤及筋骨所致的痿证。症见腰膝酸软、步行艰难、不能久立、自觉两足热气上升、头昏目眩、舌质红、脉细数等。

Flaccidity due to Yin-Deficiency　a condition of damage to the muscle and bone resulting from chronic disease, sexual overstrain, deficiency of liver-yin and kidney-yin and hyperactivity of pathogenic fire; manifested as muscular flaccidity of the legs with difficulty on walking and inability to stand for a long time, sensation of

阴虚阳浮【yīn xū yáng fú】指真阴不足，津血亏损，阳无所附而浮越于上的病理。表现为头目眩晕、面色潮红、目赤咽干、喉痛、牙痛等症。

阴虚则内热【yīn xū zé nèi rè】指阴液过度亏耗而引起的内热证。

阴癣【yīn xuǎn】股部内侧或蔓延到外阴、臀部及肛门周围的癣病，即股癣。多由风热湿邪侵于肌肤所致，初起为丘疹或小水泡，渐向周围扩大而成红斑，边缘清楚，上有簿屑，剧烈瘙痒。

阴阳【yīn yáng】阴阳属于中国古代的哲学思想。古代哲学家认为，阴阳是事物的两个方面，它的对立统一是一切事物发展、变化的根源。就事物的属性来说，在外的、向上的、功能的、兴奋的、旺盛的、强盛的、强壮的等都属于阳；相反，在内的、向下的、物质的、抑制的等属于阴。中医学运用这一理论阐明人体生理现象和病理变化规律，同时指导对疾病的诊断和治疗。

heat rising from the feet, dizziness, red tongue, small and fast pulse, etc.

floating of Yang due to Yin—Deficiency　a morbid state due to consumption of body fluid and blood and insufficiency of yin leading to the lack of support and floating up of yang; manifested as dizziness, flushed face, congestion of the eyes, dryness of the throat, sorethroat, toothache, etc.

Heat-Syndrome in the Interior Caused by Yin — Deficiency　a morbid state due to excess consumption of yin-fluid.

Tinea Inguinalis　a superficial fungal infection occurring in the medial side of the thigh or extending to the external genitals, buttock and around the anus, due to attack of wind, heat and dampness pathogens to the skin; appearing as papules or vesicles at onset, gradually spreading and forming well-demarcated, red patches covered with thin desquamation, and severe itching.

Yin Yang　a concept orginating from ancient chinese philosophy, in which yin and yang represent two contradictories in everything. The unity of opposites of yin and yang is the fundamental cause which brings about development and changes of everything. Matters which are hot, exciting, vigorous, functional, external, upward, etc, are attributive to yang, while those which are cold, inhibitiv-

阴 yin

e, weak, material, internal, downward, etc. are attributive to yin. In TCM, the theory of yin and yang is applied to interprete the law of physiological and pathological phenomena of the body. It also serves as a principle for diagnosis and treatment of diseases.

阴阳乖戾 【yīn yáng guāi lì】阴阳间失去相互协调的正常关系。疾病的发生就是由于阴阳失去协调的结果。

Dysequilibrium between Yin and Yang a morbid state in which yin and yang do not coordinate with each other and disease ensue.

阴阳互根 【yīn yáng fù gēn】阴和阳是对立统一的，二者既相互对立，又相互依存，任何一方都不能脱离另一方而单独存在。如上为阳，下为阴，没有上也就无所谓下；没有下也就无所谓上。所以说，阳依存于阴，阴依存于阳，每一方都以对方的存在为自己存在的前提。阴阳学说用此观点说明脏与腑、气与血、功能与物质在生理或病理上的密切联系。

Interdependence between Yin and Yang yin and yang are the unity of opposites. They are opposite to each other and interdependent, one cannot exist alone without the existence of the other. For instance, if upward is yang, then downward is yin; no downward without upward, and vice versa. Therefore, yin and yang are interdependent and presuppose the existence each other. This view is used to explain the physiological and pathological relationship between zang organs and fu organs, qi and blood, functions and materials.

阴阳交 【yīn yáng jiāo】指热性阳邪入于阴分，交结不解的病证。症见出汗后仍发热、狂言、不能食、脉躁疾等，多属重症。

Yin-Yang Interlocking a condition seen at the critical stage of a febrile disease, due to attack on yinfen by yang pathogen manifested as fever after sweating, crazy talk, anorexia, irritable and fast pulse, etc.

阴阳离决 【yīn yáng lí jué】即阴阳正常关系的分离决裂，是阴阳失调发展到最严重阶段。这时，生命现象也随

Separation of Yin and Yang a pathological condition manifested itself as a split of the normal relation-

之结束。

阴阳胜复 【yīn yáng shèng fù】阴阳双方交替的亢盛和衰退,用于解释某些气候变化和病理现象。

阴阳失调 【yīn yáng shī tiáo】即是阴阳消长失去平衡协调的简称。是指机体在疾病发生发展过程中,由于各种致病因素的影响,导致机体的阴阳失去相对的平衡,从而形成阴阳偏胜、偏衰,或阴不制阳、阳不制阴的病理状态。

阴阳消长 【yīn yáng xiāo zhǎng】阴阳双方是互相依存互相对立的,并总是此盛彼衰,此消彼长地变化。

阴阳转化 【yīn yáng zhuǎn huà】在一定的条件下,阴阳双方可以互相转化,阴可以转化为阳,阳可以转化为阴。如在病理上,阳证可以转化成阴证。阴证可以转化成阳证。

阴阳自和 【yīn yáng zì hé】在病理情况下,阴阳失去正常的平衡关系,经过适当的治疗,失去平衡的阴阳重新趋向平衡。表示疾病的好转或痊愈。

ship between yin and yang, which is the most serious upset between yin and yang, indicates the end of life.

Preponderance between Yin and Yang the alteration of excessiveness and deficiency between yin and yang. This view is used to interprete some climatic variations and pathological phenomena.

Incoordination between Yin and Yang a morbid state of the breakdown of yin-yang equilibrium, due to various pathogenic factors, leading to relative excessiveness or deficiency of yin and yang, or the failure of yin and yang to restrict each other.

Wane and Wax of Yin and Yang a phenomenon of the interdependence and mutual contradition of yin and yang, e. g., the excessiveness of yang may give rise to the deficiency of yin, and vice versa; the growth of yang may lead to the declination of yin, and vice versa.

Transformation between Yin and Yang yin and yang are interchangeable each other under certain circumstances. Pathologically, the yang syndrome can be transformed into yin syndrome, and vice versa.

Reestablishment of Equilibrium between Yin and Yang a condition indicating the convalescence, or recovery of a disease. The equilibrium between yin and yang is destroyed in the morbid state and is reestablished

阴痒 【yīn yáng】指外阴瘙痒。多因外阴不洁，感染或湿热蕴结，流注于下所致；也有因阴虚血燥而致。

阴液 【yīn yè】精、血、津、液等各种体液成分的通称。因其均属阴，故称。

阴脏 【yīn zàng】1、指患者的阴盛体质。2、指脾、肺、肾三脏。

阴躁 【yīn zào】指阴寒极盛所致的躁扰不安，且常伴有四肢厥冷、冷汗自出、脉微欲绝等症状。本症多由阴盛格阳所引起，常见于病情危重的患者。

阴证 【yīn zhèng】八纲中的里证、寒证、虚证。症见面色苍白或暗晦，倦卧肢冷、静而少言、语声低微、呼吸微弱、气短乏力、饮食减少、腹痛喜按、舌淡胖嫩、苔润滑、脉沉缓无力等。

by proper treatment.

Pruritus Vulvae intense itching of the external genitals of the female, caused by local infection or accumulation of dampness-heat pathogen, or by yin deficiency and blood-dryness.

Yin Fluid the components of body fluid such as essence, blood, thin and thick fluid, etc. which are attributive to yin.

Yin Organs 1. body constitution characteristic of yin hyperactivity.
2. zang-organs pertaining to yin referring to the spleen, lung and kidney.

Yin Type Irritability a syndrome usually seen in the critical stage of a disease, due to the extreme excess of yin-cold in the interior expelling the yang-qi to the superficies; manifested as irritability, and accompanied with cold limbs, profuse night sweat, impalpable pulse, etc.

Yin-Syndrome the interior, cold and deficiency syndromes among the eight principal syndromes, which are attributive to yin, and manifested as pale or lusterless complexion, cold limbs, desire for lying quietly, low voice, weak breathing, lassitude, poor appetite, flat taste in the mouth, loose stools, discharge of large amount of watery urine, abdominal pain which can be relieved by pressure, pale, enlarged and tender tongue with moist and smooth fur, sunken and slow,

阴证似阳 【yīn zhèng sì yáng】本质属阴的疾病，其临床表现却类似阳证，见于虚寒性疾病发展到严重阶段而出现的一种假象。

阴中之阳 【yīn zhōng zhī yáng】阴阳学说内容之一。指任何事物都可以分为阴阳两方面，属于阴的事物又可分两方面，其中阴性事物中又有分属阳的一方面。

阴中之阴 【yīn zhōng zhī yīn】阴阳学说内容之一。任何事物都可以分为阴阳两方面，属于阴的事物又可分为两方面，其中阴性事物中又有分属阴的一方面。

阴肿 【yīn zhǒng】妇女外阴部肿痛的一种病变。多由阴户破损，感染毒气，或肝脾二经湿热下注所致。

阴纵 【yīn zòng】 即阴茎挺长不收，或肿胀而痿的病证。本症多由肝经湿热引起。

瘖痱 【yīn fèi】指语言不利或失语，伴有四肢痿废、不能活动的病证。多由肾精亏损，或风痰阻塞经脉引起。

weak pulse, etc.

Yin-Syndrome Appearing as Yang-Syndrome a case of yin nature with some clinical manifestations of yang-syndrome, considered as a false phenomenon appearing during the critical stage of an asthenia-cold syndrome.

The Aspect of Yang within Yin one of the contents in the yin-yang theory. Anything can be divided into two aspects, yin and yang. The aspect of yin may be rediveded into two aspects, one of which is the aspect of yang within yin.

The Aspect of Yin within Yin one of the contents in the yin-yang theory. Anything can be divided into two aspects, yin and yang. The aspect of yin can be rediveded into two aspects, one of which is the aspect of yin within yin.

Swelling of Vulva a disorder accompanied with local pain, mostly due to local injury and infection, or the attack of dampness heat pathogen from the meridians of the liver and spleen.

Priapism a syndrome marked by persistent penile erection or swelling and flaccidity of the penis, mostly due to the accumulation of dampness-heat pathogen in the liver meridian.

Aphasia and Paralysis of Limbs a morbid condition mostly due to consumption of kidney essence or obstruction of meridians by wind-phlegm.

引火归原 【yǐn huǒ guī yuán】治疗肾的虚火上升的方法。肾火上升表现为上热下寒,症见面色浮红、头晕耳鸣、口舌糜烂、牙痛、腰酸腿软、两足发冷、舌质嫩红及脉虚等。

Conducting the Fire Back to its Origin (kidney) a treatment for the ascending of asthenic fire of kidney, applicable to the case with heat syndrome in the upper part but cold in the lower, manifested as flushed face, dizziness, tinnitus, erosion of the oral cavity and tongue, toothache, soreness and weakness of the loins and legs, cold feet, reddish and tender tongue, feeble pulse, etc.

引经报使 【yǐn jīng bào shǐ】指某些药物能引导其他药物到达病变所在部位,有加强药效的作用。

Guiding Drug the drug which acts as a guide of other drugs to reach the affected part and enhances their therapeutic effects.

引气 【yǐn qì】是将呼吸之气或结合内气,以意念引运到身体某一部位,现代一般称为以意敛气。

Directing Qi guiding intrinsic qi or breathing qi to a certain part of the body, also called directing qi with will.

饮 【yǐn】1、汤剂名称之一,如桑菊饮。2、指饮证,如痰饮、溢饮。3、指汤水、饮料等。

Drink 1. a decoction of Chinese medicine, such as decoction of Folium Mori and Flos Chrysanthemi. 2. **Fluid-Retention Syndrome** referring to phlegm retention syndrome, diffuse fluid retention syndrome, etc. 3. **Beverage**

饮食中毒 【yǐn shí zhòng dú】泛指误食含有毒性金属盐类的食物、毒蕈、有毒鱼类、含有细菌及毒素食物引起中毒。症见呕吐、腹痛、腹泻、发热等。严重者可致昏迷、虚脱、甚则死亡。

Food Poisoning intoxication due to taking food contaminated by poisons, or poisonous and putrefactive food; manifested as abdominal pain, diarrhea, fever, and also coma, collapse, or even death in severe case.

饮酒中毒 【yǐn jiǔ zhòng dú】(酒精中毒)由于饮酒过量,酒毒渍于脾胃,流溢经络所致。

Acute Alcoholism simple drunkenness due to attack of alcoholic poison involving the spleen, stomach, and meridians resulting from excessive in-

饮片 【yǐn piàn】指中药经过加工处理后，成为片、丝、块、段等形状，便于煎汤饮服。
Prepared Medicinal Herb the herb being processed as various forms, i. e., pieces, strips, lumps or segments, and prepared for decoction.

饮家 【yǐn jiā】患痰饮证的病人。
Patient Suffering from Phlegm Retention Syndrome

饮痫 【yǐn xián】指伴有食欲异常的痫证。多见于小儿，食欲异常，时时发生手足抽动。多因痰热食积所致。
Epilepsy with Abnormal Appetite infantile epilepsy induced by improper diet, accompanied with abnormal appetite and intermittent twitching of the extremities; usually due to phlegm-heat or indigestion.

饮证 【yǐn zhèng】指体内过量水液不得转输运化，停留或渗注于某一部位而发生的病证。属痰饮范围。见痰饮。
Fluid Retention Syndrome a type of phlegm retention syndrome due to accumulation of excessive amount of body fluid which is retained in certain part of the body.

饮心痛 【yǐn xīn tòng】因水饮停积所致的胃脘痛。症见胃脘痛、干呕或呕吐清涎或呕水、恶心烦闷、或胁下有水声、脉弦滑等。
Stomachache due to Retention of Fluid a disorder manifested as stomachache, retching or vomiting of watery fluid, nausea, sound of water bubbling in the hypochondrium, wiry and smooth pulse, etc.

饮子 【yǐn zǐ】不规定时间冷服的汤剂。
Drink a cold medicinal decoction to be taken at any time.

隐疹 【yǐn zhěn】（瘾疹、荨麻疹）因内蕴湿热、复感风寒，郁于皮腠而发；或对某些物质过敏所致。皮肤出现大小不等的风团，甚则成块成片、剧痒、时隐时现，即荨麻疹。
Urticaria a condition due to accumulation of dampness-heat pathogen and attack of wind-cold pathogen to the skin as well, or due to hypersensitivity to certain substances, marked by the intermittent occurrence of various sizes of elevated patches which are accompanied with intense itching.

樱桃痔 【yīng táo zhì】指痔形如樱桃。
Rectal Polyp

膺　【yīng】即前胸部。

迎风冷泪　【yíng fēng lěng lèi】眼部无红肿痛痒，但流泪，迎风尤甚，泪液清稀无热感。多因肝肾两虚，不能约束其液所致。

迎风流泪　【yíng fēng liú lèi】双眼遇风流泪，甚至流下频频。有冷泪和热泪之分。

迎风热泪　【yíng fēng rè lèi】由风热外袭，肝肺火炽；或肝肾阴虚，虚火上炎所致。症见遇到风则双眼热泪频流，伴有双目赤涩疼痛羞明等。

迎随补泻　【yíng suí bǔ xiè】针刺时使针尖顺着经脉循行方向进针和操作，称为随，属补法；针刺时针类逆经脉循行方向进针和操作的称为迎，属泻法。

营　【yíng】是人体生命活动所必需的物质之一。由食物经过脏腑的功能活动而成，行于经脉之中，具有营养人体各部分的作用。

Chest

Irritated Epiphora with Cold Tears an overflow of cold tears occurring after wind blow, but with no reddness, swelling, pain and itching in the eyes; usually caused by asthenia of both the liver and kidney with inability to control the flow of tears.

Epiphora an overflow of tears which may be cold or warm, as a result of irritation by wind blow.

Irritated Epiphora with Warm Tears an overflow of warm tears occurring after wind blow, accompanied with pain and congestion of the eye, and photophobia; due to attack of wind-heat and hyperactivity of liver fire and lung fire, or due to deficiency of liver-yin and kidney-yin with hyperactivity of asthenic fire.

Tonifying and Dispersing by Adjusting the Direction of Needle Insertion the acupuncture manipulation in which the tonifying effect is achieved by inserting the needle in the same direction of the meridian circulation, and the dispersing effect is achieved by inserting the needle in the opposite direction of the meridian circulation.

Nutriment one of the essential substances for body life activities. It is derived form the digested food and absorbed by the internal organs, and circulates in the vessels to nourish all parts of the boy.

营气 【yíng qì】是与血共行于脉中的精气。具有生化血液和营养全身的功能。营气属阴，故又称营阴。

Ying Qi essential substance circulating in the meridians and blood vessels, responsible for blood production and body nourishment. It is also called ying-yin, as it is attributive to yin.

营卫不和 【yíng wèi bù hé】营卫功能失调而致表证有汗的病理现象。

Disharmony between Ying and Wei a morbid state of spontaneous perspiration in the superficies syndrome due to dysfunction of ying and wei.

营分证 【yíng fèn zhèng】是温热病邪气内陷的阶段。多由气分证传变或卫分证逆传而来，以夜热甚、心烦不寐；或神昏谵语、斑疹隐现、舌质红绛、脉细数为特征。

Yingfen Syndrome a syndrome indicating the stage of pathogens invading the interior in a seasonal febrile disease, developing from qifen syndrome or weifen syndrome; marked by predominant fever at night, restlessness, insomnia, coma, delirium, invisible skin rashes, crimson tongue, small and fast pulse, etc.

营气不从 【yíng qì bù cóng】指血脉中营气运行障碍，出现痈肿的病理。

Stagnation of Ying Qi a morbid state of suppurative infection of the skin caused by circulatory disturbance of ying-qi in the blood vessels.

瘿 【yǐng】（大脖子）指颈前生长肿物，红而高突，或蒂小而下垂，有如"缨络"形状。发病与水土因素有关；或忧思郁怒，肝郁不舒，脾失健运，致气滞痰凝而成，相当于甲状腺肿大一类疾患。

Goiter a mass over the neck, referring to thyroid enlargement, an endermic disease, resulting from anxiety or anger leading to stagnation of the liver and dysfunction of the spleen, and then stagnation of qi and accumulation of phlegm.

硬下疳 【yìng xià gān】下疳的一种。症见阴茎、龟头、大小阴唇、阴道等处起硬结、不痛、不破溃。

Hard Chancre primary sore of syphilis occurring on the external genitals, manifested as indurated and painless papules.

痈 【yōng】指疮面浅而大者。多因外感六淫，过食膏粱厚味，外伤感染所

Carbuncle an abscess of the skin and subcutaneous tissue or of the vis-

致。可分内痈与外痈两类。

涌吐禁例 【yǒng tù jìn lì】禁用吐法的病例,如胸膈无痰涎壅塞、体虚、产后、病后、失血、老人、孕妇等。

忧膈 【yōu gé】因忧郁气结所致的噎膈。症见饮食噎塞不下,消瘦无力,烦闷短气等。

忧伤肺 【yōu shāng fèi】忧愁日久,可使肺气抑郁,甚而气郁化火,损伤肺阴。

幽门 【yōu mén】七冲门之一。即胃的下口,连接胃与十二指肠。

由里出表 【yóu lǐ chū biǎo】病邪从里向表透达,是病情好转的征象。

油汗 【yóu hàn】指汗出如油,粘腻不易流动。多见于亡阳虚脱的危重病人。

油灰指甲 【yóu huī zhī jiǎ】(甲癣)多由手足癣日久蔓延,以致血不荣爪而成。症见指(趾)甲增厚、变形、残缺不全、失去光泽而呈灰白色

cera, mostly caused by attack of the six pathogens, overtaking of greasy food, and trauma complicated by infection.

Cases Contraindicated for Emesis referring to the cases not suitable for emetic therapy, such as absence of accumulation of phlegm in the thorax, general debility, puerperant, convalescent, bleeding, the aged, pregnancy, etc.

Emotional Dysphagia a type of dysphagia due to melancoly and qi stagnation, manifested as difficulty in swallowing, emaciation, weakness, restlessness, shortness of breath, etc.

Grief Impairs the Lung a state of suppression lung qi due to prolonged grief or even damage of lung-yin by fire transmitted from the stagnation of qi.

Pylorus one of the seven important portals, the lower orifice of the stomach, connecting with duodenum.

From Interior to Superficies a condition in which the pathogenic factor is brough out from the interior to the superficies, showing subsidence of a disease.

Sticky Sweat a sign mostly seen in the critical condition of collapse resulting from yang depletion.

Tinea Unguium a mycotic infection of the nails spreaing from fingers and toes, with the nails becoming thickened, deformed broken, lustreless and

游风 【yóu fēng】多为脾肺燥热或表气不固，风邪袭于腠理，风热壅滞，营卫失调所致的疾病。常突然发作且游走不定，皮肤红晕、光亮、浮肿、形如云片、触之坚实、瘙痒、灼热、麻木。多发于口唇、眼睑、耳垂或胸腹、背部等处。一般无全身症状，但亦可伴有腹痛、腹泻、呕吐等症。即血管神经性水肿。

Wandering Edema a disorder due to retention of wind-heat pathogen and dysfunction of ying and wei resulting from dryness-heat in the spleen and lung, and the attack of wind pathogen to the weakened superficies; characterized by sudden onset and recurrent episodes of noninflammatory swelling of skin, mucous membrane and occasionally of viscera, often associated with erythema, urticaria and purpura, and occasionally with abdominal pain, diarrhea, vomiting, etc. syn. with giant urticaria.

有头疽 【yǒu tóu jū】指发于体表软组织之间的阳性疮疡。多因外感风湿火毒，或湿热火毒内蕴，使内脏积热，营卫不和，邪阻肌肤而成。初起患部色红发热，根束高肿，疮头如粟米，一个或多个不等，甚则疼痛剧烈、身热口渴、便秘溲赤，脉洪数。舌红苔黄。辨证分类 1、火毒凝结证 2、湿热壅滞证 3、阴虚火炽证 4、气虚毒滞证。

Carbuncle pyogenic infection of yang-type occurring between the skin and subcutaneous tissues, mostly due to exposure to wind, damp and fire pathogens or stagnation of damp, heat and fire in the interior involving the skin and muscles, and leading to disharmony between ying and wei; manifested as rednss, heat, and swelling of the affected part with multiple sinuses, or even severe pain, fever, thirst, constipation, dark urine, full and fast pulse, red tongue with yellowish fur. Types of differentiation. 1. stagnation of fire-toxin 2. retention of damp-heat 3. excessiveness of fire due to yin deficiency 4. stagnation of toxin due to qi deficiency.

瘀呃 【yū è】因瘀血阻滞胸膈所致的呃逆。症见心胸刺痛、饮水即呃、手

Hiccup due to Blood Stasis a type of hiccup due to accumulation of

足微冷、大便溏而色黑。blood stasis in the thorax, manifested as stabbing pain over the chest, hiccup induced by drinking, slightly cold limbs, loose and dark coloured stools.

瘀热 【yū rè】 1、热邪郁积在内。2、瘀血滞留引起发热的病理现象。

Stagnant Heat 1. heat pathogen retained in the interior. 2. a morbid state of fever due to blood stasis.

瘀血腹痛 【yū xuè fù tòng】指因气血瘀阻引起的腹痛。症见腹痛、痛处固定、拒按或腹痛经久不愈、舌质紫暗、脉涩等。

Abdominal Pain due to Blood Stasis abdominal pain due to stagnation of qi and blood; manifested as localized or long-standing pain and tenderness, purplish tongue, unsmooth pulse, etc.

瘀血腰痛 【yū xuè yāo tòng】因闪挫跌扑；或腰痛经久，瘀血凝积所致的腰痛。症见痛有定处、痛如锥刺、日轻夜重，伴小便赤、脉涩。

Lumbago due to Blood Stasis lumbago due to stagnation of blood resulting from sprain, trauma or prolonged pain; manifested as localized and stabbing pain over the loins, aggravated at night, accompanied with melena, darkened urine and unsmooth pulse.

瘀血 【yū xuè】指体内有血液停滞，包括离经之血积存体内，或血运不畅，阻滞于经脉及脏腑内的血液，均称为瘀血。其病证特点因瘀阻的部位和形成瘀血的原因不同而异。其临床共同特点是：疼痛，多为刺痛，痛处固定不移，拒按，夜间痛甚。

Blood Stasis a morbid condition caused by the accumulation of extravasated blood in the interior or stagnation of blood in the meridians and viscera; its characteristics varied with locations and causes; clinically manifested as localized stabbing pain, tenderness, and aggravated at night.

瘀血咳 【yū xuè ké】 指因瘀血阻于肺络所致的咳嗽。症见咳嗽、伴喉间常有腥味、吐血紫黑等。

Cough due to Blood Stasis cough due to obstruction of lung collaterals by blood stasis; accompanied with subjective stinking smell in the throat and dark purplish bloody expectoration.

瘀血头痛 【yū xuè tóu tòng】因头部外

Headache due to Blood Stasis

伤或久痛入络,瘀血阻滞脉络所致的头痛病证。症见头痛如锥刺、痛处固定、时发时止、经久不愈、舌有瘀斑、脉涩。

瘀血阻络 【yū xuè zǔ luò】因外伤或久痛不愈所致的一种病理。由于瘀血阻滞脉络,气血运行受阻,常引起以局部固定性刺痛为特点的各种痛证。如瘀血头痛、瘀血胃脘痛等。此外,某些出血性病证也被认为与瘀血阻络有关。

瘀血流注 【yū xuè liú zhù】由于跌打损伤;或产后恶露未尽,瘀滞经络,湿热毒邪乘虚而入,结肿而发生的流注病。初起局部肿胀,触之坚痛皮色微红或青紫,继则猩红灼热,并可向周围蔓延,伴有恶寒发热,骨节疼痛等症。

鱼翔脉 【yú xiáng mài】脉博极度微弱,似有似无的脉象。

headache due to obstruction of collaterals by blood stasis which is resulted from head trauma or prolonged pain; manifested as stabbing, localized, intermittent but lingering headache, ecchymosis over the tongue, and unsmooth pulse.

Obstruction of Collaterals by Blood Stasis a morbid state due to trauma or prolonged pain. Since the collaterals are obstructed by blood stasis and the flow of qi and blood is blocked, it may result in various disorders characterized by constant localized stabbing pain, such as headache due to blood stasis, stomachache due to blood stasis, etc. Furthermore, certain hemorrhagic diseases are also considered to be related to the condition.

Multiple Abscess due to Blood Stasis circumscribed collections of pus due to trauma or retention of lochia leading to the accumulation of blood stasis in the meridians and collaterals, and the invasion of virulent dampness-heat pathogen; characterized by local swelling, induration, tenderness, erythema, and cyanosis of skin, followed by red colouration, scorching heat, and involving the surrounding tissues, accompanied with aversion to cold, fever, osteodynia, arthralgia, etc.

Fish-Swimming Pulse a pulse condition which is extremely weak and

髃骨伤 【yú gú shāng】髃骨即肩胛骨。多因跌打损伤、坠撞所伤。症见疼痛肿胀，压痛明显，活动受限，触按有骨声。

Fracture of Scapula breaking of the scapula by injury, marked by local swelling, pain, tenderness, limitation of movement, and friction sound.

伛偻 【yǔ lǚ】指驼背的症候。

Hunchback

语迟 【yǔ chí】小儿至四、五岁尚不能说话。多因先天肾气不足，心气不和所致；亦可由后天脾胃亏损引起。

Retardation in Speech inability to speak up to the age of four or five years old, mostly due to congenital deficiency of the kidney qi and disorder of the heart qi, or due to acquired asthenia of the spleen and stomach.

语声重浊 【yǔ shēng zhòng zhuó】说话或咳嗽的声调重浊不清的证候。多因外感风寒或内有痰湿困阻，使气道不畅所致。

Low Raucous Voice a syndrome of hoarse and indistinct sounds in speaking or coughing, usually due to obstruction of the air passage resulting from the attack of wind-cold factors or the accumulation of phlegm-dampness.

玉翳浮睛 【yù yì fú jīng】（玉翳遮睛、玉翳浮满）即大片白翳盖满黑睛，类似全角膜白斑病。本病起病多由肝经风热引起，病久反复发作者多属肝肾不足。

Nebula Covering the Cornea a white opacity of the whole cornea, usually due to attack of wind-heat in the liver meridian, or due to asthenia of the liver and kidney in recurrent cases.

育阴潜阳 【yù yīn qián yáng】滋阴与潜阳药合用以治疗肝肾阴虚，肝阳上亢的方法。症见头痛眩晕、耳鸣耳聋、烦躁易怒、面红目赤、失眠多梦、舌质红、脉弦细数等。

Nourishing Yin and Suppressign the Excessive Yang a treatment for deficiency of liver yin and kidney yin and hyperactivity of liver yang by means of application of nourishing yin and suppressing excessive yang medicine, manifested as headache, dizziness, tinnitus, deafness, irritability, flushed face, insomnia, dreamfulness, red tongue, wiry and small, fast pulse, etc.

郁证 【yù zhèng】由于情志不畅，气机郁滞所引起的病证，症见心情抑郁、情绪不宁、胁肋窜痛、或易怒善哭、咽中如有物梗阻、咯之不出等。

郁火 【yù huǒ】 泛指阳气受抑郁而出现热盛的证候，可出现头痛、目赤、口舌生疮、腹痛、便秘、小便赤、舌红苔黄、脉数实等。

郁冒 【yù mào】1、症见胸闷、头昏、眼花、汗出、全身乏力等的病证。血虚、伤津、或肝郁等均可引起。2、见血厥。

郁热遗精 【yù rè yí jīng】由肝肾热郁，精关易于疏泄所致的遗精病证。伴有烦热、夜眠梦多、头晕、心悸等。多因肝肾阴虚，郁热内扰所致。

欲传 【yù chuán】病邪有发展的趋向。如外感风寒、发热、恶寒、无汗，微汗而发热不退、心烦口渴、脉数，是病邪将化热传里的表现。

Melancholia a syndrome due to emotional upsets and stagnation of qi, manifested as mental depression, emotional lability, hypochondriac pain, liability to be angry and crying, obstructive sensation in the throat, etc.

Stagnated Fire a syndrome of heat domination resulting from the stagnation of yang-qi; manifested as headache, congestion of conjunctiva, aphtha, abdominal pain, constipation, deep coloured urine, red tongue with yellowish fur, fast and replete pulse, etc.

Fainting a disorder marked by oppressive feeling over the chest, dizziness, sweating and fatigue, resulting from deficiency of blood, consumption of fluid, or stagnation of liver qi.

Nocturnal Emission due to Stagnated Heat a disorder due to stagnation of heat in the liver and kidney, characterized by nocturnal emission, accompanied with restlessness, dreaminess, dizziness, palpitation, etc.

Pathogenic Factors Tending to Transmit a condition indicating the further development of a disease. For instance, a disease due to exposure to wind-cold factors with symptoms such as fever, chilliness and anhidrosis, is considered to be the manifestation of the transmission of heat factor to the interior, when sweating, continuous fever, restlessness, thirst and fast pulse occur.

元气虚弱 【yuán qì xū ruò】由于元阴元阳之气不足而致脏腑功能低下的病理现象。

原（元）气 【yuán qì】是机体生命活动的源泉，包括元阴和元阳之气，由先天之精所化生，并依靠后天营养而不断滋生。

圆癣 【yuán xuǎn】（体癣）由外邪侵袭皮肤或接触传染而得。好发于面、颈、躯干、四肢等。病损为硬币状圆形红斑，边缘清楚。

圆翳内障 【yuán yì nèi zhàng】（圆翳）即白内障。多因肝肾不足或肝经风热上攻而成。症见瞳内有圆形白色翳障，瞳神外观正常。

远道刺 【yuǎn dào cì】在离病处较远部位扎针施治的刺法。

远血 【yuǎn xuè】指出血部位远离肛门，多在胃与小肠，表现为先出粪便而后便血，血色暗黑。多因饮食不节及肝气犯胃以致脾胃虚寒，脾不统血或肝郁化火，迫血妄行所致。

Deficiency of Primordial Qi a morbid condition of hypofunction of the viscera resulting from deficiency of the qi of original yin and original yang.

Primordial Qi the source of the life activities of the human body, including the qi of both primordial yin and primordial yang. It is derived from the congenital essence, and regenerated persistently by the nutrients obtained from food.

Tinea Circinata fungal infection of the skin appearing on the face, neck, trunk, extremities, etc. marked by a well defined, macular and annular lesion; caused by the attack of exogenous pathogen on the skin or by direct contact with fungus.

Cataract a disorder due to asthenia of the liver and kidney, or attack of wind-heat in the liver meridian to the eye; manifested as opacity of the crystalline lens of the eye but with normal appearance of the pupil.

Distant Puncture an acupuncture therapy by puncturing the poins far from the affected part.

Bleeding from Distant Part the passage of dark and pitchy hemaecia resulting from the bleeding far from the anus, e. g., the bleeding of the stomach and small intestine; due to inability to keep the blood in the vessels by the asthenia-cold spleen which is impaired by immoderate diet or by the sthenic liver qi, or to the extravasation of blood resulting from the stagnation of liver qi with the formation of fire factor.

约束 【yuē shù】眼睑的别称。因它有调节眼裂大小的作用。故称。

Restrainer another name for eyelid. It is so called because it has the function of regulating the width of the palpebral fissure.

哕 【yuě】1、见呃逆。2、指干呕。

1. Hiccup 2. Retching

月经过少 【yuè jīng guò shǎo】经期血量过少或经行时间过短的病证。多因血虚、血寒和肾虚所致。

Oligomenorrhea a disease marked by scanty menstrual flow or shortened menstrual cycle, usually caused by blood-asthenia, blood-cold and kidney-asthenia.

月经不调 【yuè jīng bù tiáo】泛指月经周期、经量、经色、经质异常的各种病证。

Menoxenia a general term for the disorder with abnormal menstrual amount, colour and character as well as irregular menstrual cycle.

月经过多 【yuè jīng guò duō】经期血量过多或行经时间延长的病证。多因气虚、血热、劳伤等使冲任不固所致。

Menorrhagia a disorder characterized by excessive uterine bleeding occurring at regular intervals of menstruation or prolonged duration of menstruation; usually due to debility of thoroughfare and conception vessels resulting from deficiency of qi, blood-heat, over strain, etc.

月经病 【yuè jīng bìng】指月经方面各种病证的总称。包括月经周期、经量、经色、经质的异常和经期及其前后出现的明显症状。

Menopathy referring to various menstrual disorders, including the abnormality of the cycle, amount, colour and character, as well as the symptoms appearing before, during and after the menstrual cycle.

越经传 【yuè jīng chuán】伤寒病不按六经的次序传变。如邪初犯太阳经，不传阳明而传少阳。

Skip-over Transmission through Meridians the progress of a seasonal febrile disease is not in the sequence of the six meridians, e. g. the pathogen primarily attacking taiyang meridian invades shaoyang meridian instead of yangming meridian.

晕针 【yūn zhēn】因针刺而发生的晕厥现象。多与患者体质虚弱、饥饿、疲劳、精神紧张或体位不当有关。

Fainting during Acupuncture an abnormal reaction to acupuncture, it is usually related with general debility, hunger, fatigue, mental stress, or improper posture during acupuncture.

云翳 【yún yì】即角膜出现云片状的角膜翳痕。多为黑睛损伤,消退后遗留之翳膜。相当于角膜瘢痕。

Nebula a slight corneal opacity or scar resulting from injury of the cornea.

运脾 【yùn pí】使用芳香化湿与理气健脾药以治疗湿困脾胃病证的治法。

Activating the Spleen a treatment for the accumulation of dampness in the spleen by the application of fragrant drugs with the dampness-eliminating action and drugs with the qi-regulating and spleen-invigorating action.

运气胁痛 【yùn qì xié tòng】因感受疫疠之气所致的胁痛病证。症见病起急骤、暴发寒热、胁肋刺痛、遍身作胀、脉多弦数;危重者可出现四肢厥逆、指甲紫黑、脉沉伏等。

Hypochondriac Pain due to Pestilent Pathogen a disorder manifested as sudden onset of chills and fever, hypochondriac stabbing pain, distending feeling all over the body, wiry and fast pulse, and cold limbs, purplish dark nails, sunken and impalpable pulse in serious cases.

孕悲 【yùn bēi】妇女妊娠期发生的脏躁病(类似癔病)。

Sorrowful State during Pregnancy a psychosis appearing during pregnancy, similar to hysteria.

熨法 【yùn fǎ】将药末或药物粗粒炒热,用布包后,外熨局部皮肤的一种治疗方法,适用于各种寒性痛证。

Topical Application of Heated Drugs an external therapy of applying heated medicinal powder or granules wrapped in a cloth to the affected part, applicable to the painful disorders of cold type.

杂病 【zá bìng】泛指外感病以外的内科疾病。

再逆 【zài nì】在治疗过程中又出了一次差错。

脏毒 【zàng dú】1、指内伤积久所致的便血，血色黯，多在便后。2、指脏中积毒所致的痢疾。3、指肛门痈。4、指肛门肿硬，疼痛便血。

脏气 【zàng qì】即五脏之气。指五脏的功能活动。

脏结 【zàng jié】古病名。1、指症状似结胸，心下痞硬，按之痛，时有腹泻，饮食如故，苔白腻，脉沉紧细小。多因邪气乘虚入里，与阴寒互结所致。2、指胁下素有痞块，连在脐旁，痛引少腹入筋的一种难治病证。

脏会 【zàng huì】八会之一。即章门穴，五脏精气会聚的地方。

脏真 【zàng zhēn】真气的一部分。是五脏进行生理活动的原动力。

Miscellaneous Diseases internal diseases other than those caused by exogenous pathogenic factors.

Another Mistake in Treatment

Risceral Intoxication 1. hematochezia with dark reddish bloody discharge due to prolonged visceral damage. 2. dysentery due to retention of toxin in the viscera. 3. carbuncle around the anus. 4. perianal abscess and painful hemafecia.

Zang-Qi functional activities of the zang organs.

Accumulation of Pathogenic Factors in the Viscera 1. a syndrome similar to that resulting from accumulation in the thorax, marked by epigastric tenderness, diarrhea, diet as usual, whitish and greasy fur, sunken, tense and thready pulse; due to attack of pathogens to the interior blending with yin-cold. 2. an intractable disease marked by mass in the hypochondrium down to the side of umbilicus with pain referring to the lower abdomen and external genitalia.

Convergent Point of the Zang Organs one of the eight convergent points, i. e., zhangmen point where the essential substances of the five zang organs gather.

Qi of the Five Zang Organs a part of qi serving as the motive force for physiological activities of the five

脏象 【zàng xiàng】是中医学的重要学说之一。指人体内脏表现于外的生理、病理现象。

脏痈痔 【zàng yōng zhì】指肛门肿如馒头，两边合紧，外坚而内溃，常流脓水的疾病。类似肛管直肠癌。

脏象学说 【zàng xiàng xué shuō】即是通过对人体生理、病理现象的观察，研究人体各个脏腑的生理功能、病理变化及其相互关系的学说。脏象学说对于阐明人体的生理和病理，指导临床实践具有普遍的指导意义。

脏厥 【zàng jué】古病名。指因内脏阳气衰微而引起的四肢厥冷冷。属寒厥重证。

脏腑相合 【zàng fǔ xiàng hé】指脏与腑在生理功能和病理变化的互相联系和影响。

脏腑辨证 【zàng fǔ biàn zhèng】以脏腑生理、病理特点为基础，通过四诊八纲，分析判别五脏六腑的阴阳、气血、寒热等变化的一种临床思维方法。是中医辨证的基本方法之一。

zang organs.

State of Viscera one of the major doctrines in TCM, referring to visceral outward manifestations through which physiological functions as well as pathological changes can be detected.

Anorectal Carrcinoma an indurated mass in the rectum with the blockage of the anal orifice and discharge of purulent fluid.

Viscera-State Doctrine a doctrine on the physiological functions, pathological changes of viscera, and their relationships, through the observation of the physiological and pathological phenomena of the body. It serves as a universal guide for interpreting the physiological and pathological conditions of the body and directing clinical practice.

Coldness of Extremities due to Visceral Disorder a serious cold-syndrome due to exhaustion of yang-qi in the viscera.

The Zang and Fu Organs Are in Couples the organs in couples correlate with one another physiologically and pathologically.

Differential Diagnosis according to State of Viscera one of the basic methods of differential diagnosis in TCM, i. e., to analyse and differentiate the changes of yin and yang, qi and blood, cold and heat, asthenia and sthenia of the viscera, based on the

脏躁 【zàng zào】是一种发作性的精神病,以女性多见。发作时多表现为自觉烦闷、急躁、无故叹息或悲伤欲哭等。多由心肝血虚,情志抑郁引起。

早泄 【zǎo xiè】 性交时泄精过早的证候。多由肾虚,相火过旺所致。

枣花翳内障 【zǎo huā yī nèi zhàng】(枣花翳)其翳膜形状似枣花或锯齿的病证。多见于湿热,痰火壅盛;或嗜好酒、辣之病者。

燥 【zào】(燥气)1、燥邪。六淫之一。其特点是易伤津液,可致目赤、口鼻干燥、干咳、胁痛、便秘等症。2、阴津亏损出现的内病证。见内躁。

燥火眩晕 【zào huǒ xuàn yùn】因感受燥热之邪所致的眩晕。症见身热烦躁、口渴引饮、夜卧不宁、头旋眼黑、小便赤涩、脉躁疾等。

燥剂 【zào jì】指主要由燥湿药物组成,如苍术、厚朴、赤小豆之类,具有燥湿作用的方剂。

physiological and pathological characteristics of the viscera.

Hysteria a paroxysmal psychoneurosis mostly seen in female, due to deficiency of the heart-blood and liver-blood and mental depression; manifested as subjective vexation, irritability, sighing without cause, inclination to crying due to sorrow.

Premature Ejaculation ejaculation of the semen at the beginning of the sexual intercourse, usually due to hyperactivity of the sexual life (the ministerial fire) resulting from asthenia of the kidney.

Incipient Cataract a cataract that has sectors of opacity with clear spaces intervening, usually seen in cases of accumulation of damp-heat and phlegm-fire factors or addition to alcohol and pungent food.

Dryness 1. the dryness, one of the six pathogenic factors, which tends to consume the boy fluid, and may lead to conjunctival congestion, dry mouth and nose,

Dizziness Caused by Dryness-Fire a type of dizziness manifested as fever, irritability, extreme thirst, restless sleep, vertigo, dysuria with discharge of reddish urine, fast pulse, etc.

Prescription with Drying Effect a prescription made up of drugs with the effect of expelling damp, such as Rhizoma Atractylodis, Cortex Magnoliae officinalis, Semen Phaseoli, etc.

燥痉 【zào jìng】 燥灼伤津所致的痉证。多见于热病后期,因热盛津伤,化燥动风,筋脉失养所致。症见发热、四肢痉挛、口燥咽干、皮肤干燥等。

Convlsive Seizures due to Dryness a disorder usually seen in the late stage of febrile diseases, due to consumption of body fluid and failure to nourish the muscles; manifested as fever, spasms of limbs, dryness in the mouth and throat, dryness of skin, etc.

燥可去湿 【zào kě qù shī】用燥湿的药物,能够治疗湿浊内盛,胸痞腹满之中焦湿邪。如因水湿停滞引起的水肿、小便不利,痰湿引起的咳嗽、气喘,湿阻中焦之脘腹胀满,倦怠厌食等。

Prescription with Drying Effect Can Expel the Damp prescription made up of drugs with drying effect applied for treating stuffiness in the chest and fullness in the stomach due to accumulation of damp in the middle energizer, edema and dysuria due to retention of fluid, cough and dyspnea due to damp-phlegm, fullness in epigastrium, lassitude and anorexia due to retention of damp in the middle energizer, etc.

燥气伤肺 【zào qì shāng fèi】燥邪伤于肺经,耗伤肺脏津液的病理。症见干咳、无痰或咯痰带血、咽喉疼痛、胸胁痛等。

Impairment of the Lung by Dryness a morbid state leading to the exhaustion of lung-fluid; manifested as non-productive cough, or cough with bloody sputum, sorethroat, pain in the chest and hypochondrium, etc.

燥热 【zào rè】(燥火)因感受燥邪,耗伤津液,以致化热化火的病证。症见目赤、牙龈肿痛、咽痛、口干、鼻衄、干咳、咯血等。

Dryness-Heat Syndrome a heat-syndrome resulting from consumption of body fluid after the invasion of the dryness, manifested as congestion of the eyes, swelling and pain of the gums, sorethroat, dry mouth, epistaxis, dry cough, hemoptysis, etc.

燥热咳嗽 【zào rè ké sòu】(燥咳)指外感风热燥邪,耗伤肺金所致的咳嗽。症见干咳无痰或痰少粘稠、不易咯出,鼻燥咽干,咳甚胸胁痛,或有

Cough Caused by Dryness-Heat a type of cough due to impairment of the lung by exogenous wind, heat, and dryness, manifested as non-pro-

形寒身热等表证。舌红少津。ductive cough or difficult expectoration of scanty amount of viscid sputum, dry nose and dry throat, or even chest pain, or other manifestations of superficies-syndrome with chills and fever, red tongue and deficiency of fluid, etc.

燥热痿 【zào rè wěi】由燥热伤津耗血,宗筋失于营养所致的痿证。症见手足痿软、不能行动,伴有皮毛干枯、口燥唇焦等。

Flaccidity Caused by Dryness-Heat a syndrome due to consumption of body fluid and blood by dryness-heat leading to muscular malnutrition; manifested as flaccidity of limbs with difficulty in movement, accompanied with dry skin, mouth and lips, etc.

燥胜则干 【zào shèng zé gān】燥邪偏胜,耗伤津液而出现干燥的病理。

Hyperactivity of Dryness may Cause Dehydration a morbid condition of consumption of body fluid as a result of hyperactive dryness.

燥湿 【zào shī】用味苦性燥的药物祛除湿邪的方法。适用于湿阻中焦的病证。常分为苦温燥湿和苦寒燥湿。

Drying the Damp a treatment for eliminating the damp by the application of drugs with bitter taste and dry nature, applicable to the case with retention of dampness in the middle energizer; usually accomplished by the application of drugs with bitter taste and warm nature, or drugs with bitter taste and cold nature.

燥湿化痰 【zào shī huà tán】化痰法之一。是治疗湿痰的方法。适用于脾阳不振、运化失司、聚湿生痰。症见痰白而易咯、胸闷恶心、或头眩心悸、舌苔白滑而腻等。

Drying the Damp and Eliminating Phlegm a treatment for eliminating damp-phlegm, applicable to the case with accumulation of damp and phlegm due to insufficiency of the spleen-yang, manifested as discharge of whitish sputum, feeling of oppression over the chest, nausea, dizziness, palpitation, whitish, smooth and

燥失 【zào shǐ】（燥屎）指干燥硬结的粪便。属阳明腑实证者，多伴有发热、烦渴、腹胀痛拒按等；属津虚燥结者，虽数天不大便，但无腹胀痛。

Dry Stool　　a disorder attributed to sthenia syndrome of yangming fu-organ is usually accompanied with fever, thirst, abdominal distending pain, tenderness, etc; while that due to consumption of body fluid and retention of pathogenic dryness is usually manifested as constipation but without abdominal distending pain.

燥者濡之 【zào zhě rú zhī】因燥邪所致的阴津亏损的疾病，一般宜用滋润的方药进行治疗。

Dryness Syndrome should Be Treated with Moistening Therapy　　a therapeutic principle for treating the disease with consumption of yin-fluid due to dryness factor.

燥痰 【zào tán】指由肺燥所致的一种痰症。症见痰少色白粘稠、涩而难咯，或兼见面白色枯、皮毛干焦、口干咽燥、咳嗽喘促等。

Dryness Sputum　　a syndrome due to dryness of the lung with manifestations of scanty sputum which is white and sticky, too astringent to be coughed out or complicated by pale and withered complexion, dry skin, dry mouth and throat, cough with asthma.

贼邪 【zéi xié】五邪之一。即按五行相克规律传变，以所不胜的脏传来的病邪。

Thieving Pathogens　　one of the five pathogens, i. e. pathogenic factors transmitting from the zang organ, according to the interacting relation of the five elements.

增水行舟 【zēng shuǐ xíng zhōu】属润下法。使用滋阴润燥药物，治疗属温病热结津枯所致便秘证的一种方法，犹如水涨则船行通畅，故名。

Smooth Sailing with Water Rising　　method of causing laxation by administering drugs with yin nourishing and moistening effect to treat constipation caused by accumulation of heat and exhaustion of body fluid in febrile diseases, which is compared to smooth sailing with water rising.

增液润下 【zēng yè rùn xià】属润下法。使用甘平滋阴增液的药物，治疗大肠热结津枯所致的便秘。

乍疏乍数 【zhà shū zhà shuò】脉律不整，时快时慢，散乱无序的一种脉象。多因气血即将消亡所致，常是病情垂危的反映。

痄腮 【zhà sāi】（流行性腮腺炎）为感受温毒病邪后，肠胃积热与肝胆郁火壅遏少阳经脉所致。症见一侧或先后在两侧腮腺部位肿胀，边缘不清，按之有柔韧感，并有疼痛和压痛。冬、春季节常见。辨证分类：分常证和变证。常证包括温毒在表和热毒蕴结两型，变证包括毒陷心肝和邪窜肝经两型。

谵妄 【zhān wàng】指意识模糊、胡言乱语、有错觉幻觉等证候。多因里热过盛，痰火内扰心神或热入心包所致。

Promoting the Production of Body Fluid to Relax the Bowels one of the therapeutic methods of causing laxtion, by administering drugs of sweet taste with yin-nourishing and fluid-promoting effect to treat the constipation caused by accumulation of heat and exhaustion of fluid in the large intestine.

Alternate Slowing and Acceleration of the Pulse a pulse condition with variations of frequency and totally irregular rate, usually occurring at the moment blood and qi are dying away, often considered to be the reflection of the critically ill at their last gasp.

Mumps epidemic parotitis caused by the attack of warm-toxin leading to the accumulation of heat in the intestine and stomach, and the stagnation of fire in the liver and gallbladder involving shaoyang meridian; marked by swelling of the parotid on one side or on both sides, accompanied with pain and tenderness, mostly occured in winter and spring. Differentiation types: common syndromes 1. superficial warm — toxin 2. stagnation of heat — toxin; developed syndromes 1. toxin stagnation involving the heart and liver. 2. pathogenic factor involving the liver meridian.

Delirium referring to morbid state with unconsciousness, talk nonsense and illusion, which is often caused by overabundance of internal heat, inter-

谵语 【zhān yǔ】指神志不清、胡言乱语的症状。高热、温邪入营血等扰及神明均可引起。

战栗 【zhàn lì】(振寒、寒战)自觉寒冷而躯体震颤的一种症状。多见于热病、疟疾,亦可见于阳虚证。

战汗 【zhàn hàn】指在外感热病过程中,邪盛正虚,突然战栗而后汗出的症状。是热病过程中正邪相争的表现。如正能胜邪,则疾病随汗而解;如正气不支,则气随汗脱、病趋危重。

掌骨伤 【zhǎng gǔ shāng】掌骨骨折,以第一或第五掌骨骨折为多见。伤处肿痛、畸形,可闻骨声,活动障碍。

nal interrupting mental activities, by phlegm-fire or invasion of heat into the heart.

Delirium referring to the symptom showing unconsciousness and talk nonsense, due to the stirring up of mental activities resulting from high fever or invasion of heat and warm into the blood of ying system.

Rigor a symptom showing subjective sensation of cold and trembling of the body, often seen in febrile diseases, malaria, or yang-deficiency syndrome.

Perspiration Following Chills sudden rigor and perspiration appearing in the course of exogenous febrile disease with excess of pathogenic factor and deficiency of healthy qi, as the manifestation of confrontation between healthy qi of the human body and pathogenic factors during the course of febrile disease. If the healthy qi is strong enough to suppress the pathogenic factors, the disease will be relieved along with perspiration; if healthy qi is weak, profuse perspiration will exhaust qi and contribute to the worse condition of the illness.

Fracture of Metacarpal Bone fracture of metacarpal bone usually occurring in the first or fifth metacarpal bone with local swelling and pain, deformity, hearable sound made by broken bones, and difficulty

胀 【zhàng】1、以腹部膨大胀满为主症的疾病。见鼓胀。2、指膨胀不适的自觉症状，如头胀、胁胀等。

胀后产 【zhàng hòu chǎn】相当于枕后位的异位分娩。

胀病 【zhàng bìng】即胀。以腹部膨大胀满为主症。见膨胀。

瘴 【zhàng】（瘴毒、山岚瘴气）指山林间湿热蒸郁而产生的一种病邪。

瘴气 【zhàng qì】1、古病名。指感受湿热杂毒所致的一种疫疠，2、指瘴疟。

瘴疟 【zhàng nüè】指因感受山岚瘴毒而发的一种危重疟疾。主要表现为疟发之时，神识昏迷，狂妄多言，或声音哑瘖等。

朝食暮吐 【zhāo shí mù tù】（暮食朝吐）指早晨吃的东西至黄昏时呕出的证候。是反胃的特征性症状。

折髀 【zhé bì】指股部疼痛如折的症状。

of movement.

Distention 1. a kind of disease with the chief symptom of abdominal distention and fullness. 2. feeling of distention and fullness and discomfort, such as distention of the head, hyperchondrial distention.

Occipitoposterior Position (of the fetus) a condition equivalent to the heterotopic delivery when the fetus in occipitoposterior position.

Distention Syndrome i. e. distention, which is marked by abdominal distention and fullness.

Miasma an infectious pathogen resulting from vapour-stagnancy of dampness and heat in the mountainous districts.

Miasma 1. ancient name of a disease, referring to an epidemic disease caused by exposure to the mixed toxins of dampness and heat. 2. referring to malignant malaria.

Malignant Malaria a critical malaria after exposure to miasma, marked by coma, mental confusion and delirium or hoarse voice during the attack of malaria.

Evening Vomiting with Vomitus Containing Food Eaten in the Morning referring to the syndrome characterized by afternoon vomiting of the food taken in the morning which is a special symptom of regurgitation

Severe Pain of the Thigh a pain so severe as if the thigh bone were bro-

折法 【zhé fǎ】用作用强的药物以迅速控制病情的一种治法。如热邪盛极，用大寒的方药以迅速清解热邪，控制病情。
Controlling the Disease a therapeutic method with potent drugs to control the development of disease. For example, an extreme excessiveness of heat-syndrome is cured by application of drugs of heavy cold nature.

折针 【zhé zhēn】指在针刺过程中发生针身折断于穴位内的现象。多因针体有损伤，或体位移动，或操作方法失宜引起。
Breaking of the Inserted Needle accidental breaking of the needle inserted into the body during acupuncture, which is usually due to damaged needle body, or postural movement or unusual operating method.

折疡 【zhé yáng】泛指骨折伤而成疮疡者。
Fracture Complicated by Infection generally denoting fracture of bones with the result of suppurative infection.

针灸 【zhēn jiǔ】针法和灸法两种治疗方法的合称。
Acupuncture and Moxibustion a combined term for acupuncture therapy and moxibustion therapy.

针法 【zhēn fǎ】1、针灸疗法的一大类。用一定规格病目的的方法。2、指针刺手法。简称刺法。包括进针、行针、出针过程所运用的各种手法。
Acupuncture Therapy 1. one important type of acupuncture and moxibustion by using a certain size of metal needle, most commonly used are the filiform needle, three-edged needle and plum-blossom needle, to stimulate certain superficial points of the human body for the prevention and treatment of the disease. 2. needle manipulation, including various manipulatons in the course of insertion, manipulation and withdrawal of the needle.

针刺麻醉 【zhēn cì má zuì】在针刺镇痛基础上发展起来的一种麻醉方法。即用毫针刺入特定的穴位并施以一
Acupuncture Anesthesia a method for anesthesia based on using acupuncture to induce analgesia. Af-

定手法进行刺激,以镇痛、松驰肌肉,并达到麻醉的效果,使病人能在清醒状态下接受各种手术治疗。包括体针麻醉、耳针麻醉、面针麻醉、鼻针麻醉等。

ter filiform needles are inserted into the selected acupuncture points, analgesia is induced with the muscle relaxed by manipulating the needles, so as to make the patient retain fully conscious while undergo various surgical procedures including body, auricular, facial and nasal acupuncture anesthesia.

真牙 【zhēn yá】(智齿)指生长最迟的第三臼齿,一般发育到成年,(女性约 21 岁、男性约 24 岁),智齿才能生长,也有的人终生不长。

Wisdom Tooth referring to the third molar teeth which are the last developed ones, usually not until in adult age (about 21 for female and 24 male) or not developed the whole life.

真睛破损 【zhēn jīng pò sǔn】由外伤引起眼珠穿孔或破裂,属眼外伤重症。

Perforated Wound of Eye-Ball the perforation and injury of the eye-ball caused by trauma, pertaining to serious syndrome of trauma of the eye.

真虚假实 【zhēn xū jiǎ shí】本质属虚的疾病,反而出现一些类似实证的表现。多因体质虚弱,正气不足,气血运行受阻所致。如素有脾虚气弱,运行无力,因而出现腹胀痛、脉弦等类似实证的表现。便患者腹胀是时有减轻,腹痛喜按,脉虽弦细但按之无力。

Sthenia-Syndrome in Appearance but Asthenia-Syndrome in Nature the disease itself is a deficiency but exhibits some apparently excess symptoms, mostly resulting from constitutional weakness, insufficiency of healthy qi, and obstruction of the circulation of qi and blood. For example, the patients with deficiency of the spleen and qi with the result of dibility in transportation presents some apparently excess symptoms, such as abdominal pain with fondness of pressure, and wiry pulse which feels weak by palpation.

真脏脉 【zhēn zàng mài】五脏真气败露时的脉象。即无胃、无神、无根的

Critical Pulse Condition a pulse condition revealing the exhaustion of

脉象，可见于疾病的危重阶段。对判断某些疾病的预后有一定的参考价值。如脾脏衰败时，往往出现软弱无力，节律不整，快慢不匀的脉象。qi of the zang-organs, often seen in critical cases, valuable for the referance of prognosis of certain diseases, eg. when spleen is exhausted and impaired, there may appear such pulse condition as weak, irregular, uneven.

真实假虚 【zhēn shí jiǎ xū】 本质属实邪结聚的疾病，反出现类似虚证的假象。多因邪气盛，致经络阻滞，气血不能外达所致。症见神情虽沉静但声高气粗、脉虽沉伏但按之有力等。

Asthenia — Syndrome in Appearance but Sthenia-Syndrome in Nature a morbid condition due to accumulation of pathogenic factors with pseudo-deficiency syndrome instead, mostly due to obstruction of meridians and collaterial and failure of qi and blood to resist against exopathogens because of overabunadance of pathogenic factor, marked by depressed mind with lound voice and hoarse breath, sunking and hidden pulse which feels forceful by heavy touch.

真头痛 【zhēn tóu tòng】 指以剧烈头痛，伴手足逆冷至肘膝关节为主要临床表现的一种头痛病证。本病多因邪入脑所致。

Unendurable Headache a morbid syndrome clinically characterized by severe headache, accompanied by cold clammy limbs and joints, mostly related to the invasion of pathogenic factors into the brain.

真息 【zhēn xī】（内呼吸）是指在入静中自然出现的深长、柔匀、慢细的呼吸状态，或口鼻似乎停顿的呼吸状态。

Genuine Qi also called internal breathing, referring to a slow deep and long, even and fine breathing state or to a breathing without involvment of mouth and nose which appears naturally after entering static state.

真心痛 【zhēn xīn tòng】 指心前区发作性剧烈疼痛，伴肢冷紫绀等的一种疾病。

Angina Pectoris referring to the attacking severe pain in precordial area, which is accompanied by cold

疹 【zhěn】（疹子）指温热病发疹。表现为皮肤上发现红色小点，形如粟米，抚之碍手。多由风热郁肺，内闭营分，从血络外出所致。

诊尺肤 【zhěn chǐ fū】切诊内容之一。指诊察肘关节内侧至腕部皮肤的寒热、湿润度、滑涩等变化，可以帮助判断疾病的寒热虚实。

诊法 【zhěn fǎ】诊断疾病的方法。包括四诊和辨证两个过程。即通过望、问、闻、切等方法了解病情，并据此进行辨证，对疾病作出诊断。

诊指纹 【zhěn zhǐ wén】小儿诊法之一。诊察食指掌面外侧表浅小静脉变化，以帮助判断病情。

诊胸腹 【zhěn xiōng fù】切诊内容之一。触按胸腹部以了解该部皮肤的冷热、硬度、疼痛的部位、喜按或拒按、

limbs and purpura.

Rash referring to eruption in the course of acute febrile disease, with manifestation of red spots developing over the skin shaped like granules which are in the way of touching, mostly caused by stagnancy of wind-heat in the lung which retained in yingfen with the consequence of coming out through blood collateral.

Palpation of the Chi Skin examining the skin of the part between elbow and wrist, a diagnosis method to examine the temperature, moisture and texture of the flexor aspect of the forearm by palpation, in favour of the diagnosis of the disease.

Diagnostic Method including the four diagnostics and differential diagnosis, i. e. by means of inspecton, auscultion and olfaction, interrogation, pulse feeling and palpation to obtain symptoms and signs and then to analyse and synthesize the data obtained in order to arrive at a correct diagnosis.

Inspection of the Superficial Venule of the Index Finger one of the diagnostic methods for infants to observe the changes of superficial venules on the palmar aspect of the index finger to contribute to the diagnosis of the case.

Palpation of the Thorax and Abdomen one diagnostic method of pulse-feeling and palpation, to ascertain the

有无包块、结节等情况。 temperature, rigidity, tenderness point within the area by digital palpation, to learn if it is found of pressure or resistant against it if there is any mass, node.

诊虚里 【zhěn xū lǐ】切诊内容之一。虚里相当于心尖搏动的部位,该处是宗气汇聚之处且与胃有密切关系,所以,通过触摸该处的搏动情况有助于判断胃气和宗气的盛衰。

Palpating the Cardiac Apex one of the diagnostic method of pulse-feeling and palpation, xuli is equivalent to the cardiac apex, where pectoral-qi meets closely related to the stomach, therefore, the condition of the stomach-qi and pectoral-qi can be determined by palpation on the apex of heart.

怔忡 【zhēng chóng】指自觉心跳剧烈的一种病证。多由阴血亏损,心失所养;或心阳不足,水饮上逆;或突受惊恐所致。以虚证为多。

Severe Palpitation a morbid condition presenting subjective severe palpitation, which is usually caused by impairment of yin-blood with the mal-nourishment of the heart; or by insufficiency of the heart-yang with upward flow of excessive water; or sudden panic, often seen in syndrome of deficiency type.

蒸 【zhēng】中药炮制法之一。将药物直接或加一定的辅料隔水蒸熟,以便于制剂或改变药物的性味。

Steaming one of the techniques for preparing Chinese medicine. The process of directly heating the drugs mixed with some auxiliary material for the preparation of drugs or for the purpose of changing the properties and flavours of drugs.

蒸露 【zhēng lù】中药炮制法之一。将某些药物通过蒸馏法制成药露,如金银花露、藿香露等。

Distillation one of the techniques for preparing Chines medicine. The process of vapoizing and condensing a drug to obtain volatile liquid, such as the liquid of Honeysuckle flower, the liquid of Agastache, etc.

蒸乳 【zhēng rǔ】因产妇气血壮盛,乳

Acute Mastitis a morbid state

汁壅滞不通；或产后无子饮乳，以致两乳肿硬疼痛、恶寒发热的疾病。

caused by excessive qi and blood in women after birth with the consequence of stagnation of milk; or excessive milk with no infant to feed after birth, resulting in swollon, firm and painful breasts to be followed by chill and fever.

蒸病 【zhēng bìng】以潮热为主症，其热似自内蒸发而出的病证，多由于阴虚所致。

Hectic Fever due to Yin Deficiency tide fever as chief symptom, as seemingly steam out from the interior, which is often caused by deficiency of yin.

癥瘕 【zhēng jiǎ】（癥积）指腹腔内痞块。一般以隐于腹内，按之有形，坚硬不移，痛有定处者为癥；聚散无常，推之游移不定，痛无定处者为瘕。

Mass in the Abdomen referring to the mass in the abdomen, Zheng is clinically characterized by palpable and immovable mass of a definite shape in the abdomen with pain at definite site, while Jia is characterized by the intermittent feeling of an indefinite mass in the abdomen, with pain at no definite site.

癥疝 【zhēng shàn】以骤然腹胀、有气块、胃腔疼痛为主症的一种疾病。多因饮食不节，寒温不调，肠胃气机阻滞而致。

Gastric Colic a morbid condition characterized by sudden distention and fullness of the abdomen, distention and protuberance of the stomach and intestines, and pain in the epigastrium, it often caused by the blockage of qi flow in the stomach and intestines as the consequence of improper diet with food hot and cold intermittently.

整体观念 【zhěng tǐ guān niàn】中医诊疗疾病的一种思想方法。祖国医学认为人体是一个有机的整体，构成人体的各个组成部分之间，在结构上是不可分割的，在功能上是相互协调、

Concept of Wholism It is an idea of traditional Chinese medicine in diagnosing and treating diseases. In traditional Chinese medicine a human body is regarded as an integral, with

相互为用的，在病理上是相互影响的，同时认为自然环境对人体生理、病理有不同程度的影响，既强调人体内部的协调完整性，也重视人体与外界环境的统一性。这种内外环境的统一性，机体自身整体性的思想，称之为整体观念。它是中医学基本特点之一。

various parts of this integral inseparable in structure, harmonious and coordinate in function and mutually affect in pathology, meanwhile natural environment is supposed to have effect on the physiology and pathology of the human body to a various extent; the emphasis either put on the harmony and coordination of the internal organs, or on the unity of the human body with the external environment. This unity of internal and external environments and the unity of the various parts of the integral is called concept of wholism, which is one of the basic characteristics of traditional Chinese medical theory.

正骨 【zhèng gǔ】中医诊治骨、关节、软组织和内脏损伤的一个学科。

Bone Setting a speciality of treating the injuries of bone, joints, soft tissues and internal zang organs in traditional Chinese medicine.

正骨工具 【zhèng gǔ gōng jù】治疗外伤和骨折所使用的工具，主要用于骨折的固定，如腰柱、竹帘、杉篱、夹板及绷带等。

The Tools for Bone Setting the tools used in the treatment of trauma and bone fracture for the purpose of fixation such as lumbar stick, bamboo curtain, fir fence, splint, or bandage.

正骨手法 【zhèng gǔ shǒu fǎ】骨伤治法之一。用手的一定技巧动作，治疗骨折、脱臼及软组织损伤时的各种方法。如摸、接、端、提、按、摩、推、拿等。

Manipulations of Bone Setting one of the methods to treat bone fracture, luxation or soft tissue by various manipulations, such as palpation, setting, replacement, lifting, pressing, rubbing, pushing and grasping.

正念 【zhèng niàn】指练功中思想安宁，杂念不起，能够高度集中在练功上的意念。

Correct Will referring to during the process of qi gong, the practitioner should keep peace of mind from distractions and concentrate the will

正虚邪实 【zhèng xū xié shí】指正气不足邪气过盛的病理现象。通常以正虚为本,邪实为标。

Deficiency of Healthy Qi and Sthenia of Pathogenic Factors referring to the pathological state presenting insufficiency of healthy qi and over-excess of pathogenic factor, usually with deficient body resistance as Ben (the primary) and excessive pathogenic factors as Biao (the secondary).

正气 【zhèng qì】1、真气。指人体的机能活动和抗病康复能力。2、指四季正常气候。即春温、夏热、秋凉、冬寒。

Healthy Qi 1. also called genuine qi, generally denoting the body functional activities, resistance and recovery capacity. 2. denoting the usual climate in four seasons, i. e. warmness in spring, hot in summar, cool in fall, and cold in winter.

正气存内,邪不可干 【zhèng qì cún nèi, xié bù kě gān】中医发病学很重视人体的正气,认为内脏功能正常,正气旺盛,气血充盈,卫外固密,病邪难于侵入,疾病无从发生。

The Healthy Qi Is Full inside the Body, the Pathogen Can Not Invade in in the pathological study of traditional Chinese medicine, importance is attached to healthy qi and it is considered difficult for pathogens to invade the body and cause disease as long as the internal organs function regularly, heathy qi is prosprous, qi and blood are sufficient and defensive function against exopathogens is strengthened.

正色 【zhèng sè】健康人面部的色泽。

Healthy Complexion the facial complexion of the healthy person.

正头痛 【zhèng tóu tòng】满头皆痛的一种症状,与偏头痛相对而言。

Aching all over the head a symptom characterized by headache all over the head, opposite to labial headache.

正邪相争 【zhèng xié xiāng zhēng】即致病因素侵入人体后与机体抗病功

Struggle between the Healthy Qi and the Pathogenic Factor the mutu-

能的互相作用。一般地说，一切疾病都是这种作用的反映，就个别症状来说，如恶寒发热，也是正邪斗争的反映。

al action between pathogenic factors that have invaded into the human body and the resisting function of the mechanism. Generally speaking, all the diseases are the reflection of such a action, respectively eg. chill and fever, is the reflection of the struggle between the healthy qi and the pathogenic factor.

正治　【zhèng zhì】（真反、逆从、逆取、逆治）指采用与疾病性质相反的方法和药物来治疗，是常规的治疗方法。如热者寒之，寒者热之。

Routine Treatment　treatment with recipes or drugs opposite to the nature of the disease, a routine method for the treatment eg. drugs of hot nature for cold-syndromes, drugs of cold nature for heat-syndromes.

证　【zhèng】是机体在疾病发展过程中的某一阶段的病理概括，它包括了病变的部位、原因、性质，以及邪正关系，反映了疾病发展过程中某一阶段的病理变化的本质。

Syndrome　the pathological outline of a certain stage during the course of a disease, including the position, cause, nature and relationship between pathogenic factor and healthy qi of the pathological process, which reflects the nature of pathological changes at certain stage in the course of a disease.

证候　【zhèng hòu】由一系列有内在联系的症状和体征（包括舌象、脉象等）所构成，反映一定的病变规律。

Syndrome　a term consisting of a series of internally related symptoms and signs (including the condition of the tongue, condition of the pulse and others), indicating certain developing rule of the disease.

郑声　【zhèng shēng】患者在神志不清的情况下，低声地不能自主地重复一些语句的症状。多属虚证，常是疾病后期，心气内损，精神散乱的危重征象。

Murmuring in a Unconscious State

a symptom with manifestation of uncontrolled repeating of some sentences in a low voice when the patient is in uncontiousness. It belongs to asthenic-syndrome, seen in the critical

支饮 【zhī yǐn】因饮邪滞留于胸膈,上迫于肺,肺失肃降所致的饮证。表现为胸满气短、喘咳不能平卧、浮肿等。

肢节痛 【zhī jié tòng】指肢体关节疼痛不适。多因风湿、寒湿、痰饮、瘀血留滞经络或因血虚不能养筋所致。见痹。

脂瘤 【zhī liú】(粉瘤)瘤体形圆质软,多发于头面及背部,溃后可见豆腐渣样物。多因痰气凝结所致。

直肠 【zhí cháng】大肠的末端,连结于乙状结肠,终止于肛门。

直肠泻 【zhí cháng xiè】指一进饮食就要腹泻。多由脾胃之气极虚,无力运化所致。

直接灸 【zhí jiē jiǔ】将艾炷直接放在穴位皮肤上施灸的方法。一般可分为有瘢痕灸和无瘢痕灸两种。

stage of disease with impairment of the heart-qi and mental confusion.

Fluid-Retention Syndrome the symptoms of the accumulation of fluid in the hypochondrium and epigastrium which invades the lung leading to the dysfunction of the lung in descendance, manifested by fullness in the chest with shortness of breath, cough and dyspea being confined in orthostatic posture, edema, etc.

Arthralgia of Extremities referring to the discomfort and pain in the joints of extremities, which is usually caused by wind-dampness, cold-dampness, excessive phlegm, stagnance of blood stasis in the meridian and collaterals or failure to nourish tendons due to deficiency of blood.

Lipoma a round, soft tumor of the skin frequently seen on the head or back, a smelly, beancurd like substance after rupture, it is often due to stagnation of phlegm and qi.

Rectum distal portion of the large intestine, adjoining with sigmoid colon, and ending at the anus.

Rectal Diarrhea denoting immediate diarrhea right after intake, which is mostly caused by extreme deficiency of the spleen-qi and stomach-qi and lead to disability in transportation and digestion.

Direct Contact Moxibustion application of ignited moxa cone directly on the skin surface of the selected

直视 【zhí shì】指患者在神志不清的情况下，两眼向前凝视，目睛无神的症状。多由肝风内动所致。常见于中风、惊风、癫痫等病。

直中 【zhí zhòng】病邪不经三阳经的传变而直接侵犯三阴经的一种病理现象。

直中三阴 【zhí zhòng sān yīn】病邪直接侵犯三阴经，起病即见三阴证。如腹满而吐、纳差、便溏、疲倦嗜睡、脉微细等。多见于病邪重，正气虚的情况。

直中阴经 【zhí zhòng yīn jīng】指寒邪不经过三阳经，直接侵犯三阴经，出现无热、恶寒及其他阴经的证候。

跖 【zhí】1、足底部。2、指足大趾下面。

止血 【zhǐ xuè】治疗出血症的方法。根据出血原因不同，分为清热止血、祛瘀止血、补气止血等。

point, generally in two kinds: scar-producing moxibustion and non-scar-producing moxibustion.

Staring Blandly Forward a symptom seen in unconscious patient with both eyes staring forward blandly, it is usually caused by endogenous wind stirring in the liver, often seen in patient with stroke, convulsion, epilepsy and others.

Direct Attack a pathological state in which pathogenic factors attack directly the three yin meridians instead of affecting the three yang meridians first.

Direct Attack on the Three Yin Meridians a condition with the three yin syndrome present at the onset, such as abdominal fullness, vomiting, poor appetite, watery stools, fatigue with inclination to sleep, weak and thready pulse, frequently occurring in the patient with virulent pathogenic factors and deficiency of healthy qi.

Direct Attack on the Yin Meridians direct attack on the three yin meridians without affecting the three yang meridians, exhibiting absence of heat, aversion to cold and other syndromes related to yin meridians.

Sole 1. plantar portion 2. base portion of hallux

Hemostasis a method to treat hemorrhage; it is often classified as hemostasis by clearing away heat, removing stasis and reinforcing qi,

指目 【zhǐ mù】诊脉方法之一。即利用食指、中指、无名指指尖按脉的一种方法。因为指尖感觉较灵敏,往往可以了解到脉象的微小变化。

指针 【zhǐ zhēn】是用手指按压、揉摩一定的穴位,以代替针刺的一种简便的治疗方法。

至阴 【zhì yīn】1、至,到过之意。至阴,即由阳达阴。三阴始于太阴,而脾属太阴,故称脾为至阴。2、至,作极或最解,至阴即阴气最甚者,因肾属少阴,阴气最盛,故也称肾为至阴。3、穴位名称。4、农历六月为至阴。

制化 【zhì huà】五行学说术语,即制约与生化。五脏依靠这种相互生化与相互制约的协调关系,以维持它们正常的生理功能。

制绒 【zhì róng】中药炮制法之一。将某些药物的纤维捣乱成绒状,使其容易点燃,如把艾叶制成艾绒,用于灸法。

which are considered from the angle of different causes.

Feeling the Pulse with the Finger-Tip a way of palpation with index finger, middle finger and ring finger, for the tips of the fingers are more sensitive to any minute changes of pulse condition.

Finger-Press Method a simple therapeutic method of pressing and rubbing a given point with finger nail instead of acupuncture needle.

Zhi Yin 1. Zhi means "arrive". Zhiyin means to arrive at yin from yang. The three yin originates at Taiyin while the spleen pertains to Taiyin, the spleen is so called Zhiyin. 2. Zhi means "extreme", Zhiyin means extreme yin. As the kidney pertains to shaoyin, with yin-qi extreme excessive, the kidney is so called Zhiyin. 3. an acupoint 4. June of lunar year is Zhiyin.

Inhibition and Generation (of the five elements) the term of the five elements theory, i. e. mutually inhibiting and mutuagans depend on this coordination to maintain their regular physiological functions.

Making Herbs into Wool a method which is to prepare Chinese herbal medicine by pounding the fibers of drugs into a pulp so as to make them easier to be burnt. eg. Mugwort wool made by grinding dried leaves of the Mugwort, which is used for moxibus-

制霜 【zhì shuāng】中药炮制法之一。某些药物经炮制后制成粉末,其制法有多种。如:①种子类药物去油后研成粉末,如巴豆霜、杏仁霜等;②某些药物经加工析出的结晶,如柿霜;③某些动物药去胶后的骨质粉末,如鹿角霜。

Making Drugs into Frostlike Powder a techniques of processing Chinese medicine. Some drugs are processed and ground into powder in many ways. eg. 1. removing the oils of certain medicinal seeds, and then grinding them into a fine powder such as defatted croton seed powder, apricot kernel powder. 2. crystallinzing certain drugs such as powder on the surface of a dried persimmon. 3. grinding the residue of certain animal bones after removing the glue by stewing such as deerhorn, antler powder.

炙 【zhì】中药炮制法之一。将药物与液体辅料如酒、醋、蜜、盐、姜、米泔水、童便、矾等相混后共炒,使辅料渗入药材内部,以加强药效或缓和药性。

Stir-Frying with Liquid Adjuvant technique of processing medicinal drugs, stir-frying drugs mixed with a liquid, eg. with wine, with vinegar, with honey, with salt, with ginger, with washing rice water, or with urine of child, or with vitriol so as to strengthen the action of drugs or milden the nature of drugs.

炙煿 【zhì bó】指煎烤、炸、炒等烹调方法。炙煿制成的食物,性多燥热,过食常会耗伤胃阴,发生疾病。

Cooking by Frying and Roasting the fried, stir-fried, deep-fried or roasted food is dry-heat in nature and, if overeaten, is apt to cause diseases by impairing stomach-yin.

治病必求于本 【zhì bìng bì qiú yú běn】就是治疗疾病时,必须寻找出疾病的根本原因,并针对根本原因进行治疗。这是辩证论治的一个基本原则。

Treatment must Search for the Primary Cause of Disease a major principle of diagnostic differentiation in which the primary cause of disease ought to be searched.

治法 【zhì fǎ】通常指治疗大法及运用

Therapeutic Methods generally re-

原则，也就是治则的具体化。即汗、吐、下、和、温、清、消、补等八种治疗方法。

治则 【zhì zé】即治疗疾病的法则。是用以指导治疗方法的总则。它是在整体观念和辩证论治精神指导下制定的，对临床治疗立法、处方、用药，具有普遍指导意义。如急则治其标，扶正祛邪等。

治未病 【zhì wèi bìng】1、预防疾病，包括服药预防疾病的发生和预防疾病的传变。2、有早期治疗的含意。

治削 【zhì xiāo】药物的加工、挑拣、筛、刷、刮、捣、切等。

治求其属 【zhì qiú qí shǔ】在治疗疾病时要辨别病人的一系列症状属于哪一个脏腑的病变，从而确定治法。

ferring to the key methods and principles of treatment. i. e. specified principles for the treatment, diaphoresis, emesis, purgation, regulation, warming, clearing heat, resolution and tonification.

Principle of Treatment general rules for guiding the methods of treatment. It is made under the guidance of the conception of the organism as a whole and differentiation of syndromes and plays a guiding role significantly in clinical treating methods, prescriptions and administration; eg. in emergency cases, to treat the acute symptoms first so as to strengthen the patient's resistance and dispel the invading pathogenic factors.

Preventive Treatment of Disease 1. prevention of disease including administration for keeping away of the occurance of disease and avoiding the transmission and change of disease. 2. implication of early treatment.

Processing Medicinal Herbs the process of preparing herbs by silecting, sieving, brushing, scraping, pounding or slcing.

Treating Disease according to Its Nature in treating a disease it is required to distinguish a series of symptoms of the patient and to determine the location of the pathological change so as to confirm the treating method.

痔 【zhì】1、位于肛门附近静脉曲张形成的小核。多由平素湿热内积, 过食辛辣, 久坐久立; 或临产用力, 大便秘结; 或久泻久痢引起。古代泛指多种肛门部疾病。2、指九窍中小肉突起。

痔疮 【zhì chāng】1. 泛指多种肛门部的疾病。2. 指九窍中小肉状突起物。现多指直肠下端粘膜下和肛管皮下的静脉丛, 因各种不同原因引起扩大, 曲张所致的一种疾病。按其部位不同, 分为外痔、内痔、混合痔三种。

痔瘘 【zhì lòu】即痔疮和肛瘘的合称。

蛭食 【zhì shí】指水蛭咬伤。

滞下 【zhì xià】痢疾的古称。因排便有脓血粘腻、滞涩难下, 故名。

滞气 【zhì qì】指颜面色泽晦暗、垢腻, 常是湿邪、痰浊阻滞的现象。见于暑湿、湿温、痰饮等病。

Hemorrhoid 1. a small pile forming at the anus as the result of varicose vein around the anus, mostly due to internal accumulation of dampness and heat, overeating of pungent food, long-time standing or sitting; or overexertion during parturient, constipation; or chronic diarrhea or dysentery. Anciently denoting various diseases of the anus. 2. **Nodules in the Nine Orfices**

Hemorrhoid 1. denoting various diseases at the areas of the anus. 2. referring to small fleshy prominances of the nine orificies. Presently often referring to the disease occuring in venous plexus covered by mucosa in the lower part of the rectum and in the interior of skin of anal canal, formed by enlargement and varices involving different causes. According to the different distribution, it is divided into three kinds: external, internal and mixed hemorrhoids.

Hemorrhoid and Anal Fistula

Bite by Leech

Difficulty in Defecation ancient name for dysentery, meaning difficult bowel movement with purulent and greasy and mucous blood.

Stagnation of Qi a condition with the dark and gloomy, dirty and greasy facial colour, often as the phenomenon hinting the obstruction of damp-heat and phlegm-stagnancy, it is seen in such diseases as summer

滞针 【zhì zhēn】针刺过程中出现运针困难的现象。多因病人精神紧张、局部肌肉痉挛；或捻转幅度过大，肌纤维绕针尖所致。一般在滞针部位周围轻度按摩，并将针轻轻提插；或在附近再刺一针，使肌肉松驰后，再将针拔出。

滞颐 【zhì yí】小儿口角流涎，浸渍两颐的证候。多因脾胃虚寒不能收摄；或脾胃湿热，上蒸于口而成。

中草药 【zhōng cǎo yào】中药与草药合称为中草药。

中搭手 【zhōng dā shǒu】指有头疽生于膏肓穴者。见发背条。

中丹田 【zhōng dān tián】除少数认为中丹田在脐下外，极大多数丹家都认为中丹田在两乳之间的膻中穴，其为藏气之处。

heat-dampness, damp-warmness and phlegm retention.

Sticking of the Inserted Neeled an abnormal condition during acupuncture in which needle after insertion is difficult to manipulate, usually resulting from local myospasm related to tension of the patient; twirling the needle to too great a drgree with the result of muscle fiber winding around the needle. To remove the stuck needle, gentle massage may be applied to surrounding muscle or one or two additional needles may be inserted at the nearby portion to relieve the muscular spasm.

Infantile Slobbering a condition resulting from asthenia of the spleen and stomach failure of retaining the saliva or from damp-heat in the spleen and stomach attacking the oral cavity.

Chinese Herbal Medicine a general term for herbal medicine and Chinese materia medica.

Carbuncle at the Middle Part of the Back referring to the patient with carbuncle occurring in gaohuang point (a site below the heart and above the diaphragm).

Middle Dan Tian it is an area where qi stores and generally regarded referring to the point of dan zhong between the two nipples, yet. Some people believed it referring to the region below umbilicus.

中寒 【zhōng hán】指中焦虚寒，由于脾胃阳气不足，运化功能衰退所致。常见有腹痛喜按、畏寒肢冷、口淡泛恶、食少便溏等症。

中焦 【zhōng jiāo】三焦的中部，膈以下，脐以上的上腹部，脾胃位于其中。主要功能是消化、吸收、转输营养物质。

中焦如沤 【zhōng jiāo rú ǒu】比喻中焦的功能特点。即中焦脾胃有消化、吸收、转输的作用。这种作用好象浸渍食物，使起变化。

中焦主化 【zhōng jiāo zhǔ huà】中焦的功能之一。即消化饮食物和化生营血的作用。

中满 【zhōng mǎn】腹部胀满的症状。多因气虚、食滞、寒浊上壅、湿热阻困致使脾胃运化失常、气机阻滞不畅所引起。

Asthenia-Cold of Middle-Energizer referring to hypofunction of the spleen and stomach, which is caused by insufficient yang-qi in the spleen and stomach with the result of declined function in transportation and digestion, marked by abdominal pain which is relieved by pressure, chillness, cold extremities, anorexia and loose stool.

Middle-Energizer locating in the upper abdomen in the middle region of tri-energizer which is below the diaphragm and above the umbilicus where the spleen and stomach lie; its function chiefly is digestion, absorption, transportation of nutrious material.

Middle-Energizer Is Analogized to a Soaking Pond figure of speech of the functioning characteristic of middle-energizer, i, e, digestion, absorbtion and transportation, the process of which is like soaking.

Middle-Energizer Governing Digestion one of the functions of middle energizer, by which the food is digested and the blood is produced.

Abdominal Distension a symptom of distension and fullness in the abdomen, usually caused by abnormality of the digestive and transporting functions of the spleen and stomach and disturbances of the flow of qi resulting from deficiency of qi, indigestion, upward excess of cold, accumu-

中精之腑　【zhōng jīng zhī fǔ】（中清之腑）指胆。胆所贮存的胆汁具有帮助消化的作用。

中品　【zhōng pǐn】古代把没有毒或虽有毒，只须酌量使用，能治病补虚的药物，称为中品。

中气不足　【zhōng qì bù zú】脾胃之气虚弱，运化失职，导致消化吸收功能减退的病理。症见食欲不振、腹胀、面色淡白、眩晕、急倦乏力、便溏、声低、气短、脉虚等。

中气下陷　【zhōng qì xià xiàn】（脏气下陷）指脾气虚弱引起组织弛缓不收，脏器脱垂一类病证的病理。如久泻脱肛、子宫脱垂等。

中脘　【zhōng wǎn】1、胃腔中部 2、穴位名称。

中消　【zhōng xiāo】指以多食易饥，形体消瘦为特征的消渴病。

中阳　【zhōng yáng】即脾胃的阳气。

中阳不振　【zhōmg yáng bù zhèn】指脾

lation of dampness and heat.

The Fu-Organ Containing Refined Juice (referring to the gallbladder)
the juice stored in the gallbladder aids in digestion.

Medium Drugs　an ancient name for those drugs without noxious factor or those with slightly noxious factor but those can serve as deficiency-nourishing drugs if it is used in limitation.

Deficiency of Qi in Middle-Energizer
a morbid condition showing weakened function of the spleen and stomach in digestion resulting from the debility of spleen-qi and stomach-qi with the failure to function in transportation and digestion, marked by poor appetite, abdominal distention, pallor, dizziness, fatigue, watery stool, week voice, shortness of breath, feeble pulse.

Sinking of Middle-Energizer Qi
a morbid state in which deficiency of qi of the spleen is responsible for the flaccidity of tissues and prolapse of visceral organs, eg. prolonged diarrhea, proctoptosis, prolapse of uterus, etc.

1. Middle Part of Gastric Cavity　2. An Acupoint name

Diabetes Involving Middle Energizer
diabetes marked by polyphagia and emaciation.

Middle Energizer Yang　yang qi of the spleen and stomach.

Deficience of Middle Energizer Yang

胃阳气虚弱，运化功能低下的病理。症见食欲减退、怠倦乏力、四肢清冷、便溏、面色萎黄、舌质淡、苔白、脉虚等。

a pathological change showing hypofunction of the spleen and stomach in absorption and digestion, manifested by reduced appetite, attitude and fatigue, cold limbs, loose stool, withered and yellowish complexion, pale tongue proper with whitish coating, feeble pulse, etc.

中正之官 【zhōng zhèng zhī guān】指胆。因胆具有主决断的作用。

The Official Being in Charge of Decisions referring to the gallbladder, which has something to do with one's courage in making decisions.

中指同身寸 【zhōng zhǐ tóng shēn cùn】是针灸取穴时所用一种长度标准。即以病人的中指和拇指连接成一个圆圈，以中指中节内侧两头横纹头中间的距离作为一寸。此法可用于四肢的直量和背部的横量。

Middle Finger Cun a measurement standard for acupuncture, obtained by flexing the middle finger over the thumb to form a circle, and taking the distance between folds formed by the 1st and 2nd interphalangeal joints as the standard inch (cun). It is usually used in selecting points on the back with taking crosswise measure and extremities with taking straight measure.

肿疡 【zhǒng yáng】指疮疡未出脓者。疮疡早期，由于实热蕴结、气血壅滞，体表结块肿痛者，均属此症。

Acute Skin Infection referring to the skin infection without purulent discharge. Early stage of pyogenic infection of the skin involving accumulation of sthenic heat, stagnation of qi and blood, swollen and painful masses of the body surface; mostly belongs to yang-syndrome, sthenia-syndrome and heat-syndrome.

踵 【zhǒng】足后跟着地部分。
中毒 【zhòng dú】有毒食物或毒物进入人体，因毒性作用引起的病证。
中风 【zhòng fēng】指猝然昏仆、不省

Heel hindmost part of the foot.
Poisoning a morbid condition produced by a poision.
Apoplexy a morbid condition mani-

人事，或突然口眼㖞斜，半身不遂，言语不清的病证。常发生于中年以上。病前多有头痛、眩晕、肢麻、心悸等症。多因暴怒、饮食、劳倦等诱发。辩证分类：分为中经络和中脏腑两大类，中经络分：1、风阳痰火证。2、风痰入络证。3、气虚血滞证。4、肝肾亏虚证。中脏腑又分闭证和脱证，其中闭证包括阳闭（风阳痰火证）和阴闭（痰湿证）

fested as sudden syncope, unconciousness, distortion of face, hemiplegia and dysphasia, usually seen in the middle-aged. The symptoms and signs before sudden onset are headache, dizziness, numbness of extremities, palpitation, etc. that is mostly due to irritability, food and overstrain. Types of differentiation: apoplexy involving the meridians and collaterals 1. syndrome of wind-phlegm-fire 2. syndrome of wind-phlegm involving the collaterals 3. syndrome of blood stasis due to qi-deficiency 4. syndrome of consumption of both the liver and kidney. Apoplexy involving the zang and fu organs 1. syncope syndrome, including yang-syncope and yin-syncope 2. collapse syndrome.

中腑 【zhòng fǔ】中风证的一种类型。为邪入于腑所致。以猝然昏倒、醒后出现半身不遂、口眼㖞斜、语言不利或二便不通为特征。

Apoplexy Involving the Fu Organs a type of apoplexy, which is caused by pathogenic factor invading the fu organs, with manifestation of sudden syncope, hemiplegia, deviation of the mouth and eyes, dysphasis, dysuria and dyschesia.

中寒 【zhòng hán】1、突然为寒邪侵袭的一种病证。症见突然眩晕、昏倒不知人事、口噤、身体强直、四肢战栗、恶寒、发热无汗等。2、指中焦虚寒。

Cold Stroke 1. a syndrome caused by sudden attack of cold, marked by sudden vertigo, unconsciousness, lockjaw, stiffness of the body, shiver of the limbs, aversion to cold, fever without sweat. 2. referring to the asthenic coldness in middle energizer.

中经 【zhòng jīng】病在经脉的中风证。以手足麻木、半身偏瘫、语言蹇

Apoplexy Involving the Meridian a type of stricken by wind with disease

涩而无意识障碍为特征。

中经络 【zhòng jīng luò】病在经脉和络脉的中风证的统称。以无神志改变而见口眼㖞斜、半身不遂、肢体麻木、语言不利为特征。

中络 【zhòng luò】中风证的一种类型。为邪入络脉所致。是中风的最轻型。以口眼㖞斜、肌肤不仁为特征。

中湿 【zhòng shī】1、即湿痹。2、泛指外感或内伤于湿邪引起的一些症状。如皮肤麻木、胸胁胀满、气喘、浮肿、腰痛而重坠、肢节不利等。

中食 【zhòng shí】类中风的一种类型。

中暑 【zhòng shǔ】（中喝、暍）指夏季炎热高温环境中感受暑邪而突然昏厥的病证。多伴见身热烦躁、气喘、大汗或无汗、牙关紧闭、四肢抽搐等。

developing in the meridian, characterized by numbness of the hands and feet, hemiplegia, divagation without mental disturbance.

Apoplexy Involving the Meridian and Collateral a general term for apoplexy with the disease located in the meridian and collateral, characterized by absence of emotional disorder but deviation of the face, hemiplegia, numbness of the body, dysarthria.

Apoplexy Involving the Collaterals a midest type of apoplexy caused by pathogenic factor invading collaterals, characterized by deviation of the face, numbness of the skin and muscles.

Syndrome due to Damp 1. arthralgia caused by damp. 2. denoting the symptoms caused by external pathogenic factors or internal exhaustion of damp, marked by numbness of the skin, distention and fullness of the chest and hyperchondrium, ethma, swelling, lumbago with heavy feeling, and limitations of movement of joints.

Syncope of Crapulence a type of apoplexy disease, which is caused by crapulence.

Sunstroke a morbid state exhibiting sudden faintness caused by prolonged exposure to hot environment in summer, which is accompanied with fever, restlessness, dyspnea, profuse sweating or no sweating at all,

中暑眩晕 【zhòng shǔ xuán yún】(感冒眩晕) 因中暑邪所致的一种病证。表现为眩晕欲倒、身热烦躁、口渴、脉虚, 严重者可出现昏不知人。

中恶 【zhòng wù】因突然受大惊而引起的病状。如手足逆冷、面色发青、精神错乱、头晕目眩、牙关紧闭、甚至昏厥等。

中脏 【zhòng zàng】中风证的一种类型。为邪入于脏所致。是中风的最重型。以神昏不语、口角流涎为特征, 按其症状不同又分为闭证和脱证。

重剂 【zhòng jì】指用质量重、有镇坠、镇静作用的药物如磁石、朱砂之类组成的方剂。

重可去怯 【zhòng kě qù qiè】重剂有镇静作用, 可以治疗精神紊乱、惊怯等症。

重舌 【zhòng shé】由心脾湿热, 复感风邪, 邪气相搏, 循经上结于舌所致的病证。症见舌下血脉胀起, 形如小舌, 或红或紫, 或连贯而生, 状如莲花, 身发潮热, 头痛项强, 饮食难下,

trismus and spasm of extremities.

Dizziness Caused by Summer-Heat a dizziness syndrome due to exposure to summer heat with symptoms of dizziness tending to fall, feverish body with restlessness, thirst, feeble pulse, even loss of consciousness.

Fright a disorder resulting from sudden frightening, which is marked by coldness of extremities, pallor, mental disturbance, dizziness, trismus and even syncope.

Apoplexy Involving the Zang Organs the most serious case of apoplexy caused by invasion of pathogenic factor into the viscera characterized by coma, salivation; according to different symptoms, it is classified into sthenia-syndrome and collapse-syndrome.

The Prescription Composed Of Heavy Drugs a prescription containing mineral remedy with tranquilizing action such as those composed of magnet, cinnabar, etc.

Prescription Containing Minerals Can Calm the Patient a prescription of heave weight has the sedative action and is applied for the treatment of mental disturbance, frightening, etc.

Sublingual Swelling Tongue a morbid condition resulting from damp-heat in the heart and spleen, with repeated affecting of wind; the pathogenic factors upwards along the

言语不清，口流清涎，日久溃腐。 meridian stagnate in the tongue. Marked by congestion of sublingual vein, show the appearance of a small tongue in red or purple in colour, or continuous congestion shaped-like lotus flower, tider fever, headache, stiffy neck, difficult swollow, disturbance of speech, salivation and becoming ulceration if prolonged.

重阳必阴 【zhòng yáng bì yīn】即阳极转阴。当阳气过盛达到一定限度时，会向阴的方面转化。

Overabundance of Yang Transforming to Yin on the basis of the transformation between yin and yang, if the overabundance of yang reaches a certain limit, yang will transform into its opposite, yin.

重阴必阳 【zhòng yīn bì yáng】即阴极转阳，当阴气过盛达到一定限度时，会向阳的方面转化。

Overabundance of Yin Transforming to Yang on the basis of the transformation between yin and yang, if the overabundance of yin reaches a certain limit, yin will transform into its oppsite, yang.

重镇安神 【zhòng zhèn ān shén】（镇心）使用质重具有镇静作用的金石类或贝壳类药物，以治疗心神不安的方法。常用于惊狂、失眠、心悸等症。

Tranquilization with Sedatives of Heavy Weight a method for the treatment of restlessness with sedatives of heavy weight such as minerals and shells; it is usually applied for the cases manifested with mania, insomnia, palpitation, etc.

重症鼻渊 【zhòng zhèng bí yuān】（脑崩、脑漏）即以鼻塞鼻酸、浊涕不止，腥臭难闻、甚则头晕目眩，头痛健忘为主要临床表现的一种病证。多因胆移热于脑所致。

Serious Nasosinusitis a morbid condition due to attack of gallbladder-heat to the brain, marked by stuffy nose, nasal irritation, profuse discharge of foul, purulent fluid, even dizziness, headache, amnesia, etc.

州都之官 【zhōu dū zhī guān】指膀胱。因膀胱是尿液聚集的地方。

The Official Managing the Reservoir referring to the bladder as is the

肘 【zhǒu】连接上臂与前臂的关节。

肘痈 【zhǒu yōng】生于肘部之痈。多由心肺两经风火毒邪凝结而成。

诸虫 【zhū chóng】泛指寄生于人体内，可致病的各种虫类。

诸阳之会 【zhū yáng zhī huì】指头部。因人体清阳之气皆上注于头；十二经脉中手三阳经和足三阳经也均经头部。

诸痫瘖 【zhū xián yīn】小儿痫证发作后，发音不出。

铢 【zhū】我国古代衡制中的重量单位，在唐代以前常用它作为药量单位。一铢合当时的 1/24 两。

猪胆汁导法 【zhū dǎn zhī dǎo fǎ】导便法之一。用猪胆汁加适量醋和匀，灌入肛门内，达到通便目的。一般适用于里热重、大便干结难解之证。

猪癫 【zhū diān】癫痫的俗称。

逐水 【zhú shuǐ】使用具有峻烈泻水作用的药物，以攻逐水饮的方法。适用于腹水、胸胁积水等实证。

逐寒开窍 【zhú hán kāi qiào】（温开法）是用性温而芳香的药物治疗寒湿痰浊阻闭心包、神志昏迷的方法。适

place for the storage of urine.

Elbow the joint connecting the upper arm and the forearm.

Carbuncle around Elbow carbuncle occurring in the area of elbow, which is caused by accumulation of toxin, and of wind and fire in the heart and lung meridians.

Parasites denoting parasites living in the human body, that may cause disease.

Convergence of All Yang (Qi or Meridians) the head, where all of yang-qi converges into the head, and all yang-meridians pass through the head.

Aphonia after an Attack of Epilepsy of Infants

Zhu a weigh unit in ancient China, often used as an apothecary weight early before Tang Dynasty, one zhu was equivalent to 1/24 liang at the time.

Pig-Bile Enema an enema with solution of pig's bile and vinegar, applicable to the case of constipation due to serious heat-syndrome in the interior.

Epilepsy

Hydragogue Method eliminating retained fluid with drastic purgatives, indicated for excess syndrome such as ascites, pleural effusion, etc.

Eliminating Cold-Phlegm for Resuscitation using drugs of warm nature and fragrant odour to treat

用于中风、突然昏倒、不省人事、面色青白、手足冷、脉沉等。 blockage of the heart by cold phlegm and coma, indicated for stroke, sudden syncope, loss of consciousness, palor, cold limbs, sunken pulse.

主证 【zhǔ zhèng】指疾病过程中表现出的主要症状和体征,是辨证论治的主要依据。

Principal Symptom and Sign referring to the chief symptoms and signs manifested in the course of disease, as important indications for diagnostic differentiation of syndromes.

煮 【zhǔ】中药炮制法之一。将某些药物放在清水内或其他液体辅料内略煮,以减少药物的毒性或使药物纯净。

Decoct one technique of preparing Chinese drugs by boiling the drugs in water along or with other adjuvants for decreasing its toxicity or for purifying.

注车注船 【zhù chē zhù chuán】(晕车晕船)指乘车船时出现头晕呕吐的症状。

Car Sickness and Sea Sickness referring to the symptom of dizziness and vomiting while taking car or ship.

疰夏 【zhù xià】(注夏)由脾胃虚弱或气阴不足,不能适应夏令炎热所致的病证。因有明显的季节性,每于夏令发病,故名。症见入夏之后,精神萎靡,倦怠乏力,微热,食欲不振,大便时见溏薄,形体消瘦等。辨证分类:1、湿困脾胃 2、脾胃气虚。

Summer Fever a disease due to unaccomodation to the hot weather resulting from asthenia of the spleen and stomach or that of qi and yin; manifested as listlessness, fatigue, fever, poor appetite, diarrhea, emaciation, etc. Types of differentiation 1. dampness involving the spleen and stomach 2. deficiency of both the spleen-qi and stomach-qi.

助阳解表 【zhù yáng jiě biǎo】用补阳药与解表药组成的方,以治疗阳虚外感之证的方法,是扶正祛邪治则的具体应用。

Restoring Yang and Expelling Superficial Factors a treatment for the case with yang-deficiency exposed to the exogenous factors by the application of drugs for restoring yang and for expelling superficial factors, which is a combination of supporting the healthy-qi and eliminating factors.

转胞 【zhuǎn bāo】(转脬、胞转) 以脐下急痛、小便不通为主症的病证。多由肾气虚、气化不利所致。

转筋 【zhuǎn jīn】(抽筋) 多由气血不足,阴液亏损,风冷或寒湿侵袭所致。症见肢体筋脉牵掣拘挛。好发于小腿腓肠肌,甚则牵连腹部拘急。

壮火 【zhuàng huǒ】是指阳热亢盛的实火,最易损伤人体的正气,而使全身性的机能衰退。

壮火食气 【zhuàng huǒ shí qì】指阳热亢盛之实火。能消耗正气,使正气衰竭,机能衰退。

壮热 【zhuàng rè】指实证中出现的高热。

壮数 【zhuàng shù】即每次施灸所燃的艾炷数。凡施灸时燃一个艾炷,称为一壮。

壮水之主,以制阳光 【zhuàng shuǐ zhī zhǔ, yǐ zhì yáng guāng】用滋阴壮水的方法,抑制阳亢火盛,以治疗属阴虚阳亢的虚热病证。

壮阳 【zhuàng yáng】用性温有补益作用的药物以强壮阳气的方法,主要治疗心肾阳气虚衰的病证。

Bladder Colic a condition marked by acute colic of the lower abdomen and dysuria, which is due to deficiency of kidney qi leading to hypofunction of qi activity.

Crapm a sudden painful contraction caused by the attack of wind-cold or cold-dampness as the result of insufficiency of qi and blood and impairment of yin-fluid, which is marked by spasm of the limbs frequently occurring in the calf muscle, even involving abdominal muscle spasms.

Sthenic-Fire an abnormally hyperactive fire, being harmful to the healthy qi and leading to general hypofunction.

Sthenic Fire Consumes Qi referring to sthenic fire of yang-heat overabundance which is able to consume vital qi and impair functions.

High Fever referring to the high fever which is present in the case with sthenia syndrome.

Cone Number number of ignited cones which is used during a moxibustion treatment.

Restraining Yang by Nourishing Yin a principle for treating the disease of asthenic-heat with yin-deficiency and yang-excess.

Strengthening Yang the method for strengthening yang, esp. for treating the case with the tonics of warm nature, which is deficiency of yang-qi of the heart and kidney.

灼痛 【zhuó tòng】指痛处有烧灼感。多见于郁火伤阴引起的胃脘痛或热毒亢盛的疮疡、烫火伤等。

Burning Pain a symptom which is seen in gastric pain due to impairment of yin by the retention of fire, or seen in the pyogenic infection of the skin due to hyperactivity of the virulent heat and burn.

浊气 【zhuó qì】1、指水谷精华的浓浊部分,与清气相对而言。2、指排出体外的污浊之气。如呼出之气及肛门排出的矢气。

Turbid Qi 1. referring to the thick part of food essence, opposite to the clear qi. 2. referring to the turbid qi discharged from the body such as air exhaled and gas flatus discharged.

浊气归心 【zhuó qì guī xīn】指食物精华的浓浊部分,通常是先运行到心,然后再由心脏通过经脉输送到全身组织器官。

Conveyance of Turbid Essence to the Heart the concentrated and turbid part of food essence is collected by the heart through circulation of the blood, and from the heart distributed to the different parts of the whole body through the blood vessels.

浊邪 【zhuó xié】指湿浊之邪,是重浊、粘腻的一类致病因素。

Turbid Pathogenic Factor referring to such factors causing disease as damp and turbid, which are heavy, turbid, sticky and greasy.

浊邪害清 【zhuó xié hài qīng】指湿浊之邪容易阻抑清阳,蒙蔽清窍,引起神志和感官障碍的病理。症见神志昏蒙、听觉障碍等。

Dampness Involving the Orifices of Head a disorder of the inhibition of lucid yang by damp, which results in mental disorder and dysfunction of sences organs, marked by semiconsciousness, impairment of hearing, etc.

浊阴 【zhuó yīn】1、与清阳相对的概念,一般指体内具有营养作用的重浊物质。2、体内代谢产生的污浊之物。

Turbid-Yin a concept opposite to clear yang, generally referring to 1. heavy, turbid and nourishing substance in the body. 2. dirty and turbid matter as the result of metabolism in the body.

浊阴不降 【zhuó yīn bù jiàng】由于脾

Turbid-Yin Failure in Sending Down

胃功能紊乱，水谷的营养物质与糟粕物质不能正常被消化、吸收和排泄的病理。症见胸闷、腹胀、便溏、小便黄及食欲减退等。
a pathological change with disturbance in regular digestion, absorption and discharge of nutritive matter and waste matter in food essenses, marked by stuffy chest, abdominal distention, loose stool, yellowish urine and poor appetite.

浊阴出下窍 【zhuó yīn chū xià qiào】阴主形主降，故浊阴多出于前后阴等下窍，如大小便从前后阴排出等。
Turbid-Yin Is Eliminated through the Lower Orifices as yin is in charge of form and desending, turbid yin is discharged through the anus and urethra, eg. in the form of urine and stool.

浊阴归六腑 【zhuó yīn guī fǔ】六腑的主要功能之一是转化水谷以供养全身，饮食水谷都归流于六腑，故称。
Turbid-Yin Moving toward the Six Fu Organs a physiological function in which the six fu organs store up the digested food and provide nutrients to the whole body.

浊阴走五脏 【zhuó yīn zǒu wǔ zàng】指水谷精微较浓浊部分，内走于五脏的生理现象。
Turbid-Yin Distributing to the Five-Zang Organs a physical phenomennon in which the thick and turbid part of digested food essence is distributed to the five-zang organs.

滋涯 【zī ái】指小儿躁动。因心经有风邪所致。
Infantile Restlessness a morbid condition caused by pathogenic wind in the heart meridian.

滋水涵木 【zī shuǐ hán mù】（滋肾养肝）是根据五行相生理论在治法上的运用，即滋养肾阴以养肝阴的方法。适用于肾阴亏损，肝阴不足，肝阳偏亢之证。
Providing Water for the Growth of Wood a theory of generation in the five elements applied to the treatment, i, e., a treatment for restoring the liver-yin by nourishing the kidney-yin, suitable for the cases of the consumption of kidney-yin, asthenia of the liver-yin and hyperactivity of the liver-yang.

滋肾 【zī shèn】（补肾阴）是治疗肾阴
Nourishing the Kidney a method of

不足的方法。适用于肾阴虚。症见腰酸腿软、遗精盗汗、头晕耳鸣、五心烦热、失眠、健忘、口干、舌红少苔、脉细等。

treating insufficiency of the kidney-yin, indicated for the deficiency of the kidney-yin, marked by distress of the loin, weakness of the legs, spermatorrhea, night sweat, dizziness, tinnitus, dysphoria with feverish sensation in the chest, palms and soles, amnesia, dry mouth, insomnia, red tongue with little coating, thready pulse, etc.

滋养肝肾 【zī yǎng gān shèn】1、用滋补肝肾的药物，以治疗肝阴虚的方法。适用于肝肾阴虚。症见头晕、耳鸣、腰部酸痛、咽干、夜卧不安或盗汗、舌红苔少、脉弦细等。2、滋肾阴以养肝阴的方法。见滋水涵木。

Nourishing the Liver and Kiney 1. a method to treat deficiency of the liver-yin and kidney-yin with drugs for nourishing the liver and kidney which is indicated for deficiency of the liver-yin and kidney-yin, marked by dizziness, tinnitus, distress and pain in the loin, dry throat, sleeplessness at night, or night sweat, red tongue with little coating, wiry and thready pulse. 2. a method to nourish the liver-yin by tonifying the kidndy-yin.

滋养胃阴 【zī yǎng wèi yīn】用甘寒滋润的药物，以治疗胃阴不足的方法，适用于胃阴不足。症见胃部有灼热感、胃中不舒、易饥、口干咽燥、大便干结、舌红少苔、脉细数等。

Nourishing the Stomach-Yin a method to treat deficiency of vital essence in the stomach with the moist drugs sweet in flavour and cold in nature, indicated for insufficiency of stomach-yin, marked by burning sensation in gastric area, discomfort in the stomach, inclination to hunger, dry mouth and throat, constipation, red tongue with little coating, thready and fast pulse.

滋阴利湿 【zī yīn lì shī】治疗湿热伤阴，小便不利的方法。常用滋阴养血药与利水而不伤阴的同用，以达到

Nourishing Yin and Promoting Diuresis a method of using yin-nourishing drugs combined with diuretics to

既滋阴又利湿的目的。 treat disturbance of urinary excretion caused by pathogenic damp-heat with impairment of yin for the purpose of both nourishing yin and promoting diuresis.

滋阴平肝潜阳 【zī yīn píng gān qiǎn yǎng】见育阴潜阳。 **Nourishing Yin, Restraining the Hyperactivity of the Liver Yang syn. and Suppressing Sthenic Yang.**

滋阴熄风 【zī yīn xī fēng】以滋阴为主的方药，治疗因阴虚动风的方法。一般用于热性病后期，热伤真阴。症见发热不甚但久留不退、手足心热、虚烦不眠、咽干口燥、神倦心慌、甚或耳聋、手足有轻微的不自主运动或抽搐、舌干深红、脉虚数或细数等。 **Nourishing Yin to Calm the Wind-Syndrome** a method to treat wind syndrome due to yin deficiency chiefly with yin-nourishing drugs. It is generally used at the late stage of febrile disease with the vital essence impaired by heat with such symptoms as slight fever but insistant, heat sensation of palms and solse, restlessness, insomnia, dry throat and mouth, mental fatigue, palpitation, even tinnitus, tremor or convulsion, dark red tongue, weak and fast or thready and fast pulse.

子盗母气 【zǐ dào mǔ qì】五行学说术语。用五行相生的母子关系说明五脏病变的相互影响。具有母子关系的两个脏，当子（脏）发生病变时，常可以累及母（脏）。如脾土为母，肺金为子，肺气虚弱可以导致脾脏虚弱。 **Illness of the Child Organ May Involve the Mother Organ** a term for the five elements theory mutual influence in the pathology of the five-zang organs according to the relationship between mother organ and child organ based on the theory of the interpromoting relation of the five elements. A diseased child organ may invole mother organ. eg. the spleen, the mother，the lung, the child, the deficiency of the lung-qi may result in the deficiency of the spleen.

紫癜 【zǐ diàn】以皮肤、粘膜出现瘀 **Purpura** a disease marked by pe-

点或瘀斑，颜色或红或紫或青，压之不褪色为特征的病证。常呈对称分布，数日后渐变为紫色、棕色而消失。可伴有鼻衄、齿衄，大小便出血等症。多因风热外侵，伤及脉络，或脾气虚弱，不能摄血所致。辨证分类：1、风热伤络 2、血热妄行 3、气不摄血。

techia or ecchymcsis in the skin or mucous membrane, reddish, violet or dark in colour, and never disappeared after press, symmetry distribution; accompanied with epistaxis, bleeding from gum, hematochezia, hematruia, etc, mostly due to exogenous wind and heat involving the meridians and collaterals, or due to asthenia of the spleen-qi failure to control the blood circulation. Types of differentiation 1. wind-heat attacking the collaterals 2. the disorder of blood circulation caused by blood-heat 3. qi failure to control blood.

子烦 【zī fán】指孕妇出现心惊胆怯、烦闷不安的病证。多因阴血不足或痰火扰心神志不宁所致。

Restlessness during Pregnancy a condition due to insufficiency of yin-blood or involvement of the heart by phlegm-fire.

子宫脱垂 【zī gōng tuō chuí】（子宫脱出）由气虚下陷，带脉失约，冲任虚损，或多产、难产、产时用力过度伤及胞络及肾气虚而使胞宫失于维系所致的疾病。症见子宫位置下垂或脱出阴道口外，甚者连同阴道壁、膀胱或直肠一并膨出。根据子宫下垂的程度，一般分为三度。辨证分类：1、气虚证 2、肾虚证。

Hysteroptosis a morbid condition marked by falling down of the uterus into the vagina from its normal position or protrusion of the uterus through the viginal orifice, even the protrusion involving the vagina wall, bladder and rectum; which is caused by down-collapse of qi, dysfunction of belt vessel, consumption of the thoroughfare and conception vessels, multigravida, dystocia, overstrain, damage of uterus and deficiency of the kidney-qi. Types of differentiation 1. syndrome of qi-deficiency 2. syndrome of the kidney-asthenia.

子宫外妊娠 【zī gōng wài rèn shēn】即子宫腔以外部位的妊娠。症见停经、

Extrauterine Pregnancy a condition of development of the fertilized ovum

小腹发作性剧痛,阴道出血、腹腔内出血、贫血、休克等。多属瘀血内停,气机阻滞的实证。

子户肿胀 【zǐ hù zhǒng zhàng】妇女外阴部肿胀的病证。

子淋 【zǐ lín】孕女出现的淋证。因阴虚、实热、湿气或气虚引起膀胱气化不利所致。

子气 【zǐ qì】1、妇女怀孕后由于脾肾阳虚,水湿停聚,流注于下,出现下肢浮肿,小便清长的病证。2、在五行具有相生关系的二行中,被生者称为子气。如木生火,火为木之子气。

子死腹中 【zǐ sǐ fù zhōng】妊娠过程中,胎儿死于腹中的病证。可因母体虚弱、跌扑闪挫、热病、药物等引起。

子嗽 【zǐ sòu】孕妇出现咳嗽的病证。因阴虚火动或痰饮上逆,外感风寒等

outside of the uterine cavity, which is caused by the retention of blood stasis and the weak qi activity, marked by sthenia-syndrome: as menolipsis, abdominal colicky pain, vaginal bleeding, intraabdominal hemorrhage, anemia, shock, etc.

Swelling of the Vulva a morbid condition with swelling and distention of the women's vulva.

Stranguria during Pregnancy stranguria occurring in a pregnant woman which is caused by dysfunction of the urinary bladder resulting from yin-deficiency, sthenia-heat, damp or qi-deficiency.

Qi of the Child Organ 1. a morbid state in pregnant women marked by edema in the lower limbs, profuse urine due to descending of the stagnated water-damp which is related to deficiency of the spleen-yang and kidney-yang. 2. the five elements in interelationship, any one being generated is known as the child, eg. wood generates fire and so fire is the child-qi of wood.

Dead Fetus in the Uterus a morbid condition occurring during the pregnancy when fetus is dead in the wolva, which may be caused by general weakness of the mother's body, traumatic injury or sprain, febrile disease, drugs.

Intractable Cough during Pregnancy referring to cought occurring in

引起肺失肃降，气机不畅所致。
pregnant women, in which the lungs loses its clearing and descending function leading to disturbances of qi which is caused by the stirring of fire as the result of yin-deficiency, or upper adverseness of retention phlegm, exposure to wind-cold.

子痫 【zǐ xián】（子冒）孕妇出现癫痫样发作的病证。多因平素肝肾阴虚，阴虚阳亢、肝风内扰、虚火上炎、引动心火，内火相煽所致。

Eclampsia Gravidarum a morbid condition of puerperal eclampsia attack in the pregnant woman, usually caused by the heat in the heart in contact with wind which is produced by internal stirring up of the liver-wind, upwarm flaming of asthenic fire, which are related to general deficiency of the liver-yin and kidney-yin with hyperfunction of yang.

子悬 【zǐ xuán】（胎上逼心）孕妇出现胸胁胀满的病证。多因肾阴不足，肝失所养，阴亏于下，气浮于上，冲逆胸胁所致。

Fullness over the Chest during Pregnance a symptom of feeling of distension in the thorax during pregnancy, which is usually due to insufficiency of the kidney-yin, mal-nourishment of the liver, downward impairment of yin, upward floating of qi which attacks the thorax.

子瘖 【zǐ yīn】孕妇出现声音嘶哑或失音的一种病证。因妊娠后期，胞脉受阻，肾阴不能上荣于舌本所致。

Aphonia during Pregnancy a morbid condition due to blockage of bao vessel which is resulted in the failure of the kindney-yin reaching tongue in the later period of pregnancy.

子痈 【zǐ yōng】指生于睾丸的痈。多由湿热下注或阴虚湿痰凝滞而成。症见起病急聚，初起仅感一侧睾丸或附睾胀痛和下坠感，迅速出现肿胀和剧烈疼痛，阴囊红肿热痛。可伴有寒热、头痛、口渴、恶心、小便短赤、舌苔

Carbuncle Occuring in the Testicle a disease characterized by sudden onset, distending pain and heavier sensation on one side of the testide or epidiaymis, swelling, sharp pain, local redness and accompanied with chilli-

黄腻、脉滑数等症。辨证分类：1、湿热下注证 2、痄腮余毒证

子肿 【zǐ zhǒng】怀孕后期全身水肿的病证。因孕妇平素脾肾阳虚，胎儿日渐长大后，母体的运化输布功能失调，以致水湿泛滥，流于四肢。症见足面浮肿，遍及下肢，渐至周身，头面俱肿，小便短少。

紫白癜风 【zī bái diàn fēng】（汗斑）症见局部皮肤有紫褐色或灰色斑点，并可逐渐扩大互相融合成片，表面光滑、边缘清楚、有时微痒、夏重冬轻。多由脏腑积热，感受暑湿、气滞血凝而成。

自汗 【zì hàn】在清醒状态下，不因活动、厚衣或发热而汗自出的一种症状。多因气虚、阳虚所致，血瘀痰阻或伤湿亦可引起。

ness, fever, headache, thirst, nausea, oliguria with dark urine, yellow and greasy tongue coating, slippery and fast pulse. Types of differentiation 1. syndrome of damp-heat involving the lower energizer 2. syndrome due to persisting toxin of mumps.

Edema during Pregnancy a disorder occuring in the pregnant women with deficiency of the spleen-yang and kidney-yang, which is caused by the retention of the body fluid due to the further functional disorder of the spleen and kidney. Manifested as edema of the foot, of the lower limbs, gradually of the general body, the head and face and oliguria.

Tines Versicolor a superficial fungal infection of the skin marked by purple and brown or grey and white patches in local skin, which may gradually expand and coalesce with esch other, with their surface smooth and border clear, occasionally accompanied by slight itching feeling occurring more in summer than in winter, mostly produced by accumulated heat in the zang-fu organs, affection from summer dampness, a

Spontaneous Perspiration a symptom appearing in the state of consciousness, which is never produced by exertion, over clothing or fever, it is mostly caused by blood stasis, phlegm blockage or pathogenic dampness as the result of qi-deficiency, and

自衄 【zì nù】指急性热病在高热无汗的情况下，忽然鼻衄不止，鼻衄后而热退身凉，起到汗出而解的同样作用，故称自衄。

眦赤烂 【zì chì làn】（眦帏赤烂）为眼弦赤烂之一种，局限于眼眦赤烂。多因内有湿热蕴结，外感风邪所致。

渍 【zì】用水将药物渐渐浸透、变软、又能保持药性的一种炮制方法。

宗筋 【zōng jīn】1、指前阴部。2、指阴茎。

宗筋之会 【zōng jīn zhī huì】1、若干肌腱集合之处。2、男性外生殖器。

宗脉 【zōng mài】泛指经脉汇集之处。通常分布于眼、耳等重要器官上。

宗气 【zōng qì】气的一种。它来源于水谷之气和吸入的空气，运行于胸中，以保证呼吸和循环功能的正常。

总按 【zǒng àn】诊脉方法之一。用食、中、无名指同时按寸、关、尺三个部位的脉搏。

yang-deficiency.
Spontaneous Epistaxis a sudden onset of bleeding from the nose with the result of subsidence of high fever, which is seen in an acute febrile disease with absence of perspiration.
Blepharitis Angularis an eye disease marked by redness, pain and erosion of the canthus, which is due to the retention of damp-heat in the body and the attack of wind.
Soaking a technique of soaking the crude drugs in water to soften them and the medical nature is still preserved.
Urogenital Region 1. referring to the front pudendum 2. referring to the penis.
1. Convergence Of Tendons 2. Male Genitals.
Converging Meridians the major or large meridians formed by the convergence of small meridians, which distributes over the important organs, such as the eyes and ears.
Pectoral Qi a combination of the air inhaled and the nutritive qi which originates from the essence of food, this pectoral qi circulates in the chest to ensure the normal respiration and circlation.
Feeling the Pulse with Three Fingers Simultaneously a way of pulse palpation with the index, middle and ring fingers putting on the cun, guan and chi sites simultaneously.

走马喉风 【zǒu mǎ hóu fēng】喉风之发病急骤，病情迅速发展者。

走马牙疳 【zǒu mǎ yá gān】以急剧发展的齿龈硬结、红肿疼痛，甚则坏死、溃烂为特征的一种疾病。多由病后或感受时行疫疠之邪。积毒上攻齿龈所致。

足发背 【zǔ fā bèi】（足背发）多因湿热下注或外伤瘀血化热所致的病证。初起整个足面结毒肿痛、坚硬、继而成脓。

足疔 【zú dīng】生于足部疔疮的总称。

足跟痛 【zú gēn tòng】（脚跟痛）多由肾亏、精血不足所致。症见足跟一侧或两侧疼痛、不红不肿、行走不便。

足踝疽 【zú huái jū】发于足踝部的疽。多因脾经寒湿下注，气血瘀滞；或先有疮毒，外伤余毒留于关节所致。症见局部红肿疼痛，常伴发热恶寒等全身症状，继则化脓溃破。

Acute Pyogenic Infection of Pharynx an acute and serious pharynx disease with sudden onset and swift development.

Acute Gangrenous Stomatitis a disease characterized by rapidly spreading induration, redness, pain, even necrosis ulceration on the gum, frequently caused by invasion of pathogenic factor and accumulated toxins upwardly attacking the gum.

Carbuncle on the Dorsum of the Foot an infection of the skin and subcutaneous tissue due to attack of damp-heat and formation of heat by blood stasis after injury, at the onset indurated swelling and pain on the dorsum of foot and soon with pus formation.

Furuncle on the Fool

Heel Pain a symptom mostly caused by impairment of the kidney and insufficiency of the essence and blood, which is marked by pain in one or both sides of the foot, difficulty in walking, but without red swelling.

Chronic Pyogenic or Tuberculous Arthritis of Ankle Joint an infection frequently caused by descending of cold-dampness in the spleen-meridian with stagnation of qi and blood; or ulcers and residual toxions in ankle joint; marked by local red, swelling pain, often accompanied by fever, chilliness and then followed by rupture with discharge of pus.

足心痈 【zǔ xīn yōng】（涌泉痈）即脚心涌泉穴处生痈。多因肾虚湿热下注所致。

佐金平木 【zuǒ jīn píng mù】用清肃肺气以抑肝的方法。常用于肝气上冲于肺，肺气不得下降而上逆的病证。症见两胁疼痛、气喘、脉弦者。

坐板疮 【zuò bǎn chuāng】 臀部的痱疮。

坐药 【zuò yào】用药制成丸剂、片剂或用纱布包裹药末，塞入阴道内，以治疗白带、阴痒等。

Abscess over the Center of the Sole abscess over the yongquan point, which is caused by descending of damp-heat due to deficiency of the kidney.

Supporting "Metal" to Suppress "Wood" a therapeutic method for keeping the adverse lung-qi downward to suppress the liver-qi, usually applicable for the case with failure of descending of the lung-qi resulting from the attack of the liver-qi to the lung, which is marked by hypochondriac pain, dyspnea, wiry pulse, etc.

Furunculosis Of Buttock

Vaginal Suppository a pharmaceutical preparation made of medicinal pills, tablets or powder wrapped in gauze, which is inserted into the vagina, for the treatment of leuckorrhea, itching in vaginal cavity.

附录1　中医病案书写格式

（一）门诊病案

1. 初诊记录

姓名：　　　性别：　　　年龄：　　　病案号：
科别：　　　＿＿年＿＿月＿＿日
问诊：
主诉：病人最痛苦的主要症状（或体征）及持续时间。
病史：主症发生的时间、病情发展变化的情况、诊治经过及必要的既往病史等。
望、闻、切诊：
与诊断有关的望、闻、切诊的阳性所见，必要的体格检查等。
舌象（舌体、舌质、舌苔、舌底脉络）。
脉象（两周岁以下小儿需察指纹）。
实验室检查及特殊检查结果。
辨证分析：
归纳四诊所得的主症、阳性体征、舌象、脉象等，扼要分析病位、病因、证候属性、病机转化。
诊断：
含中医病（证）名，证候及西医病名诊断。可写疑似诊断，但门诊三次仍未确诊者，应请上级医师会诊，协助诊断。
治法：
根据辨证写出指导用药的立法。
方药：
运用成方可写方名及加减，自拟方可不写方名。每行写四味药，药物名称右上角写特殊煎、服法，右下角写剂量"克"，亦可写"g"。
医嘱：
进一步诊治建议、护理、饮食宜忌等。

　　　　　　　　　　　　　　　　　　　　医师签全名：×××

2. 复诊记录

科别：　　　＿＿年＿＿月＿＿日
记录前次诊疗后四诊变化情况，如治法及方药发生变动，应做简要辨证分析。如有上级医师的诊治意见亦应记录在案。也可按病情变化，望闻切诊，简要病机，治法，方药，修改诊断等分项书写。右下方正楷签全名。

（二）急诊病案

1. 急诊初诊记录

除同门诊病案初诊记录的书写格式外，还应记录：

（1）病人急诊时间和医师检查时间，附上述年、月、日外，要加上时刻，如08：30；15：20；22：30等。

（2）急救措施、实施时间、用药及药物剂量、使用方法等。

（3）向家属交代病情及家属意见。

（4）会诊及上级医师诊查时间、所提的诊治意见。

（5）抢救无效或死亡者，应记录抢救措施、经过、用药情况（剂量及用法）及参加抢救的医师护士姓名。

2. 急诊留观记录

急诊留观记录书写格式同住院记录。

（三）住院病案

1. 住院病历

姓名：　　　　性别：　　　　病案号：
年龄：　　　　婚况：
职业：　　　　出生地：
民族：　　　　国籍：
家庭地址：　　　　　邮政编码：
入院时间：　　　　　病史采集时间：
病史陈述者：　　　　可靠程度：
发病节气：记录急性疾患发病或慢性疾患急性发作时的节气。
问诊：
主诉：简要记录患者感觉最痛苦的主要症状（部位、性质）或体征、持续时间，一般不宜用诊断或检查结果来代替。多项主诉者，应按发生顺序分别列出，如心悸三年，浮肿一天，喘息四小时。

现病史：围绕主诉详细询问疾病发生发展及诊治过程，重点写明起病诱因、原因、时间、形式、始发症状，主要症状和伴随症状（部位、性质），病情发展与演变过程，检查、诊断、治疗经过，所用过的中、西药物的名称、剂量、用法和用药时间以及其它特殊疗法，治疗反应及症状、体征等病情变化情况，发病以来精神、饮食、睡眠、二便等变化及现在症状（结合"十问"加以记录），对有鉴别诊断意义的阴性表现也应列入。

既往史：记录既往健康状况，按时间顺序系统回顾过去曾患疾病的情况，及传染病接触史等。

个人史：记录出生地、居留地、居住环境和条件、生活和工作情况、饮食习惯、情志状态、特殊嗜好等。

　　婚育史：女性患者要记录经带胎产情况,月经史包括初潮年龄、行经期/周期、绝经年龄；生育史包括孕、胎、产情况,配偶及子女的健康状况。

　　过敏史：记载药物、食物及其它过敏情况。

　　家族史：记录直系亲属和与本人生活密切相关的亲属的健康状况,如亲属已死亡则应记录其死因、死亡时间及年龄。

　　望、闻、切诊：

　　神色形态：包括神志、精神、体态及气色。

　　声息气味：包括语言、呼吸、咳喘、呕恶、太息、呻吟、腹鸣吸各种气味。

　　皮肤毛发：毛发的疏密、色泽、分布；肌肤温度、湿度、弹性以及有无斑疹、疮疡、瘰疬、肿块、浮肿等。

　　舌象：舌苔（苔形、苔色、津液）,舌质（色、瘀点、瘀斑）,舌体（形、态）,舌底脉络（颜色、形态）。

　　脉象：寸口脉,必要时切人迎、趺阳脉,两周岁以下小儿可写指纹情况。

　　头面、五官、颈项的望、闻、切诊：

　　胸腹部的望、闻、切诊：

　　腰背、四肢、爪甲的望、闻、切诊：

　　前后二阴及排泄物的望、闻、切诊：

　　体格检查：

　　记录西医查体的阳性体征及有鉴别诊断意义的阴性体征。各科或专科专病特殊检查情况均可记录在此。

　　实验室检查：（包括特殊检查）

　　记录入院时已取得的各种实验室检查结果及特殊检查结果,如血、尿、便常规,肝功、HB_sA_g、胸透、心电图、内窥镜、CT 等。

　　四诊摘要：

　　把四诊所得的资料（与辨证论治有密切关系的）进行全面、系统、扼要的归纳。

　　辨证分析：

　　要求从四诊、病因病机、证候分析、病证鉴别、病势演变等方面进行书写。

　　西医诊断依据：

　　指主要疾病的诊断诊据,并非所有疾病。

　　入院诊断：

　　　　　中医诊断：病（证）名
　　　　　　　　　　　证候
　　　　　西医诊断：病　　名

　　有几个病（证）写几个病（证）,病类与证类名称当另行写出,并与病（证）名错过一格,以示从属本病的病类、证类名称；西医诊断写在中医诊断的下方,有几个病写几个病,病名参照 ICD—9,凡超过 2 种以上诊断者,按主次先后顺序排列。
治则治法:
治则是治疗的指导原则,治法指具体的治疗方法。
方药:
运用成方要写出方名及加减,自拟方可不写方名。处方药物要求每行写四味药,药物名称右上角注明特殊煎服法,右下角写剂量,必要时写明煎法与服法。
辨证调护:
指医师对调养、给药、及食疗、及食疗、护理等方面的要求。

实习医师签全名:×××
住院医师签全名:×××
主治医师签全名:×××

2. **住院记录**
姓名: 性别: 病案号:
年龄: 婚况:
职业: 出生地:
民族: 国籍:
家庭地址: 邮政编码:
入院时间: 病史采集时间:
病史陈述者: 可靠程度:
发病节气:同住院病历要求。
问诊:
主诉:同住院病历要求。
现病史:同住院病历要求。
既往史:按住院病历要求书写,但可不系统回顾。
其它情况:记录重要的个人史、婚育史、过敏史和家族史内容(特别是与此次疾病的发生和治疗有关者)。
望、闻、切诊:
阳性所见及有鉴别诊断意义的阴性所见。
体格检查:记录阳性体征及有鉴别意义的阴性体征。
实验室检查:(包括特殊检查)
已有的各种实验室检查结果。
辨证分析:
按住院病历要求简明书写。
入院诊断:有几个病(证)写几个病(证),按主次排列。
中医诊断:病(证)名
证候

西医诊断：病　名
（参照 ICD—9）

诊疗计划：

医师签全名：×××

住院记录举例：

住　院　记　录

姓名：王××　　性别：男　　病案号：21753
年龄：63岁　　婚况：已婚
职业：工人　　出生地：北京
民族：汉　　国籍：中国
家庭地址：××××××5号　邮政编码：100023
入院时间：1988年2月22日15时
病史采集时间：1988年2月22日15时
病史陈述者：患者本人　　可靠程度：可靠
发病节气：雨水前一天
问诊：
主诉：左半身不遂五天。
现病史：1988年2月17日由于家庭纠纷而生闷气，次日10时许在车间劳动时，突感心慌，胸部闷痛，微喘，头痛，即去医务室就诊，肌注"氨茶碱0.25g"，半小时后症状略有好转，下楼时，骤然心慌加重，头晕仆地，被扶起时，发现左侧肢体完全不能活动，说话不流利，诉头痛头晕，右侧跳胀痛，同时冷汗频出，双手发凉，喘促，烦躁不安，急送××医院就诊，当时查BP16/10.1Kpa，意识清，双瞳孔直径3mm，等大圆。心率102次/分，心律不齐，心尖部可闻及双期杂音，心电图描记为心房纤颤。两眼向左凝视，口角歪向右侧，伸舌偏左，左上下肢肌力0级，左侧腱反射亢进，左巴氏征及夏道克氏征阳性，颈无抵抗。诊为："左侧偏瘫，脑栓塞；风湿性心脏病，二尖瓣狭窄及闭锁不全，心房纤颤"。当时予扩张血管药物"烟酸"静脉点滴，剂量不详。下午六时眼球已无偏斜，但心慌、半身不遂仍无好转。中医会诊认为"气虚血瘀，心阳不振"，予补阳还五汤合桂枝甘草汤加减治疗。三天后，半身不遂仍无好转，来我科住院治疗。现左侧肢体不能活动，说话欠流利，头痛沉胀如裹，心悸，胸闷脘痞，咳嗽，咯痰，痰稠色白，腹胀热敷后稍减，食少泛呕，下肢浮肿，难于平卧，夜寐不安，尿少而赤，大便五日未解。
既往史：咽痛反复发作，有痹证（风湿性关节炎）病史20余年，但近年无关节肿痛。10年前因心慌气短，曾诊为"风湿性心脏病"。
其它情况：无特殊。
望、闻、切诊：
神清合作，表情痛苦，神情倦怠，面色苍白，形体消瘦，肌肤少华，目珠不黄，眼睑微浮,唇干色暗,声低语怯,呼吸短促,咳声偶作,痰白粘稠,较难咯出,颈部青筋暴露,双下肢浮肿,口角右歪,伸舌偏左,左侧肢体软瘫。

舌象:舌体偏胖,伸舌向左侧歪斜。舌质暗淡,苔中心淡黄而腻。

脉象:脉弦滑,左寸重取无力,两尺兼沉,乍疏乍数。

体格检查:

T36.5℃　P96次/分　R24次/分　BP16/10Kpa

发育正常,营养较差,浅表淋巴结未触及,颈静脉怒张,两肺底散在中小水泡音。心率116次/分,心律不齐,心音强弱不等,心浊音界向左右两侧扩大,心尖部可闻及雷鸣样舒张期杂音及Ⅲ粗糙吹风样收缩期杂音,肝大,右锁骨中线肋下4cm,剑突下6cm,质地中等偏软,轻度压痛,双下肢可凹性水肿。神经系统检查:左鼻唇沟变浅,示齿左侧力弱,伸舌偏左,左上下肢肌力0级,肌张力低。左侧肢体痛觉、音叉震动觉减弱,腱反射左侧亢进,左侧可引出巴氏征及夏道克氏征,余无异常发现。

实验室检查:

血、尿、便常规,肝功、HBsAg均正常。

余未回报。

辨证分析:

此患者起病急,主要表现为头晕倒地,口舌歪斜,左半身不遂,发病前曾有生闷气的诱因,因此可拟诊为中风,以半身不遂为主而意识清,故属中经。虽然患者有四肢关节游走性疼痛史二十余年,但近年关节疼痛不重,故目前不作痹证诊断而有痹证史;发病时虽有头晕倒地,但神志清楚,又无四肢逆冷,故不能诊断为厥证;头晕倒地时无四肢抽搐、两目上视、口吐涎沫、昏不知人等,故与痫证不同。

风寒湿邪内侵,流注经脉,合而为痹,脉痹舍心,痹久耗气,心阳不振,则见心悸胸闷气短;心病日久,由心及脾,心脾气虚,脾失健运,痰浊内生,又久痹入络,瘀血内阻,津液外渗,亦可成痰;痰阻肺络,气失清肃,则微喘而咳;痰壅化热,则痰粘稠;移热膀胱则尿少而赤;扰动心神则夜寐不安;痰结火郁,腑气不通则苔转黄腻,大便五日未解;痰浊内阻,阻遏气机,清阳不升,则头痛沉胀如裹,胸闷脘痞;气机失调,胃气上逆,故食少而呕。水气内停,泛溢肌肤,发为水肿。患者病程日久,瘀血内阻,痰浊内壅,加之情志相激,肝阳上扰内风旋动,气血逆乱在脑,风痰瘀血阻滞经脉,而发为中风,因无神志障碍,故为中经。综观舌脉症,主病在心(脑),涉及肺、肝、脾、胃,证属本虚标实。

入院诊断:

中医诊断:1. 中风

中经

痰热腑实　风痰上扰

2. 心悸

心阳不振　气虚血瘀
西医诊断：1. 左侧偏瘫
　　　　　　　脑栓塞
　　　　　　　右颈内动脉系统
　　　　　2. 风湿性心脏瓣膜病
　　　　　　　二尖瓣狭窄及关闭不全
　　　　　　　全心功能衰竭Ⅱ°
　　　　　　　心房纤颤

诊疗计划：
1. 完善各项入院检查。尽早查头部CT，以求进一步确诊。
2. 急则治标，先宜化痰通腑为主，尔后当标本同治，益气活血。
3. 针对心功能不全及快速房颤，必要时给予强心利尿药治疗并记出入量。

　　　　　　　　　　　　　　　　　　　医师签全名：×××

3. 出院记录

　　　年　　月　　日　　时　科或病区，床号，病案号
　　姓名、性别、年龄、职业。于　　年　　月　　日　　时入院　　年　　月　　日　出院，共住院　　天。
入院情况：入院时四诊情况及体检要点。
入院诊断
　　　　中医诊断：病（证）名
　　　　　　　　　证候
　　　　西医诊断：病　名
住院期间诊疗及结果，主要的实验室检查阳性发现。
出院诊断：
　　　　中医诊断：病（证）名
　　　　　　　　　证候
　　　　西医诊断：病　名
出院医嘱：治疗、调摄的要求，出院带药。

　　　　　　　　　　　　　　　　　　　医师签全名：×××

出院记录举例：

出　院　记　录

　　89—3—5　2pm
　　胡××，男性，45岁，工人。于89年3月21日15时入院，经治痊愈，于89年4月16日10am出院，共住院25天。
　　病人以发热、恶寒、咳嗽2天，右胸掣痛半天入院，伴有周身酸楚，用解表药则汗出，头痛连脑，鼻塞涕浊，间有咳嗽，痰黄而粘，咳之易出，气粗微喘，右胸

掣痛，深息加剧。舌红，苔黄微腻，脉弦滑略数。T38℃，P82次/分，R20次/分，BP17.3/12KPa。右肺中部可闻及中、小水泡音，左肺呼吸音粗，心界不扩大，心率82次/分，律齐，各瓣膜听诊区未闻及病理性杂音。化验：血WBC22800个/mm^3（$2.98×10^{10}$/L），N97%，L3%。胸透：右中叶大叶性肺炎征象。

入院诊断：
   中医诊断：风温
      卫气同病，痰热蕴肺
   西医诊断：大叶性肺炎，右中肺

住院期间，依据症舌脉表现，辨证为外感风热病邪，痰浊风蕴化热。治以疏风解表，清化痰热，佐以通腑。汤药以银翘散合麻杏石甘汤加减治疗，配合静点清开灵注射液而痊愈。

出院诊断：
   中医诊断：风温
      肺阴不足 痰热未净
   西医诊断：大叶性肺炎，右中肺

出院带药：
1. 川贝枇杷露 3瓶 10ml/次 3/日
2. 养阴清肺膏 3瓶 10ml/次 3/日

嘱：避风寒，调饮食，注意休息。

       医师签全名：×××

The Standard Forms of Medical Record—Writing in Traditional Chinese Medicine

（一）Out-patient Clinic Medical Records（门诊病案）

1. The Medical Record at the First Visit（初诊记录）

Name：   Sex：   Age：   Clinic record No.：
Dept：   day   month   year
Inquiring：
Chief Complaint：The most suffering symptoms or signs and their duration.
Medical History：The occurence and development of chief syndromes and process of the diagnosis and treatment and relevant past medical history, etc.
Inspection, Auscultation and Olfaction, Pulse-feeling and Palpation：
  The positive findings related to the above diagnostic methods and the negative findings which is of significance in identifying diagnosis, necessary physical examination.

Picture of the Tongue (the size, property of the tongue, the fur, and the superficial veins beneath the tongue):

Pulse Condition:

(Superficial veins of the fingers for infants below two years old).

Various results of laboratory tests as well as special tests.

Diagnostic differentiation and analysis:

Based on the four diagnostic methods, synthesize the chief symptoms, positive signs, picture of the tongue and pulse condition, etc, analyse the diseased location, cause, the property of syndromes, and the development of the mechanism of disease.

Diagnosis:

Name of disease (zheng), syndrome form of TCM, and it of WM. A doubt diagnosis may be written, however, as for cases having been consulted for three times but still failed to get definitive diagnosis, it is necessary to call in a superior doctor for consultation to help with the identification of the disease.

Method of Treatment:

List the principles for guiding the medicine usage based on the diagnostic differentiation of syndromes.

Formula:

The name of the formula and its modification can be written out except the name of recipe prescribed personally. Four ingredients are written in one line with the note of special decoction and oral administration in the right-hand above each ingredient, and below it is the dosage "g".

Medical order:

Suggestions for further treatment, advisable nursing and prohibition in diet.

Doctor's signature (regular script)

2. **The Medical Record of Return Visit（复诊记录）**

Dept: _____ day _____ month _____ year

Take notes of the changes of four diagnostic methods after the first visit, the chief diagnostic differentiation and analysis ought to be made if there is any change in the medical treatment principle and prscription. The consulting opinions from superior doctors ought to be included in the record. They are also written separately in the light of the changes of the disease, the four diagnostic methods, chief mechanism of the disease, principle, formular and revised diagnosis. In the lower right-hand space is the signature of the doctor's full name in regular script.

（二）Emergency Medical Record（急诊病案）

1. **The Emergency Medical Record at the First Visit**（急诊初诊记录）

It is written in the same form as Out-patient Clinic Record. Furthermore, it also includes the followings:

(1) The time of emergency call and doctor's examination, exact time such as 8:30; 15:20; 22:30 should be added except day, month, year mentioned above.

(2) The measure of first-aid treatment and the time of adopting it, the administration, the dosage and the usage of drugs.

(3) Explaining the case condition to the patient's relatives and soliciting opinios from them.

(4) The time of consultation, superior doctor's consulting hour as well as the opinion of their diagnosis and treatment.

(5) Necessary notes of the measure for emergency treatment, process, administraiton (dosage and usage) and the signatures of the doctors and nurse on the spot in cases who failed to respond to emergency treatment and died.

2. **The Emergency Medical Record of Admission and Observation** （急诊留观记录）

It is written in the same form as In-patient Clinic Record.

（三）Admission Medical Record （住院病案）

1. **In-patient Medical Record** （住院病历）

Name:　　　　　Sex:　　　　　Admission record No.

Age:　　　　　　Marriage:

Occupation:　　　Place of birth:

Nation:　　　　　Nationality:

Family address:　Post code:

Date of admission:

The hour of collecting medical history:

Teller of medical history:　　　Reliability degree:

Solar term of the onset: take notes of the solar term of the acute onset or it of chronic disease.

Inquiring:

Chief Complaint:

take brief notes of the patient's most suffering symptoms and signs subjectively (location, property), or and their continuous duration. It is not advisable to use results of diagnosis and examination as substitution. Multiple complaints are separately listed in accordance with their order of occurence. For instance, palpitaion for three years, edema for one day, asthma for four hours.

History of Present Illness:

Around the chief complaint, inquire in detail about the onset, development and precedure of diagnosis and treatment of the disease. The major points to be recorded are the predisposing cause of invasion, cause, time, form, initiative symptom, chief symptoms and concomitant symptoms (location, property), the development of the case condition and change process, examination, diagnosis, the course of treatment, the prescribed traditional Chinese and western medicines and their dosage, usage and in-take hours, as well as other special therapy; the response to the treatment and the changes of symptoms and signs, the changes since onset in energy, diet, sleep, urination and defecation (in combination with" Ten Aspects"). The negative sign providing identification in diagnosis should be listed.

History of Past Illness: take notes of general health condition and occurence of illness in the past as well as its time, and any contract with contagious and epidemic diseases.

Personal History: make a record of the place of birth, the place of residence, the surroundings and conditions of living, working condition, diet habit, the state of emotion, special hobby, etc.

Marriage History: for the female case, the record includes menstruation, Leukorrhea, gynecopathy and obstetrics, the history of menstruation related to the age of menophania, the duration/period of menstruation, the age of amenorrhea; child bearing history related to pregnancy, fetus and delivery, the health conditions of spouse and children.

Allergic History: record of drug, food and other allergic factors.

Family History: take notes of health condition of patient's lineal and close relatives. If any of the relatives is dead, add to the record about his cause and time of death and age.

Inspection, Auscultation and Olfaction, Pulse-feeling and Palpation:

Appearance: including consciousness, mental state, carriage and complexion.

Voice and Smell:

including speech, respiration, dyspnea, vomiting and nausea, sigh, moan and groan, peristaltic sound and various smells.

Skin and Hair: the density, color and distribution of hair; the temperature humidity and elasticity of the skin; the presence of maculopapulae, sore, scrofula, mass and dropsy, etc.

The Picture of the Tongue: tongue fur (its shape, colour and moisture), tongue property (its colour, petechiae and ecchymosis), tongue body (shape and state), sublingual vessels and ligament of tongue (colour and state).

Pulse Conditon:

cun, guan and chi both left and right, and renying pulse and fuyang pulse are to be felt if necessary; examination of venules of the fingers is applicable for infants below two years old.

Inspection, Auscultation and Olfaction, Pulse—feeling and Palpation of the head, facial five organs and neck:

Inspection, Auscultation and Olfaction, Pulse—feeling and Palpation of the chest and abdomen:

Inspection, Auscultation and Olfaction, Pulse—feeling and Palpation of the lumber, back, the extremities and nails.

Inspection, Auscultation and Olfaction, Pulse—feeling and Palpation of the vulva, anus and excreta:

Physical Examination:

Take notes of those positive signs and those negative signs that are of significance in identification of diagnosis, including the reports of special examination of every departments or special subject.

Laboratory test: (including special tests)

Place on record of all kinds of the results and special test results since admission, such as blood, urine, routine bowl test, liver function, HBsAg, Chest X—ray, ECG, endoscopy and CT, etc.

Abstract of Four Diagnostic Methods:

Make a general systematic and brief induction on the basis of all the informations drawn from the four diagnostic methods (related to differential diagnosis closely)

Diagnostic differentiation and analysis:

It is required to write out from the aspects of the four diagnostic methods, etiology, pathogen, analysis of syndrome form, differentiation of syndrome, development of disease.

Identification of Diagnosis in WM:

Referring the identification for the main disease, not meaning of all the diseases.

Diagnosis of admission:

        Diagnosis of TCM: the name of disease (zheng)

                    syndrome form

        Diagnosis of WM: the name of disease

Write out as many diseases as there are, with the names of disease and syndrome forms being written in alternate line, the first word of syndrome form being directly under the second word of the name to indicate the both names of the disease. The diagnosis of WM is under that of TCM with all diseases being listed out in the same form. the ICD—9 is for reference, if there are two diagnosis or more, it is required to write them out in order of priority of primary and secondary.

The principal and method of treatment: principle is the guide of treatment, method is the way of treatment.

Formula:

It is necessary to write out the name of the formula and its modification, but not necessarily for personal prescription. Four ingredients are written in one line with the note of special decoction and administration in the right-hand above ech ingredient, and below it is the dosage "g". The decoction and administration should be written if necessarily.

Syndrome differentiation for the nursing:

It includes the requirements of doctor in prohibition、administration、dietotherapy and nursing, etc.

signature of intern (regular script)
signature of resident (regular script)
signature of attending doctor (regular script)

2. Admission Note（住院记录）

Name:　　　　　Sex:　　　　　Admission record No.:
Age:　　　　　Marriage:
Occupation:　　　　　Place of birth:
Nation:　　　　　Nationality:
Family address:　　　　　Post code:
Date of admission:
The hour of coller of medical history:
Teller of medical history:
Reliability degree:
Solar terms of the onset: the same as the requirements of In-patient Medical Record.
Inquiring:
Chief Complaint: the same as the requirements of In—patient Medical Record. History of Present Illness: the same as the requirements of In-patient Medical Record.
History of Past illness: the same as the requirements of In-patient Medical Record.

Others: records of important personal history, history of marriage and pregnancy, allergic history and family history (especially those related to the occurence and treatment of the present illness).

Inspection, Auscultation and Olfaction Pulse-feeling and Palpation: All the positive fingings and those negative findings that are of significance in indentifying diagnosis.

Physical Examination:

All the positive findings and those negative findings that are of significance in indentifying diagnosis.

Laboratory tests: (including special tests)

All the reports available.

Diagnostic differentiation and analysis:

Brief note according to the requirements of In-patient Medical Record.

Diagnosis of admission: (write out all the diseases (zheng) present in order of primary and secondary)

      Diagnosis of TCM: the name of disease (zheng)
               syndrome form
      Diagnosis of WM: the name of disease
            (ICD—9 for reference)

Plan of treatment: signature of doctor's full name
              (regular script)

Model of Admission Note: （住院记录举例）

Admission Note （住院记录）

Name: Wang Sex: male Admission record No. 21753
Age: 63   Marriage: married
Occupation: worker Place of birth: Beijing
Nation: Han   Nationality: China
Family address: No. 5…… Post code: 100023
Hour of admission: 15: 00 February 22, 1988
Hour of collecting disease history: 15: 00 February 22, 1988
Teller of medical history: the patient himself
Reliability degree: be reliable
Solar terms of the onset: the previous day of Rain water
Inquiring:
Chief Complaint: disability of movement on the left-side of the body for five days.

History of present illness: On Feb. 17, 1988, the patient went to see doctor with the complatint of sudden palpitation, oppressed feeling and pain in the chest, a slight short breath, and headache which attacked him at 10:00 am. while he was working in the workshop, being, in the dumps owing to family trouble yesterday. Having been given im "aminophylline 0.25g", the patient felt better half an hour later; an attack of aggravated palpitation when he walked downstairs, and then fell into a dead faint. When held up, he was found to have complete disability on the left-side of body and slurred speech. The symptoms present at the time were headache, dizziness, jumping and distending pain on the right side of the head accompanied by frequent cold sweating, cold hands, gasping breath, irritability and then was hurriedly sent to a hospital for consultation. Under the medication with BP 16/10 lKpa, clear consciousness, with two pupils equal and their diameter 3mm; heart rate 102 beats/min, arrhythmia, diastolic and systolic murmur at the area of the heart, the tracing of ECG indicated atrial fibrillation; both eyes strabismal towards the left and labial angle deviated to the right side; the tongue protruded in the left side, muscle strength testing was graded as grade 0 in the left upper and lower extremities. Reflexes were extension on the left, Babinski's and Chaddook signs were positive on the left, there was no resistance on the neck. The case was diagnosed as "left hemiplegia, cerebral embolism, rheumatic heart disease, mitral stenosis and insufficiency, atrial fibrillation," and medicated with Nicotinic acid for intravenous drip to expand the blood vessels, the dosage is uncertain. The deviation of eye balls disappeared at six in the afternoon, but palpitation and hemiplegia did not get better. The consultaton of TCM arrived at the diagnosis of "the deficiency of qi resulting in blood stasis and insufficiency of the heart-yang," using the modified prescription of Buyang Huanwa Tang (Invigoration Yang for Recuperation Decoction) and Gui Zhi Gan Cao Tang (Cinnamon Twigs and Licoric root Decoction). Three days late, his hemiplegia didn't improve, the patient was hospitalized in our department for treatment. The present manifestations are left hemiplegia and dysarthria, headache, heavy and swollen feeling in the head, palpitation, oppressed feeling in chest, epigastric fullness and pain, cough with thick and whitish sputum, abdominal distenion was lightly relieved with hot compress, poor appetite with frequent vomiting, edema in the low limbs, difficulty in lying flat, restlessness in the sleep, scanty and deep colored urine, absence of bowel movement for five days. History of past illness: the patient has had recurrent sorethroat, rheumatic arthritis for 20 years, but there was no swelling joints for late years and was once diagnosed as "rheumatic heart disease" due to palpitation and shortness of breath ten years before.

Others: nothing unusual has happened.

Inspection, Auscultation and olfaction, Pulse-feeling and Palpation:

clear consciousness and cooperation, painful expression, emotional fatigue, pallor complexion, pathologic leanness, dim complexion, eyeballs without icterus, puffy eyelid, dry lips with dim colour, weak voice, short breath, occasional attacks of cough with sticky and whitish sputum which being difficult to expectorate, fully distending jugular vein, edema in the lower extremities, labial angle deviated to the right side, the tongue protruded in the left side, hemiplegia on the left-side of the body.

Picture of the tongue: enlarged body of the tongue, it protruded in the left side, dark and pale tongue with light yellow and greasy fur on the central part.

Pulse condition: wiry and slippery, sunken pulse at both chi regions, irregularity in sequence of pulse beat.

Physical examination: T: 36.5°C P: 96beats/min R: 24/min BP: 16/10k pa., normal development, poor nourishment, unpalpation of superficial lymph node, distending jugular vein, scattering bubbling sound in the base of the lung; heart rate 116 beats/min, arrhythmia, unequal intensity of heart sounds, laterally extending cardiac dullness area, thunder-like diastolic murmur audible in the cardiac apix and harsh and blowing systolic murmur of third degree, hepatomegaly by 4cm inferior to the rib, 6cm inferior to the xiphoid process, midding soft, slight press pain, pitting edema in the low extremities.

Examination of nervous system: shallow nasolabial sulcus on the left and the strength of facial muscle on the left neveals weakness when exhibiting teeth, tongue protruded in the left, zero degree of muscle strength on the left extremities with lower muscular tension, pain sensation, weakened vibratory sense to the tuning fork in the left extremities, tendon reflex indicating more hyperactivity on the left. Left-side Babinskis and Chaddook signs (+), others (−).

Laboratory tests: routine tests of blood, urine, stool, liver function, and HBsAg are normal.

Diagnostic differentiation and analysis:

apoplexy (zhongfen) may be confirmed as the sudden onset manifested as dizziness, fall down on the ground, deviation of the mouth and tongue, hemiplegia on the left side of the body and the presence of dumps before the onset; the main symptom and signs of hemiplegia with clear consciousness, which indicated the attack involving the meridian (zhongjing). The presence of history of bizheng but not a diagnosis of bizheng, as the patient has suffered from moving pain in the four extremities for twenty years, but no joints pain later years; diagnosis of jiuzheng could not be made because of clear consciousness, and no cold extremities; it differs from xianzheng as no spasms of extremities, up-looking of the eyes, and no unconsciousness.

Invadation of pathogenic wind, cold and damp involved the meridians and vessels to form bi of the meridian and vessels consumped qi leading to hypoactivity of the heart-yang, marked by palpitation, depress feeling over the chest and shortness of breath; prolonged heart disease affected the spleen resulting in qi-deficiency of the heart and spleen, and failure of digestion and transportation, so leading to interiorly production of phlegm; as well as prolonged bi attacked collaterals, interiorly blood stasis and exteriorly of the body fluid produced phlegm; the phlegm obstructed the lung meridian result in failure of clear and descending marked by cough with slight athsma; retention of phlegm transmitted to heat, marked by sticky and thick sputum; heat transmitted to the gall—bladder marked by dark and scanty urine; disturbing the mind marked by night restlessness; retention of phlegm and heat leading to obstruction of fu-organ qi marked by yellow and greasy fur coating and no movement abowl for five days; retention of phlegm obstructed qi activity, clear-yang failure to rise up marked by headache with heavy and distending sensation, and depress feeling over the chest and palpitation; disorder of qi circulation leading to upwards of the stomach-qi, marked by poor appetite with nausea, retention of qi and interiorly of water distributed the skin and muscle leading to edema. The case has prolonged disease course with the condition of interior blockade of blood stasis and retention of phlegm, added emotional upsets, resulting in the upward disturbing of the liver-yang and hyperactivity of the interior wind, all the disorder of qi and blood involved the brain, and all the wind, phlegm and blood stasis obstructed the meridians and vessels, apoplexy occured; involvment of meridians is confirmed as no mental trouble. Sythmetic observation of the tongue, and pulse, and syndrome, the main diseased part is the brain and related to the lung, liver, spleen and stomach, the syndromes belongs to deficiency of the healthy qi and excess of pathogenic factors.

Diagnosis for admission:

diagnosis of TCM: 1. Apoplexy

    Involvment of meridian

        heat-phlegm resulting in excessive factors in fu-organs,

        upward disturbing of wind-phlegm·

  2. Palpitation

    hypoactivity of heart-yang, qi-deficiency blood stasis

diagnosis of WM: 1. left-side hemiplegia cerebral thrombosis right-side internal carotid artery

2. Rheumatic cardiac vovlu disease mitral stenosis and insufficiency heart failure Ⅱ° atrial fibrillation

Arrangement for medication.

    1. To perfect all kinds of examination for hospital admission, make examination of CT on the head soon for furthermore certificant diagnosis.

    2. For emergency, to treat the biao (superficiality aspect first by desolving phlegm and get the fu-organ qi off obstruction, and then treat both biao (superficiality) and ben (origin) aspects simultaneously by replenishing qi and activating blood circulation.

    3. In order to treat cardiac insufficiency and fast atrial fibrillation, giving cardiac diuretics for administration if necessary and to take notes of the inflow and outflow amounts.

doctor's signature

3. **Discharge Note** （出院记录）

_____hour _____day _____month _____year

Dept. _____bed No. _____medical record No. _____

Name _____Sex _____Age _____Occupation _____hour _____day _____month _____year be admitted _____day _____month _____year be discharged, total stay days in hospital _____.

Admission condition: about Four Diagnostic methods, and the main points of physical examination.

Admission diagnosis:

    diagnosis of TCM: the name of disease (zheng)

                  syndrome form

    diagnosis of WM: the name of disease

Medicating process and its results, important positive Lab. findings during the stay in hospital.

Diagnosis for being discharged:

    diagnosis of TCM: the name of disease (zheng)

                  syndrome form

    diagnosis of WM: the name of disease

Medical order for discharge: requirements of treatment, recuperations and drugs for discharge.

doctor's signature

Model of Discharge Note: (出院记录举例)

Discharge Note

2pm. 5/3/1989

Hu xx, male, 45years old, worker, was admitted at 3:00/pm, March, 21, 1989. He has completely recovered after medication and was discharged at 10:00am, April 16, 1989, he has been in hospital for 25 days totally.

The patient was hospitalized with the complaints of fever, chillness, cough, and referred pain in the right chest for half a day accompanied by distress all over. Following administration of diaphoretic, there is the manifestation of sweat, headache related to the brain, stuffy nose with thick running, intermittent cough with easy expectoration of yellow and thick sputum, dyspnea with a slight gasp, and aggravation of referred pain in the right chest by deep breath. Red tongue, yellow fur and slight greasy, wiry slippery and fast pulse. T 38°C, P 82 beats/min, R 20 beats/min, BP 17.3/12kpa. Mediate and light bubbling sound was audible from the right middle area of the lung, in the left lobe there was respiratory harshness, no enlargement of the heart area, the heart rate was 82 beats/min, the heart rhythm were regular, there was no pathogenic murmur from auscultaory area of all valves. Laboratory test: blood WBC 29800/mm^3, (2.98 x 10^{10}/L), N97%, L3%. Chest X—ray: signs of lobar pneumonia in the right middle lobe.

Admission diagnosis:

    diagnosis of TCM: wind-warm syndrome involvement of both wei and qi, stagnation of phlegm-heat in the lung.

    diagnosis of WM: lobar pheumonia, in the right middle lobe.

In the duration of hospitalization, the syndrome was differentiated as affection by wind-heat exopathogens and stagnation of phlegm in the interior transmitted to heat in accordance with the manifestations of the syndrome, tongue and pulse. the medication is dispelling exopathogenic wind from the exteroior, clearing away phlegm-heat and keeping the fu organs from obstruction. The prescriptions chosen for the treatment is Yinqiao San (powder of Lonicera and Forsythia) and modified Ma Xing Shi Gan Tang in combination with subordinative Qing Kai Ling for intravenous injection. The patient responded well to the treatment and recovered completely.

Diagnosis for being discharged:

    diagnosis of TCM: wind-warm insufficiency of the lung-yin, retention of the phlegm-heat.

diagnosis of WM: lobar pneumonia, the right middle lobe.

Prescription for discharge:

1. Syrup of Sichuan Fritillary Bulb and Loquat Leaf 3 bottles, 10ml per time, 3times per day.

2. Semifluid Extract for nourihing yin and clearing the lung-heat, 3 bottles, 10ml/per time, 3times per day.

Doctor's instruction: avoid wind and cold, proper diet and take a good rest.

dotor's signature

附录2 常用中草药
Appendix Ⅱ Common Chinese Materia Medica

解表药 【jiě biǎo yào】
Drugs for Treating Exterior Syndromes

发散风寒药 【Fā sàn fēng hán yào】
Drugs for Dispersing Pathogenic Wind—Cold

麻黄	【má huáng】	HERBA EPHEDRAE	Ephedra
桂枝	【Guì zhī】	RAMULUS CINNAMOMI	Cassia twig
香薷	【xiāng rú】	HERBA ELSHOLTZIAE	Herb of cimnamon twig elsholtzia
荆芥	【jīng jiè】	HERBA SCHIZONEPETAE	Herb of fineleaf schizonepeta
防风	【Fáng fēng】	RDIX LEDEBOURIELLAE	Root of saposhnikowia divavicata
羌活	【Qiāng huó】	NOTOPTERYGIUM IMCISIUM TING	Rhizome or root of notopteryginm
白芷	【Bái zhǐ】	RADIX ANGELICAE DAHURICAE	Root of dahurian angelica
细辛	【Xì xīn】	HERBA ASARI	Herb of Manchurian wildginger
藁本	【Gǎo běn】	RHIZOMALIGVSTTCI	Rhizome of Chinese Ligusticum
辛夷	【Xīn yí】	FLOS MAGNOLIAE	Flowerbud of biond Magnolia Li
苍耳子	【Cāng ěr zǐ】	HERBA XANTHII	Ripe fruit of Siberian Cocklebur
鹅不食草	【E bù shí cǎo】	HERBA CENTIPEDAE	Herb of Smallcen-

tipeda
生姜	【Shēng jiāng】	RHIZOMAZINGIBRIS RECENC	Fresh Ginger
柽柳	【Chēng liǔ】	RESINA TAMARICIS	Resin of Chinese Tamarisk
葱白	【Cōng bái】	BULBVS ALLIIFISTVLOSI	Fistular Onion Stalk

发散风热药 【Fā sàn fēng rè yào】
Drugs for Dispersing Pathogenic Wind—Heat

薄荷	【Bò hè】	HERBA MENTHAE	Herb of field Mint
牛蒡子	【Niú bàng zǐ】	FRVCTUS ARCTII	Achene of great Burdock
桑叶	【Sāng yè】	FOLIUM MORI	Mulberry Leaf
葛根	【Gě gēn】	RADIX PUERARIAE	Root of Lobed Kudzuvine
柴胡	【Chái hú】	RADIX BUPLEVRI	Root of Chinese Thorowax
升麻	【Shēng má】	RHIZOMA CIMICIFUGAE	Rhizome of Largetrifoliolious Bugbane
蔓荆子	【Màn jīng zǐ】	FRVCTVS VITICIS	Fruit of Simpleleaf shastetree
淡豆豉	【Dàn dòu chǐ】	SEMEN SOJAE PREPARATUM	Fermented Soybean
蝉蜕	【Chán tuì】	PRRIOSTRACVM CICADAE	Cicada Slough
浮萍	【Fú píng】	HERBA SPIRODELAE	Herb of Common Ducksmeat

清热药 【Gīng rè yào】
Drugs for Heat—Clearing and Fire—Purging

石膏	【Shí gāo】	GYPSUM FIBROSUM	Gypsum
知母	【zhī mǔ】	RHIZOMA ANEMARRHENAE	Rhizome of Common Anemarrhena
栀子	【Zhī zǐ】	FRUTVS GARDENIAE	Fruit of Cape Jasmine
天花粉	【Tiān huā fěn】	RADIX TRICHOSANTHIS	Snakegourd Root
芦根	【Lú gēn】	RHIZOMA PHRAGMITIS	Reed Rhizome
淡竹叶	【Dàn zhú yè】	HERBA LOPHATHERI	Herb of Common Lophatherum
莲子心	【Lián zǐ xīn】	PLUMULA NELUMBINIS	Lotus P Lumule
黄芩	【Huáng qín】	RADIX SCUTELLARIAE	Root of Baikal Skullcap
黄连	【Huáng lián】	RHIZOMA COPTIDIS	Coptis Root
黄柏	【Huáng bó】	CORTEX PHELLODENDRI	Bark of Chinese Corktree
龙胆草	【Lóng dǎn cǎo】	RADIX GENTIANAE	Gentian Root

苦参　　【Kǔ shēn】RADIX SOPHORAE FLAVESCEN-TIS　　Root of Lightyellow Sophoua

清热凉血药【Qīng rè liàng xùè yào】
Drugs for Heat—Clearing and Blood—Cooling

犀角　　【Xī jiǎo】　　CORNV RHINOCEROTIS　　Rhinoceros Horn Horn of Asiatic Rhinoceros
生地黄　　【Shēng dì huáng】　　RADIX REHMANNIDE　　Dired Rehmannia Root
玄参　　【Xuán shēn】　　RADIX RCROPHBLARIA　　Scrophularia Root
牡丹皮　　【Mǔ dān pí】　　CORTEX MOUTAN RADICIS　　Tree Peony Bart
赤芍　　【Chì sháo】　　RADIX PAEONIAE RVBRA　　Red Peony Root
紫草　　【Zǐ cǎo】　　RADIX ARNERIAE　　Root of Sinkiang Arnebia
　　　　　　RADIX LITHOSPERMI FLAVESCEN—TIS　　Root of Lightyellow Sophoua

清虚热药【Qīng xū rè yào】
Drugs for Clear the Asthenic fever

地骨皮　　【dì gǔ pí】　　CORTEX LYCII RADICIS　　Root—Bark of Chinese Wolfberry
白薇　　【Bái wēi】　　RADIX CYNANCHI ATRATI　　Root of Blackend Swallowwort
银柴胡　　【Yín chái hú】　　RADIX STELLARIAE　　Starwort Root
胡黄连　　【Hú huáng lián】　　RHIZOMA PICRORHIZAE　　Rhizome of Figwortflower picrorhiza

清热解毒药【Qīng rè jiě dú yào】
Drugs for Heat—Clearing and Detoxicating

金银花　　【Jīn yín huā】　　FLOSLONICERAE　　Honeysuckle Flower
连翘　　【Lián qiào】　　FRUCTUS FORSYTHIAE　　Capsule of Weeping Forsythia
大青叶　　【Dà qīng yè】　　FOLIUM ISATIDIS　　Leaf of Indigowood
板蓝根　　【Bǎn lán gēn】　　RADIX ISATIDIS　　Root of Indigowood
紫花地丁　　【Zǐ huā dì dīng】　　HERBAYIOLAE　　Herb of Tokyo Violet
蒲公英　　【Pú gōng yīng】　　HERBATARAXACI　　Dandelion
白蔹　　【Bái liǎn】　　RADIX AMPELOPSIS　　Root of Japanese Ampelopsis
土茯苓　　【Tǔ fú líng】　　RHIZOMA SMILACISGLABRAE　　Rhizome of Glabrous Greebrier

败酱	【Bài jiàng】	HERBA PATRINIAE	Herb of Dahurian patrinia
白鲜皮	【Bái xiān pí】	CORTEX DICTAMNI RADICIS	Root—Bark of Densefruitpittany
马齿苋	【Mǎ chǐ xiàn】	HERBA PORTVLACAE	Herb of purslane
白头翁	【Bái tóu wēng】	RADIX PULSATILLAE	Root of Chinese pulsatilla
秦皮	【Qín pí】	CORTEX FRAXINI	Ash Bark
山豆根	【Shān dòu gēn】	RADIX SOPHORAE TONKINENSIS	Root of Tonkin Sophora
射干	【Shè gān】	HHIZOMA BELAMCANDAE	Rhizome of Blackberrylily
马勃	【Mǎ bó】	LASIOSPHAERA SEV CALVATIA	Puff—Ball

清热明目药【Qīng rè míng mù yào】
Drugl for Clearing—Heat and Improving Eyesight

决明子	【Jué míng zǐ】	SEMEN CASSIAE	Cassia Seed
夏枯草	【Xià kū cǎo】	SPICA PRVNELLAE	Fruit—spirke of common Selfheal
青箱子	【Qīng xiāng zǐ】	SEMEN CELOSIAE	Seed of Feather Cockscomb
密蒙花	【Mì méng huā】	FLOS BUDDLEJAE	Flower of Pale Butterf Lybush
谷精草	【Gǔ jīng cǎo】	FLOSERIOCAULI	Flower of Buerger Pipewort
木贼	【Mù zéi】	HERBAEQUISETIHIEMALIS	Herb of Common Scouring Rush

抗疟药【Kàng nüè yào】
Antimalarial

青蒿	【Qīng hāo】	HERBA ARTEMISIAE ANNVAE	Herb of sweet Wormwood
常山	【Cháng shān】	RADIX DICHROAE	Root of Antifebrile Dichroa
鸦胆子	【Yā dǎn zǐ】	FEVCTVS BRVCEAE	Fruit of Jaua Brucea

化痰、止咳、平喘药【Huà tán zhǐ ké píng chuǎn yào】
Drugs for Resolving Phlegm, Relieving Cough and Asthma

温化寒痰药【Wēn huà hán tán yào】
Drugs for Resolving Cold—Phlegm

半夏	【Bàn xià】	RHIZOMA PINELLIAE	Tuber of Pinellia
天南星	【Tiān nán xīng】	RHIZOMA ARISAEMATIS	Jackinthe Pulpit

Tuber

白附子	【Bái fù zǐ】	RHIZOMA TYPHNII	Rhizome of Giant typhonium
白芥子	【Bái jiè zǐ】	SEMEN SINAPIS ALBAE	White Mustard Seed
旋复花	【Xuán fù huā】	FLOSINULAE	Inula Flower

清热化痰药 【Qīng rè huà tán yào】
Drugs for Resolving1 Heat—Phlegm

桔梗	【Jié gěng】	RADIX PLATYCODI	Platycodon Root
贝母	【Bèi mǔ】	BULBUS FRITILARIAE	Fritillary Bulb
前胡	【Qián hú】	RADIX PEUCEDANI	Root of white flower Hogfennel
瓜蒌	【Guā lóu】	FRUCTUS TRICHOSANTHIS	Fruit of trichosanthis
竹茹	【Zhú rú】	CAVLIS BAMBUSAEIN TAENIAM	Bsmboo Shavings
礞石	【méng shí】	LAPIS CHLORITI	Chlorite—schist
浮海石	【Fú hǎi shí】	PVMFX	Pumice Stone
海藻	【Hǎi zǎo】	SARGASSUM	Scaweed
昆布	【Kūn bù】	THALLUSLAMINARIA	Tangle

止咳平喘药 【Zhǐ ké píng chuǎn yào】
Drugs for Relieving Cough and Asthma

马兜铃	【Mǎ dōu líng】	FRUCTUS ARISTOLOCHIAE	Dutchmanspipe Fruit
桑白皮	【Sāng bái pí】	CORTEX MORI RADICIS	Root—Bark of Morus albs
荠苧	【Jì níng】	HERBA MOSLAEGROSSESERRA—TAE	Herb of Largeserrate Mosla
葶苈子	【Tíng lì zǐ】	SEMEN LEPIDII	Seed of Pepperweed
紫苏子	【Zǐ sū zǐ】	FRUCTUS PERILLAE	Perilla Seed
苦杏仁	【Kǔ xìng rén】	SEMEN ARMENIACAE AMARUM	Bitter Apricot Seed
百部	【Bǎi bù】	RADIX STEMONAE	Root of sessile stemona
紫菀	【Zǐ yuǎn】	RADIX ASTERIS	Root of Tatarian Aster
款冬花	【Kuǎn dōng huā】	FLOSFARFARE	Flower of Common Coltsfoot

芳香化湿药 【Fāng xiāng huà shī yào】
Aromatic Drugs for Resolving Dampness

藿香	【Huò xiāng】	HERBA AGASTACHES	Herb of wrinkled Gianthyssop
佩兰	【Pèi lán】	HERBA EUPATORII	Herb of Fortune Eupatorium

| 白豆蔻 | 【Bái dòu kòu】 | FRUCTUS AMDMI RDTUNKUS | Round cardamom |

砂仁　　【Shā rén】　FRUCTUS AMOMI　　Fruit of Villous Amomum
草豆蔻　【Cǎo dòu kòu】　SEMEN ALPINIAEKATSUMADAI　Seed of Katsumada Galangal
草果　　【Cǎo guǒ】　FRUCTUS TSAOKO　Caoguo
石菖蒲　【Shí chāng pú】　RHIZOMA ACORIGRAMINEI　Rhizome of Grassleaf Sweetflag
苍术　　【Cāng zhù】　RHIZOMA ATRACTYLODIS　Rhizome of Swordlike Atractylodes

消导药【Xiāo dǎo yào】
Drugs for promoting Digestion and Removing stasis

鸡内金　【Jī nèi jīn】　ENDOTHELIUM CORNEUM GIGERIAE GALLI　Membrane of Chicken Gizzard
麦芽　　【Mài yá】　FRUCTUS HORDEI GERMINATUS　Malt
谷芽　　【Gǔ yá】　FRUCTUS SETARIAE GERMINA—TUS　Millet Sprout
六曲　　【Liù qū】　MASSA MEDICATA FERMENTATA　Medicated Leaven
山楂　　【Shān zhā】　FRUCTUS CRATAEGI　Hawthorn Fruit
莱菔子　【Lái fú zǐ】　SEMEN RAPHANI　Radish Seed

行气药【Xíng qì yào】
Drugs for Promoting vital energy (Qi) circulation

枳实　　【Zhǐ shí】　FRUCTUS AURANTII IMMATURUS　Immature bitter Orange
橘皮　　【Jú pí】　PERICARPIUM CITRI RETICUATAE　Tangerine Peel
青皮　　【Qīng pí】　PERICARPIUMCITRI RETICULA—TAEUIRIDE　Green Tangerine Peel
佛手　　【Fó shǒu】　FRUCTUS CITRI SARCODACTYLIS　Finger Cirtron
厚朴　　【Hòu pǔ】　CORTEX MAGNOLIAE OFFICINALIS　Barkof official Magnolia
木香　　【Mù xiāng】　RADIX AUCKLANDIAE　Costusroot
香附　　【Xiāng fù】　RHIZOMA CYPERI　Rhizome of Nutgrass Galingale
乌药　　【Wū yào】　RADIX LINDERAE　Root of Combined Spicebush

泻下药【Xiè xià yào】

Purgative Drugs
攻下药【Gōng xià yào】
Purgatives

大黄	【Dài huáng】	RADIX ETRHIZOMARHEI	Rhubarb
芒硝	【Máng xiāo】	NATRII SULFAS	Mirabilite
番泻叶	【Fān xiè yè】	FOLIVM SENNAE	Senna Leaf

润下药【Rùn xià yào】
Laxatives

火麻仁	【Huǒ má rén】	FRUCTUS CANNABIS	Hemp Seed
郁李仁	【Yù lǐ rén】	SEMEN PRUNI	Seed of Chinese Dwarf Cherry

峻下逐水药【Jùn xià zhú shuǐ yào】
Drastic Hydragogues

甘遂	【Gān suì】	RADIX KANSRI	Root of Gansui
大戟	【Dà jǐ】	RADIX KNOXIAE	Knoxia Root
芫花	【Yuán huā】	FLOSGENK WA	Flower bud of Lilac Daphne

驱虫药【Qū chóng yào】
Anthelmintics

使君子	【Shǐ jūn zi】	FRUCTUS QUISQUASIS	Fruit of Rangooncreeper
苦楝皮	【Kǔ liàn pí】	CORTEX MELIAE	Bark of Szechwan Chinaberry Bark of Chinaberry—Tree
川楝子	【Chuān liàn zǐ】	FRUCTUS TOOSENDAN	Fruit of Szechwan Chinaberry
槟榔	【Bīng láng】	SEMEN ARECAE	Areca Seed

开窍药【Kāi qiào yào】
Drugs for Inducing Resuscitation

麝香	【Shè xiāng】	MOSCHUS	Musk
冰片	【Bīng piàn】	BORNEOLUM SYNTHETICUM	Borneol

温里药【Wēn lǐ yào】
Drugs for Dispelling interal cold

附子	【Fù zi】	RADIX ACONITI LATERALIS PREPARATA	Prepared lateral Root of Common Monkshood
干姜	【Gān jiāng】	RHIZOMA ZINGIBERIS	Dried Ginger
肉桂	【Ròu guì】	CORTEX CINNAMOMI	Cinnamomum Bark
小茴香	【Xiǎo huí xiāng】	FRUCTUSFOENICULI	Fennel, Fennel Fruit

荜澄茄	【Bì chéng qié】	FRUCTUSLITSEAE	Fruit of Morntain Specy Tree
高良姜	【Gāo liáng jiāng】	RHIZOMA ALPINIAE OFFICINARUM	Rhizome of Lesser galangal
吴茱萸	【Wú zhū yú】	FRUCTUS EUODIAE	Fruit of Medicinal Evodia
丁香	【Dīng xiāng】	FLOSCARYOPHYLLI	Clove

平肝药 【Píng gān yào】
Drugs for Calming the Liver

平肝熄风药 【Píng gān xī fēng yào】
Drugs for Calming the Liver to Check Endogenous Wind

羚羊角	【Líng yáng jiǎo】	CORNU SAIGAE TATARICAE	Antelope's Horn
牛黄	【Niú huáng】	CALCULRS BOVIS	Cow—bezoare
地龙	【Dì lóng】	LUMBRICUS	Earth Worm
钩藤	【Gōu téng】	RAMULUS UNCARIAE CUM RNCIS	Gambir Plant
天麻	【Tiān má】	RHIZOMA GASTRODIAE	Turber of Tall Gastrodia
僵蚕	【Jiāng cán】	BOMBYX BATRYTICATUS	Larua of a Silkworm with Batrytis
全蝎	【Quán xiē】	SCORPIO	Scropion
蜈蚣	【Wú gōng】	SCOLOPENDRA	Centipede

平肝潜阳药 【Píng gāng qián yáng yào】
Drugs for Calming the Liver and Suppressing Hyperactivity of the Liver—Yang

石决明	【Shí jué míng】	CONCHAHALITOTIDIS	Sea—ear Shell
代赭石	【Dài zhě shí】	OCHRA HAEMATITUM	Red Ochre
珍珠母	【Zhēn zhū mǔ】	CONCHA MARAARITIFERAUSTA	Nacre
白芍	【Bái sháo】	RADIX PAEONIAEALBA	White Peony Root
龙骨	【Lóng gǔ】	OS DRACONIS	Dragon's Bone
牡蛎	【Mǔ lì】	GONCHA OSTREAE	Oyster Shell
磁石	【Cí shí】	MAGNETITUM	Magnetite
罗布麻	【Luó bù má】	FOLIUA APOCYNI VENETI	Leaf of dogbane

安神药 【ān sén yào】
Tranquilizers

朱砂	【Zhū shā】	CINNABARIS	Cinnabar
琥珀	【Hǔ pò】	SUCCINUM	Amber
酸枣仁	【Suān zǎo rén】	SEMEN ZIZIPHI SPINOSAE	Seed of Sprine Date

柏子仁	【Bǎi zǐ rén】	SEMEN BIOTAE	Seed of Chinese Arboruitae
首乌藤	【Shǒu wū téng】	CAULIS POLYGDNI MULTIFLORI	Stem of Tuber Fleeceflower
远志	【Yuǎn zhì】	RADIX POLYGALAE	Root of Thinleaf Milkwort
合欢	【Hé huān】	FLOS ALBIZZIAE	Silktree Albizzia

利水渗湿药【Lì shuǐ shèn shī yào】
Drugs of Inducing Diruesis and Excreting Dampness

利水退肿药【Lì shuǐ tuì zhǒng yào】
Drugs for Inducing Diuresis and Subduing Swelling

茯苓	【Fú líng】	PORIA	Indian Bread
猪苓	【Zhū líng】	POLYPORUS	Umbellate Pore Fungus
泽泻	【Zé xiè】	RHIZOMA ALTSMATIS	Rhizome of oriental Water Plantatin
赤小豆	【Chì xiǎo dòu】	SEMEN PHASEOLI	Rice Bean
薏苡仁	【Yì yǐ rén】	SEMENCOICIS	Coix Seed
半边莲	【Bàn biān lián】	HERBALOBELIAE CHINENSIS	Herb of Chinese Lobelia
泽漆	【Zé qī】	HERBA EUPHORBIAE HELIOSCO—PIAE	Herb of Sun Euphorbia

利水通淋药【Lì shuǐ tōng lín yào】
Drugs for Inducing Diuresis to Treat Stranguria

车前子	【Chē qián zi】	SEMEN PLANTAGINIS	Pllantain Steeed
木通	【Mù tōng】	CAULIS AKEBIAE	Akcbia Stem
滑石	【Huá shí】	TALCUM	Talc
萹蓄	【Biǎn xù】	HERBA POLYGONI AVICULARIS	Herb of Common Knotgrass
瞿麦	【Qú mài】	HERBA DIANTHI	Herb of Lilac pink
石韦	【Shí wěi】	FOLIUM PYRROSIAE	Leaf of Shearer's pyrrosia

利湿退黄药【Lì shuǐ tuì huáng yào】
Drugs for Inducing Diuresis to Relieving Jaundice

茵陈	【Yīn chén】	HERBA ARTEMISEAE SCOPARIAE	Herb of Virgate Wormwood
金钱草	【Jīn qián cǎo】	HERBA LYSIMACHIAE	Her of Christina Loosestrife
地耳草	【Dì ěr cǎo】	HERBAHYPERICI JAPONICI	Herb of Japanese St. John'Swort

| 垂盆草 | 【Chuí pén cǎo】 | HERBA SEDISARMENTOSI | Herb of Stringy Stonecrop |
| 虎杖 | 【Hǔ zhàng】 | RHIZOMA POLYGONICUSPIDATI | Rhizome of Giant Knotweed |

祛风湿药【Qù fēng shī yào】
Antirheumatics

祛风湿止痹痛药【Qù fēng shī zhǐ bì tòng yào】
Drugs for Expelling Wind—Damp to Relieving Pain

| 独活 | 【Dú huó】 | RADIX ANGELICAE PUBESCENTIS | Root of Doubleteeth Pubescent Angelica |
| 威灵仙 | 【Wēi líng xiān】 | RADIX CLEMATIDIS | Root of Chinese Clematis |

舒筋活络药【Shū jīn huó luò yào】
Drugs for Dredging the Tendons and Activiting the Meridians

木瓜	【Mù guā】	FRUCTUS CHAENOMELIS	Fruit of Common Floweringquince
伸筋草	【Shēn jīn cǎo】	HERBA LYCOPODII	Herd of Common Clubmoss
络石藤	【Luò shí téng】	CAULIS TRACHELOSPERMI	Stem of Chinese Starjasmine
海风藤	【Hǎi fēng téng】	CAULIS PIPERIS FUTOKADSURAE	Stem of Kadsura Pep per
桑枝	【Sāng zhī】	RAMULUS MORI	Mulberry Twig
豨莶草	【Xī xiān cǎo】	HERBA SIEGESBECKIAE	Herb of Commom St. Paulswort
路路通	【Lù lù tōng】	FRUCTUS LIQUIDAMBARIS	Fruit of Beartiful Sweetgum

祛风湿强筋骨药【Qù fēng shī qiáng jīn gǔ yào】
Drugs for Expelling Wind—Damp and Strenthening the Tendons, Muscles and Bones

五加皮	【Wǔ jiā pí】	CORTEX ACATHOPANACIS RADICIS	Root—Bark of Slenderstyle Acanthopanax
骨碎补	【Gǔ suì bǔ】	RHIZOMA DRYNARIAE	Rhizome of Fortune's Drynaria
续断	【Xù duàn】	RADIX DIPSACI	Root of Himalayan Teasel
桑寄生	【Sāng jì shēng】	RAMULUS TAXILLI	Twig of Chinese Taxil-

lus

狗脊　【Gǒu jǐ】　RHIZOMA CIBOTII　Rhizome of East Asian Tree Fern

止血药 【Zhǐ xuè yào】
Hemostics

收敛止血药　【Shōu liǎn zhǐ xuè yào】
Drugs for Inducing Astringency to Arrest Hemorrhage

仙鹤草　【Xiān hè cǎo】　HERBA AGRIMONIAE　Herb of Hair Yuein Agrimonia
白芨　【Bái jí】　RHIZOMA BLETILLAE　Tuber of Common Bletilla
血余炭　【Xuè yú tàn】　CRINIS CARBONISATUS　Charrid Human Hair

凉血止血药 【Liáng xuè zhǐ xuè yào】
Drugs for Stopping Bleeding by Cool the Blood

小蓟　【xiǎo jì】　HERBA CEPHALANOPLORIS　Herb of common Cephalanoplos
大蓟　【Dà jì】　HERBA CIRSII JAPONICI　Herb of Japanese Thistle
地榆　【Dì yú】　RADIX SANGUISORBAE　Root of sangaisorba
槐花　【Huái huā】　FLOS SOPHORAE　Flower of Japanese Pagodatree
侧柏叶　【Cè bǎi yè】　CACUMEN BIOTAE　Leafy Twigs of Chinese Arboruitae
白茅根　【Bái máo gēn】　RHIZOMA IMPERATAE　Rhizome of Lalang Grass

化瘀止血药 【Huē yū zhǐ xuè yào】
Drugs for Stopping Bleeding by Resolving Blood Stasis

三七　【Sān qi】　RADIX NOTOGINSENG　Notoginseng
蒲黄　【Pú huáng】　POLLENTYPHAE　Cattail pollen
茜草根　【Qiàn cǎo gēn】　RADIX RUBIAE　Root of India madde

温经止血药 【Wēn jīn zhǐ xuè yào】
Drugs for Warming Meridians to Arrest Bleeding

艾叶　【Ai yè】　FOLIUM ARTEMISIAE ARGYI　Leaf of Argy Wormwood
炮姜　【Pào jiāng】　RHIZOMA ZINGBERIS　Dried Ginger

活血祛瘀药 【Huó xuè qù yū yào】
Drugs for Promoting Blood Circulation and Removing Blood Stasis

川芎　【Chuāng xiōng】　RHIZOMA CHUANXIONG　Rhizome of Chuanxiong

丹参	【Dān shēn】	RADIX SALVIAE MILTIORRHIZAE	Root of Red sage
月季花	【Yuè jì huā】	FLOS ROSAE CHINENSIS	Flower of Chinese Rose
泽兰	【Zé lán】	HERBA LYCOPI	Herb of Hirsute Shiny Bugleweed
王不留行	【Wáng bù liú xíng】	SEMEN VACCARIAE	Seed of Cowherb
益母草	【Yì mǔ cǎo】	HERBA LEONURI	Motherwort Herb
牛膝	【Niú xī】	RADIX ACHYRANTIS BIDENTATAE	Root of Twotooth Achyrantes
红花	【Hóng huā】	FLOS CARIHAMI	Safflower
桃仁	【Táo rén】	SEMEN PETSICAE	Peach Seed
血竭	【Xuè jié】	RESINA DRACONIS	Dragon's Blood
苏木	【Sū mù】	LIGNUM SAPPAN	Sappan Wood
郁金	【Yù jīn】	RADIX CURCUMAE	Root — Tuber of Aromatic Turmeric
穿山甲	【Chuān shān jiǎ】	SQUAMA MANITIS	Pangolin Scales
乳香	【Rǔ xiāng】	OLIBANUM	Frankincense
没药	【Mò yào】	MYRRHA	Myrrh
五灵指	【Wǔ líng zhī】	FAECES TROGOPTERORI	Trogopterus Drng
三棱	【Sān léng】	RHIZOMA SPARGANII	Rhizome of common Burreed
水蛭	【Shuǐ zhì】	HIRUDO	Leech

抗肿瘤药【Kàng zhǒng liú yào】
Anticarcinogen

长春花	【Cháng chūn huā】	HERBA CATHARANTHI ROSEI	Herb of Madagascar Periwinkle
喜树	【Xǐ shù】	FRUCTUS SEU RADIX CAMPTO—THECAEACUMINATAE	Fruit of Root of Common Camptotheca
莪术	【é zhú】	RHIZOMA ZEKOARIAE	Zedoray
农吉利	【Nóng jí lì】	HERBA CROTALARIAE	Herb of Purpleflower Crotalaria
半枝莲	【Bàn zhī lián】	HERBA SCUTELLARIAE BARBATAE	Herb of Barbed Skrllcap
白花蛇舌草	【Bái huā shé shé cǎo】	HERBA HEDYOTIS DIFFUSAE	Herb of Spreading Hedyotis

麻醉、止痛药【Má zuì zhǐ tòng yào】
Anesthetic and Analgesic

| 川乌 | 【Chuān wū】 | RADIX ACONITI | Mother Root of Common Monkshood |

雪上一枝蒿　【Xuě shàng yì shi hāo】　RADIX ACONITI KONGBOENSIS Root of Kongpo Monkshood

祖司麻	【Zǔ sī mǎ】	CORTEX DAPHNES	Bark of Girald Daphne
天仙子	【Tiān xiān zǐ】	SEMEN HYOSCYAMI	Henbane Seed
洋金花	【Yáng jīn huā】	FLDS DATURAE	Datura Flower
延胡索	【Yán hú suǒ】	RHIZOMA CORYDALIS	Yanhusuo
夏天无	【Xià tiān wú】	RHIZONA CORYDALIS DECUMBE NTIS	Rhizome of Decumbent corydalis
八角枫	【Bā jiǎo fēng】	RADIX ALANGII	Root of Chinese Alangium
两面针	【Liǎng miàn shēn】	RADIX ZANTHOXYLI NITIDI	Root of Shiny Leaf Prick Lyash
徐长卿	【Xú cháng qīng】	RADIX CYNANCHI PANICULATI	Root of Paniculate Swallowwort
雪胆	【Xuě dǎn】	RADIX HEMSL EYAE	Root of Lovely Hemsleya

补益药 【Bǔ yì yào】
Tonics
补气药 【Bǔ qì yào】
Drugs for Tonifying Qi (vital energy)

人参	【Rén shēn】	RADIX GINSENG	Ginseng
党参	【Dǎng shēn】	RADIX CODONOPSIS PILOSULAE	Root of Pilose Asiabell
五味子	【Wǔ wèi zǐ】	FRUCTUS SCHISANDRAE	Fruit of Chinese Magnoliaving
太子参	【Tài zǐ shēn】	RADIX PSERDOS TELLARIAE	Root of Heterophylly Falsestarwort
黄芪	【Huáng qí】	RADIX ASTRAGALI	Root of Mongolian Milkuetch
白术	【Bái zhú】	RHIZOMA ATRACTYLODIS MACROCEPHALAE	Rhizome of Largehead Atract Ylodes
山药	【Shān yào】	RHIZOMA DIOSCOREAE	Rhizome of Common Yam
大枣	【Dà zǎo】	FRUCTUS JUJUBAE	Jujube
饴糖	【Yí táng】	SACCHARUM GRANORUN	Maltose
甘草	【Gān cǎo】	RADIX GLYCYRRHIZAE	Liquorice Root

补阳药 【Bǔ yáng yào】
Drugs for Yang—Tonifying

| 鹿茸 | 【Lù róng】 | CORNU CERVU PANTOTRICHUM | Hairy Deerhorn |

补骨脂 【Bǔ gǔ zhī】 FRUCTUS PSORALAE Fruit of Malaytea Scurfpea

巴戟天 【Bā jǐ tiān】 RADIX MORINDAR OFFICINALIS Root of Medicinal Indianmulberry

淫羊藿 【Yín yáng huò】 HERBA EPIMEDII Herb of Shorthorned Epimedium

仙茅 【Xiān máo】 RHIZOMA CURCULIGINIS Rhizome of Common Curculigo

海马 【Hǎi mǎ】 HIPPOCAMPUS Sea—horse

山茱萸 【Shān zhū yú】 FRUCTUS CORNI Fruit of Asiatic Cornelian cherry

杜仲 【Dù zhòng】 CORTEX EUCOMMIAE Eucommia Bark

肉苁蓉 【Ròu cōng róng】 HERBA CISTANCHES Desertliving Cistanche

锁阳 【Suǒ yáng】 HERBA CYNOMORII Herb of Songaria Cynommorium

沙苑子 【Shā yuàn zǐ】 SEMEN ASTRAGALI COMPLANATI Seed of Flatstem Milkvetch

菟丝子 【Tù sī zǐ】 SEMEN CUSCUTAE Dodder Seed

冬虫夏草 【Dōng chóng xià cǎo】 CORDYCEPS Chinese Cater Pillar Fungus

蛤蚧 【Gé jiè】 GECKO Tokay

紫河车 【Zǐ hé chē】 PLACENTA HOMINIS Dired Human Placenta

补血药 【Bǔ xuè yào】
Drugs for Blood—Tonifying

当归 【Dāng guī】 RADIX ANGELICAE SINESIS Root of Chinese Angelica

鸡血藤 【Jī xuè téng】 CAULIS SPATHOLOBI Stem of Suberect Spatholobus

熟地 【Shú dì】 RADIX REHMANNIAE PRAEPARATA Prepared Rehmannia Root

阿胶 【ē jiāo】 COLLA CORII ASINI Donkey—hide Gelatin

何首乌 【Hé shǒu wū】 RADIX POLYGONI MULIFLORI Root of Tuver Fleeceflower

枸杞子 【Gǒu qǐ zǐ】 FRUCTUS LYCII Fruit of Barbary Wolfberry

补阴药 【Bǔ yīn yào】
Drugs for Yin—Tonifying

北沙参	【Běi shān shēn】	RADIX GLEHNIAE	Root of Coastal Glehnia
明党参	【Míng dǎng shēn】	RADIX CHANGII	Root of Medicinal Changium
麦门冬	【Mài mén dōng】	RADIX OPHIOPOGDNIS	Ophiopogon Root
天门冬	【Tiān mén dōng】	RADIX ASPARAGI	Root of Cochinchinese Asparagus
百合	【Bǎi hé】	BULBUS LILII	Lily Bulb
玉竹	【Yù zhú】	RHIZOMA POLYGONATI ODORATI	Rhizome of Fragrant Solomonseal
黄精	【Huáng jīng】	RHIZOMA POLYGONATI	Rhizome of King Solomonseal
石斛	【Shí hú】	HERBA DENDROBII	Dendrobium Stem
女贞子	【Nǚ zhēn zǐ】	FRUCTUS LIGUSTRUM LUCIOOM	Fruit of Glossy Priuet
龟板	【Guī bǎn】	PLASTRUM TESTUDINIS	Tortoise Plastron
鳖甲	【Biē jiǎ】	CARAPAX TRIONYCIS	Turtle Shell

收涩药 【Shōu sè yào】
Astringents

止汗药 【Zhǐ hàn yào】
Antiperspirant

麻黄根	【Má huáng gēn】	RADIX EPHEDRAE	Ephedra Root
浮小麦	【Fú xiǎo mài】	FRUCTUS TEITICI LEVIS	Shriveled Wheat

止泻药 【Zhǐ xiè yào】
Antidiarrheal

赤石脂	【Chì shí zhǐ】	HALLOYSITUM RUBRUM	Red Halloysite
禹粮石	【Yǔ liáng shí】	LIMONITUM	Limonite
肉豆蔻	【Ròu dòu kòu】	SEMEN MYRISTICAE	Nutmeg
诃子	【Hē zǐ】	FRUCTUS CHEBULAE	Fruit of Medicine Terminalia
罂粟壳	【Yīng sù qiào】	PERICARPIMI PAPAUERIS	Poppy Capsule
乌梅	【Wū méi】	FRUCTUS MUME	Smoked Plum
石榴皮	【Shí liú pí】	PUNICA RPIUMGRANATI	Pomegranate Rind
明矾	【Míng fán】	ALUMEN	Alum
五倍子	【Wǔ bèi zǐ】	GALLA CHINESIS	Chinese Nut—Gall
椿皮	【Chūn pí】	CORTEX AILANTHI	Bark of Tree—of—heaven

Ailanthus

涩精、缩尿、止带药【Sè jīng suō niào zhǐ dài yào】
Drugs for Nocturnal Emission, Reducing Urination and Curign Leukorrhagia

金樱子	【Jīn yīng zǐ】	FRUCTUS ROSAE LAEVIGATAE	Fruit of Cherokee Rose
桑螵蛸	【Sāng piāo xiāo】	OOTHECA MANTIDIS	Mantis Egg—Case
益智仁	【Yì zhì rén】	FRUCTUS ALPINIAE OXYPHYLLAE	Bitter Cardamon
乌贼骨	【Wū zéi gú】	OS SEPIELLA SEU SEPIAE	Cuttle—Bone
银杏	【Yín xìng】	SEMEN GINKGO	Guinkgo Seed
芡实	【Qiàn shí】	SEMEN EURYALES	Seed of Gordon Euryale
莲子	【Lián zǐ】	SEMEN NELUMBINIS	Lotus Seed
复盆子	【Fù pén zǐ】	FRUCTUS RUBI	Fruit of Palmleaf Radpberry

外用药【Wài yòng yào】
External Application

硫黄	【Liú huáng】	SULPUUR	Sulfur
铅丹	【Qiān dān】	MINIUM	Red Lead
水银	【Shuǐ yín】	HYDRARGYRVM	Mercuy Quicksilver
轻粉	【Qīng fěng】	CALOMELAS	Calomel
雄黄	【Xióng huáng】	REALGAR	Realgar
胆矾	【Dǎn fán】	CHALCANTHITUM	Chalcanthite
炉甘石	【Lú gān shí】	CALAMINA	Calamine
硼砂	【Péng shā】	BORAX	Borax
大枫子	【Dà fēng zǐ】	SEMEN HYDNOCARPI	Chaulmoogra Seed
木槿皮	【Mù jīn pí】	CORTEX HIBISCI	Bark of Shrubalthea

附录 3 药用衡量折算表

Appendix Ⅲ Table of Apothecaries' Weights Eguivalents

Ancient Market System (旧市制)	Metric System (公制)	Modern Market System (市制)	Metric System (公制)
I Jin (斤)	500g (克)	I Jin (斤)	500g (克)
I Liang (两)	31.25g (克)	I Liang (两)	50 (克)
I Qian (钱)	3.125 (克)	I Qian (钱)	5g (克)
I Fen (分)	0.3125 (克)	I Fen (分)	0.5 (克)

附录4　天干地支

Appendix IV Ten Heavenly Stems and Twelve Earthly Branches

天干　Ten Heavenly Stems
甲　the first of the ten Heavenly Stems
乙　the second of the ten Heavenly Stems
丙　the third of the ten Heavenly Stems
丁　the fourth of the ten Heavenly Stems
戊　the fifth of the ten Heavenly Stems
己　the sixth of the ten Heavenly Stems
庚　the seventh of the ten Heavenly Stems
辛　the eighth of the ten Heavenly Stems
壬　the ninth of the ten Heavenly Stems
癸　the last of the ten Heavenly Stems

地支　Twelve Earthly Branches
子　the first of the twelve Earthly Branches
丑　the second of the twelve Earthly Branches
寅　the third of the twelve Earthly Branches
卯　the fourth of the twelve Earthly Branches
辰　the fifth of the twesve Earthly Branches
己　the sixth of the twelve Earthly Branches
午　the seventh of the twelve Earthly Branches
未　the eighth of the twelve Earthly Branches
申　the ninth of the twelve Earthly Branches
酉　the tenth of the twelve Earthly Branches
戌　the eleventh of the twelve Earthly Branches
亥　the last of twelve Earthly Branches

附录5　二十四节气

Appendix V　The Twenty—four Solar Terms

立春　Beginning of Spring
　　　(1st solar term)
雨水　Rain Water
　　　(2nd solar term)
惊蛰　Waking of Insects
　　　(3rd solar term)
春分　Spring Equinox
　　　(4th solar term)
清明　Pure Brightness
　　　(5th solar term)
谷雨　Grain Rain
　　　(6th solar term
立夏　Beginning of Summer
　　　(7th solar term)
小满　Grain Full
　　　(8th solar term
芒种　Grain in Ear
　　　(9th solar term)
夏至　Summer Solstice
　　　(10th solar term)
小暑　Slight Heat
　　　(11th solar term)
大暑　Great Heat
　　　(12th solar term)

立秋　Beginning of Autumn
　　　(13th solar term)
处暑　Limit of Heat
　　　(14th solar term)
白露　White Dew
　　　(15th solar term)
秋分　the Autumnal Equinox
　　　(16th solar term)
寒露　Cold Dew
　　　(17th solar term)
霜降　Frost's Dew
　　　(18th solar term)
立冬　Beginning of Winter
　　　(19th solar term)
小雪　Slight Snow
　　　(20th solar term)
大雪　Great Snow
　　　(21st solar term)
冬至　Winter Solstice
　　　(22nd solar term)
小寒　Slight Cold
　　　(23rd solar term)
大寒　Great Cold
　　　(24th solar term)

条目汉语拼音音节索引

A

ā shì xué 阿是穴 ……………（1）
ái 癌 ………………………（1）
ài jiǔ bǔ xiè 艾灸补泻 ……（1）
ài róng 艾绒 ………………（1）
ài tiáo (juǎn) 艾条（卷）…（1）
ài zhù 艾炷 ………………（2）
ài zhù jiǔ 艾炷灸 …………（2）
ài fǔ 嗳腐 …………………（2）
ài qì 嗳气 …………………（2）
ài nǎi 嗌奶 …………………（3）
ān shén 安神 ………………（3）
ān zhōng 安中 ……………（3）
ān mó 按摩 …………………（3）
àn chǎn 暗产 ………………（3）
áo 熬 ………………………（3）

B

bā fǎ 八法 …………………（4）
bā gāng 八纲 ………………（4）
bā gāng biàn zhèng 八纲辨证
………………………………（4）
bā huì 八会 …………………（4）
bā kuò 八廓 …………………（4）
bā xī 八溪 …………………（5）
bā huǒ guàn 拔火罐 ………（5）
bái 白 ………………………（5）
bái bēng 白崩 ………………（5）
bái dài 白带 …………………（5）
bái diàn fēng 白癜风 ………（6）
bái hóu 白喉 ………………（6）
bái hóu huá tāi 白厚滑苔 …（6）
bái jīng 白睛 ………………（7）
bái lì 白痢 …………………（7）
bái lòu 白喉 ………………（7）
bái méi tāi 白霉苔 …………（7）
bái mó qīn jīng 白膜侵睛 …（7）
bái nèi zhàng 白内障 ………（7）
bái nián nì tāi 白粘腻苔 …（8）
bái pēi 白痦 …………………（8）
bái rèn dīng 白刃疔 ………（8）
bái tāi 白苔 …………………（8）
bái tū chuāng 白秃疮 ………（8）
bái xiè fēng 白屑风 ………（8）

bái zhuó 白浊	(9)	bēn tún 奔豚	(14)
bǎi hé bìng 百合病	(9)	bēn mén 贲门	(14)
bǎi rì ké 百日咳	(9)	běn cǎo 本草	(14)
bǎi zuì sòu 百晬嗽	(9)	bēng lòu 崩漏	(15)
bān 斑	(9)	bí 鼻	(15)
bān shā 斑痧	(9)	bí chuāng 鼻疮	(15)
bān tū 斑秃	(10)	bí dīng 鼻疔	(15)
bān zhěn 斑疹	(10)	bí fēng 鼻风	(15)
bàn biǎo bàn lǐ zhèng 半表半里证	(10)	bí gān zào 鼻干燥	(16)
bàn cì 半刺	(10)	bí gān 鼻疳	(16)
bàn shēn bù suí 半身不遂	(10)	bí jū 鼻疽	(16)
bàn shēn hàn chū 半身汗出	(11)	bí kǒng 鼻孔	(16)
bàn shēn má mù 半身麻木	(11)	bí nǜ 鼻衄	(16)
bàn zhī fēng 半肢风	(11)	bí sāi 鼻塞	(16)
bāo jiān 包煎	(11)	bí zhì 鼻痔	(17)
bāo 胞	(11)	bí yuān 鼻渊	(17)
bāo bì 胞痹	(11)	bí zhēn liáo fǎ 鼻针疗法	(17)
bāo hán bù yùn 胞寒不孕	(11)	bí zhǒng 鼻肿	(17)
bāo xì liǎo lì 胞系了戾	(12)	bì 闭	(17)
bāo yī bù xià 胞衣不下	(12)	bì jīng 闭经	(17)
bāo zhǒng 胞肿	(12)	bì zhèng 闭证	(18)
bāo zǔ 胞阻	(12)	bì qì 闭气	(18)
báo pí chuāng 薄皮疮	(12)	bì 痹	(18)
bào wén cì 豹文刺	(12)	bì qì 痹气	(19)
bào bēng 暴崩	(13)	bì zhèng 痹证	(19)
bào lóng 暴聋	(13)	bì 髀	(19)
bào jué 暴厥	(13)	bì shū 髀枢	(19)
bào máng 暴盲	(13)	biān shí 砭石	(19)
bào xián 暴痫	(13)	biàn bì 便秘	(19)
bào yīn 暴瘖	(13)	biàn nóng xuè 便浓血	(19)
bào zhù 暴注	(13)	biàn táng 便溏	(19)
bēi zé qì xiāo 悲则气消	(13)	biàn xuè 便血	(20)
bèi tòng 背痛	(13)	biàn zhèng 变证	(20)
bèi wù hán 背恶寒	(14)	biàn bān zhě 辨斑疹	(20)
bèi 焙	(14)	biàn chuāng yáng 辨疮疡	(20)
		biàn luò mài 辨络脉	(20)

biàn zhèng 辨证 …… (21)	bìng néng 病能…… (26)
biàn zhèng lùn zhì 辨证论治 …… (21)	bìng qì biāo běn 病气标本 …… (27)
biàn zhèng qiú yīn 辨证求因 …… (21)	bìng rù gāo huāng 病入膏盲 … (27)
biāo běn 标本 …… (21)	bìng sè 病色…… (27)
biāo běn tóng zhì 标本同治 … (21)	bìng tuí 病㿗 …… (27)
biǎo jū 瘭疽 …… (22)	bìng wēn 病温 …… (27)
biǎo hán 表寒 …… (22)	bìng yīn biàn shèng 病因辨证 …… (27)
biǎo hán lǐ rè 表寒里热 …… (22)	bìng zài zhōng páng qǔ zhī 病在中旁取之 …… (27)
biǎo jiě lǐ wèi hé 表解里未和 …… (22)	bó tāi 剥苔 …… (27)
biǎo lǐ 表里 …… (22)	bó jué 薄厥 …… (28)
biǎo lǐ chuán 表里传 …… (23)	bǔ fǎ 补法 …… (28)
biǎo lǐ jù hán 表里俱寒 …… (23)	bǔ jì 补剂 …… (28)
biǎo lǐ jù rè 表里俱热 …… (23)	bǔ pí 补脾 …… (28)
biǎo lǐ jù shí 表里俱实 …… (23)	bǔ pí yì fèi 补脾益肺 …… (28)
biǎo lǐ jù xū 表里俱虚 …… (23)	bǔ qì 补气 …… (28)
biǎo lǐ shuāng jiě 表里双解 … (24)	bǔ qì gù biǎo 补气固表 …… (29)
biǎo lǐ tóng bìng 表里同病 … (24)	bǔ qì shè xuè 补气摄血 …… (29)
biǎo rè 表热 …… (24)	bǔ shèn 补肾 …… (29)
biǎo rè lǐ hán 表热里寒 …… (24)	bǔ shèn nà qì 补肾纳气 …… (29)
biǎo shí 表实 …… (24)	bǔ tuō 补托 …… (29)
biǎo xié 表邪 …… (25)	bǔ xuè 补血 …… (29)
biǎo xié nèi xiàn 表邪内陷 …… (25)	bǔ yáng 补阳 …… (29)
biǎo xū 表虚 …… (25)	bǔ yīn 补阴 …… (30)
biǎo zhèng 表证 …… (25)	bù chuán 不传 …… (30)
biǎo zhèng rù lǐ 表证入里 …… (26)	bù mèi 不寐 …… (30)
bīng xiá yì 冰瑕瞖 …… (26)	bù nèi wài yīn 不内外因 …… (30)
bìng bìng 并病 …… (26)	bù shí 不食 …… (30)
bìng chuán 病传 …… (26)	bù yù 不育 …… (31)
bìng jī 病机 …… (26)	bù yùn zhèng 不孕证 …… (31)
bìng mài 病脉 …… (26)	bù zhǐ 布指 …… (31)

C

cāng lǐn zhī guān　仓廪之官 …（32）
cáo zá　嘈杂 ……………………（32）
cǎo yào　草药 …………………（32）
cēn wǔ bù tiáo　参伍不调 ……（32）
chā yào　插药 …………………（32）
chā jīng　差经 …………………（32）
chā tuí　差㿗 …………………（32）
chá　茶 …………………………（32）
chá mù　察目 …………………（33）
chān yào　掺药 …………………（33）
chán yāo huǒ dān　缠腰火丹 …（33）
chǎn hòu bì zhèng　产后痹证
　………………………………（33）
chǎn hòu biàn shēn téng tòng　产
　后遍身疼痛…………………（33）
chǎn hòu bìng jìng　产后病痉
　………………………………（34）
chǎn hòu bù yǔ　产后不语 ……（34）
chǎn hòu chì zòng　产后瘛疭 …（34）
chǎn hòu chuāng yáng　产后疮疡
　………………………………（34）
chǎn hòu dà biàn nán　产后大便难
　………………………………（35）
chǎn hòu dào hàn　产后盗汗 …（35）
chǎn hòu è lù bù jué　产后恶露不
　绝……………………………（35）
chǎn hòu fù tòng　产后腹痛 …（35）
chǎn hòu gǎn rǎn fā rè　产后感染
　发热…………………………（35）
chǎn hòu jiāo cháng bìng　产后交肠
　病……………………………（36）
chǎn hòu jīng jì　产后惊悸 …（36）
chǎn hòu jū luán　产后拘挛 …（36）
chǎn hòu kǒu kě　产后口渴 …（36）
chǎn hòu má mào　产后麻瞀 …（37）
chǎn hòu rǔ zhī zì chū　产后乳汁
　自出…………………………（37）
chǎn hòu sān chōng　产后三冲
　………………………………（37）
chǎn hòu sān tuō　产后三脱 …（37）
chǎn hòu shāng shí　产后伤食
　………………………………（37）
chǎn hòu sì zhī xū zhǒng　产后四
　肢虚肿………………………（38）
chǎn hòu tóu tòng　产后头痛 …（38）
chǎn hòu xiǎo biàn bù lì　产后小
　便不利………………………（38）
chǎn hòu xū fán　产后虚烦 …（38）
chǎn hòu xuè bēng　产后血崩
　………………………………（38）
chǎn hòu xuè yūn　产后血晕 …（39）
chǎn hòu yāo tòng　产后腰痛
　………………………………（39）
chǎn hòu yí niào　产后遗尿 …（39）
chǎn hòu yīn　产后瘖 …………（39）
chǎn hòu zhà hàn zhà rè　产后乍寒乍
　热……………………………（39）
chǎn hòu zhòng shǔ　产后中暑
　………………………………（39）
chǎn mén　产门 …………………（40）
cháng mài　长脉 ………………（40）
cháng zhēn　长针 ………………（40）
cháng bì　肠痹 …………………（40）
cháng fēng　肠风 ………………（40）
cháng míng　肠鸣 ………………（40）
cháng yōng　肠痈 ………………（40）

cháng zhì 肠痔	(41)
cháng dú 肠毒	(41)
cháo rè 潮热	(41)
cháo chǎo 炒	(41)
chēn zhàng 䐜胀	(42)
chén mài 沉脉	(42)
chéng fāng 成方	(42)
chí mài 迟脉	(42)
chǐ mài 尺脉	(42)
chǐ 齿	(42)
chǐ gǎo 齿槁	(43)
chǐ hén shé 齿痕舌	(43)
chǐ jiāo 齿焦	(43)
chǐ nǜ 齿衄	(43)
chǐ qǔ 齿龋	(43)
chǐ xiè 齿龂	(43)
chǐ yín zhǒng tòng 齿龈肿痛	(44)
chì 赤	(44)
chì bái dài xià 赤白带下	(44)
chì bái lì 赤白痢	(44)
chì bái zhuó 赤白浊	(44)
chì dài 赤带	(44)
chì miàn fēng 赤面风	(44)
chì rú pèi xuè 赤如衃血	(45)
chì zhuó 赤浊	(45)
chì zòng 瘛疭	(45)
chōng fú 冲服	(45)
chōng qì 冲气	(45)
chōng rèn bù gù 冲任不固	(45)
chōng rèn sǔn shāng 冲任损伤	(46)
chóng jī 虫积	(46)
chóng shòu shāng 虫兽伤	(46)
chóng xián 虫痫	(46)
chóng yáng 重阳	(46)
chóng yīn 重阴	(46)
chōu fēng 抽风	(47)
chōu jīn shā 抽筋痧	(47)
chū zhēn 出针	(47)
chū cháo 初潮	(47)
chū chí 初持	(47)
chū shēng bù niào 初生不尿	(47)
chū shēng bù rǔ 初生不乳	(48)
chù bí 嚃鼻	(48)
chù zhěn 触诊	(48)
chuán biàn 传变	(48)
chuán dào zhī guān 传导之官	(48)
chuán jīng 传经	(48)
chuǎn 喘	(48)
chuǎn míng 喘鸣	(49)
chuǎn zhàng 喘胀	(49)
chuǎn zhèng 喘证	(49)
chuàn 串	(49)
chuāng 疮	(49)
chuāng dú gōng xīn 疮毒攻心	(49)
chuāng yáng 疮疡	(49)
chuī yào 吹药	(50)
chún xián 春弦	(50)
chún yáng zhī tǐ 纯阳之体	(50)
chún 唇	(50)
chún chuāng 唇疮	(50)
chún dīng 唇疔	(50)
chún jū 唇疽	(50)
chún liè 唇裂	(50)
chún zǐ 唇紫	(51)
cóng wài cè nèi 从外测内	(51)
còu lǐ 腠理	(51)
cù bìng 卒病	(51)
cù yāo tòng 卒腰痛	(51)
cù zhòng 卒中	(51)

cù mài 促脉 ……………… (51)
cuī rǔ 催乳 ……………… (52)
cuī tù fǎ 催吐法 ………… (52)
cuì 淬 …………………… (52)
cùn bái chóng bìng 寸白虫病 … (52)
cùn、guān、chǐ 寸、关、尺

………………………… (52)
cùn kǒu 寸口 …………… (52)
cùn mài 寸脉 …………… (52)
cuō zhēn 搓针 ………… (53)
cuò shāng 挫伤 ………… (53)
cuò yǔ 错语 …………… (53)

D

dà biàn bù tōng 大便不通 … (53)
dà biàn gān jié 大便干结 …… (53)
dà cháng 大肠 …………… (53)
dà cháng hán jié 大肠寒结 … (53)
dà cháng rè jié 大肠热结 …… (54)
dà cháng shī rè 大肠湿热 … (54)
dà cháng xū hán 大肠虚寒 … (54)
dà cháng yè kuī 大肠液亏 … (54)
dà cháng zhǔ chuán dǎo 大肠主
　传导 ………………… (55)
dà dú 大毒 ……………… (55)
dà fāng 大方 …………… (55)
dà gǔ kū gǎo 大骨枯槁 …… (55)
dà hàn 大汗 …………… (55)
dà jié xiōng 大结胸 ……… (56)
dà kě yǐn yǐn 大渴引饮 …… (56)
dà mài 大脉 …………… (56)
dà nù 大衄 ……………… (56)
dà tóu wēn 大头瘟 ……… (56)
dà xiè 大泻 …………… (57)
dà zhēn 大针 …………… (57)
dà zì lòu 大眦漏 ………… (57)
dāi bìng 呆病 …………… (57)
dài mài 代脉 …………… (57)
dài zhǐ 代指 …………… (57)
dài xià 带下 …………… (57)
dài xià bìng 带下病 ……… (58)
dài xià yī 带下医 ………… (58)
dài yǎn 戴眼 …………… (58)
dài yáng 戴阳 …………… (58)
dān 丹 ………………… (58)
dān dú 丹毒 …………… (58)
dān tián 单田 …………… (59)
dān àn 单按 …………… (59)
dān é 单蛾 ……………… (59)
dān fāng 单方 …………… (59)
dān fù zhàng 单腹胀 …… (59)
dān rǔ é 单乳蛾 ………… (60)
dān shǒu jìn zhēn fǎ 单手进针
　法 …………………… (60)
dān xíng 单行 …………… (60)
dǎn 胆 ………………… (60)
dǎn huáng 胆黄 ………… (60)
dǎn ké 胆咳 …………… (60)
dǎn qì 胆气 …………… (61)
dǎn rè 胆热 …………… (61)
dǎn rè duō shuì 胆热多睡 … (61)
dǎn shí 胆实 …………… (61)
dǎn xū 胆虚 …………… (61)
dǎn xū bù dé mián 胆虚不得眠 …
………………………… (61)
dǎn zhàng 胆胀 ………… (62)

dǎn zhǔ jué duàn 胆主决断 ………… (62)
dàn yù mèi 但欲寐 ………… (62)
dàn shèn lì shī 淡渗利湿 …… (62)
dàn wèi shèn xiè wéi yáng 淡味渗泄为阳 ………… (63)
dāo fǔ shāng 刀斧伤 ………… (63)
dāo yūn 刀晕 ………… (63)
dǎo fǎ 导法 ………… (63)
dǎo qì 导气 ………… (63)
dǎo yǐn 导引 ………… (63)
dǎo zhì tōng fǔ 导滞通腑 …… (63)
dǎo zhēn 捣针 ………… (63)
dào jié quán máo 倒睫拳毛 ………… (64)
dào hàn 盗汗 ………… (64)
dé qì 得气 ………… (64)
dé shén 得神 ………… (64)
dí tán 涤痰 ………… (64)
diān 巅 ………… (64)
diān jí 巅疾 ………… (64)
diān 癫 ………… (65)
diān kuáng 癫狂 ………… (65)
diān xián fā zuò 癫痫发作 … (65)
diǎn cì 点刺 ………… (65)
diàn zhēn liáo fǎ 电针疗法 … (65)
diào jiǎo shā 吊脚痧 ………… (65)
diào xuàn 掉眩 ………… (66)
diē dǎ sǔn shāng 跌打损伤 … (66)
diē pū shāng tāi 跌仆伤胎 … (66)
dīng chuāng 疔疮 ………… (66)
dīng ěr 耵耳 ………… (66)

dīng níng 耵聍 ………… (67)
dǐng 顶 ………… (67)
dìng fēng 定风 ………… (67)
dìng 锭 ………… (67)
dōng shí 冬石 ………… (67)
dōng wēn 冬温 ………… (67)
dòng mài 动脉 ………… (68)
dòng gōng 动功 ………… (68)
dòng shāng 冻伤 ………… (68)
dú yáng 独阳 ………… (68)
dú yǔ 独语 ………… (68)
dú lì 毒痢 ………… (69)
dú shé yǎo shāng 毒蛇咬伤 ………… (69)
dú yào gōng xié 毒药攻邪 … (69)
dù rǔ 妒乳 ………… (69)
duǎn mài 短脉 ………… (69)
duǎn qì 短气 ………… (70)
duàn 煅 ………… (70)
duì kǒu chuāng 对口疮 ……… (70)
dùn fú 顿服 ………… (70)
dùn ké 顿咳 ………… (70)
dùn 燉 ………… (71)
duō hàn 多汗 ………… (71)
duō mèng 多梦 ………… (71)
duō wàng 多忘 ………… (71)
duó hàn zhě wú xuè 夺汗者无血 ………… (71)
duó jīng 夺精 ………… (71)
duó xuè zhě wú hàn 夺血者无汗 ………… (71)

E

é kǒu chuāng 鹅口疮	(71)	ěr kuò 耳廓	(75)
é zhǎng fēng 鹅掌风	(72)	ěr làn 耳烂	(75)
é jú 额疽	(72)	ěr lóng 耳聋	(75)
ě xīn 恶心	(72)	ěr mì 耳泌	(76)
è chuāng 恶疮	(72)	ěr míng 耳鸣	(76)
è lù 恶露	(73)	ěr mó 耳膜	(76)
è sè 恶色	(73)	ěr nèi yì wù 耳内异物	(76)
è xuè 恶血	(73)	ěr nù 耳衄	(76)
è niàn 恶念	(73)	ěr tǐng 耳挺	(76)
è nì 呃逆	(73)	ěr tòng 耳痛	(76)
ér zhěn tòng 儿枕痛	(73)	ěr yǎng 耳痒	(76)
ěr 耳	(73)	ěr yōng 耳痈	(77)
ěr díng 耳疔	(74)	ěr zhēn 耳针	(77)
ěr dìng 耳定	(74)	ěr zhēn liáo fǎ 耳针疗法	(77)
ěr fáng fēng 耳防风	(74)	èr shí bā mài 二十八脉	(77)
ěr gēn dú 耳根毒	(74)	èr yáng bìng bìng 二阳并病	(77)
ěr hòu jū 耳后疽	(75)	èr yīn 二阴	(78)
èr jūn 耳菌	(75)		

F

fā bèi 发背	(78)	fà chí 发迟	(80)
fā biǎo bù yuǎn rè 发表不远热	(78)	fà jì chuāng 发际疮	(80)
fā hàn jìn lì 发汗禁例	(78)	fà kū 发枯	(80)
fā huáng 发黄	(78)	fà luò 发落	(80)
fā nǎo 发脑	(78)	fà wèi xuè zhī yú 发为血之余	(80)
fā pào 发泡	(78)	fān huā zì 翻花痔	(80)
fā pào jiǔ 发泡灸	(78)	fán kě 烦渴	(81)
fā rè 发热	(79)	fán rè 烦热	(81)
fā rè wù hán 发热恶寒	(79)	fán zào 烦躁	(81)
fā yí 发颐	(79)	fǎn guān mài 反关脉	(81)
fá gān 伐肝	(79)	fǎn zhì 反治	(81)
fà 发	(79)	fàn běn 犯本	(82)
fà bái 发白	(79)	fàn hòu fú 饭后服	(82)

fàn qián fú 饭前服 ……(82)	fèi shèn tóng zhì 肺肾同治……(88)
fàn ě 泛恶 ……(82)	fèi shèn xiāng shēng 肺肾相生 …… (89)
fāng 方 ……(82)	fèi shī qīng sù 肺失清肃……(89)
fāng jì pèi wǔ 方剂配伍 ……(82)	fèi wéi jiāo zàng 肺为娇脏……(89)
fāng xiāng huà zhuó 芳香化浊 …… (82)	fèi wěi 肺痿……(89)
fáng láo 房劳 ……(83)	fèi xì 肺系 ……(89)
fēi dòu 飞痘 ……(83)	fèi xián 肺痫 ……(89)
fēi yáng hóu 飞扬喉 ……(83)	fèi xié xié tòng 肺邪胁痛 ……(90)
fēi fēng 非风 ……(83)	fèi xū 肺虚 ……(90)
féi nián chuāng 肥粘疮 ……(83)	fèi xū chuǎn jí 肺虚喘急……(90)
fèi 肺 ……(83)	fèi xū ké sòu 肺虚咳嗽 ……(90)
fèi bì 肺痹 ……(84)	fèi yán chuǎn sòu 肺炎喘嗽 …(90)
fèi bìng 肺病 ……(84)	fèi yīn 肺阴 ……(91)
fèi cháo bǎi mài 肺朝百脉……(84)	fèi yīn xū 肺阴虚 ……(91)
fèi gān 肺疳 ……(84)	fèi yōng 肺痈 ……(91)
fèi hé dà cháng 肺合大肠 ……(84)	fèi zào 肺燥 ……(92)
fèi hé pí máo 肺和皮毛 ……(85)	fèi zhàng 肺胀 ……(92)
fèi huǒ 肺火 ……(85)	fèi zhǔ qì 肺主气 ……(92)
fèi kāi qiào yú bí 肺开窍于鼻 …… (85)	fèi zhǔ shēng 肺主声 ……(92)
fèi ké 肺咳 ……(86)	fèi zhǔ sù jiàng 肺主肃降……(93)
fèi láo 肺痨 ……(86)	fèi zhǔ xíng shuǐ 肺主行水 …(93)
fèi luò sǔn shāng 肺络损伤……(86)	fèi zhǔ zhì jié 肺主治节 ……(93)
fèi, qí huá zài máo, qí chōng zài pí 肺，其华在毛，其充在皮…… (86)	fèi chuāng 痱疮 ……(93)
	fēn miǎn 分娩 ……(93)
fèi qì 肺气 ……(87)	fěn cì 粉刺 ……(93)
fèi qì bù lì 肺气不利 ……(87)	fěn liú 粉瘤 ……(94)
fèi qì bù xuān 肺气不宣 ……(87)	fēng 风 ……(94)
fèi qì bù zú 肺气不足 ……(87)	fēng bì 风秘 ……(94)
fèi qì shàng nì 肺气上逆 ……(87)	fēng bì 风痹 ……(94)
fèi qì xū 肺气虚 ……(87)	fēng chù 风搐 ……(94)
fèi rè ké sòu 肺热咳嗽 ……(87)	fēng fèi 风痱 ……(95)
fèi rè bìng 肺热病 ……(88)	fēng guān 风关 ……(95)
fèi shèn liǎng xū 肺肾两虚 ……(88)	fēng hán chuǎn jí 风寒喘急 …(95)
	fēng hán ěr lóng 风寒耳聋 ……(95)
	fēng hán gǎn mào 风寒感冒 …(95)

fēng hán ké sòu 风寒咳嗽 …… (96)	fēng tán xuàn yūn 风痰眩晕
fēng hàn shī bì 风寒湿痹 …… (96)	…………………………… (103)
fēng hán shù fèi 风寒束肺 …… (96)	fēng wēn 风温 ………… (104)
fēng hán tóu tòng 风寒头痛 …… (96)	fēng wēn yìng 风温痉 …… (104)
fēng hán xié tòng 风寒胁痛 … (97)	fēng xián 风痫 ………… (104)
fēng huǒ lì 风火疬 …………… (97)	fēng xiāo 风消 ………… (104)
fēng huǒ yǎn tòng 风火眼痛 … (97)	fēng xiè 风泻 ………… (104)
fēng huǒ xiāng shàn 风火相煽	fēng xīn tòng 风心痛 … (104)
…………………………… (97)	fēng xuàn 风眩 ………… (105)
fēng jiā 风家 ……………… (98)	fēng yì 风懿 ………… (105)
fēng jìng 风痉 ……………… (98)	fēng cáng shī zhí 封藏失职 …… (105)
fēng jū 风疽 ……………… (98)	fēng quǎn yǎo shāng 疯犬咬伤
fēng lì 风疬 ……………… (98)	…………………………… (105)
fēng lún 风轮 ……………… (98)	fēng lòu 蜂瘘 ………… (105)
fēng nüè 风疟 ……………… (98)	fēng shì shāng 蜂螫伤 … (105)
fēng qǐ wāi xié 风起㖞斜 …… (98)	fū zhàng 肤胀 ………… (106)
fēng qì nèi dòng 风气内动 …… (99)	fū yáng mài 跗阳脉 …… (106)
fēng rè 风热 ……………… (99)	fū gǔ shāng 跗骨伤 …… (106)
fēng rè ěr lǒng 风热耳聋 …… (99)	fū zhǒng 跗肿 ………… (106)
fēng rè gǎn mào 风热感冒 …… (99)	fū 敷
fēng rè hóu bì 风热喉痹 …… (100)	fú chóng bìng 伏虫病 …… (106)
fēng rè jīng jì 风热惊悸 …… (100)	fú jiǎ 伏瘕 …………… (106)
fēng rè ké sòu 风热咳嗽 …… (100)	fú liáng 伏梁 ………… (106)
fēng rè tóu tòng 风热头痛 …… (100)	fú mài 伏脉 …………… (107)
fēng rè xuàn yūn 风热眩晕 …… (100)	fú qì 伏气 …………… (107)
fēng rè yá gān 风热牙疳 …… (101)	fú rè 伏热 …………… (107)
fēng rè yāo tòng 风热腰痛 …… (101)	fú shǔ 伏暑 …………… (107)
fēng shā 风痧 ……………… (101)	fú tán 伏痰 …………… (107)
fēng shī 风湿 ……………… (102)	fú yǐn 伏饮 …………… (107)
fēng shī tóu tòng 风湿头痛 …… (102)	fú zhèng gù běn 扶正固本 …… (108)
fēng shī xiāng bó 风湿相搏 … (102)	fú zhèng qū xié 扶正祛邪 …… (108)
fēng shī yāo tòng 风湿腰痛 …… (102)	fú mài 浮脉 …………… (108)
fēng shuǐ 风水 ……………… (102)	fú zhōng chén 浮中沉 …… (108)
fēng tán 风痰 ……………… (103)	fǔ dǐ chōu xīn 釜底抽薪 …… (108)
fēng tán cì 风痰痓 …… (103)	fǔ fèi mài 釜沸脉 …… (109)
fēng tán tóu tòng 风痰头痛 … (103)	fǔ huì 腑会 …………… (109)

fǔ jīng 腑精 ……… (109)
fǔ zhèng 腑证 ……… (109)
fǔ tāi 腐苔 ……… (109)
fù gǔ jū 附骨疽 ……… (109)
fù fāng 复方 ……… (110)
fù 腹 ……… (110)
fù mǎn 腹满 ……… (110)
fù tòng 腹痛 ……… (110)
fù yōng 腹痈 ……… (111)
fù zhàng 腹胀 ……… (111)

G

gān huò luàn 干霍乱 ……… (111)
gān jiǎo qì 干脚气 ……… (111)
gān ké 干咳 ……… (112)
gān ǒu 干呕 ……… (112)
gān xuǎn 干癣 ……… (112)
gān xuè láo 干血痨 ……… (112)
gān 甘 ……… (112)
gān gān 甘疳 ……… (112)
gān hán shēng jīn 甘寒生津 ……… (113)
gān shǒu jīn huán 甘守津还 ……… (113)
gān hán zī yùn 甘寒滋润 ……… (113)
gān wēn chú rè 甘温除热 ……… (114)
gān xīn wú jiàng 甘辛无降 ……… (114)
gān 肝 ……… (114)
gān bìng 肝病 ……… (115)
gān cáng xuè 肝藏血 ……… (115)
gān dǎn shī rè 肝胆湿热 ……… (115)
gān fēng nèi dòng 肝风内动 ……… (115)
gān gān 肝疳 ……… (115)
gān hán 肝寒 ……… (116)
gān hé dǎn 肝合胆 ……… (116)
gān huǒ 肝火 ……… (116)
gān huǒ bù dé wò 肝火不得卧 ……… (116)
gān huǒ ěr lóng 肝火耳聋 ……… (117)
gān huǒ ěr míng 肝火耳鸣 ……… (117)
gān huǒ shàng yán 肝火上炎 ……… (117)
gān huǒ xuǎn yūn 肝火弦晕 ……… (117)
gān jīng shī rè dài xià 肝经湿热带下 ……… (117)
gān jué 肝厥 ……… (118)
gān ké 肝咳 ……… (118)
gān láo 肝劳 ……… (118)
gān pí bù hé 肝脾不和 ……… (118)
gān, qí huá zài zhǎo 肝,其华在爪 ……… (118)
gān qì 肝气 ……… (119)
gān qì fàn wèi (pí) 肝气犯胃(脾) ……… (119)
gān qì xié tòng 肝气胁痛 ……… (119)
gān qì xū 肝气虚 ……… (119)
gān qì yù jié bù yùn 肝气郁结不孕 ……… (119)
gān rè wù zǔ 肝热恶阻 ……… (120)
gān rè zì hàn 肝热自汗 ……… (120)
gān shèn kuī sǔn tòng jīng 肝肾亏损痛经 ……… (120)
gān shèn tóng yuán 肝肾同源(肝肾相生) ……… (120)
gān shèn yīn xū 肝肾阴虚(肝肾亏损) ……… (121)
gān shèn yīn xū bēng lòu 肝肾阴虚崩漏 ……… (121)

gān shēng yú zuǒ	肝生于左 …(121)	gāng jìng	刚痉 …(127)
gān, tǐ yīn ér yòng yáng	肝, 体阴而用阳 …(122)	gāng liè	肛裂 …(128)
		gāng lòu	肛漏 …(128)
gān wéi gāng zàng	肝为刚脏 …(122)	gāng mén	肛门 …(128)
		gāng mén yōng	肛门痈 …(128)
gān wèi qì tòng	肝胃气痛 …(122)	gāo fēng què mù nèi zhàng	高风雀目内障 …(128)
gān wù fēng	肝恶风 …(122)		
gān xuè	肝血 …(122)	gāo zhě yì zhī	高者抑之 …(128)
gān xuè xū	肝血虚 …(122)	gāo	膏 …(129)
gān yáng huà huǒ	肝阳化火 …(123)	gāo huāng	膏肓 …(129)
gān yáng shàng kàng	肝阳上亢 …(123)	gāo liáng hòu wèi	膏粱厚味 …(129)
		gāo lìn	膏淋 …(129)
gān yáng tóu tòng	肝阳头痛 …(123)	gāo mó	膏摩 …(130)
gān yáng xuàn yùn	肝阳眩晕 …(123)	gāo yào	膏药 …(130)
		gé mài	革脉 …(130)
gān yīn	肝阴 …(123)	gé bǐng jiǔ	隔饼灸 …(130)
gān yīn xū	肝阴虚 …(124)	gé jiāng jiǔ	隔姜灸 …(130)
gān yōng	肝痈 …(124)	gé suàn jiǔ	隔蒜灸 …(130)
gān yù	肝郁 …(124)	gé yán jiǔ	隔盐灸 …(130)
gān yù jīng xíng xiān qī	肝郁经行先期 …(124)	gé chuāng	瘑疮 …(131)
		gé	膈 …(131)
gān yù pí xū	肝郁脾虚 …(125)	gé tán	膈痰 …(131)
gān yù xié tòng	肝郁胁痛 …(125)	gé xián	膈痫 …(131)
gān zhǔ jīn	肝主筋 …(125)	gēng yī	更衣 …(131)
gān zhǔ móu lù	肝主谋虑 …(125)	gōng bǔ jiān shī	攻补兼施 …(131)
gān zhǔ shū xiè	肝主疏泄 …(126)	gōng kuì	攻溃 …(132)
gān zhǔ xiè hǎi	肝主血海 …(126)	gōng lǐ bù yuǎn hán	攻里不远寒 …(132)
gān jī	疳积 …(126)		
gān kě	疳渴 …(126)	gōng	肱 …(132)
gān láo	疳痨 …(126)	gū fǔ	孤腑 …(132)
gān lì	疳痢 …(126)	gū yáng shàng fú	孤阳上浮 …(132)
gān rè	疳热 …(127)	gū yīn	孤阴 …(132)
gān xiè	疳泻 …(127)	gū zhàng	孤脏 …(132)
gān zhèng	疳证 …(127)	gū wéi yào	箍围药 …(132)
gǎn mào	感冒 …(127)	gǔ dǎn	谷疸 …(132)
gǎn mào tóu tòng	感冒头痛 …(127)	gǔ dào	谷道 …(133)

gǔ qì 谷气 ……… (133)	guā xiàn fǎ 挂线法 ……… (137)
gǔ bì 骨痹 ……… (133)	guān gé 关格 ……… (137)
gǔ cáo fēng 骨槽风 ……… (133)	guān mài 关脉 ……… (137)
gǔ gěng 骨鲠 ……… (133)	guān mén bù lì 关门不利 ……… (137)
gǔ huì 骨会 ……… (134)	guān shén sè 观神色 ……… (138)
gǔ liú 骨瘤 ……… (134)	guàn kǒu jū 鹳口疽 ……… (138)
gǔ tòng 骨痛 ……… (134)	guāng bō tāi 光剥苔 ……… (138)
gǔ wěi 骨痿 ……… (134)	guǎng cháng 广肠 ……… (138)
gǔ zhé 骨折 ……… (135)	guī běi 归经 ……… (138)
gǔ zhēng 骨蒸 ……… (135)	guī bèi 龟背 ……… (139)
gǔ 蛊 ……… (135)	guī bèi tuó 龟背驼 ……… (139)
gǔ dú 蛊毒 ……… (135)	guī bèi tán 龟背痰 ……… (139)
gǔ zhù 蛊注 ……… (135)	guī tóu zhǒng tòng 龟头肿痛
gǔ zhàng 鼓胀 ……… (136)	……… (139)
gù bēng zhǐ dài 固崩止带 ……… (136)	guǐ jī 鬼击 ……… (139)
gù jiǎ 固瘕 ……… (136)	guǐ tāi 鬼胎 ……… (139)
gù shèn sè jīng 固肾涩精 ……… (136)	guó 腘 ……… (140)
gù jí 痼疾 ……… (137)	guò jīng 过经 ……… (140)
gù lěng 痼冷 ……… (137)	guò qī liú chǎn 过期流产 ……… (140)
guā cháng 刮肠 ……… (137)	

H

hǎi dǐ lòu 海底漏 ……… (140)	hán jì 寒剂 ……… (143)
hān shēng 鼾声 ……… (140)	hán jié 寒结 ……… (143)
hán 寒 ……… (140)	hán jìng 寒痉 ……… (143)
hán bāo huǒ 寒包火 ……… (141)	hán jué 寒厥 ……… (143)
hán bì 寒痹 ……… (141)	hán lěng fù tòng 寒冷腹痛 ……… (143)
hán chuǎn 寒喘 ……… (141)	hán lì gǔ hàn 寒栗鼓颔 ……… (144)
hán è 寒呃 ……… (141)	hán lì 寒痢 ……… (144)
hán gé 寒膈 ……… (142)	hán néng qù rè 寒能去热 ……… (144)
hán huà 寒化 ……… (142)	hán néng zhì rè 寒能制热 ……… (144)
hán huò luàn 寒霍乱 ……… (142)	hán níng qì zhì 寒凝气滞 ……… (144)
hán jī fù tòng 寒积腹痛 ……… (142)	hán nüè 寒疟 ……… (144)
hán jī shēng rè 寒极生热 ……… (143)	hán ǒu 寒呕 ……… (145)

hán pǐ 寒癖	(145)		(152)
hán rè 寒热	(145)	hàn chū rú yóu 汗出如油	(152)
hán rè cuò zá 寒热错杂	(145)	hàn fǎ 汗法	(152)
hán rè wǎng lái 寒热往来	(145)	hàn kōng 汗空	(153)
hán shān 寒疝	(146)	hàn kǒng 汗孔	(153)
hán shāng xíng 寒伤形	(146)	hàn zhèng 汗证	(153)
hán shèng zé fú 寒胜则浮	(146)	háo zhēn 毫针	(153)
hán shī jiǎo qì 寒湿脚气	(146)	hé bìng 合病	(153)
hán shī jiǔ bì 寒湿久痹	(146)	hé jì 合剂	(153)
hán shī lì 寒湿痢	(147)	hé 和	(153)
hán shī níng zhì jīng bì 寒湿凝滞经闭	(147)	hé fǎ 和法	(154)
hán shī tóu tòng 寒湿头痛	(147)	hé gān 和肝	(154)
hán shī xuàn yūn 寒湿眩晕	(147)	hé huǎn 和缓	(154)
hán shī yāo tòng 寒湿腰痛	(148)	hé jiě shào yáng 和解少阳	(155)
hán shí 寒实	(148)	hé wèi 和胃	(155)
hán sòu 寒嗽	(148)	hé wèi lǐ qì 和胃理气	(155)
hán tán 寒痰	(148)	hé xuè xī fēng 和血熄风	(155)
hán wú fàn hán 寒无犯寒	(149)	hé 颌	(156)
hán wú fú 寒无浮	(149)	hè xī fēng 鹤膝风	(156)
hán xià 寒下	(149)	hēi 黑	(156)
hán xián 寒痫	(149)	hēi dài 黑带	(156)
hán xié xuàn yùn 寒邪眩晕	(149)	hēi dǎn 黑疸	(156)
hán xiè 寒泄	(149)	hēi jīng 黑睛	(156)
hán yè tí 寒夜啼	(150)	hēi rú tái 黑如炱	(157)
hán yì 寒疫	(150)	hēi tāi 黑苔	(157)
hán yīn hán yòng 寒因寒用	(150)	hēi zǐ 黑子	(157)
hán yīn rè yòng 寒因热用	(150)	héng gǔ shāng 胻骨伤	(157)
hán zé qì shōu 寒则气收	(150)	héng xuán 横痃	(157)
hán zé shōu yǐn 寒则收引	(151)	hōng 烘	(157)
hán chàng 寒胀	(151)	hóng sī dīng 红丝疔	(157)
hán zhě rè zhī 寒者热之	(151)	hóng tún 红臀	(158)
hán zhèng 寒证	(151)	hóng mài 洪脉	(158)
hán zhì gān mài 寒滞肝脉	(152)	hōu chuǎn 齁喘	(158)
hàn 汗	(152)	hóu bì 喉痹	(158)
hàn chū jí jí rán 汗出汲汲然		hóu dīng 喉疔	(158)
		hóu fēng 喉风	(158)

hóu gān 喉疳	(159)	huà zào 化燥	(166)
hóu guān 喉关	(159)	huái yùn 怀孕	(166)
hóu hé 喉核	(159)	huài bìng 坏病	(166)
hóu jiān kuì làn 喉间溃烂	(159)	huán gāng lòu 环肛漏	(166)
hóu xuǎn 喉癣	(160)	huán tiào jū 环跳疽	(166)
hóu yǎng 喉痒	(160)	huán tiào liú tán 环跳流痰	(166)
hóu yīn 喉音	(160)	huǎn fāng 缓方	(166)
hóu yōng 喉痈	(160)	huǎn jū 缓疽	(167)
hóu zhōng shuǐ jī shēng 喉中水鸡声	(160)	huǎn mài 缓脉	(167)
		huǎn xià 缓下	(167)
hòu yīn 后阴	(161)	huǎn zé zhì běn 缓则治本	(167)
hòu qì 候气	(161)	huāng 肓	(167)
hū xī bǔ xiè 呼吸补泻	(161)	huáng dài 黄带	(167)
hú chòu 狐臭	(161)	huáng dǎn 黄疸	(167)
hú huò 狐惑	(161)	huáng fēng nèi zhàng 黄风内障	(168)
hú niào cì 狐尿刺	(162)		
hú shàn 狐疝	(162)	huáng gān tāi 黄干苔	(168)
hú sūn gān 猢狲疳	(162)	huáng guā yōng 黄瓜痈	(168)
hǔ kǒu dīng 虎口疔	(162)	huáng hàn 黄汗	(168)
huā diān 花癫	(162)	huáng jiā 黄家	(169)
huā xuǎn 花癣	(163)	huáng nì tāi 黄腻苔	(169)
huá jì 滑剂	(163)	huáng pàng 黄胖	(169)
huá jīng 滑精	(163)	huáng rú zhǐ shí 黄如枳实	(169)
huá kě qù zhuó 滑可去着	(163)	huáng shuǐ chuāng 黄水疮	(169)
huá mài 滑脉	(163)	huáng tāi 黄苔	(169)
huá tāi 滑胎	(163)	huáng yè shàng chōng 黄液上冲	(170)
huá xiè 滑泄	(164)		
huà bān 化斑	(164)	huī tāi 灰苔	(170)
huà fēng 化风	(164)	huī cì 恢刺	(170)
huà huǒ 化火	(164)	huí cháng 回肠	(170)
huà nóng jiǔ 化脓灸	(164)	huí xuán jiǔ 回旋灸	(170)
huà rè 化热	(165)	huí yáng jiù nì 回阳救逆	(170)
huà shī 化湿	(165)	huí dòng wǎn tòng 蛔动脘痛	
huà tán 化痰	(165)		(171)
huà tán kāi qiào 化痰开窍	(165)	huí jué 蛔厥	(171)
huà yǐn jiě biǎo 化饮解表	(165)	huí chóng 蛔虫	(171)

huí chóng bìng 蛔虫病	(171)	
huí gān 蛔疳	(171)	
huí jué 蛔厥	(171)	
huì yàn 会厌	(172)	
huì yīn 会阴	(172)	
huì gé 恚膈	(172)	
hūn jué 昏厥	(172)	
hūn kuì 昏愦	(172)	
hūn mí 昏迷	(172)	
hūn shuì 昏睡	(172)	
hùn hé zhì 混合痔	(173)	
hún jīng zhàng 混睛障	(173)	
huó xuè huà yū 活血化瘀	(173)	
huǒ 火	(173)	
huǒ bù shēng tǔ 火不生土	(173)	
huǒ dú 火毒	(173)	
huǒ gān 火疳	(174)	
huǒ guàn 火罐	(174)	
huǒ ké 火咳	(174)	
huǒ nì 火逆	(174)	
huǒ shèng xíng jīn 火盛刑金	(174)	
huǒ tóu tòng 火头痛	(174)	
huǒ xiàn 火陷	(175)	
huǒ xìng yán shàng 火性炎上	(175)	
huǒ yù chuǎn 火郁喘	(175)	
huǒ zhēn liáo fǎ 火针疗法	(175)	
huǒ zhēn 火针	(175)	
huǒ zhū chuāng 火珠疮	(176)	
huò luàn 霍乱	(176)	
huò luàn zhuǎn jīn 霍乱转筋	(176)	

J

jī pū 击仆	(176)	
jī bù yù shí 饥不欲食	(176)	
jī 肌	(176)	
jī bì 肌痹	(176)	
jī còu 肌腠	(177)	
jī fū jiǎ cuò 肌肤甲错	(177)	
jī nǜ 肌衄	(177)	
jī ròu bù rén 肌肉不仁	(177)	
jī ròu ruǎn 肌肉软	(177)	
jī xiōng 鸡胸	(177)	
jī fāng 奇方	(177)	
jī jù 积聚	(177)	
jī jīng 激经	(178)	
jí fāng 急方	(178)	
jí hóu bì 急喉	(178)	
jí hóu fēng 急喉风	(178)	
jí huáng 急黄	(178)	
jí jīng fēng 急惊风	(179)	
jí láo 急劳	(179)	
jí rǔ é 急乳蛾	(179)	
jí xià cún yīn 急下存阴	(179)	
jí zhě huǎn zhī 急者缓之	(179)	
jí zhě zhì biāo 急者治标	(180)	
jí xú bǔ xiè 疾徐补泻	(180)	
jí yī 疾医	(180)	
jǐ 脊	(180)	
jǐ gān 脊疳	(180)	
jì kǒu 忌口	(180)	
jì xíng 剂型	(180)	
jì lèi bù 季肋部	(181)	

拼音	词条	页码	拼音	词条	页码
jì xié tòng	季胁痛	(181)	jiāo	胶	(186)
jì xīn tòng	悸心痛	(181)	jiāo chuāng	椒疮	(186)
jiā bǎn	夹板	(181)	jiāo yuán	焦原	(185)
jiá	颊	(181)	jiǎo gōng fǎn zhāng	角弓反张	(186)
jiǎ jū	甲疽	(181)	jiǎo gēn gǔ shāng	脚跟骨伤	(186)
jiǎ hán	假寒	(181)	jiǎo pàn chū jù	脚盘出臼	(186)
jiǎ rè	假热	(181)	jiǎo qì	脚气	(187)
jiān yīn	坚阴	(181)	jiǎo qì chuāng	脚气疮	(187)
jiān zhě xiāo zhī	坚者消之	(182)	jiǎo xīn tòng	脚心痛	(187)
jiān	肩	(182)	jiǎo zhǐ jiè shī	脚趾龄失	(187)
jiān bèi tòng	肩背痛	(182)	jiǎo zhǒng	脚肿	(187)
jiān dú	肩毒	(182)	jiē	疖	(187)
jiān guān jié tuō jiù	肩关节脱臼	(182)	jié qì	节气	(188)
jiān jiǎ	肩胛	(182)	jié jìng fǔ	洁净腑	(188)
jiān jiǎ jū	肩胛疽	(182)	jié hé	结核	(188)
jiān tòng	肩痛	(182)	jié mài	结脉	(188)
jiān xī	肩息	(182)	jié xiōng	结胸	(188)
jiān yú	肩髃	(183)	jié yīn	结阴	(189)
jiān fāng	兼方	(183)	jié yáng	结阳	(189)
jiān zhèng	兼证	(183)	jié zā fǎ	结扎法	(189)
jiān	煎	(183)	jié zhě sàn zhī	结者散之	(189)
jiān yào fǎ	煎药法	(183)	jié máo	睫毛	(189)
jiǎn chún	茧唇	(183)	jié nuè	截疟	(189)
jiàn jiē jiǔ	间接灸	(184)	jiě biǎo	解表	(189)
jiàn rì nüè	间日疟	(184)	jiě biǎo fǎ	解表法	(190)
jiàn zhě bìng xíng	间者并行	(184)	jiě dú	解毒	(190)
jiàn pí	健脾	(184)	jiě jī	解肌	(190)
jiàn pí shū gān	健脾疏肝	(184)	jiě jìng	解痉	(190)
jiàn wàng	健忘	(185)	jiě lú	解颅	(190)
jiàn wèi	健胃	(185)	jiě suǒ mài	解索脉	(190)
jiàng jì	降剂	(185)	jiè chuāng	疥疮	(191)
jiàng kě qù shēng	降可去升	(185)	jīn chuāng	金创	(191)
jiàng nì xià qì	降逆下气	(185)	jīn gān	金疳	(191)
jiàng qì	降气	(185)	jīn pò bù míng	金破不鸣	(191)
jiāo tōng xīn shèn	交通心肾	(185)	jīn zhēn bō zhàng fǎ	金针拨障法	

	………… (191)		………… (197)
jīn 津	………… (191)	jīng xíng fā rè 经行发热	……(197)
jīn xuè tóng yuán 津血同源	…(192)	jīng xíng hòu qī 经行后期	……(197)
jīn yè 津液	………… (192)	jīng xíng nǜ xuè 经行衄血	……(197)
jīn 筋	………… (192)	jīng xíng tù xuè 经行吐血	……(197)
jīn bì 筋痹	………… (192)	jīng xíng xiān hòu wú dìng qī 经行先后无定期	……(197)
jīn huǎn 筋缓	………… (192)		
jīn huì 筋会	………… (192)	jīng xíng xiān qī 经行先期	……(197)
jīn mó 筋膜	………… (192)	jīng xíng xiè xiè 经行泄泻	……(198)
jīn tì ròu rún 筋惕肉瞤	…(192)	jīng zhèng 经证	………… (198)
jīn wěi 筋痿	………… (193)	jīng fēng 惊风	………… (198)
jīn yǐng 筋瘿	………… (193)	jīng gé sòu 惊膈嗽	………… (198)
jǐn mài 紧脉	………… (193)	jīng hòu tóng xié 惊后瞳斜	…(198)
jìn zhēn 进针	………… (193)	jīng jī 惊积	………… (198)
jìn xuè 近血	………… (193)	jīng jué 惊厥	………… (199)
jìn xǐ jì 浸洗剂	………… (193)	jīng lì 惊痢	………… (199)
jìn yín chuāng 浸淫疮	……(193)	jīng rè 惊热	………… (199)
jìn cì 禁刺	………… (194)	jīng shāng xié tòng 惊伤胁痛	………… (199)
jìn fāng 禁方	………… (194)		
jìn kǒu lì 禁口痢	………… (194)	jīng shuǐ 惊水	………… (199)
jīng bì fā zhǒng 经闭发肿	…(194)	jīng tān 惊瘫	………… (200)
jīng cì 经刺	………… (195)	jīng tí 惊啼	………… (200)
jīng duàn qián hòu zhū zhèng 经断前后诸证	……(195)	jīng xián 惊痫	………… (200)
		jīng zé qì luàn 惊则气乱	…(200)
jīng fāng 经方	………… (195)	jīng zhě píng zhī 惊者平之	…(200)
jīng hòu tǔ nǜ 经后吐衄	…(195)	jīng zhèn nèi zhàng 惊震内障	(200)
jīng jìn 经尽	………… (195)	jīng 睛	………… (200)
jīng jué 经绝	………… (195)	jīng 精	………… (201)
jīng lái fú zhǒng 经来浮肿	…(196)	jīng cháo 精巢	………… (201)
jīng lái kuáng yán zhān yǔ 经来狂言谵语	……(196)	jīng qì duó zé xū 精气夺则虚	……… (201)
		jīng qiào 精窍	………… (201)
jīng lái ǒu tù 经来呕吐	…(196)	jīng míng zhī fǔ 精明之府	…(201)
jīng luò 经络	………… (196)	jīng shén nèi shǒu 精神内守	
jīng mài 经脉	………… (196)		………… (201)
jīng qì 经气	………… (196)		
jīng rú xiā má zǐ 经如虾蟆子		jīng wēi 精微	………… (201)

jīng xuě tóng yuán	精血同源 …… (201)	jiù lǐ	救里 …… (206)
jīng zhī	精汁 …… (201)	jiù tuō	救脱 …… (206)
jǐng jū	井疽 …… (202)	jū jí	拘急 …… (206)
jǐng yōng	颈痈 …… (202)	jū	疽 …… (206)
jìng fǔ	净腑 …… (202)	jú fú	焗服 …… (206)
jìng gōng	净功 …… (202)	jǔ àn	举按 …… (207)
jìng	痉 …… (203)	jǔ àn xún	举、按、寻 …… (207)
jiǒng yào	炅药 …… (203)	jú fēn	巨分 …… (207)
jiǒng zé qì xiè	炅则气泄 …… (203)	jù àn	拒按 …… (207)
jiǒng	䐃 …… (203)	jú sàn zhàng	聚散障 …… (207)
jiǔ qiào	九窍 …… (203)	jú xīng zhàng	聚星障 …… (207)
jiǔ zàng	九脏 …… (203)	jué dú zhī guān	决渎之官 …… (208)
jiǔ zhēn	九针 …… (203)	jué hàn	绝汗 …… (208)
jiǔ ké	久咳 …… (204)	jué nì	厥逆 …… (208)
jiǔ lì	久痢 …… (204)	jué nì tóu tòng	厥逆头痛 …… (208)
jiǔ nüè	久疟 …… (204)	jué qì	阙气 …… (208)
jiǔ rè shāng yīn	久热伤阴 …… (204)	jué xīn tòng	厥心痛 …… (208)
jiǔ xiè bù zhǐ	久泻不止 …… (204)	jué yáng	厥阳 …… (209)
jiǔ yīn	久瘖 …… (204)	jué yáng dú xíng	厥阳独行 …… (209)
jiǔ fǎ	灸法 …… (204)	jué yīn	厥阴 …… (209)
jiǔ bèi	酒悖 …… (205)	jué yīn bìng	厥阴病 …… (209)
jiǔ dǎn	酒疸 …… (205)	jué yīn tóu tòng	厥阴头痛 …… (209)
jiǔ jì	酒剂 …… (205)	jué zhèng	厥证 …… (209)
jiǔ kè	酒客 …… (205)	jūn zhén zuǒ shǐ	君臣佐使 …… (210)
jiǔ pǐ	酒癖 …… (205)	jūn huǒ	君火 …… (210)
jiǔ zhā bí	酒齄（渣）鼻 …… (205)	jūn liè chuāng	皲裂疮 …… (210)
jiǔ zhàng	酒胀 …… (206)	jùn xià	峻下 …… (210)

K

kǎ xuè	咯血 …… (211)	kāi qiào	开窍 …… (211)
kāi hé bǔ xiè	开阖补泻 …… (211)	kāi wèi	开胃 …… (211)
kāi jìn tōng guān	开噤通关 …… (211)	kàng hài chéng zhì	亢害承制 …… (212)
kāi pǐ	开痞 …… (211)		

kàng yáng 亢阳	(212)	kǒu kǔ 口苦	(216)
kāo 尻	(212)	kǒu kǔ yān gān 口苦咽干	(216)
kē 颏	(212)	kǒu mí 口糜	(217)
ké chuǎn 咳喘	(212)	kǒu ruǎn 口软	(217)
ké nì shàng qì 咳逆上气	(212)	kǒu suān 口酸	(217)
ké sōu 咳嗽	(213)	kǒu tián 口甜	(217)
ké sōu shī yīn 咳嗽失音	(213)	kǒu xián 口咸	(217)
ké sōu tán shèng 咳嗽痰盛	(213)	kǒu yǎn wāi xié 口眼歪斜	(217)
ké xuè 咳血	(213)	kǒu zhōng hé 口中和	(217)
kè zhě chú zhī 客者除之	(214)	kǒu zhōng wú wèi 口中无味	(218)
kōng fù fú 空腹服	(214)	kū pēi 枯痞	(218)
kōng qiào 空窍	(214)	kū zhì fǎ 枯痔法	(218)
kǒng shāng shèn 恐伤肾	(214)	kǔ hán qīng qì 苦寒清气	(218)
kǒng zé qì xià 恐则气下	(215)	kǔ hán qīng rè 苦寒清热	(218)
kòng nǎo shā 控脑痧	(215)	kǔ hán zào shī 苦寒燥湿	(219)
kōng mài 芤脉	(215)	kǔ wēn píng zào 苦温平燥	(219)
kǒu 口	(215)	kǔ wēn zào shī 苦温燥湿	(219)
kǒu bù rén 口不仁	(215)	kuà yōng 胯痈	(219)
kǒu chuāng 口疮	(215)	kuáng 狂	(220)
kǒu chún xiǎn zhèng 口唇险症		kuáng yán 狂言	(220)
	(216)	kuí duó qí héng 揆度奇恒	(220)
kǒu dàn 口淡	(216)	kuì yáng 溃疡	(220)
kǒu gān fēng 口疳风	(216)	kuì yáng bù liǎn 溃疡不敛	(220)

L

lán mén 阑门	(220)	láo zhài 劳瘵	(222)
làn dīng 烂疔	(220)	láo zhě wēn zhī 劳者温之	(222)
làn hóu fēng 烂喉风	(221)	láo mài 牢脉	(223)
láo fù 劳复	(221)	láo chuāng 痨疮	(223)
láo juàn 劳倦	(222)	lǎo fù xíng jīng 老妇行经	(223)
láo lín 劳淋	(222)	lǎo huáng tāi 老黄苔	(223)
láo rè 劳热	(222)	lǎo lín 老淋	(223)
láo sòu 劳嗽	(222)	lǎo tán 老痰	(223)
láo zé qì hào 劳则气耗	(222)	lào fǎ 烙法	(223)

léi tóu fēng 雷头风	(224)	lì qīng chuāng 沥青疮	(231)
lèi jū 肋疽	(224)	lì 疠	(231)
lèi 泪	(224)	lì fēng 疠风	(231)
lèi qiào 泪窍	(224)	lì zǐ zhì 栗子痔	(231)
lèi jīng 类经	(224)	lì fēng 疬风	(232)
lèi xiāo zhèng 类消症	(224)	lì jì 痢疾	(232)
lèi zhòng fēng 类中风	(225)	lián zǐ fā 莲子发	(232)
lěng bì 冷秘	(225)	lián zǐ lì 莲子疬	(232)
lěng fú 冷服	(225)	lián chuāng 臁疮	(232)
lěng hàn 冷汗	(225)	liǎn fèi zhǐ ké 敛肺止咳	(233)
lěng lín 冷淋	(226)	liǎn hàn gù biǎo 敛汗固表	(233)
lěng rè gān 冷热疳	(226)	liǎn yīn 敛阴	(233)
lěng tòng 冷痛	(226)	liàn gōng fǎn yìng 练功反应	
lěng xiāo 冷哮	(226)		(233)
lěng xīn tòng 冷心痛	(227)	liàn gōng yào lǐng 练功要令	(233)
lěng yùn fǎ 冷熨法	(227)	liàn gōng zá niàn 练功杂念	(234)
lí hēi bān 黧黑斑	(227)	liàn méi chuāng 恋眉疮	(234)
lǐ hán 里寒	(227)	liàn yì 炼意	(234)
lǐ hán gé rè 里寒格热	(228)	liáng xuè 凉血	(234)
lǐ jí hòu zhòng 里急后重	(228)	liáng xuè jiě dú 凉血解毒	(234)
lǐ rè 里热	(228)	liǎng gǎn shāng hán 两感伤寒	
lǐ shí 里实	(228)		(235)
lǐ xū 里虚	(229)	liǎng xié jū jí 两胁拘急	(235)
lǐ zhèng 里证	(229)	liǎng xū xiāng dé 两虚相得	(235)
lǐ qì 理气	(229)	lín shuì qián fú 临睡前服	(235)
lǐ fǎ 理法	(229)	lín 淋	(235)
lǐ xuè 理血	(229)	lín jiā 淋家	(235)
lǐ zhōng 理中	(230)	lín zhuó 淋浊	(235)
lì jié fēng 历节风	(230)	liú yǐn 留饮	(235)
lì chí 立迟	(230)	liú zhě gōng zhī 留者攻之	(236)
lì fǎ chǔ fāng 立法处方	(230)	liú zhēn 留针	(236)
lì shī 利湿	(230)	liú chǎn 流产	(236)
lì shuǐ tōng lín 利水通淋	(230)	liú tán 流痰	(236)
lì xiǎo biàn, shí dà biàn 利小便,		liú xián 流涎	(237)
实大便	(231)	liú zhù 流注	(237)
lì jiāng shēng 沥浆生	(231)	liú zhù lì 流注疬	(237)

liú 瘤 (238)	lóng bì 癃闭 (240)
liù fǔ 六腑 (238)	lóng shàn 癃疝 (240)
liù jīng 六经 (238)	lóu fù 偻附 (240)
liù jí 六极 (238)	lóu gū cuàn 蝼蛄窜 (240)
liù jīng biàn zhèng 六经辨证 (238)	lòu dǐ shāng hán 漏底伤寒 (241)
	lòu hàn 漏汗 (241)
liù jīng bìng 六经病 (239)	lòu jīng 漏睛 (241)
liù qì 六气 (239)	lòu lì 漏疬 (241)
liù shén zhī fǔ 六神之府 (239)	lòu xiàng 漏项 (241)
liù yáng mài 六阳脉 (239)	lù shí xiè 禄食泄 (241)
liù yīn mài 六阴脉 (239)	lù 露 (241)
liù yín 六淫 (239)	lǚ 膂 (241)
liù yù 六郁 (239)	lù fēng nèi zhàng 绿风内障 (241)
liù zàng 六脏 (240)	luó dīng 螺疔 (242)
lóng yǎ 聋哑 (240)	luǒ lì 瘰疬 (242)
lóng 癃 (240)	luò cì 络刺 (242)

M

má zhěn 麻疹 (242)	mài huì 脉会 (245)
má zhěn bì zhèng 麻疹闭证 (243)	mài jìng 脉静 (245)
má zhěn hóu tòng 麻疹喉痛 (243)	mài kǒu 脉口 (245)
má zhěn nì zhèng 麻疹逆证 (243)	mài nì sì shí 脉逆四时 (245)
má zhěn shī yīn 麻疹失音 (244)	mài wēi zhī lěng 脉微肢冷 (245)
má zhěn shùn zhèng 麻疹顺证 (244)	mài wěi 脉痿 (246)
má zhèng hōu hē 麻证齁䶎 (244)	mài wú wèi qì 脉无胃气 (246)
má mù 麻木 (244)	mài xiàng 脉象 (246)
mǎ tǒng xuǎn 马桶癣 (244)	mài xiàng zhǔ bìng 脉象主病 (246)
mǎ yá 马牙 (244)	
mài 脉 (244)	mài yīn yáng jù fú 脉阴阳俱浮 (246)
mài bào chū 脉暴出 (244)	
mài bì 脉痹 (245)	mài yīn yáng jù jǐn 脉阴阳俱紧 (246)
mài guǎn 脉管 (245)	mài yǒu wèi qì 脉有胃气 (247)
mài hé sì shí 脉合四时 (245)	mài zhèng hé cān 脉证合参 (247)

màn gān fēng 慢肝风 (247)
màn gān jīng fēng 慢肝惊风 (248)
màn jīng fēng 慢惊风 (248)
màn pí fēng 慢脾风 (248)
māo yǎn chuāng 猫眼疮 (248)
máo jì 毛际 (248)
mào jiā 冒家 (248)
mào chì 瞀瘛 (248)
méi dú 梅毒 (248)
méi hé qì 梅核气 (249)
měng jū 猛疽 (249)
mèng yí 梦遗 (249)
mì bié qīng zhuó 泌别清浊 (249)
mì jiān dǎo fǎ 蜜煎导法 (249)
miàn bù dīng chuāng 面部疔疮 (250)
miàn chén 面尘 (250)
miàn dīng 面疔 (250)
miàn gòu 面垢 (250)
miàn huáng jī shòu 面黄肌瘦 (250)
miàn mù fú zhǒng 面目浮肿 (250)
miàn sè cāng bái 面色苍白 (251)
miàn sè cāng hēi 面色苍黑 (251)
miàn sè wěi huáng 面色萎黄 (251)
miàn sè yuán yuán zhèng chì 面色缘缘正赤 (251)
miàn tuō 面脱 (251)
miàn yóu fēng 面游风 (251)
miàn zhēn liáo fǎ 面针疗法 (252)
miàn zhǒng 面肿 (252)
míng táng 明堂 (252)
mìng guān 命关 (252)
mó 膜 (252)
mó rù shuǐ lún 膜入水轮 (252)
mǔ bìng jí zǐ 母病及子 (252)
mǔ qì 母气 (253)
mǔ zàng 牡脏 (253)
mù huǒ xíng jīn 木火刑金 (253)
mù kè tǔ 木克土 (253)
mù shé 木舌 (253)
mù shèn 木肾 (253)
mù xǐ tiáo dá 木喜条达 (254)
mù yù dá zhī 木郁达之 (254)
mù yù huà fēng 木郁化风 (254)
mù yù huà huǒ 木郁化火 (254)
mù bù míng 目不瞑 (254)
mù fēi xuè 目飞血 (254)
mù fēng sāi 目封塞 (254)
mù gān sè 目干涩 (255)
mù gāng 目纲 (255)
mù hūn 目昏 (255)
mù kē 目窠 (255)
mù dē shàng wēi zhǒng 目窠上微肿 (255)
mù sè 目涩 (255)
mù shāng sè 目沙涩 (255)
mù shàng bāo 目上胞 (256)
mù shàng gāng 目上纲 (256)
mù xià gāng 目下纲 (256)
mù yǎng 目疡 (256)
mù yǎng 目痒 (256)
mù yūn 目晕 (256)
mù zhí 目直 (256)
mù zhōng bù liǎo liǎo 目中不了了 (256)
mù zì 目眦 (256)
mù yuán 幕原 (256)

N

nà dāi 纳呆 ……………… (257)	脘痛 …………………… (261)
nǎi xuǎn 奶癣 ……………… (257)	nèi shāng yāo tòng 内伤腰痛
nán chǎn 难产 ……………… (257)	………………………… (261)
nán rǔ 难乳 ……………… (257)	nèi shāng yǐn shí jīng 内伤饮食
náng suō 囊缩 ……………… (257)	痉 …………………… (261)
náng yōng 囊痈 ……………… (257)	nèi shī 内湿 ……………… (261)
náo chóng bìng 蛲虫病 …… (258)	nèi tuō 内托 ……………… (262)
nǎo 脑 …………………… (258)	nèi xiāo 内消 …………… (262)
nǎo fēng 脑风 …………… (258)	nèi yīn 内因 …………… (262)
nǎo gān 脑疳 …………… (258)	nèi yōng 内痈 …………… (262)
nǎo gǔ shāng 脑骨伤 …… (258)	nèi zào 内燥 …………… (262)
nǎo jù 脑疽 …………… (258)	nèi zhì 内治 …………… (262)
nǎo míng 脑鸣 ………… (259)	nèi zhì 内痔 …………… (263)
nǎo suǐ 脑髓 …………… (259)	néng yuǎn qiè jìn zhèng 能远怯近症
nào gǔ shāng 臑骨伤 …… (259)	………………………… (263)
nào yōng 臑痈 …………… (259)	néng jìn qiè yuǎn zhèng 能近怯
nèi chuī 内吹 …………… (259)	远症 ………………… (263)
nèi diào 内钓 …………… (259)	ní qiū jū 泥鳅疽 ………… (263)
nèi dú 内毒 …………… (259)	nì chuán 逆传 …………… (263)
nèi fēng 内风 …………… (259)	nì chuán xīn bāo 逆传心包 … (263)
nèi hán 内寒 …………… (260)	nì liú wǎn zhōu 逆流挽舟 … (263)
nèi huái jū 内踝疽 …… (260)	nì zhèng 逆证 …………… (264)
nèi lòu 内漏 …………… (260)	nì tāi 腻苔 …………… (264)
nèi qǔ 内取 …………… (260)	nì chuāng 懿疮 ………… (264)
nèi rè 内热 …………… (260)	niǎn zhēn 捻针 ………… (264)
nèi shāng 内伤 …………… (260)	niào 尿 ………………… (264)
nèi shāng bù dé wò 内伤不得卧	niào xuè 尿血 …………… (264)
………………………… (261)	niào zhuó 尿浊 …………… (265)
nèi shāng fā rè 内伤发热 … (261)	niē jī 捏脊 …………… (265)
nèi shāng tóu tòng 内伤头痛 ……	niē rú 颞颥 …………… (265)
………………………… (261)	níng zhī yì 凝脂翳 ……… (265)
nèi shāng wèi wǎn tòng 内伤胃	niú pí xuǎn 牛皮癣 …… (266)

niǔ shāng 扭伤	(266)	nǚ láo dǎn 女劳疸	(268)
nóng ěr 脓耳	(266)	nǚ láo fù 女劳复	(268)
nóng wō chuāng 脓窝疮	(266)	nǚ zǐ bāo 女子胞	(268)
nóng xuè lì 脓血痢	(266)	nǜ jiā 衄家	(268)
nòng chǎn 弄产	(267)	nǜ xuè 衄血	(269)
nòng shé 弄舌	(267)	nüè jí 疟疾	(269)
nú ròu pān jīng 胬肉攀睛	(267)	nüè mǔ 疟母	(269)
nù shāng gān 怒伤肝	(267)	nüè xié 疟邪	(269)
nù zé qì shàng 怒则气上	(267)		

O

ǒu jiā 呕家	(269)	ǒu tù kǔ shuǐ 呕吐苦水	(269)
ǒu rǔ 呕乳	(269)	ǒu xuè 呕血	(269)
ǒu tù 呕吐	(269)	ǒu fāng 偶方	(270)

P

pán cháng chǎn 盘肠产	(270)	pào fú 泡服	(272)
pán gāng yōng 盘肛痈	(270)	pēi xuè 衃血	(272)
pán shàn 盘疝	(270)	péi tǔ 培土	(272)
pán shé lì 蟠蛇疬	(270)	pī jiān 披肩	(272)
páng guāng 膀胱	(270)	pī shuāng zhòng dú 砒霜中毒	(272)
páng guāng ké 膀胱咳	(270)		
páng guāng qì bì 膀胱气闭	(270)	pí bì 皮痹	(273)
pàng guāng shī rè 膀胱湿热	(271)	pí còu 皮腠	(273)
páng guāng xū hán 膀胱虚寒	(271)	pí fū zhēn 皮肤针	(273)
		pí máo 皮毛	(273)
páng guāng zhàng 膀胱胀	(271)	pí máo wěi 皮毛痿	(273)
pāo qì bù gù 脬气不固	(271)	pí nèi zhēn 皮内针	(273)
páo 炮	(271)	pí shuǐ 皮水	(273)
páo zhì 炮炙	(271)	pí jí zhī běn 罢极之本	(273)
pào zhì 炮制	(271)	pí 脾	(274)
pào 泡	(272)	pí bì 脾痹	(274)

pí bìng 脾病 …… (274)	pí zhǔ hòu tiān 脾主后天 …… (281)
pí bù tǒng xuè 脾不统血 …… (275)	pí zhǔ jī ròu 脾主肌肉 …… (281)
pí fèi liǎng xū 脾肺两虚 …… (275)	pí zhǔ shēng qīng 脾主升清 …… (282)
pí fēng 脾风 …… (275)	pí zhǔ sí zhī 脾主四肢 …… (282)
pí gān 脾疳 …… (275)	pí zhǔ wéi wèi xíng pí jīn yè 脾主为胃行其津液 …… (282)
pí hé wèi 脾和胃 …… (275)	pí zhǔ yùn huà 脾主运化 …… (282)
pí jīng 脾精 …… (276)	pí zhǔ zhōng yáng 脾主中央 …… (283)
pí kāi qiào yú kǒu 脾开窍于口 …… (276)	pí jī 痞积 …… (283)
pí ké 脾咳 …… (276)	pǐ kuài 痞块 …… (283)
pí láo 脾劳 …… (276)	pǐ mǎn 痞满 …… (283)
pí, qí huá zài chún sì bái 脾，其华在唇四白 …… (276)	pǐ qì 痞气 …… (283)
pí qì 脾气 …… (277)	piān fāng 偏方 …… (284)
pí qì bù shēng 脾气不升 …… (277)	piān jù 偏沮 …… (284)
pí qì bù shū 脾气不舒 …… (277)	piān tān 偏瘫 …… (284)
pí rè 脾热 …… (277)	piān tóu fēng 偏头风 …… (284)
pí rè duō xián 脾热多涎 …… (277)	piān zhuì 偏坠 …… (284)
pí shèn liǎng xū 脾肾两虚 …… (278)	pián zhī 胼胝 …… (284)
pí shī jiàn yùn 脾失健运 …… (278)	piàn 片 …… (285)
pí tǒng xuè 脾统血 …… (278)	piǎo 漂 …… (285)
pí wèi shī rè 脾胃湿热 …… (278)	pín fú 频服 …… (285)
pí wù shī 脾恶湿 …… (279)	pìn nüè 牝疟 …… (285)
pí xiāo 脾消 …… (279)	pìn zàng 牝脏 …… (285)
pí xiè 脾泄 …… (279)	pìn zhì 牝痔 …… (285)
pí xū 脾虚 …… (279)	píng dàn fú 平旦服 …… (285)
pí xū dài xià 脾虚带下 …… (279)	píng gān xī fēng 平肝熄风 …… (285)
pí xū duō xián 脾虚多涎 …… (280)	píng mài 平脉 …… (286)
pí xū jīng bì 脾虚经闭 …… (280)	píng rén 平人 …… (286)
pí xū shī kùn 脾虚湿困 …… (280)	pò qì 破气 …… (286)
pí xū xiè xiè 脾虚泄泻 …… (280)	pò shāng fēng 破伤风 …… (286)
pí yáng 脾阳 …… (280)	pò tóu chuāng 破头疮 …… (286)
pí yáng xū 脾阳虚 …… (281)	pò xuè 破血 …… (287)
pí yīn 脾阴 …… (281)	pò yū xiāo zhēng 破瘀消癥 …… (287)
pí yīn xū 脾阴虚 …… (281)	pò 魄 …… (287)
pí yuē 脾约 …… (281)	pò hàn 魄汗 …… (287)

pò mén 魄门 …………… (287)	pú táo yì 葡萄疫 …………… (287)
pū fěn 扑粉 …………… (287)	

Q

qī chōng mén 七冲门 …………… (288)	qì gǔ 气鼓 …………… (292)
qī fāng 七方 …………… (288)	qì gǔ 气臌 …………… (292)
qī guài mài 七怪脉 …………… (288)	qì guān 气关 …………… (292)
qī qiào 七窍 …………… (288)	qì hǎi 气海 …………… (292)
qī qíng 七情 …………… (288)	qì huà 气化 …………… (293)
qī rì fēng 七日风 …………… (289)	qì huì 气会 …………… (293)
qī chuāng 漆疮 …………… (289)	qì jī 气积 …………… (293)
qí héng zhī fǔ 奇恒之腑 …………… (289)	qì jī 气机 …………… (293)
qí 脐 …………… (289)	qì jī bù lì 气机不利 …………… (293)
qí chuāng 脐疮 …………… (289)	qì jué 气绝 …………… (293)
qí fēng 脐风 …………… (289)	qì jué 气厥 …………… (293)
qí lòu 脐漏 …………… (289)	qì lì 气疬 …………… (293)
qí shàn 脐疝 …………… (289)	qì lì 气痢 …………… (293)
qí shī 脐湿 …………… (290)	qì lín 气淋 …………… (294)
qí xià jì 脐下悸 …………… (290)	qì liú 气瘤 …………… (294)
qí xuè 脐血 …………… (290)	qì lún 气轮 …………… (294)
qí yōng 脐痈 …………… (290)	qì mén 气门 …………… (294)
qì 气 …………… (290)	qì nì 气逆 …………… (294)
qì mì 气秘 …………… (290)	qì ǒu 气呕 …………… (294)
qì bì 气痹 …………… (291)	qì pǐ 气痞 …………… (295)
qì chuǎn 气喘 …………… (291)	qì qiè 气怯 …………… (295)
qì duǎn 气短 …………… (291)	qì shàn 气疝 …………… (295)
qì è 气呃 …………… (291)	qì shàng chōng xīn 气上冲心 …………… (295)
qì fēn zhèng 气分证 …………… (291)	
qì gé 气膈 …………… (291)	qì sòu 气嗽 …………… (295)
qì gōng 气功 …………… (291)	qì suí xuè tuō 气随血脱 …………… (295)
qì gōng gōng néng tài 气功功能态 …………… (292)	qì tán 气痰 …………… (296)
	qì tòng 气痛 …………… (296)
qì gōng liáo fǎ 气功疗法 …………… (292)	qì wéi xuè shuài 气为血帅 …………… (296)
qì gōng xué 气功学 …………… (292)	qì wèi 气味 …………… (296)

qì wèi yīn yáng 气味阴阳 …… (296)	qì yóu zàng fā 气由脏发 …… (302)
qì xiè 气泻 …………………… (297)	qì yǒu yú biàn shì huǒ 气有余便
qì xīn tòng 气心痛 …………… (297)	是火 ……………………… (303)
qì xū 气虚 …………………… (297)	qì yù 气郁 …………………… (303)
qì xū bēng lòu 气虚崩漏 ……… (297)	qì yù wǎn tòng 气郁脘痛 …… (303)
qì xū bì 气虚痹 ……………… (297)	qì yù xié tòng 气郁胁痛 …… (303)
qì xū biàn bì 气虚便秘 ……… (297)	qì yù xuàn rūn 气郁眩晕 …… (303)
qì xū bù shè 气虚不摄 ……… (298)	qì yù xuè bēng 气郁血崩 …… (303)
qì xū chuǎn 气虚喘 …………… (298)	qì zhàng 气胀 ……………… (304)
qì xū ěr lóng 气虚耳聋 ……… (298)	qì zhì 气痔 ………………… (304)
qì xū ěr míng 气虚耳鸣 ……… (298)	qì zhì 气滞 ………………… (304)
qì xū fù tòng 气虚腹痛 ……… (298)	qì zhì fù tòng 气滞腹痛 …… (304)
qì xū huá tāi 气虚滑胎 ……… (299)	qì zhì jīng xíng hòu qī 气滞经行
qì xū rè 气虚热 ……………… (299)	后期 ……………………… (304)
qì xū tóu tòng 气虚头痛 …… (299)	qì zhì tòng jīng 气滞痛经 …… (305)
qì xū wěi 气虚痿 …………… (299)	qì zhì xuè yū jīng bì 气滞血瘀
qì xū xīn jì 气虚心悸 ……… (299)	经闭 ……………………… (305)
qì xū xuàn yūn 气虚眩晕 …… (299)	qì zhì xuè yū xīn jì 气滞血瘀
qì xū yuè jīng guò duō 气虚月经	心悸 ……………………… (305)
过多 ……………………… (299)	qì zhì yāo tòng 气滞腰痛 …… (305)
qì xū yuè jīng xiān qī 气虚月经	qì zhǒng 气肿 ……………… (305)
先期 ……………………… (300)	qì qì 泣 …………………… (305)
qì xū zé hán 气虚则寒 ……… (300)	qiān rì chuāng 千日疮 ……… (305)
qì xū zhōng mǎn 气虚中满 …… (300)	qiān suì chuāng 千岁疮 …… (306)
qì xū zì hàn 气虚自汗 ……… (300)	qián hòu bù tōng 前后不通 … (306)
qì xuè biàn zhèng 气血辨证 … (300)	qián yīn 前阴 ……………… (306)
qì xuè chōng hé 气血冲和 …… (301)	qián yáng 潜阳 ……………… (306)
qì xuè shī tiáo 气血失调 …… (301)	qián zhèn 潜镇 ……………… (306)
qì xuè tán shí biàn zhèng 气血痰	qiáng yīn 强阴 ……………… (306)
食辨证 …………………… (301)	qiáng zhōng 强中 …………… (307)
qì xuè xū ruò tòng jīng 气血虚弱	qiē mài 切脉 ……………… (307)
痛经 ……………………… (301)	qiē zhěn 切诊 ……………… (307)
qì xuè liǎng xū 气血两虚 …… (301)	qín huà 噙化 ……………… (307)
qì yíng liǎng fán 气营两燔 … (302)	qín zhēn 撳针 ……………… (307)
qì yíng liǎng qīng 气营两清 … (302)	qīng 青 …………………… (307)
qì yǐng 气瘿 ………………… (302)	qīng dài 青带 ……………… (307)

qīng fēng nèi zhàng 青风内障 ……… (308)	……………………………………… (314)
qīng máng 青盲 ……………… (308)	qīng yáng chū shàng qiào 清阳出上窍 ……………………………… (314)
qīng rú cǎo zī 青如草兹 ………… (308)	qīng yáng fā còu lǐ 清阳发腠理 ……………………………………… (315)
qīng fāng 轻方 ………………… (308)	
qīng jì 轻剂 …………………… (308)	qīng yáng shí sì zhī 清阳实四肢 ……………………………………… (315)
qīng kě qù shí 轻可去实 ……… (309)	
qīng qīng shū jiě 轻清疏解 …… (309)	qīng yíng 清营 ………………… (315)
qīng qīng xuān fèi 轻清宣肺 ……………………………………… (309)	qīng yíng tòu zhěn 清营透疹 ……………………………………… (315)
qīng xuān rùn zào 轻宣润燥 ……………………………………… (309)	qiū máo 秋毛 …………………… (316)
qīng cháng rùn zào 清肠润燥 ……………………………………… (310)	qiú mài zòng héng 虬脉纵横 ……………………………………… (316)
	qiú pán juǎn qū 虬蟠卷曲 …… (316)
qīng fǎ 清法 …………………… (310)	qiú qiú 軱 ……………………… (316)
qīng luò bǎo yīn 清络保阴 …… (310)	qū 曲 …………………………… (316)
qīng qì 清气 …………………… (310)	qū chóng 驱虫 ………………… (316)
qīng rè huà shī 清热化湿 …… (311)	qū fēng 祛风 ………………… (316)
qīng rè huà tán 清热化痰 …… (311)	qū fēng chú shī 祛风除湿 …… (317)
qīng rè huà tán kāi qiào 清热化痰开窍 …………………… (311)	qū fēng yǎng xuè 祛风养血 …… (317)
	qū hán huà tán 祛寒化痰 …… (317)
qīng rè jiě biǎo 清热解表 …… (311)	qū tán 祛痰 …………………… (317)
qīng rè jiě dú 清热解毒 …… (312)	qū xié fū zhèng 祛邪扶正 …… (317)
qīng rè jiě shǔ 清热解暑 …… (312)	qū yū huó xuè 祛瘀活血 …… (318)
qīng rè kāi qiào 清热开窍 …… (312)	qū yū xiāo zhǒng 祛瘀消肿 …… (318)
qīng rè lì shī 清热利湿 …… (312)	qū yū zhǐ xuè 祛瘀止血 …… (318)
qīng rè zhǐ xuè 清热止血 …… (313)	qù huǒ dú 去火毒 …………… (318)
qīng shǔ lì shī 清暑利湿 …… (313)	qù yù chén cuò 去菀陈莝 …… (319)
qīng shǔ yì qì 清暑益气 …… (313)	qù yóu 去油 …………………… (319)
qīng sù fèi qì 清肃肺气 …… (313)	quán shēn fú zhǒng 全身浮肿 ……………………………………… (319)
qīng wèi jiàng nì 清胃降逆 …… (314)	
qīng xiè shào yáng 清泄少阳 ……………………………………… (314)	quán shēn tòng 全身痛 ……… (319)
	quán shēn wú lì 全身无力 …… (319)
qīng xīn 清心 ………………… (314)	quán chì 颧赤 ………………… (320)
qīng yáng 清阳 ………………… (314)	quē pén 缺盆 ………………… (320)
qīng yáng bù shēng 清阳不升	quē rǔ 缺乳 …………………… (320)

què bān 雀斑	(320)	què shàng 阙上	(320)
què zhuó mài 雀啄脉	(320)	rǎn tāi 染苔	(321)
què 阙	(320)		

R

rè 热	(321)	rè rù xīn bāo 热入心包	(327)
rè bì 热秘	(321)	rè rù xuè fēn 热入血分	(327)
rè bì 热痹	(321)	rè shāng fèi luò 热伤肺络	(327)
rè chǎn 热产	(321)	rè rù xuè shì 热入血室	(328)
rè chuǎn 热喘	(322)	rè shāng jīn mài 热伤筋脉	(328)
rè chuāng 热疮	(322)	rè shāng qì 热伤气	(328)
rè dú 热毒	(322)	rè shāng shén míng 热伤神明	(328)
rè è 热呃	(322)	rè shēn jué shēn 热深厥深	(328)
rè fū zhǐ tòng fǎ 热敷止痛法	(322)	rè shèn fā jìng 热甚发痉	(329)
rè fú chōng rèn 热伏冲任	(323)	rè shèng zé zhǒng 热胜则肿	(329)
rè fú 热服	(323)	rè shèng fēng dòng 热盛风动	(329)
rè gé 热膈	(323)	rè shèng qì fēn 热盛气分	(329)
rè hōng 热烘	(323)	rè sòu 热嗽	(329)
rè huà 热化	(323)	rè tán 热痰	(330)
rè huò luàn 热霍乱	(324)	rè wú chén 热无沉	(330)
rè jí shēng hán 热极生寒	(324)	rè wú fàn rè 热无犯热	(330)
rè jì 热剂	(324)	rè xián 热痫	(330)
rè jié 热结	(324)	rè xié 热邪	(331)
rè jié páng guāng 热结膀胱	(324)	rè xié zǔ fèi 热邪阻肺	(331)
rè jié xià jiāo 热结下焦	(325)	rè xiè 热泻	(331)
rè jié xiōng 热结胸	(325)	rè xīn tòng 热心痛	(331)
rè jué 热厥	(325)	rè yàn fǎ 热熨法	(332)
rè lèi 热泪	(325)	rè yè tí 热夜啼	(332)
rè lì 热痢	(326)	rè yīn hán yòng 热因寒用	(332)
rè lín 热淋	(326)	rè yīn rè yòng 热因热用	(332)
rè néng qù hán 热能去寒	(326)	rè yù 热郁	(332)
rè ǒu 热呕	(326)	rè zhàng 热胀	(333)
rè pò dà cháng 热迫大肠	(327)		

rè zhě hán zhī 热者寒之	(333)
rè zhèng 热证	(333)
rè zhōng 热中	(334)
rè zhuó shèn yīn 热灼肾阴	(334)
rén dòu jiē zhòng (fǎ) 人痘接种（法）	(334)
rén shì bù xǐng 人事不省	(334)
rén yíng 人迎	(334)
rén zhōng dīng 人中疔	(335)
rèn shēn chuǎn 妊娠喘	(335)
rèn shēn chuāng yáng 妊娠疮疡	(335)
rèn shēn e zǔ 妊娠恶阻	(335)
rèn shēn xiǎo biàn bú lì 妊娠小便不利	(335)
rèn shēn xīn fán 妊娠心烦	(336)
rèn shēn xīn fù zhàng mǎn 妊娠心腹胀满	(336)
rèn shēn xuàn yūn 妊娠眩晕	(336)
rèn shēn yāo tòng 妊娠腰痛	(336)
rèn shēn yào jì 妊娠药忌	(337)
rèn shēn zhǒng zhàng 妊娠肿胀	(337)
rèn shēn zhòng fēng 妊娠中风	(337)
rì bū fā rè 日晡发热	(337)
rì shài chuāng 日晒疮	(337)
róu jìng 柔痉	(338)
ròu cì 肉刺	(338)
ròu fèn 肉分	(338)
ròu liú 肉瘤	(338)
ròu lún 肉轮	(338)
ròu tuō 肉脱	(338)
ròu wěi 肉痿	(338)
ròu yǐng 肉瘿	(339)
rú sàng shén shǒu 如丧神守	(339)
rú mài 濡脉	(339)
rǔ é 乳蛾	(339)
rǔ fā 乳发	(340)
rǔ fáng zhàng tòng 乳房胀痛	(340)
rǔ gān 乳疳	(340)
rǔ jiē 乳疖	(340)
rǔ láo 乳痨	(340)
rǔ lòu 乳瘘	(341)
rǔ nù 乳衄	(341)
rǔ shí jī zhì 乳食积滞	(341)
rǔ tóu jūn liè 乳头皲裂	(342)
rǔ xì 乳细	(342)
rǔ xiàn zēng shēng bìng 乳腺增生病	(342)
rǔ yán 乳岩	(342)
rǔ yōng 乳痈	(343)
rǔ zhī bù zú 乳汁不足	(343)
rǔ zǐ 乳子	(344)
rù fēng 蓐风	(344)
rù jìng 入静	(344)
rù láo 蓐劳	(344)
ruǎn jiān chú mǎn 软坚除满	(344)
ruǎn jiān sàn jié 软坚散结	(344)
ruǎn tān 软瘫	(345)
ruǎn xià gān 软下疳	(345)
rùn xià 润下	(345)
rùn zào 润燥	(345)
rùn zào huà tán 润燥化痰	(345)
ruò mài 弱脉	(345)
ruò 爇	(345)

S

sāi fǎ 塞法 …………… (346)
sāi yīn sāi yòng 塞因塞用 …… (346)
sān bǎo 三宝 …………… (346)
sān bì 三痹 …………… (346)
sān bù 三部 …………… (346)
sān bù jiǔ hóu 三部九候 …… (346)
sān fǎ 三法 …………… (347)
sān fú 三伏 …………… (347)
sān jiāo 三焦 …………… (347)
sān jiāo biàn zhèng 三焦辨证
  ………………………… (347)
sān jiāo ké 三焦咳 …… (348)
sān jiāo shí rè 三焦实热 …… (348)
sān jiāo zhǔ jué dú 三焦主决渎
  ………………………… (348)
sān pǐn 三品 …………… (348)
sān rì nuè 三日疟 …… (348)
sān tiáo 三调 …………… (348)
sān xiāo 三消 …………… (348)
sān yáng bìng 三阳病 …… (349)
sān yīn jìng 三阴痉 …… (349)
sān yáng hé bìng 三阳合病 …… (349)
sān yīn 三因 …………… (349)
sān yīn bìng 三阴病 …… (350)
sān yīn nuè 三阴疟 …… (350)
sǎn 散 …………… (350)
sǎn mài 散脉 …………… (350)
sàn zhě shōu zhī 散者收之 …… (350)
sè bù 色部 …………… (350)
sè cuì 色悴 …………… (351)
sè mài hé cān 色脉合参 …… (351)
sè suí qì huá 色随气华 …… (351)
sè zhěn 色诊 …………… (351)
sè cháng zhǐ xiè 涩肠止泻 …… (351)
sè jì 涩剂 …………… (352)
sè kě qù tuō 涩可去脱 …… (352)
sè mài 涩脉 …………… (352)
shā xuè xīn tòng 杀血心痛 …… (352)
shā shī bìng 杀虱病 …… (352)
shā shí lìn 砂石淋 …… (352)
shā 痧 …………… (353)
shā kuài 痧块 …………… (353)
shā zhàng 痧胀 …………… (353)
shǎn cuò 闪挫 …………… (353)
shǎn diē xuè bēng 闪跌血崩 …… (353)
shǎn guàn fǎ 闪罐法 …… (353)
shǎn shāng 闪伤 …………… (353)
shǎn 疝 …………… (353)
shàn jī 善饥 …………… (354)
shàn kǒng 善恐 …………… (354)
shàn jīng 善惊 …………… (354)
shàn nù 善怒 …………… (354)
shàn sè 善色 …………… (354)
shàn lòu 鳝漏 …………… (354)
shāng fēng 伤风 …………… (355)
shāng fēng fā jìng 伤风发痉
  ………………………… (355)
shāng fēng ké sòu 伤风咳嗽 …… (355)
shāng hán 伤寒 …………… (355)
shāng hán biǎo zhèng 伤寒表证
  ………………………… (355)
shāng hán lǐ zhèng 伤寒里证 …
  ………………………… (355)
shāng hán xù shuǐ zhèng 伤寒蓄
  水证 …………………… (356)
shāng hán xù xuè zhèng 伤寒蓄

血证	(356)	shàng qì 上气	(361)
shāng jīn 伤津	(356)	shàng qiào 上窍	(362)
shāng jīn 伤筋	(356)	shàng rè xià hán 上热下寒	(362)
shāng jiǔ sóu gòng 伤酒头痛	(357)	shàng shèng 上盛	(362)
shāng kē 伤科	(357)	shàng shí xià xū 上实下虚	(362)
shāng lì zhèng 伤力症	(357)	shàng sǔn jí xià 上损及下	(362)
shāng rǔ shí 伤乳食	(357)	shàng tù xià xiè 上吐下泻	(363)
shāng rǔ shí tù 伤乳食吐	(357)	shàng wǎn 上脘	(363)
shāng shī 伤湿	(357)	shàng xiāo 上消	(363)
shāng shī ké sòu 伤湿咳嗽	(357)	shàng xū xià shí 上虚下实	(363)
shāng shī yāo tòng 伤湿腰痛	(358)	shāo cún xìng 烧存性	(363)
shāng shī zì hàn 伤湿自汗	(358)	shāo shān huǒ 烧山火	(363)
shāng shí 伤食	(358)	shāo shāng 烧伤	(364)
shāhg shí góu tòng 伤食头痛	(358)	shào fù jū jí 少腹拘急	(364)
shang shí tù 伤食吐	(359)	shào fù rú shàn 少腹如扇	(364)
shāng shǔ 伤暑	(359)	shào fù yīng mǎn 少腹硬满	(364)
shāng shǔ yāo tòng 伤损腰痛	(359)	shào huǒ 少火	(365)
shang yáng 伤阳	(359)	shào yáng 少阳	(365)
shāng yīn 伤阴	(359)	shào yàng bìng 少阳病	(365)
shāng zào ké sòu 伤燥咳嗽	(359)	shào yáng fǔ bìng 少阳腑病	(365)
shàng bāo xià chuí 上胞下垂	(360)	shào yáng jīng bìng 少阳经病	(365)
shàng bìng xià qǔ 上病下取	(360)	shào yáng tóu tòng 少阳头痛	(365)
shàng dān tián 上丹田	(360)	shào yīn 少阴	(366)
shàng è yōng 上腭痈	(360)	shào yīn bìng 少阴病	(366)
shàng fā bèi 上发背	(360)	shào yīn hán huà 少阴寒化	(366)
shàng hán xià rè 上寒下热	(360)	shào yīn rè huà 少阴热化	(366)
shàng jiāo 上焦	(361)	shào yīn tóu tòng 少阴头痛	(367)
shàng jiāo rú wù 上焦如雾	(361)	shé 舌	(367)
shàng jiāo zhǔ nà 上焦主纳	(361)	shé běn 舌本	(367)
shàng juē xià jié 上厥下竭	(361)	shé bì 舌痹	(367)
shàng pǐn 上品	(361)	shé biān 舌边	(367)
		shé chàn 舌颤	(368)
		shé chū 舌出	(368)
		shé chuāng 舌疮	(368)

shé dǐ shàng é 舌抵上腭 …… (368)	shé fù dīng 蛇腹疔 …… (374)
shé dīng 舌疔 …… (368)	shé jié dīng 蛇节疔 …… (374)
shé duǎn 舌短 …… (368)	shé kē chuāng 蛇窠疮 …… (374)
shé gēn 舌根 …… (368)	shé tóu dīng 蛇头疔 …… (375)
shé gēn yōng 舌根痈 …… (369)	shēn shé 伸舌 …… (375)
shé hóng 舌红 …… (369)	shēn rè 身热 …… (375)
shé jiān 舌尖 …… (369)	shēn shòu bù yùn 身瘦不孕 …… (375)
shé jiǎn 舌謇 …… (369)	shēn yǎng 身痒 …… (375)
shé jiàng 舌绛 …… (369)	shēn zhòng 身重 …… (375)
shé juǎn 舌卷 …… (369)	shén 神 …… (375)
shé juǎn náng suō 舌卷囊缩 … (370)	shén bù shǒu shè 神不守舍 …… (376)
shé jūn 舌菌 …… (370)	shén hūn 神昏 …… (376)
shé làn 舌烂 …… (370)	shén mén mài 神门脉 …… (376)
shé liè 舌裂 …… (370)	shén què 神阙 …… (376)
shé mián rú jìng 舌面如镜 …… (370)	shén zàng 神脏 …… (376)
shé nǜ 舌衄 …… (370)	shén zhì bù qīng 神志不清 …… (376)
shé pàng 舌胖 …… (371)	shěn miáo qiào 审苗窍 …… (376)
shé pàng chǐ xíng 舌胖齿形 … (371)	shèn 肾 …… (376)
shé qǐ máng cì 舌起芒刺 …… (371)	shèn bì 肾痹 …… (377)
shé qiáng 舌强 …… (371)	shèn bìng 肾病 …… (377)
shé sè 舌色 …… (371)	shèn cáng jīng 肾藏精 …… (377)
shé shén 舌神 …… (372)	shèn chuǎn 肾喘 …… (377)
shé shēng pào 舌生泡 …… (372)	shèn gān 肾疳 …… (378)
shé sǔn 舌笋 …… (372)	shèn hé páng guāng 肾合膀胱 …… (378)
shé tāi 舌苔 …… (372)	
shé tāi hòu 舌苔厚 …… (372)	shèn huǒ piān kàng 肾火偏亢 …… (378)
shé tǐ 舌体 …… (372)	
shé wāi 舌歪 …… (373)	shèn jiān dòng qì 肾间动气 … (378)
shé wěi 舌痿 …… (373)	shèn jīng 肾精 …… (379)
shé xíng 舌形 …… (373)	shèn jué tóu tòng 肾厥头痛 … (379)
shé yīn 舌瘖 …… (373)	shèn kāi qiào yú ěr 肾开窍于耳 …… (379)
shé yōng 舌痈 …… (373)	
shé zhàng dà 舌胀大 …… (374)	shèn kāi qiào yú èr yīn 肾开窍于二阴 …… (379)
shé zhěn 舌诊 …… (374)	
shé zhōng 舌中 …… (374)	shèn ké 肾咳 …… (379)
shé zhǒng 舌肿 …… (374)	shèn láo 肾劳 …… (380)

shèn náng fēng	肾囊风	(380)
shèn, qí huá zài fà	肾,其华在发	(380)
shèn qì	肾气	(380)
shèn shēng gǔ suǐ	肾生骨髓	(380)
shèn shù lòu	肾俞漏	(381)
shèn shù xū tán	肾俞虚痰	(381)
shèn xiào	肾哮	(381)
shèn xiāo	肾消	(381)
shèn xiè	肾泄	(381)
shèn xū	肾虚	(382)
shèn xū bù yùn	肾虚不孕	(382)
shèn xū huá tāi	肾虚滑胎	(382)
shèn xū jīng bì	肾虚经闭	(382)
shèn xū jīng xíng hòu qī	肾虚经行后期	(382)
shèn xū shuǐ fàn	肾虚水泛	(383)
shèn xū tóu tòng	肾虚头痛	(383)
shèn xū xuàn yūn	肾虚眩晕	(383)
shèn xū yáng wěi	肾虚阳萎	(384)
shèn xū yāo tòng	肾虚腰痛	(384)
shèn xu yī jīng	肾虚遗精	(384)
shèn xū yuè jīng guò shǎo	肾虚月经过少	(384)
shèn yán	肾岩	(385)
shèn yáng	肾阳	(385)
shèn yáng shuāi wēi	肾阳衰微	(385)
shèn yáng xū	肾阳虚	(385)
shèn yīn	肾阴	(385)
shèn yīn xū	肾阴虚	(386)
shèn yǔ páng guāng xiāng biǎo lǐ	肾与膀胱相表里	(386)
shèn zhī fǔ	肾之府	(386)
shèn zhǔ gǔ	肾主骨	(386)
shèn zhǔ jì qiǎo	肾主伎巧	(386)
shèn zhǔ ná qì	肾主纳气	(386)
shèn zhǔ shuǐ	肾主水	(387)
shèn zhǔ xiān tiān	肾主先天	(387)
shèn zháo	肾着	(387)
shèn zhě cóng zhī	甚者从之	(387)
shèn zhě dú xíng	甚者独行	(387)
shèn zhǒng	肾肿	(387)
shēng jì	升剂	(387)
shēng jiàng fú chén	升降浮沉	(388)
shēng jiàng shī cháng	升降失常	(388)
shēng kě qù jiàng	升可去降	(388)
shēng tí zhōng qì	升提中气	(388)
shēng jīn	生津	(389)
shēng zhí zhī jīng	生殖之精	(389)
shēng rú zhuài jù	声如拽锯	(389)
shèng qì	胜气	(389)
shī jué	尸厥	(389)
shī jīng jiā	失精家	(389)
shī mián	失眠	(389)
shī qì	失气	(390)
shī róng	失荣	(390)
shī shén	失神	(390)
shī xuè	失血	(390)
shī xuè xīn tòng	失血心痛	(390)
shī xuè xuàn yūn	失血眩晕	(390)
shī yīn	失音	(390)
shī zhěn	失枕	(391)
shī bì	湿痹	(391)
shī bìng	湿病	(391)
shī dú	湿毒	(391)
shī dú dài xià	湿毒带下	(391)
shī dú xià xuè	湿毒下血	(392)

shī jì	湿剂	(392)
shī jiā	湿家	(392)
shī jiǎo qì	湿脚气	(392)
shī jiè	湿疥	(392)
shī jìng	湿痉	(393)
shī ké	湿咳	(393)
shī kě qù kū	湿可去枯	(393)
shī kùn pí yáng	湿困脾阳	(393)
shī nüè	湿疟	(393)
shī rè	湿热	(393)
shī rè fù tòng	湿热腹痛	(394)
shī rè huáng dǎn	湿热黄疸	(394)
shī rè nèi yùn	湿热内蕴	(394)
shī rè tóu tòng	湿热头痛	(395)
shī rè wěi	湿热痿	(395)
shī rè xià zhù	湿热下注	(395)
shī rè xié tòng	湿热胁痛	(395)
shī rè xuàn yūn	湿热眩晕	(396)
shī rè yāo tòng	湿热腰痛	(396)
shī shèng yáng wēi	湿胜阳微	(396)
shī shèng zé rú xiè	湿胜则濡泻	(396)
shī tán	湿痰	(396)
shī tán jiǎo qì	湿痰脚气	(397)
shī tán liú zhù	湿痰流注	(397)
shī tán wěi	湿痰痿	(397)
shī wēn bìng	湿温病	(397)
shī xiè	湿泻	(397)
shī xuǎn	湿癣	(398)
shī yù	湿郁	(398)
shī yù rè fú	湿郁热伏	(398)
shī zhuó	湿浊	(398)
shī zǔ qì fēn	湿阻气分	(398)
shī zǔ zhōng jiāo	湿阻中焦	(399)
shí bā fǎn	十八反	(399)
shí èr jì	十二剂	(399)
shí èr shí	十二时	(399)
shí èr zàng	十二脏	(400)
shí juǔ wèi	十九畏	(400)
shí wèn	十问	(400)
shí é	石蛾	(400)
shí jiǎ	石瘕	(400)
shí jū	石疽	(401)
shí lín	石淋	(401)
shí nǚ	石女	(401)
shí shuǐ	石水	(401)
shí yǐng	石瘿	(402)
shí bìng	时病	(402)
shí dú	时毒	(402)
shí dú fā yí	时毒发颐	(402)
shí fāng	时方	(402)
shí lìng	时令	(403)
shí xié	时邪	(403)
shí xíng gǎn mào	时行感冒	(403)
shí xíng hán yì	时行寒疫	(403)
shí xíng lì qì	时行疠气	(403)
shí xíng sòu	时行嗽	(403)
shí yì	时疫	(403)
shí yì fā bān	时疫发斑	(403)
shí bì	实秘	(404)
shí chuǎn	实喘	(404)
shí huǒ	实火	(404)
shí mài	实脉	(404)
shí pǐ	实痞	(404)
shí rè	实热	(405)
shí zé tài yáng, xú zé shào yīn	实则太阳，虚则少阴	(405)
shí zhàng	实胀	(405)
shí zhě xiè qí zǐ	实者泻其子	(406)
shí zhě xiè zhī	实者泻之	(406)
shí zèng	实证	(406)

shí zhōng jiá xū 实中夹虚 …… (407)	shōu sè 收涩 ………… (412)
shí bì 食痹 ……………… (407)	shǒu bù dīng chuāng 手部疔疮
shí fù 食复 ……………… (407)	………… (412)
shí jī 食积 ……………… (407)	shǒu fā bèi 手发背 ……… (412)
shí jī fù tòng 食积腹痛 …… (408)	shǒu xīn dú 手心毒 ……… (412)
shí nüè 食疟 …………… (408)	shǒu zhǐ má mù 手指麻木 … (412)
shí ǒu 食呕 …………… (408)	shǒu zhǐ tuō jiè 手指脱骱 … (413)
shí qì 食气 …………… (408)	shǒu zú hàn 手足汗 ……… (413)
shí ròu zé fù 食肉则复 …… (408)	shǒu zú jué lěng 手足厥冷 … (413)
shí xián 食痫 …………… (409)	shǒu zú xīn rè 手足心热 …… (413)
shí xiè zhòng dú 食蟹中毒 … (409)	shǒu fēng 首风 ………… (413)
shí xīn tòng 食心痛 ……… (409)	shòu yāo 寿夭 ………… (413)
shí xùn jùn zhòng dú 食蕈菌中毒 …	shòu shèng zhī fǔ 受盛之腑 … (414)
………… (409)	shòu shèng zhī guān 受盛之官
shí yī 食医 …………… (409)	………… (414)
shí yì 食亦 …………… (409)	shū biǎo 疏表 ………… (414)
shí yù 食郁 …………… (410)	shū biǎo huà shī 疏表化湿 …… (414)
shí yù ròu zhòng dú 食郁肉中毒	shū fēng 疏风 ………… (414)
………… (410)	shū fēng xiè rè 疏风泄热 …… (414)
shí yuǎn fú 食远服 ……… (410)	shū gān 疏肝 ………… (415)
shí zhàng 食胀 ………… (410)	shū tōng jīng luò 疏通经络 …… (415)
shí zhì 食治 …………… (410)	shū yù lǐ qì 疏郁理气 …… (415)
shí zhī wèi wǎn 食滞胃脘 … (410)	shǔ 暑 ……………… (415)
shí zhū yú zhòng dú 食诸鱼中毒	shǔ bìng 暑病 ………… (416)
………… (411)	shǔ fēng 暑风 ………… (416)
shì chì rú bái 视赤如白 …… (411)	shǔ jué 暑厥 ………… (416)
shì yī wèi èr zhèng 视一为二症	shǔ ké 暑咳 ………… (416)
………… (411)	shǔ lì 暑痢 ………… (416)
shì yī 视衣 …………… (411)	shǔ nüè 暑疟 ………… (417)
shì zhān hūn miǎo 视瞻昏渺	shǔ rè 暑热 ………… (417)
………… (411)	shǔ rè nié tòng 暑热胁痛
shì nǚ 室女 …………… (411)	shǔ rè zhèng 暑热证 …… (417)
shì nǚ jīng bì 室女经闭 …… (411)	shǔ shā 暑痧 ………… (417)
shì piān shí 嗜偏食 ……… (411)	shǔ shī 暑湿 ………… (417)
shì wò 嗜卧 …………… (412)	shǔ shī xuàn yūn 暑湿眩晕 … (417)
shì wò yù mèi 嗜卧欲寐 … (412)	shǔ wēn 暑温 ………… (418)

shǔ xián 暑痫 …………………（418）	shuǐ xìng liú xià 水性流下 ……（424）
shǔ xiè 暑泻 …………………（418）	shuǐ zhēn liáo fǎ 水针疗法 ……（424）
shǔ zhài 暑瘵 …………………（418）	shuǐ zhǒng 水肿 ………………（424）
shǔ yì 鼠疫 …………………（418）	shuǐ zì chuāng 水渍疮 …………（424）
shù dí 漱涤 …………………（419）	shùn chuán 顺传 ………………（424）
shuāi zhě bǔ zhī 衰者补之 ……（419）	shùn zhèng 顺证 ………………（424）
shuāng rǔ é 双乳蛾 …………（419）	shùn 瞤 ………………………（425）
shuǐ bù hán mù 水不涵木 ……（419）	shuò mài 数脉 …………………（425）
shuǐ bù huà qì 水不化气………（419）	sī shāng pí 思伤脾 ……………（425）
shuǐ chuǎn 水喘 ………………（419）	sī zé qì jié 思则气结 …………（425）
shuǐ dòu 水痘 …………………（419）	sī shà 嘶嗄 ……………………（425）
shuǐ dú 水毒 …………………（420）	sǐ shé yōng 死舌痈 ……………（425）
shuǐ dú bìng 水毒病 …………（420）	sǐ tāi 死胎 ……………………（425）
shuǐ fēi 水飞 …………………（420）	sǐ tāi bù xià 死胎不下 ………（426）
shuǐ fǔ 水府 …………………（420）	sǐ xuè xié tòng 死血胁痛 ……（426）
shuǐ gǔ zhī sǎi 水谷之海………（420）	sì pàng 四傍 …………………（426）
shuǐ gǔ zhī jīng 水谷之精 ……（420）	sì hǎi 四海 ……………………（426）
shuǐ gǔ 水臌 …………………（420）	sì jí 四极 ……………………（426）
shuǐ guàn fǎ 水罐法 …………（421）	sì mò 四末 ……………………（427）
shuǐ hán shè fèi 水寒射肺 ……（421）	sì nì 四逆 ……………………（427）
shuǐ huǒ bù jì 水火不济 ………（421）	sì qì 四气 ……………………（427）
shuǐ huǒ tàng shāng 水火烫伤 …………………………（421）	sì shí 四时 ……………………（427）
shuǐ huǒ xiāng jì 水火相济……（422）	sì shí bù zhèng zhī qì 四时不正之气…………………………（427）
shuǐ huǒ zhī záng 水火之脏 …（422）	sì shí zhī mài 四时之脉 ………（427）
shuǐ jié xiōng 水结胸 …………（422）	sì wéi 四维 ……………………（427）
shuǐ jīng 水精 …………………（422）	sì yǐn 四饮 ……………………（427）
shuǐ kuī huǒ wáng 水亏火旺 …………………………（422）	sì zhěn 四诊 …………………（427）
shuǐ lún 水轮 …………………（423）	sì zhěn hé cān 四诊合参 ……（427）
shuǐ nì 水逆 …………………（423）	sì zhī jū jí 四肢拘急 …………（428）
shuǐ qì 水气 …………………（423）	sì zhī má mù 四肢麻木 ………（428）
shuǐ qì líng xīn 水气凌心 ……（423）	sì zhī pí juàn 四肢疲倦 ………（428）
shuǐ shàn 水疝 ………………（423）	sì zhī wú lì 四肢无力 …………（428）
shuǐ tǔ bù fú 水土不服 ………（424）	sōng pí xuǎn 松皮癣 …………（428）
shuǐ xiè 水泻 …………………（424）	sòng fú 送服 …………………（429）
	sōu fēng zhú hán 搜风逐寒 ……（429）

sōu shuò 溲数 ……… (429)
sù chuāng 粟疮 ……… (429)
suān 酸 ……… (430)
suàn gān huà yīn 酸甘化阴 … (430)
suān kǔ yǒng xiè wéi yīn 酸苦涌
　　泄为阴 ……… (430)
suān xián wú shēng 酸咸无升 …
　　……… (430)
suǐ 髓 ……… (430)
suǐ hǎi 髓海 ……… (430)
suǐ huì 髓会 ……… (431)
suǐ tì 髓涕 ……… (431)
sūn xiè 飧泄 ……… (431)
sǔn shàng yū xuè 损伤瘀血 … (431)
suō jiǎo liú zhù 缩脚流注 …… (431)
suǒ gāng zhì 锁肛痔 ……… (432)
suǒ hóu yōng 锁喉痈 ……… (432)
suǒ kǒu 锁口 ……… (432)
suǒ zǐ gǔ shāng 锁子骨伤 …… (432)

T

tà pí chuāng 溻皮疮 ……… (432)
tà yù 溻浴 ……… (433)
tāi gòu 苔垢 ……… (433)
tāi huá 苔滑 ……… (433)
tāi yùn 苔润 ……… (433)
tāi bìng 胎病 ……… (433)
tāi bù zhǎng 胎不长 ……… (433)
tāi bù zhèng 胎不正 ……… (433)
tāi chì 胎赤 ……… (434)
tāi dòng bù ān 胎动不安 …… (434)
tāi dòng xià xuè 胎动下血 …… (434)
tāi dú 胎毒 ……… (434)
tāi féi 胎肥 ……… (434)
tāi fēng 胎风 ……… (435)
tāi fēng chì làn 胎风赤烂 …… (435)
tāi hán 胎寒 ……… (435)
tāi huàn nèi zhàng 胎患内障 …
　　……… (435)
tāi huáng 胎黄 ……… (435)
tāi jí 胎疾 ……… (435)
tāi lòu 胎漏 ……… (436)
tāi qì 胎气 ……… (436)
tāi yè 胎热 ……… (436)
tāi shàn 胎疝 ……… (436)
tāi shuǐ zhǒng mǎn 胎水肿满
　　……… (436)
tāi xián 胎痫 ……… (436)
tāi yuán 胎元 ……… (437)
tāi zì duò 胎自堕 ……… (437)
tài chōng mài 太冲脉 ……… (437)
tài xī 太息 ……… (437)
tài yáng 太阳 ……… (437)
tài yáng bìng 太阳病 ……… (437)
tài yáng fǔ bìng 太阳腑病 …… (438)
tài yáng jīng bìng 太阳经病 … (438)
tài yáng sháng hán 太阳伤寒
　　……… (438)
tài yáng tóu tòng 太阳头痛 … (438)
tài yáng yǔ shào yáng hé bìng 太
　　阳与少阳合病 ……… (439)
tài yáng yǔ yáng míng hé bìng
　　太阳与阳明合病 ……… (439)
tài yáng zhòng fēng 太阳中风
　　……… (439)

tài yīn 太阴	(439)	tán shī tóu tòng 痰湿头痛	(446)
tài yīn bìng 太阴病	(439)	tán shī zǔ fèi 痰湿阻肺	(447)
tài yīn jū 太阴疽	(440)	tán xī bái 痰稀白	(447)
tài yīn tóu tòng 太阴头痛	(440)	tán xiāo 痰哮	(447)
tāi huàn 瘫痪	(440)	tán xiè 痰泻	(447)
tái shí mài 弹石脉	(440)	tán yǐn 痰饮	(447)
tái zhēn 弹针	(440)	tán yǐn ké sòu 痰饮咳嗽	(448)
tái 痰	(441)	tán yǐn wèi wǎn tòng 痰饮胃脘痛	(448)
tái báo 痰包	(441)	tán yǐn xuàn yūn 痰饮眩晕	(448)
tái bì 痰秘	(441)	tán yōng yí jīng 痰壅遗精	(448)
tái chuǎn 痰喘	(441)	tán zhì è zǔ 痰滞恶阻	(448)
tán duō mò 痰多沫	(442)	tán zhòng 痰中	(449)
tán è 痰呃	(442)	tán zhuó nèi bì 痰浊内闭	(449)
tán hé 痰核	(442)	tán zǔ fèi luò 痰阻肺络	(449)
tán huǒ jìng 痰火痉	(442)	tán zhōng 膻中	(449)
tán huǒ ěr míng 痰火耳鸣	(442)	tàn tǔ 探吐	(450)
tán huǒ yǎo xīn 痰火扰心	(442)	tàng yè 汤液	(450)
tán huǒ tóu tòng 痰火头痛	(443)	táng xiè 溏泄	(450)
tán huǒ xuàn yūn 痰火眩晕	(443)	táng xiāo 糖哮	(450)
tán huǒ zhèng chōng 痰火怔忡	(443)	tàng huǒ shāng 烫火伤	(450)
tán jī 痰积	(443)	tàng shāng 烫伤	(450)
tán jué 痰厥	(443)	tí chā bǔ xiè 提插补泻	(450)
tán jué tóu tòng 痰厥头痛	(443)	tǐ jué 体厥	(451)
tán lì 痰疠	(444)	tǐ zhēn liáo fǎ 体针疗法	(451)
tán tán mí xīn qiào 痰迷心窍	(444)	tiān guǐ 天癸	(451)
tán nián chóu 痰粘稠	(444)	tiān huā 天花	(451)
tán müè 痰疟	(444)	tiān páo chuāng 天泡疮	(451)
tán ǒu 痰呕	(445)	tiān yén xiāng yìng 天人相应	(451)
tán pǐ 痰痞	(445)	tiān tíng 天庭	(452)
tán pǐ 痰癖	(445)	tiān xíng chì yǎn 天行赤眼	(452)
tán yè zǔ fèi 痰热阻肺	(445)	tiān zhù gǔ dǎo 天柱骨倒	(452)
tán shī 痰湿	(445)	tiān zhù gǔ zhé 天柱骨折	(452)
tán shī bù yùn 痰湿不孕	(446)	tiáo jì 条剂	(452)
tán shī nèi zǔ 痰湿内阻	(446)	tiáo fú 调服	(452)

tiáo hé gān pí 调和肝脾	(452)	tóu ruǎn 头软	(459)
tiáo hé yíng wèi 调和营卫	(453)	tóu tòng 头痛	(459)
tiáo jīng 调经	(453)	tóu tòng rú pí 头痛如劈	(460)
tiáo shēn 调身	(453)	tóu xiàng qiáng tòng 头项强痛	(460)
tiáo xī 调息	(453)	tóu yáo 头摇	(460)
tiáo xīn 调心	(454)	tóu zhàng 头胀	(460)
tīng shēng yīn 听声音	(454)	tóu zhòng 头重	(461)
tíng jīng 停经	(454)	tóu zhū dīng 头珠疔	(461)
tíng yǐn xié tòng 停饮胁痛	(454)	tòu bān 透斑	(461)
tíng yǐn xīn jì 停饮心悸	(454)	tòu guān shè jiǎ 透关射甲	(461)
tíng yǐn xuàn yùn 停饮眩晕	(454)	tòu tiān liáng 透天凉	(461)
tōng fǔ xiè rè 通腑泄热	(455)	tòu xié 透邪	(462)
tōng jì 通剂	(455)	tòu xiè 透泄	(462)
tōng jīng 通经	(455)	tòu zhēn 透针	(462)
tōng kě qù zhì 通可去滞	(455)	tòu zhěn 透疹	(462)
tōng mài 通脉	(455)	tǔ bù zhì shuǐ 土不制水	(462)
tōng yáng 通阳	(456)	tǔ lì 土粟	(463)
tōng yīn tōng yòng 通因通用	(456)	tǔ shēng wàn wù 土生万物	(463)
tóng bìng yì zhì 同病异治	(456)	tù fǎ 吐法	(463)
tóng nán 童男	(456)	tù fèn 吐粪	(463)
tóng nǚ 童女	(456)	tǔ nà fǎ 吐纳法	(463)
tóng yén gān quē 瞳人干缺	(456)	tǔ nòng shé 吐弄舌	(463)
tóng shén 瞳神	(456)	tǔ qīng shuǐ 吐清水	(464)
tóng shén qī cè 瞳神欹侧	(457)	tù rǔ 吐乳	(464)
tóng shén sàn dà 瞳神散大	(457)	tù suān 吐酸	(464)
tóng shén suō xiǎo 瞳神缩小	(457)	tù xián 吐涎	(464)
tòng fēng 痛风	(458)	tù xuè 吐血	(464)
tòng jīng 痛经	(458)	tù chún 兔唇	(464)
tòng yǒu dìng chù 痛有定处	(458)	tuī ná 推拿	(464)
tóu fēng 头风	(458)	tuī xún 推寻	(465)
tóu fēng bái xiè 头风白屑	(458)	tuǐ tòng 腿痛	(465)
tóu hàn 头汗	(459)	tuì shàn 癞疝	(465)
tóu qiáng 头强	(459)	tuì yīn 瘄阴	(465)
tóu rè 头热	(459)	tuì zhēn 退针	(465)
		tūn suān 吞酸	(465)

tún　臀 …………………………（465）	tuō jiù　脱臼 ………………………（467）
tún yōng　臀痈 ……………………（465）	tuō jū　脱疽 ………………………（467）
tuō dú tòu nóng fǎ　托毒透脓法	tuō qì　脱气 ………………………（468）
…………………………………（466）	tuō ròu pò jiǒng　脱肉破䐃 ……（468）
tuō jū　托疽 ………………………（466）	tuō yáng　脱阳 ……………………（468）
tuō pán dìng　托盘疔 ……………（466）	tuō yīn　脱阴 ………………………（468）
tuō gāng　脱肛 ……………………（466）	tuō zhèng　脱证 …………………（468）
tuō gāng zhì　脱肛痔 ……………（466）	

W

wāi pì bù suí　㖞僻不遂 …………（469）	wài zhèng　外证 ……………………（472）
wài chuī　外吹 ……………………（469）	wài zhì fǎ　外治法 ………………（472）
wài gǎn　外感 ……………………（469）	wài zhì　外痔 ………………………（472）
wài gǎn bù dé wò　外感不得卧	wān zhēn　弯针 ……………………（472）
…………………………………（469）	wán chuāng　顽疮 …………………（472）
wài gǎn fā yè　外感发热 …………（469）	wán tán　顽痰 ……………………（472）
wài gǎn tón tòng　外感头痛 ……（469）	wán xuǎn　顽癣 ……………………（472）
wài gǎn wèi wǎn tòng　外感胃脘	wán zhèng　顽症 …………………（473）
痛…………………………………（469）	wǎn　丸 ……………………………（473）
wài gǎn yāo tòng　外感腰痛 ……（470）	wàn gǔ zhé　腕骨折 ………………（473）
wài hán　外寒 ……………………（470）	wáng jīn　亡津 ……………………（473）
wài huái jū　外踝疽 ………………（470）	wáng xuè　亡血 ……………………（473）
wài kē bǔ fǎ　外科补法 …………（470）	wáng xuè jiā　亡血家 ……………（473）
wài kē xiāo fǎ　外科消法 ………（470）	wáng yáng　亡阳 …………………（474）
wài lián　外廉 ……………………（471）	wáng yīn　亡阴 ……………………（474）
wài shāng　外伤 …………………（471）	wáng lán chuāng　王烂疮 ………（474）
wài shèn diào tòng　外肾吊痛	wàng chǐ　望齿 ……………………（474）
…………………………………（471）	wàng huí chóng zhèng　望蛔虫证
wài shèn zhǒng yìng　外肾肿硬	…………………………………（475）
…………………………………（471）	wàng xíng tài　望形态 ……………（475）
wài shī　外湿 ……………………（471）	wàng yǎn biàn shāng　望眼辨伤
wài yǎn jiǎo　外眼角 ……………（471）	…………………………………（475）
wài yīn　外因 ……………………（471）	wàng zhěn　望诊 …………………（475）
wài yōng　外痈 ……………………（471）	wēi huáng tāi　微黄苔 ……………（475）

wēi huǒ 微火 …… (475)	wèi qì bù hé 胃气不和 …… (481)
wēi mài 微脉 …… (475)	wèi qì bù jiàng 胃气不降 …… (481)
wēi zhě nì zhī 微者逆之 …… (475)	wèi qì xū 胃气虚 …… (481)
wēi 煨 …… (475)	wèi rè 胃热 …… (481)
wěi dǐ gǔ shāng 尾骶骨伤 …… (476)	wèi rè è zǔ 胃热恶阻 …… (481)
wěi zhōng yōng 委中痈 …… (476)	wèi rè shā gǔ 胃热杀谷 …… (482)
wěi huáng 萎黄 …… (476)	wèi rè yōng shèng 胃热壅盛 …… (482)
wěi bì 痿躄 …… (476)	wèi ruò è zǔ 胃弱恶阻 …… (482)
wěi jué 痿厥 …… (476)	wèi shí 胃实 …… (482)
wěi zhèng 痿证 …… (476)	wèi wǎn 胃脘 …… (483)
wèi fēn zhèng 卫分证 …… (477)	wèi wǎn tòng 胃脘痛 …… (483)
wèi qì 卫气 …… (477)	wèi xū 胃虚 …… (483)
wèi qì bù gù 卫气不固 …… (477)	wèi yīn 胃阴 …… (483)
wèi qì tóng bìng 卫气同病 …… (477)	wèi yīn xū 胃阴虚 …… (483)
wèi qì yíng xuè biàn zhèng 卫气营血辨证 …… (478)	wèi zhàng 胃胀 …… (484)
	wèi zhōng zào shǐ 胃中躁矢 …… (484)
wèi qiáng yíng yuò 卫强营弱 …… (478)	wèi zhǔ fǔ shú 胃主腐熟 …… (484)
wèi yuò yíng qiáng 卫弱营强 …… (478)	wèi zhǔ jiàng zhuó 胃主降浊 …… (484)
wèi yíng dóng bìng 卫营同病 …… (478)	wèn zhǔ shòu nà 胃主受纳 …… (484)
wèi fā bìng qián fú 未发病前服 …… (479)	wēn bìng 温病 …… (484)
	wēn bìng pài 温病派 …… (485)
wèi lǎo jīng duàn 未老经断 …… (479)	wēn bìng xué 温病学 …… (485)
wèi guāng 畏光 …… (479)	wēn bìng xué shuō 温病学说 …… (485)
wèi 胃 …… (479)	wēn bǔ mìng mén 温补命门 …… (485)
wèi bìng 胃病 …… (479)	wēn dú 温毒 …… (485)
wèi cháng 胃肠 …… (480)	wēn dú fā bān 温毒发斑 …… (486)
wèi hán 胃寒 …… (480)	wēn fǎ 温法 …… (486)
wèi hán è zǔ 胃寒恶阻 …… (480)	wēn fú 温服 …… (486)
wèi huǒ shàng shēng 胃火上升 …… (480)	wēn hé jiǔ 温和灸 …… (486)
	wēn jīng qù hán 温经祛寒 …… (486)
wèi jiā 胃家 …… (480)	wēn má 温麻 …… (487)
wèi jiā shí 胃家实 …… (480)	wēn nüè 温疟 …… (487)
wèi qì 胃气 …… (480)	wēn pí 温脾 …… (487)
	wēn rè 温热 …… (487)

拼音	词条	页码
wēn rè jìng	温热痉	(487)
wēn shèn	温肾	(487)
wēn shèn lì shuǐ	温肾利水	(488)
wēn shèn zhù yáng	温肾助阳	(488)
wēn wèi jiàn zhōng	温胃健中	(488)
wēn xià	温下	(488)
wēn xié	温邪	(489)
wēn xié fàn fèi	温邪犯肺	(489)
wēn xuè	温血	(489)
wēn yáng	温阳	(489)
wēn yáng lì shī	温阳利湿	(490)
wēn yáng lì shuǐ	温阳利水	(490)
wēn yǎng	温养	(490)
wēn yì	温疫	(490)
wēn zhēn	温针	(490)
wēn zhōng qū hán	温中祛寒	(490)
wēn huáng	瘟黄	(491)
wēn shā	瘟痧	(491)
wēn yì	瘟疫	(491)
wén huǒ	文火	(491)
wén chén	纹沉	(491)
wén fú	纹浮	(492)
wén zhì	纹滞	(492)
wén zhěn	闻诊	(492)
wèn ěr mù	问耳目	(492)
wèn èr biàn	问二便	(492)
wèn fù nǚ	问妇女	(492)
wèn hán rè	问寒热	(493)
wèn hàn	问汗	(493)
wèn qǐ bìng	问起病	(493)
wèn shuì mián	问睡眠	(493)
wèn tóu shēn	问头身	(494)
wèn xiǎo ér	问小儿	(494)
wèn xiōng fù	问胸腹	(494)
wèn yǐn shí kǒu wèi	问饮食口味	(494)
wèn zhěn	问诊	(495)
wò bù ān	卧不安	(495)
wū fēng nèi zhàng	乌风内障	(495)
wū lài	乌癞	(495)
wū shà	乌痧	(495)
wū shà jīng fēng	乌痧惊风	(496)
wū tóu lèi zhòng dú	乌头类中毒	(496)
wū lòu mài	屋漏脉	(496)
wú bān hén jiǔ	无瘢痕灸	(496)
wú dú	无毒	(496)
wú hàn	无汗	(496)
wú míng zhǒng dú	无名肿毒	(496)
wú tán gān ké	无痰干咳	(497)
wú tóu jū	无头疽	(497)
wú fàn wèi qì	毋犯胃气	(497)
wú shí shí	毋实实	(497)
wú xū xū	毋虚虚	(497)
wú gōng yǎo shāng	蜈蚣咬伤	(497)
wǔ bài	五败	(497)
wǔ bēng	五崩	(498)
wǔ bù nán	五不男	(498)
wǔ bù nǚ	五不女	(498)
wǔ cái	五裁	(498)
wǔ cháng	五常	(498)
wǔ chí	五迟	(498)
wǔ chù	五畜	(499)
wǔ chuǎn è hòu	五喘恶候	(499)
wǔ dǎn	五疸	(499)
wǔ dīng	五疔	(499)
wǔ duó	五夺	(499)

wǔ dù 五度	(499)	wǔ wèi suǒ jìn 五味所禁	(505)
wǔ fǔ 五腑	(500)	wǔ wèi suǒ shāng 五味所伤	(505)
wǔ gān 五疳	(500)	wǔ wèi suǒ yù 五味所入	(505)
wǔ gēng sòu 五更嗽	(500)	wǔ xiè 五泄	(505)
wǔ gēng xiè 五更泄	(500)	wǔ xīn fán yè 五心烦热	(505)
wǔ gǔ 五谷	(500)	wǔ xíng xué shuō 五行学说	(506)
wǔ guān 五官	(501)	wǔ xū 五虚	(506)
wǔ ruǎn 五软	(501)	wǔ yè 五液	(506)
wǔ guǒ 五果	(501)	wǔ yí 五宜	(506)
wǔ jī 五积	(501)	wǔ yīng 五瘿	(506)
wǔ jīng 五精	(501)	wǔ yìng 五硬	(507)
wǔ jué 五绝	(501)	wǔ yǒu yú 五有余	(507)
wǔ láo 五劳	(501)	wǔ yùn liù qì 五运六气	(507)
wǔ láo suǒ shāng 五劳所伤	(501)	wǔ zàng 五脏	(507)
wǔ lín 五淋	(501)	wǔ zàng bì 五脏痹	(507)
wǔ lún 五轮	(502)	wǔ zàng huà yè 五脏化液	(508)
wǔ mài 五脉	(502)	wǔ zàng liù fǔ ké 五脏六腑咳	(508)
wǔ sè 五色	(502)	wǔ zàng suǒ cáng 五脏所藏	(508)
wǔ sè dài xià 五色带下	(502)	wǔ zàng suǒ wù 五脏所恶	(508)
wǔ sè lì 五色痢	(502)	wǔ zàng suǒ zhǔ 五脏所主	(508)
wǔ sè wǔ wèi suǒ rù 五色五味所入	(502)	wǔ zhì huà huǒ 五志化火	(509)
wǔ sè zhěn 五色诊	(503)	wǔ zhì guò jí 五志过极	(509)
wǔ sè zhǔ bìng 五色主病	(503)	wǔ zhǒng è hòu 五种恶候	(509)
wǔ shàn 五善	(503)	wǔ zǒu 五走	(509)
wǔ shēng 五声	(504)	wǔ huǒ 武火	(510)
wǔ shí dòng 五十动	(504)	wù ǒu rù jīng 物偶入睛	(510)
wǔ shí 五实	(504)	wù xià 误下	(510)
wǔ shuǐ 五水	(504)	wù fēng 恶风	(510)
wǔ tǐ 五体	(504)	wù hán 恶寒	(510)
wǔ wèi 五味	(504)	wù rè 恶热	(510)
wǔ wèi piān shì 五味偏嗜	(504)	wù shí 恶食	(510)
wǔ wèi suǒ hé 五味所合	(504)	wù táng 鹜溏	(510)

X

xī cù 吸促 ……………………（510）	xià jiāo yú dú 下焦如渎 ………（515）
xī ér wēi shuò 吸而微数 ………（511）	xià jué sháng mào 下厥上冒 …（515）
xī yù 吸入 ………………………（511）	xià jué shàng jié 下厥上竭 …（515）
xī yuǎn 吸远 ……………………（511）	xià lì 下利 ……………………（515）
xī 息 ……………………………（511）	xià lì qīng gǔ 下利清谷 ……（515）
xī cū 息粗 ………………………（511）	xià pǐn 下品 …………………（516）
xī bēn 息贲 ……………………（511）	xià pò 下迫 …………………（516）
xī gāo 息高 ……………………（511）	xià quán 下泉 ………………（516）
xī wēi 息微 ……………………（511）	xià qiào 下窍 ………………（516）
xī ròu zhì 息肉痔 ………………（512）	xià sǔn jí shàng 下损及上 …（516）
xī gǔ 溪谷 ……………………（512）	xià wǎn 下脘 ………………（516）
xī fēng 熄风 ……………………（512）	xià xiāo 下消 ………………（516）
xī gài sǔn duàn 膝盖损断 ……（512）	xià zhě jǔ zhī 下者举之 ……（516）
xī 膝 ……………………………（512）	xià zhù chuāng 下注疮 ……（517）
xī tòng 膝痛 ……………………（512）	xià lìng má zhěn 夏令麻疹 …（517）
xí chuāng 席疮 …………………（512）	xià jì rè 夏季热 ……………（517）
xǐ 洗 ……………………………（513）	xià hóng 夏洪 ………………（517）
xǐ rè yǐn 喜热饮 ………………（513）	xiān tiān 先天 ………………（517）
xǐ lěng yǐn 喜冷饮 ……………（513）	xiān gōng hòu bǔ 先攻后补 …（518）
xǐ àn 喜按 ……………………（513）	xiān bié yīn yáng 先别阴阳 …（518）
xǐ shāng xīn 喜伤心 …………（513）	xián bìng 痫病 ………………（518）
xǐ zé qì huǎn 喜则气缓 ………（513）	xiān bǔ hòu gōng 先补后攻 …（518）
xì mài 细脉 ……………………（513）	xiān zhào zǐ xián 先兆子痫 …（519）
xiā yóu mài 虾游脉 ……………（513）	xiān zhào liú chǎn 先兆流产
xiā má wēn 虾蟆瘟 ……………（513）	……………………………（519）
xià bìng shàng qǔ 下病上取 …（513）	xián wèi yǒng xiè wèi yīn 咸味涌
xià fǎ 下法 ……………………（514）	泄为阴 ………………………（519）
xià fā bèi 下发背 ……………（514）	xián hán zēng yè 咸寒增液 …（519）
xià dān tián 下丹田 …………（514）	xián 咸 ………………………（520）
xià gān 下疳 …………………（514）	xián mài 弦脉 ………………（520）
xià jí shèn yīn 下汲肾阴 ……（514）	xián rǔ 乳 ……………………（520）
xià jiāo 下焦 …………………（515）	xiāng chéng 相乘 ……………（520）
xià jiāo zhǔ chū 下焦主出 …（515）	xiāng fǎn 相反 ………………（520）

xiāng kè 相克 (520)	xiǎo biàn sè tòng 小便涩痛 (527)
xiāng shēng 相生 (520)	xiǎo chǎn 小产 (527)
xiāng shǐ 相使 (521)	xiǎo cháng 小肠 (527)
xiāng wù 相恶 (521)	xiǎo cháng bìng 小肠病 (528)
xiāng wèi 相畏 (521)	xiǎo cháng ké 小肠咳 (528)
xiāng xū 相须 (521)	xiǎo cháng shàn 小肠疝 (528)
xiāng wǔ 相侮 (521)	xiǎo cháng shí rè 小肠实热 (528)
xiàng huǒ 相火 (522)	xiǎo cháng xū hán 小肠虚寒 (528)
xiàng huǒ wàng dòng 相火妄动 (522)	xiǎo chǎng zhàng 小肠胀 (529)
xiàng qiáng 项强 (522)	xiǎo cháng zhǔ shòu shèng 小肠主受盛 (529)
xiàng ruǎn 项软 (522)	xiǎo dú 小毒 (529)
xiàng bèi qiáng 项背强 (522)	xiǎo ér bào jīng 小儿暴惊 (529)
xiāo bìng 哮病 (523)	xiǎo ér fá shā 小儿发痧 (529)
xiāo chuǎn 哮喘 (523)	xiǎo ér chóng tù 小儿虫吐 (529)
xiāo bǔ jiān shī 消补兼施 (523)	xiǎo ér cù lì 小儿卒利 (530)
xiāo dǎo 消导 (524)	xiǎo ér biǎo rè 小儿表热 (530)
xiāo fǎ 消法 (524)	xiǎo ér gān yǎn 小儿疳眼 (530)
xiāo gǔ shàn jī 消谷善饥 (524)	xiǎo ér gǎn mào 小儿感冒 (530)
xiāo dān 消瘅 (524)	xiǎo ér hán tù 小儿寒吐 (531)
xiāo kě 消渴 (524)	xiǎo ér jīng tù 小儿惊吐 (531)
xiāo pǐ 消痞 (525)	xiǎo ér jiǎo luán 小儿脚挛 (531)
xiāo pǐ huà jī 消痞化积 (525)	xiǎo ér kè wǔ 小儿客忤 (531)
xiāo shí dǎo zhì 消食导滞 (525)	xiǎo ér ké nì 小儿咳逆 (531)
xiāo tán 消痰 (525)	xiǎo ér ké sòu 小儿咳嗽 (532)
xiāo tán píng chuǎn 消痰平喘 (526)	xiǎo ér shí rè 小儿实热 (532)
xiāo tán ruǎn jiān 消痰软坚 (526)	xiǎo ér léi shòu 小儿羸瘦 (532)
xiǎo biàn bù lì 小便不利 (526)	xiǎo ér shǔ wēn 小儿暑温 (532)
xiǎo biàn bù jìn 小便不禁 (526)	xiǎo ér shuǐ zhǒng 小儿水肿 (533)
xiǎo biàn lín lì 小便淋沥 (526)	xiǎo ér xiāo chuǎn 小儿哮喘 (534)
xiǎo biàn huáng chì 小便黄赤 (527)	xiǎo ér xiè xiè 小儿泄泻 (534)
xiǎo biàn pín shuò 小便频数 (527)	xiǎo ér xū rè 小儿虚热 (535)
	xiǎo fāng 小方 (535)

xiǎo fù 小腹	(535)
xiǎo fù jū 小腹疽	(535)
xiǎo fù tòng 小腹痛	(536)
xiǎo fù mǎn 小腹满	(536)
xiǎo jiā bǎn 小夹板	(536)
xiǎo hù jià tòng 小户嫁痛	(536)
xiǎo nì 小逆	(536)
xiǎo jié xiōng 小结胸	(536)
xiǎo shāng hán 小伤寒	(537)
xiǎo shé 小舌	(537)
xiǎo xī 小溪	(537)
xiǎo tuǐ zhuǎn jīn 小腿转筋	(537)
xiǎo xīn 小心	(537)
xiǎo zhōng fēng 小中风	(537)
xié rè xiá lì 协热下利	(537)
xié 邪	(538)
xié hài kōng qiào 邪害空窍	(538)
xié liàn xīn bāo 邪恋心包	(538)
xié liú sān jiāo 邪留三焦	(538)
xié qì shèng zé shí 邪气盛则实	(538)
xié zhī suǒ còu, qí qì bì xū 邪之所凑，其气必虚	(539)
xié 胁	(539)
xié lèi jū 胁肋疽	(539)
xié lèi zhàng tòng 胁肋胀痛	(539)
xié tòng 胁痛	(539)
xié xiá pǐ yìng 胁下痞鞕	(539)
xié yōng 胁痈	(540)
xié fēi mài 斜飞脉	(540)
xiè jì 泻剂	(540)
xiè kě qù bì 泻可去闭	(540)
xiè xiè 泄泻	(540)
xiè gān 泻肝	(541)
xiè fèi 泄肺	(541)
xiè huǒ xī fēng 泻火熄风	(541)
xiè xià jìn lì 泻下禁例	(541)
xié jīng 蟹睛	(542)
xīn bāo luò 心包络	(542)
xīn bì 心痹	(542)
xīn bìng 心病	(542)
xīn dòng jì 心动悸	(542)
xīn fán 心烦	(543)
xīn gān 心疳	(543)
xīn hàn 心汗	(543)
xīn hé mài 心合脉	(543)
xīn hé xiǎo cháng 心合小肠	(543)
xīn huǒ shàng yán 心火上炎	(543)
xīn huǒ nèi chì 心火内炽	(544)
xīn kāi qiào yú shé 心开窍于舌	(544)
xīn jì 心悸	(544)
xīn ké 心咳	(544)
xīn láo 心劳	(544)
xīn pí liǎng xū 心脾两虚	(545)
xīn, qí huá zài miàn 心，其华在面	(545)
xīn qì 心气	(545)
xīn qì bù gù 心气不固	(545)
xīn qì bù níng 心气不宁	(545)
xīn qì shèng 心气盛	(545)
xīn qì xū 心气虚	(546)
xīn qì xū bù dé wò 心气虚不得卧	(546)
xīn rè 心热	(546)
xīn shàn 心疝	(546)
xīn shèn xiāng jiāo 心肾相交	(546)
xīn shén fán luàn 心神烦乱	(547)
xīn tòng 心痛	(547)
xīn tòng chè bèi 心痛彻背	(547)

xīn wū rè 心恶热 …… (547)	xīn wēn jiě biǎo 辛温解表 …… (553)
xīn xì 心系 …… (548)	xīn gǎn 新感 …… (554)
xīn xià jì 心下悸 …… (548)	xīn gǎn wēn bìng 新感温病 …… (554)
xīn xià pǐ tòng 心下痞痛 …… (548)	xīn rèn zhī xié 馨饪之邪 …… (554)
xīn xià pǐ mǎn 心下痞满 …… (548)	xīn mén 囟门 …… (554)
xīn xià zhī jié 心下支结 …… (548)	xīn xiàn 囟陷 …… (554)
xīn xū 心虚 …… (548)	xīn tián 囟填 …… (555)
xīn xū dǎn qiè 心虚胆怯 …… (548)	xīng chòu qì 腥臭气 …… (555)
xīn xuè 心血 …… (548)	xíng chí 行迟 …… (555)
xīn xuè xū 心血虚 …… (548)	xíng jīng fù tòng 行经腹痛 …… (555)
xīn xuè xū bù dé wò 心血虚不得卧 …… (549)	xíng qì 行气 …… (555)
xīn yáng 心阳 …… (549)	xíng qì huó xuè 行气活血 …… (555)
xīn yáng xu 心阳虚 …… (549)	xíng zhēn 行针 …… (556)
xīn yí rè yú xiǎo cháng 心移热于小肠 …… (549)	xíng féi jīng shǎo 形肥经少 …… (556)
xīn yīn 心阴 …… (550)	xíng tǐ 形体 …… (556)
xīn yīn xū 心阴虚 …… (550)	xíng qì 形气 …… (556)
xīn yíng guò hào 心营过耗 …… (550)	xíng qì xiāng shī 形气相失 …… (557)
xīn zhě, jūn zhǔ zhī guān 心者，君主之官 …… (550)	xíng qì xhāng dé 形气相得 …… (557)
xīn zhōng dǎn dǎn dà dòng 心中憺憺大动 …… (551)	xíng zàng 形脏 …… (557)
xīn zhǔ shén míng 心主神明 …… (551)	xǐng pí 醒脾 …… (557)
xīn zhǔ hàn 心主汗 …… (551)	xìng néng 性能 …… (558)
xīn zhǔ yán 心主言 …… (551)	xiōng gǔ shāng 胸骨伤 …… (558)
xīn zhǔ xuè mài 心主血脉 …… (551)	xiōng bì 胸痹 …… (558)
xīn 辛 …… (552)	xiòng pǐ 胸痞 …… (558)
xīn gan fā sàn wéi yáng 辛甘发散为阳 …… (552)	xiōng mǎn 胸满 …… (559)
xīn gān huà yáng 辛甘化阳 …… (552)	xiōng tòng 胸痛 …… (559)
xīn hán shēng jīn 辛寒生津 …… (552)	xiōng wéi 胸围 …… (559)
xīn kai kǔ xiè 辛开苦泄 …… (552)	xiōng xié kǔ mǎn 胸胁苦满 …… (559)
xīn liáng jiě biǎo 辛凉解表 …… (553)	xiōng xià jié yìng 胸下结硬 …… (559)
xīn liáng qīng qì 辛凉清气 …… (553)	xiōng zhōng pǐ yìng 胸中痞鞭 …… (560)
	xiōng zhōng fán rè 胸中烦热 …… (560)
	xiōng yīng 胸膺 …… (560)
	xiōng zhōng zhī fǔ 胸中之府 …… (560)

xiū xī lì 休息痢 …… (560)	xū zhōng jiá shí 虚中夹实 …… (568)
xiù qì wèi 嗅气味 …… (560)	xù xuè 蓄血 …… (569)
xū bì 虚秘 …… (561)	xù xuè fā huáng 蓄血发黄 …… (569)
xū lì 虚痢 …… (561)	xuān bì tōng yáng 宣痹通阳 …… (569)
xū chuǎn 虚喘 …… (561)	
xū cè 虚痤 …… (561)	xuān fèi 宣肺 …… (569)
xū fán 虚烦 …… (562)	xuān jì 宣剂 …… (569)
xū fēng nèi dòng 虚风内动 …… (562)	xuān fèi huà tán 宣肺化痰 …… (570)
xū huǒ 虚火 …… (562)	xuān kě qù yōng 宣可去壅 …… (570)
xū huǒ shàng yán 虚火上炎 …… (563)	xuān tōng shuǐ dào 宣通水道 …… (570)
xū hán 虚寒 …… (563)	
xū hán dòng xiè 虚寒洞泄 …… (563)	xuán pǐ 痃癖 …… (570)
xū huáng 虚黄 …… (563)	xuán ěr chuāng 旋耳疮 …… (571)
xū jiǎ 虚瘕 …… (564)	xuán luó tū qǐ 旋螺突起 …… (571)
xū láo 虚劳 …… (564)	xuán pǐ 悬癖 …… (571)
xū láo yāo tòng 虚劳腰痛 …… (564)	xuán qí fēng 悬旗风 …… (571)
xū láo dào hàn 虚劳盗汗 …… (564)	xuán yǐn 悬饮 …… (571)
xū jī lì 虚积痢 …… (564)	xuán yōng 悬痈 …… (572)
xū mài 虚脉 …… (565)	xuán yōng chuí 悬雍垂 …… (572)
xū nüè 虚疟 …… (565)	xuán yūn 眩晕 …… (572)
xū rè 虚热 …… (565)	xuàn pū 胸仆 …… (572)
xū pǐ 虚痞 …… (565)	xué wèi mái xiàn liáo fǎ 穴位埋线疗法 …… (572)
xū yè jīng xíng xiān qī 虚热经行先期 …… (566)	xué wèi fēng bì liáo fǎ 穴位封闭疗法 …… (572)
xū shí 虚实 …… (566)	
xū xián 虚痫 …… (566)	xué wèi zhù shè liáo fǎ 穴位注射疗法 …… (573)
xū tán 虚痰 …… (566)	
xū xiàn 虚陷 …… (567)	xué wèi cì jī jié zhā liáo fǎ 穴位刺激结扎疗法 …… (573)
xū xié 虚邪 …… (567)	
xū yáng shàng fú 虚阳上浮 …… (567)	xuè 血 …… (573)
xū zhàng 虚胀 …… (567)	xuè bēng 血崩 …… (573)
xū zhě bǔ qí mǔ 虚者补其母 …… (568)	xuè bēng fù tòng 血崩腹痛 …… (573)
	xuè bēng hūn àn 血崩昏暗 …… (574)
xū zhě bǔ zhī 虚者补之 …… (568)	xuè bì 血痹 …… (574)
xū zhèng 虚证 …… (568)	xuè bù guī jīng 血不归经 …… (574)
xū zuò nǔ zé 虚坐努责 …… (568)	xuè bù xún jīng 血不循经 …… (574)

xuè bù yǎng jīn 血不养筋 …… (574)	xuè tuō 血脱 …… (582)
xuè fēn rè dú 血分热毒 …… (575)	xuè wèi qì mǔ 血为气母 …… (582)
xuè fēn zhèng 血分证 …… (575)	xuè xīn tòng 血心痛 …… (582)
xuè fēn yū rè 血分瘀热 …… (575)	xuè xū 血虚 …… (583)
xuè fēng chuāng 血风疮 …… (575)	xuè xū bì 血虚痹 …… (583)
xuè gān chuāng 血疳疮 …… (576)	xuè xū bù yùn 血虚不孕 …… (583)
xuè gōng zhì 血攻痔 …… (576)	xuè xū ěr lóng 血虚耳聋 …… (584)
xuè gǔ 血蛊 …… (576)	xuè xū fā rè 血虚发热 …… (584)
xuè hǎi 血海 …… (576)	xuè xū fù tòng 血虚发痛 …… (584)
xuè hán jīng xíng hòu qī 血寒经行后期 …… (577)	xuè xū huá tāi 血虚滑胎 …… (584)
xuè hán yuè jīng guò shǎo 血寒月经过少 …… (577)	xuè xū jīng xíng hòu qī 血虚经行后期 …… (585)
xuè hàn 血汗 …… (577)	xuè xū shēng fēng 血虚生风 … (585)
xuè huì 血会 …… (577)	xuè xū tóu tòng 血虚头痛 …… (585)
xuè jī 血积 …… (577)	xuè xū shǒu jiǎo má mù 血虚手脚麻木
xuè jiàn 血箭 …… (578)	xuè xū xīn jì 血虚心悸 …… (586)
xuè jiàn zhì 血箭痔 …… (578)	xuè xū wěi 血虚痿 …… (586)
xuè jiǎ 血瘕 …… (578)	xuè xū xuàn yūn 血虚眩晕 …… (586)
xuè jué 血厥 …… (578)	xuè xū yāo tòng 血虚腰痛 …… (586)
xuè kū jīng bì 血枯经闭 …… (578)	xuè xū yuè jīng guò shǎo 血虚月经过少 …… (587)
xuè kuī jīng bì 血亏经闭 …… (579)	xuè xū zì hàn 血虚自汗 …… (587)
xuè lì 血疬 …… (579)	xuè yǐng 血瘿 …… (587)
xuè lì 血痢 …… (579)	xuè yū 血瘀 …… (587)
xuè lín 血淋 …… (579)	xuè yū bēng lòu 血瘀崩漏 …… (587)
xuè liú 血瘤 …… (580)	xuè yū jīng xíng hòu qī 血瘀经行后期 …… (588)
xuè lún 血轮 …… (580)	xuè yū bù yùn 血瘀不孕 …… (588)
xuè niào 血尿 …… (580)	xuè yū tòng jīng 血瘀痛经 …… (589)
xuè rè chuāng 血热疮 …… (580)	xuè yū wěi 血瘀痿 …… (589)
xuè rè huá tāi 血热滑胎 …… (580)	xuè zhèng 血证 …… (589)
xuè rè yuè jīng guò duō 血热月经过多 …… (581)	xuè zhì 血痔 …… (589)
xuè shàn 血疝 …… (581)	xuè zhì 血痣 …… (589)
xuè shì 血室 …… (581)	xuè zhì fù tòng 血滞腹痛 …… (590)
xuè shuān zhì 血栓痔 …… (582)	xuè zhì jīng bì 血滞经闭 …… (590)
xuè suí qì xiàn 血随气陷 …… (582)	

xuè zhǒng 血肿 …… (590)	xún zhēng 熏蒸 …… (591)
xún jīng chuán 循经传 …… (590)	

Y

yà diàn 压垫 …… (591)	yáng bìng 阳病 …… (596)
yá 牙 …… (591)	yáng bìng zhì yīn 阳病治阴 …… (596)
yá dīng 牙疔 …… (591)	yáng cháng yǒu yú, yīn cháng bù zú 阳常有余,阴常不足 …… (596)
yá gān 牙疳 …… (591)	
yá tòng 牙痛 …… (591)	yáng huà qì, yīn chéng xíng 阳化气,阴成形 …… (596)
yá yín 牙龈 …… (591)	
yá xuān 牙宣 …… (592)	yáng huáng 阳黄 …… (596)
yá yōng 牙痈 …… (592)	yáng jié 阳结 …… (597)
yān 咽 …… (592)	yáng jìng 阳痉 …… (597)
yān hóu 咽喉 …… (592)	yáng jué 阳绝 …… (597)
yān mén 咽门 …… (592)	yáng jué 阳厥 …… (597)
yán xiāo 盐哮 …… (592)	yáng luò shāng zé xuè wài yì 阳络伤则血外溢 …… (597)
yán 颜 …… (593)	
yǎn 眼 …… (593)	yáng míng 阳明 …… (597)
yǎn xì 眼系 …… (593)	yáng míng bìng 阳明病 …… (598)
yǎn bāo tán hé 眼胞痰核 …… (593)	yáng míng jīng bìng 阳明经病 …… (598)
yǎn xián chì làn 眼弦赤烂 …… (593)	
yǎn tōu zhēn 眼偷针 …… (594)	yáng míng fǔ bìng 阳明腑病 …… (598)
yǎn zhū 眼珠 …… (594)	
yǎn zhū qiān xié 眼珠牵斜 …… (594)	yáng míng tóu tòng 阳明头痛 …… (598)
yǎn 罨 …… (594)	
yàn fāng 验方 …… (594)	yáng míng yǔ shào yáng hé bìng 阳明与少阳合病 …… (599)
yàn shí 厌食 …… (594)	
yáng shuǐ 羊水 …… (595)	yáng qì 阳气 …… (599)
yáng shuǐ guò duō 羊水过多 …… (595)	yáng qiào 阳窍 …… (599)
	yáng shā yīn cáng 阳杀阴藏 …… (599)
yáng xián fēng 羊痫风 …… (595)	yáng shēng yīn zhǎng 阳生阴长 …… (599)
yáng xū chuāng 羊须疮 …… (595)	
yáng 阳 …… (595)	yáng shēng yú yīn 阳生于阴 …… (600)
yáng bān 阳斑 …… (595)	

yáng shèng zé rè 阳盛则热 …… (600)	yáng yī 疡医 ……………… (606)
yáng shèng zé yīn bìng 阳盛则阴病 ……………………… (600)	yǎng gān 养肝 ……………… (606)
	yǎng xīn ān shén 养心安神 … (606)
yáng shèng 阳盛 …………… (600)	yǎng xuè jiě biǎo 养血解表 …… (606)
yáng shèng gé yīn 阳盛格阴 … (600)	yǎng xuè yùn zào 养血润燥 … (607)
yáng shèng yīn shāng 阳盛阴伤 ……………………… (600)	yǎng yīn jiě biǎo 养阴解表 …… (607)
	yǎng yīn yùn zào 养阴润燥 … (607)
yáng shèng zé wài rè 阳盛则外热 ………………… (601)	yǎng yīn qīng fèi 养阴清肺 …… (607)
	yǎng fēng 痒风 ……………… (608)
yáng shǔ 阳暑 ……………… (601)	yáo jū 夭疽 ………………… (608)
yáng shuǐ 阳水 ……………… (601)	yāo bèi tòng 腰背痛 ………… (608)
yáng sǔn jí yīn 阳损及阴 …… (601)	yāo kāo tòng 腰尻痛 ………… (608)
yáng wěi 阳萎 ……………… (601)	yāo gǔ sǔn duàn 腰骨损断 …… (608)
yáng xié 阳邪 ……………… (602)	yāo jǐ tòng 腰脊痛 ………… (609)
yáng xū 阳虚 ……………… (602)	yāo suān 腰酸 ……………… (609)
yáng xū fā rè 阳虚发热 …… (602)	yāo tòng 腰痛 ……………… (609)
yáng xū shuǐ fàn 阳虚水泛 … (602)	yáo zhēn 摇针 ……………… (609)
yáng xū tóu tòng 阳虚头痛 … (603)	yào ài tiáo 药艾条 ………… (609)
yáng xū shī zǔ 阳虚湿阻 …… (603)	yào gāo 药膏 ……………… (610)
yáng xū wù hán 阳虚恶寒 …… (603)	yào guàn 药罐 ……………… (610)
yáng xū xuàn yūn 阳虚眩晕 ……………………… (603)	yào tǒng bá fǎ 药筒拔法 …… (610)
	yào xiàn yǐn liú 药线引流 … (610)
yáng xū yīn shèng 阳虚阴盛 ……………………… (604)	yào yùn 药熨 ……………… (610)
	yē gé 噎膈 ………………… (611)
yáng xū zé wài hán 阳虚则外寒 ………………… (604)	yè máng 夜盲 ……………… (611)
	yè sòu 液嗽 ………………… (611)
yáng xū zì hàn 阳虚自汗 …… (604)	yè tí 夜啼 ………………… (611)
yáng zàng 阳脏 …………… (604)	yè dào 液道 ……………… (612)
yáng zhèng 阳证 …………… (604)	yè zào shēng fēng 液燥生风 … (612)
yáng zhèng sì yīn 阳证似阴 … (605)	yè tòng 腋痛 ……………… (612)
yáng zhèng zhī yáng 阳中之阳 ……………………… (605)	yè yōng 腋痈 ……………… (612)
	yī nì 一逆 ………………… (612)
yáng zhèng zhī yīn 阳中之阴 ……………………… (605)	yí zhǐ 移指 ………………… (612)
	yí dú 遗毒 ………………… (612)
yáng cì 杨刺 ……………… (605)	yí jīng 遗精 ……………… (613)
yáng méi chuāng 杨梅疮 …… (606)	yí niào 遗尿 ……………… (613)

yǐ dú gōng dú 以毒攻毒 …… (613)	伤则血内溢 …… (620)
yì bìng tóng zhì 异病同治 …… (613)	yīn píng yáng bì 阴平阳秘 …… (620)
yì qì 异气 …… (614)	yīn qì 阴气 …… (621)
yì lì 疫疬 …… (614)	yīn qiào 阴窍 …… (621)
yì nüè 疫疟 …… (614)	yīn rè 阴热 …… (621)
yì dīng 疫疔 …… (614)	yīn shàn 阴疝 …… (621)
yì lì 疫痢 …… (614)	yīn shēng yú yáng 阴生于阳 …… (621)
yì hóu shā 疫喉痧 …… (614)	yīn shèng zé yáng bìng 阴胜则阳病 …… (621)
yì zhěn 疫疹 …… (615)	yīn shèng 阴盛 …… (621)
yì qì yǎng xuè 益气养血 …… (615)	yīn shèng gé yáng 阴盛格阳 …… (622)
yì qì shēng jīn 益气生津 …… (615)	yīn shèng yáng xū 阴盛阳虚 …… (622)
yì qì jiàn Pí 益气健脾 …… (615)	yīn shèng zé hán 阴盛则寒 …… (622)
yì qì jiě biǎo 益气解表 …… (616)	yīn shī chuāng 阴虱疮 …… (622)
yì shǒu 意守 …… (616)	yīn shí 阴蚀 …… (622)
yì wèi 益胃 …… (616)	yīn shǔ 阴暑 …… (622)
yì 嗌 …… (616)	yīn shuǐ 阴水 …… (623)
yì rǔ 溢乳 …… (616)	yīn sǔn jí yáng 阴损及阳 …… (623)
yì yǐn 溢饮 …… (616)	yīn suō 阴缩 …… (623)
yì xuè 溢血 …… (617)	yīn tǐng 阴挺 …… (623)
yì 瘱 …… (617)	yīn tóu yōng 阴头痛 …… (624)
yīn rén zhì yí 因人制宜 …… (617)	yīn tuō 阴脱 …… (624)
yīn dì zhì yí 因地制宜 …… (617)	yīn xián 阴痫 …… (624)
yīn shí zhì yí 因时制宜 …… (617)	yīn xié 阴邪 …… (624)
yīn 阴 …… (618)	yīn xū 阴虚 …… (624)
yīn cì 阴刺 …… (618)	yīn xū chuǎn 阴虚喘 …… (624)
yīn hàn 阴汗 …… (618)	yīn xū dào hàn 阴虚盗汗 …… (625)
yīn hú shàn 阴狐疝 …… (618)	yīn xū fā rè 阴虚发热 …… (625)
yīn hù 阴户 …… (618)	yīn xū fèi zào 阴虚肺燥 …… (625)
yīn hù zhǒng tòng 阴户肿痛 …… (618)	yīn xū ké sòu 阴虚咳嗽 …… (625)
yīn huáng 阴黄 …… (619)	yīn xū hóu bì 阴虚喉痹 …… (626)
yīn huǒ 阴火 …… (619)	yīn xū huǒ wàng 阴虚火旺 …… (626)
yīn jié 阴结 …… (619)	yīn xū tóu tòng 阴虚头痛 …… (626)
yīn jié yáng tuō 阴竭阳脱 …… (619)	yīn xū wěi 阴虚痿 …… (626)
yīn jué 阴绝 …… (620)	yīn xū yáng fú 阴虚阳浮 …… (627)
yīn lěng 阴冷 …… (620)	
yīn luò shāng zé xuè nèi yì 阴络	

yīn xū zé nèi rè 阴虚则内热 … (627)	yǐn xīn tòng 饮心痛 … (633)
yīn xuǎn 阴癣 … (627)	yǐn zǐ 饮子 … (633)
yīn yáng 阴阳 … (627)	yǐn zhěn 隐疹 … (633)
yīn yáng guāi lì 阴阳乖戾 … (628)	yīng táo zhì 樱桃痔 … (633)
yīn yáng hù gēn 阴阳互根 … (628)	yīng 膺 … (634)
yīn yáng jiāo 阴阳交 … (628)	yíng fēng lěng lèi 迎风冷泪 … (634)
yīn yáng lí jué 阴阳离决 … (628)	yíng fēng liú lèi 迎风流泪 … (634)
yīn yáng shèng fù 阴阳胜复 … (629)	yíng fēng rè lèi 迎风热泪 … (634)
yīn yáng shī tiáo 阴阳失调 … (629)	yíng suí bǔ xiè 迎随补泻 … (634)
yīn yáng xiāo zhǎng 阴阳消长 … (629)	yíng 营 … (634)
yīn yáng zhuǎn huà 阴阳转化 … (629)	yíng qì 营气 … (635)
yīn yáng zì hé 阴阳自和 … (629)	yíng wèi bù hé 营卫不和 … (635)
yīn yǎng 阴痒 … (630)	yíng fèn zhèng 营分证 … (635)
yīn yè 阴液 … (630)	yíng qì bù cóng 营气不从 … (635)
yīn zàng 阴脏 … (630)	yǐng 瘿 … (635)
yīn zào 阴躁 … (630)	yìng xià gān 硬下疳 … (635)
yīn zhèng 阴证 … (630)	yōng 痈 … (635)
yīn zhèng sì yáng 阴证似阳 … (631)	yǒng tù jìn lì 涌吐禁例 … (636)
yīn zhōng zhī yáng 阴中之阳 … (631)	yōu gé 忧膈 … (636)
yīn zhōng zhī yīn 阴中之阴 … (631)	yōu shāng fèi 忧伤肺 … (636)
yīn zhǒng 阴肿 … (631)	yōu mén 幽门 … (636)
yīn zòng 阴纵 … (631)	yóu lǐ chū biǎo 由里出表 … (636)
yīn fèi 瘖痱 … (631)	yóu hàn 油汗 … (636)
yǐn huǒ guī yuán 引火归原 … (632)	yóu huī zhī jiǎ 油灰指甲 … (636)
yǐn jīng bào shǐ 引经报使 … (632)	yóu fēng 游风 … (637)
yǐn qì 引气 … (632)	yǒu gōu jū 有头疽 … (637)
yǐn 饮 … (632)	yū è 瘀呃 … (637)
yǐn shí zhòng dú 饮食中毒 … (632)	yū rè 瘀热 … (638)
yǐn jiǔ zhòng dú 饮酒中毒 … (632)	yū xuè fù tòng 瘀血腹痛 … (638)
yǐn piàn 饮片 … (633)	yū xuè yāo tòng 瘀血腰痛 … (638)
yǐn jiā 饮家 … (633)	yū xuè 瘀血 … (638)
yǐn xián 饮痫 … (633)	yū xuè ké 瘀血咳 … (638)
yǐn zhèng 饮证 … (633)	yū xuè tóu tòng 瘀血头痛 … (638)
	yū xuè zǔ luò 瘀血阻络 … (639)
	yū xuè liú zhù 瘀血流注 … (639)
	yú xiáng mài 鱼翔脉 … (639)

yú gú shāng 髃骨伤	(640)		(642)
yǔ lǔ 伛偻	(640)	yuǎn dào cì 远道刺	(642)
yǔ chí 语迟	(640)	yuǎn xuè 远血	(642)
yǔ shēng zhòng zhuó 语声重浊	(640)	yuē shù 约束	(643)
		yuě 哕	(643)
yù yì fú jīng 玉翳浮睛	(640)	yuè jīng guò shǎo 月经过少	(643)
yù yīn qián yáng 育阴潜阳	(640)	yuè jīng bù tiáo 月经不调	(643)
yù zhèng 郁证	(641)	yuè jīng guò duō 月经过多	(643)
yù huǒ 郁火	(641)	yuè jīng bìng 月经病	(643)
yù mào 郁冒	(641)	yuè jīng chuán 越经传	(643)
yù rè yí jīng 郁热遗精	(641)	yūn zhēn 晕针	(644)
yù chuán 欲传	(641)	yún yì 云翳	(644)
yuán qì xū yuò 元气虚弱	(642)	yùn pí 运脾	(644)
yuán qì 原（元）气	(642)	yùn qì xié tòng 运气胁痛	(644)
yuán xuǎn 圆癣	(642)	yùn bèi 孕悲	(644)
yuán yì mèi zhàng 圆翳内障		yùn fǎ 熨法	(644)

Z

zá bìng 杂病	(645)	zǎo xiè 早泄	(647)
zái nì 再逆	(645)	zǎo huā yì nèi zhàng 枣花翳内障	
zàng dú 脏毒	(645)		(647)
zàng qì 脏气	(645)	zào 燥	(647)
zàng jié 脏结	(645)	zào huǒ xuàn yùn 燥火眩晕	(647)
zàng huì 脏会	(645)	zào jì 燥剂	(647)
zàng zhēn 脏真	(645)	zào jìng 燥痉	(648)
zàng xiàng 脏象	(646)	zào kě qù shī 燥可去湿	(648)
zàng yōng zhì 脏痈痔	(646)	zào qì shāng fèi 燥气伤肺	(648)
zàng xiàng xué shuō 脏象学说		zào rè 燥热	(648)
	(646)	zào rè ké sòu 燥热咳嗽	(648)
zàng jué 脏厥	(646)	zào rè wěi 燥热痿	(649)
zàng fǔ xiāng hé 脏腑相合	(646)	zào shèng zé gān 燥胜则干	(649)
zàng fǔ biàn zhèng 脏腑辨证		zào shī 燥湿	(649)
	(646)	zào shī huà tán 燥湿化痰	(649)
zàng zào 脏燥	(647)	zào shǐ 燥矢	(650)

zào zhě rú zhī 燥者濡之 …… （650）	zhěn chǐ fū 诊尺肤 …… （657）
zào tán 燥痰 …… （650）	zhěn fǎ 诊法 …… （657）
zéi xié 贼邪 …… （650）	zhěn zhǐ wén 诊指纹 …… （657）
zēng shuǐ xíng zhōu 增水行舟 …… （650）	zhěn xiōng fù 诊胸腹 …… （657）
zēng yè yùn xià 增液润下 …… （651）	zhěn xū lǐ 诊虚里 …… （658）
zhà shū zhà shuò 乍疏乍数 …… （651）	zhēng chōng 怔忡 …… （658）
zhà sāi 痄腮 …… （651）	zhēng 蒸 …… （658）
zhàn wàng 谵忘 …… （651）	zhēng lù 蒸露 …… （658）
zhān yǔ 谵语 …… （652）	zhēng rǔ 蒸乳 …… （658）
zhàn lì 战栗 …… （652）	zhēng bìng 蒸病 …… （659）
zhàn hàn 战汗 …… （652）	zhēng jiǎ 癥瘕 …… （659）
zhǎng gǔ shāng 掌骨伤 …… （652）	zhēng shàn 癥疝 …… （659）
zhàng 胀 …… （653）	zhěng tǐ guān niàn 整体观念 …… （659）
zhàng hòu chǎn 胀后产 …… （653）	zhèng gǔ 正骨 …… （660）
zhàng bìng 胀病 …… （653）	zhèng gǔ gōng jù 正骨工具 …… （660）
zhàng 瘴 …… （653）	zhèng gǔ shǒu fǎ 正骨手法 …… （660）
zhàng qì 瘴气 …… （653）	zhèng niàn 正念 …… （660）
zhàng nüè 瘴疟 …… （653）	zhèng xū xié shí 正虚邪实 …… （661）
zhāo shí mù tǔ 朝食暮吐 …… （653）	zhèng qì 正气 …… （661）
zhé bì 折髀 …… （653）	zhèng qì cún nèi, xié bù kě gān 正气存内，邪不可干 …… （661）
zhé fǎ 折法 …… （654）	zhèng sè 正色 …… （661）
zhé zhēn 折针 …… （654）	zhèng tóu tòng 正头痛 …… （661）
zhé yáng 折疡 …… （654）	zhèng xié xiāng zhēng 正邪相争 …… （661）
zhēn jiǔ 针灸 …… （654）	
zhēn fǎ 针法 …… （654）	zhèng zhì 正治 …… （662）
zhēn cì má zuì 针刺麻醉 …… （654）	zhèng zhèng 正证 …… （662）
zhēn yá 真牙 …… （655）	zhèng hòu 证候 …… （662）
zhēn jīng pò sǔn 真睛破损 …… （655）	zhèng shēng 郑声 …… （662）
zhēn xū jiǎ shí 真虚假实 …… （655）	zhī yǐn 支饮 …… （663）
zhēn zàng mài 真脏脉 …… （655）	zhī jié tòng 肢节痛 …… （663）
zhēn shí jiǎ xū 真实假虚 …… （656）	zhī liú 脂瘤 …… （663）
zhēn tóu tòng 真头痛 …… （656）	zhí cháng 直肠 …… （663）
zhēn xī 真息 …… （656）	zhí cháng xiè 直肠泻 …… （663）
zhēn xīn tòng 真心痛 …… （656）	zhí jiē jiǔ 直接灸 …… （663）
zhěn 疹 …… （657）	

zhí shì 直视	(664)		(670)
zhí zhòng 直中	(664)	zhōng mǎn 中满	(670)
zhí zhòng sān yīn 直中三阴	(664)	zhōng jīng zhī fǔ 中精之腑	(671)
zhí zhòng yīn jīng 直中阴经	(664)	zhōng pǐn 中品	(671)
zhǐ 跖	(664)	zhōng qì bù zú 中气不足	(671)
zhǐ xuè 止血	(664)	zhōng qì xià xiàn 中气下陷	(671)
zhǐ mù 指目	(665)	zhōng wǎn 中脘	(671)
zhǐ zhēn 指针	(665)	zhōng xiāo 中消	(671)
zhì yīn 至阴	(665)	zhōng yáng 中阳	(671)
zhì huà 制化	(665)	zhōng yáng bù zhèn 中阳不振	(671)
zhì róng 制绒	(665)	zhōng zhèng zhī guān 中正之官	(672)
zhì shuāng 制霜	(666)	zhōng zhǐ tóng shēn cùn 中指同身寸	(672)
zhì jiǔ 炙	(666)	zhǒng yáng 肿疡	(672)
zhì bó 炙礴	(666)	zhǒng 踵	(672)
zhì bìng bì qiú yú běn 治病必求于本	(666)	zhòng dú 中毒	(672)
zhì fǎ 治法	(666)	zhòng fēng 中风	(672)
zhì zé 治则	(667)	zhòng fǔ 中腑	(673)
zhì wèi bìng 治未病	(667)	zhòng hán 中寒	(673)
zhì xiāo 治削	(667)	zhòng jīng 中经	(673)
zhì qiú qí shǔ 治求其属	(667)	zhòng jīng luò 中经络	(674)
zhì 痔	(668)	zhòng luò 中络	(674)
zhì chuāng 痔疮	(668)	zhòng shī 中湿	(674)
zhì lòu 痔瘘	(668)	zhòng shí 中食	(674)
zhì shí 蛭食	(668)	zhòng shǔ 中暑	(674)
zhì xià 滞下	(668)	zhòng shǔ xuán yūn 中暑眩晕	(675)
zhì qì 滞气	(667)	zhòng wù 中恶	(675)
zhì zhēn 滞针	(669)	zhòng zàng 中脏	(675)
zhì yí 滞颐	(669)	zhòng jì 重剂	(675)
zhōng cǎo yào 中草药	(669)	zhòng kě qù qiè 重可去怯	(675)
zhōng dā shǒu 中搭手	(669)	zhòng shé 重舌	(675)
zhōng dān tián 中丹田	(669)	zhòng yáng bì yīn 重阳必阴	(676)
zhōng hán 中寒	(670)	zhòng yīn bì yáng 重阴必阳	(676)
zhōng jiāo 中焦	(670)		
zhōng jiāo rú òu 中焦如沤	(670)		
zhōng jiāo zhǔ huà 中焦主化			

zhòng zhèn ān shén 重镇安神 ……(676)	zhuó xié 浊邪 ……(680)
zhòng zhèng bí yuān 重症鼻渊 ……(676)	zhuó xié hài qīng 浊邪害清 …(680)
zhōu dū zhī guān 州都之官 ……(676)	zhuó yīn 浊阴 ……(680)
zhǒu 肘 ……(677)	zhuó yīn bù jiàng 浊阴不降 …(680)
zhǒu yōng 肘痈 ……(677)	zhuó yīn chū xià qiào 浊阴出下窍 ……(681)
zhū chóng 诸虫 ……(677)	zhuó yīn guī liù fǔ 浊阴归六腑 ……(681)
zhū yáng zhī huì 诸阳之会 …(677)	zhuó yīn zǒu wǔ zàng 浊阴走五脏 ……(681)
zhū xián yīn 诸痫喑 ……(677)	zī ái 嗌嗳 ……(681)
zhū zhū 诸铢 ……(677)	zī shuǐ hán mù 滋水涵木 ……(681)
zhū dǎn zhī dǎo fǎ 猪胆汁导法 ……(677)	zī shèn 滋肾 ……(681)
zhū diān 猪癫 ……(677)	zī yǎng gān shèn 滋养肝肾 …(682)
zhú shuǐ 逐水 ……(677)	zī yǎng wèi yīn 滋养胃阴 …(682)
zhú hán kāi qiào 逐寒开窍 …(677)	zī yīn lì shī 滋阴利湿 …(682)
zhǔ zhèng 主证 ……(678)	zī yīn píng gān qián yáng 滋阴平肝潜阳 ……(683)
zhǔ zhǔ 煮 ……(678)	
zhù chē zhù chuán 注车注船 ……(678)	zī yīn xī fēng 滋阴熄风 ……(683)
zhù xià 疰夏 ……(678)	zī dào mǔ qì 子盗母气 ……(683)
zhù yáng jiě biǎo 助阳解表 ……(678)	zī diàn 紫癜 ……(683)
zhuǎn bāo 转胞 ……(679)	zī fán 子烦 ……(684)
zhuǎn jīn 转筋 ……(679)	zī gōng tuō chuí 子宫脱垂 …(684)
zhuàng huǒ 壮火 ……(679)	zī gōng wài rèn shēn 子宫外妊娠 ……(684)
zhuàng huǒ shí qì 壮火食气 …(679)	zī hù zhǒng zhàng 子户肿胀 …(685)
zhuàng rè 壮热 ……(679)	zī lìn 子淋 ……(685)
zhuàng shù 壮数 ……(679)	zī qì 子气 ……(685)
zhuàng shuǐ zhī zhǔ, yǐ zhì yáng guāng 壮水之主,以制阳光 ……(679)	zī sǐ fù zhōng 子死腹中 …(685)
	zī sòu 子嗽 ……(685)
	zī xián 子痫 ……(686)
zhuàng yáng 壮阳 ……(679)	zī xuán 子悬 ……(686)
zhuó tòng 灼痛 ……(680)	zī yīn 子喑 ……(686)
zhuó qì 浊气 ……(680)	zī yōng 子痈 ……(686)
	zī zhǒng 子肿 ……(687)
zhuó qì guī xīn 浊气归心 …(680)	zī bái diàn fēng 紫白癜风 …(687)

zì hàn 自汗 …… (687)	zǒu mǎ yá gān 走马牙疳 …… (689)
zì nǜ 自衄 …… (688)	zú fā bèi 足发背 …… (689)
zì chī làn 眦赤烂 …… (688)	zú dīng 足疔 …… (689)
zì 渍 …… (688)	zú gēn tòng 足跟痛 …… (689)
zōng jīn 宗筋 …… (688)	zú huái jū 足踝疽 …… (689)
zōng jīn zhī huì 宗筋之会 …… (688)	zú xīn yōng 足心痈 …… (690)
zōng mài 宗脉 …… (688)	zuǒ jīn píng mù 佐金平木 …… (690)
zōng qì 宗气 …… (688)	zuò bǎn chuāng 坐板疮 …… (690)
zǒng àn 总按 …… (688)	zuò yào 坐药 …… (690)
zǒu mǎ hóu fēng 走马喉风 …… (689)	